inside the body. You can focus your gaze on the third eye, the heart, the tip of the nose, or the movement of *prana* (life-force energy). How you use your drishti can help bring moment-to-moment meditative awareness of your self. Whenever possible in your practice, try closing your eyes to draw your attention within.

Practical Considerations of Yoga

Yoga has many healing benefits, but it is important to have the guidance of an experienced teacher to gain the most from your practice and to avoid injury. Always keep a balanced practice in mind, including: intention (*sankalpa*), sound work (*mantra*, or sounding), breath work (*pranayama*), meditation, relaxation, and every category of asana (standing, seated, on the belly, on the back, balancing, backbending, side bending, and inversions). The body is a holistic system that operates as a unified organism, and your practice should focus on the alignment of your whole being.

Whenever possible, it is best to do yoga in a natural setting where there is fresh air and prana flowing. Wear simple, comfortable, and light-colored natural fabrics that embody the uplifting spirit of yoga.

The time of day and the way in which you practice affects your entire physiological and energetic systems: your circulation, hormone secretion, the flow of lunar and solar energies in the *nadis* (the energy pathways of the body), and your state of mind. Traditionally, it is understood that yoga practice should be done facing the rising sun to absorb its physical and energetic benefits. It is ideal to practice in the morning on an empty stomach.

If you are practicing at anoth carefully. Be aware of the nature or stimulating? Observe the effec mind, and emotions to find the be balance that is in harmony with the daily, monthly, and yearly cycles of nature.

Learn about your unique Ayurvedic constitution, not only to discover what to eat and how to optimize your health, but also to help choose the appropriate asana and pranayama practice for you. I often say that yoga is a lifestyle that begins in the kitchen.

Most important is the attitude and intention with which you practice. The Hatha Yoga sage Gorakhnatha said, "hasobha karobha dhyanam." *Hasobha* means joy, *karo* means action, and *dhyanam* means meditation. We must do our meditation with joy. I often tell my students, "happy breathing" or "happy toes" to remind them to bring that joyful attitude to every cell of their body.

Right here, right now, you are whole and complete. Let yogasana bring you light and peace. Hari Om.

Sanskrit to English Transliteration & Pronunciation Guide

अक्षर (letter)		Trans-literated Script	Phonetic Sound	English Word
अ		a	a	apple
आ	ा	ā	a/aa	car
इ	ि	i	i	in
ई	ी	T	ee	deep
उ	ु	u	u	pun
ऊ	ू	ū	oo	pool
ऋ		ṛ	ri	rig
ॠ	ॄ	ṝ	rea	reach
ऌ		Ḷ	l	late
ए		e	a-e	fate
ऐ		ai	ai	aisle
ओ	ो	o	o	yoga
औ	ौ	au	ow	ounce
अं		m	m/n	nap
अः	:	ḥ	(silent)	heir
क् / क		k	k	link
ख् / ख		kh	kh	bronchitis
ग् / ग		g	g	girl
घ् / घ		gn	gh	ghost
ङ् / ङ		ṅ	ng	hunger

अक्षर (letter)		Trans-literated Script	Phonetic Sound	English Word
च् / च		c	ch	church
छ् / छ		ch	chh	Churchill
ज् / ज		j	j	judge
झ् / झ		jh	z	azure
ञ् / ञ		ñ	n	pinch
ट् / ट		ṭ	t	tub
ठ् / ठ		ṭh	th	thunder
ड् / ड		ḍ	d	odd
ढ् / ढ		ḍh	dh	redhead
ण् / ण		ṇ	n	gone
त् / त		t	t	pasta
थ् / थ		th	th	thumb
द् / द		d	th	other
ध् / ध		dh	dh	Buddha
न् / न		n	n	no
प् / प		p	p	paw
फ् / फ		pn	f	photo
ब् / ब		b	b	bubble
भ् / भ		bh	bh	clubhouse
म् / म		m	m	mug

अक्षर (letter)		Trans-literated Script	Phonetic Sound	English Word
य् / य		y	y	yes
र् / र		r	r	rub
ल् / ल		l	l	love
व् / व		v	v	variety
श् / श		ś	sh	shall
ष् / ष		ṣ	s	west
स् / स		s	s	Sun
ह् / ह		h	h	hug
क्ष् / क्ष		kṣ	ksh	rickshaw
त्र् / त्र		tr	tr	tree
ज्ञ् / ज्ञ		Jñ	jn	jñana

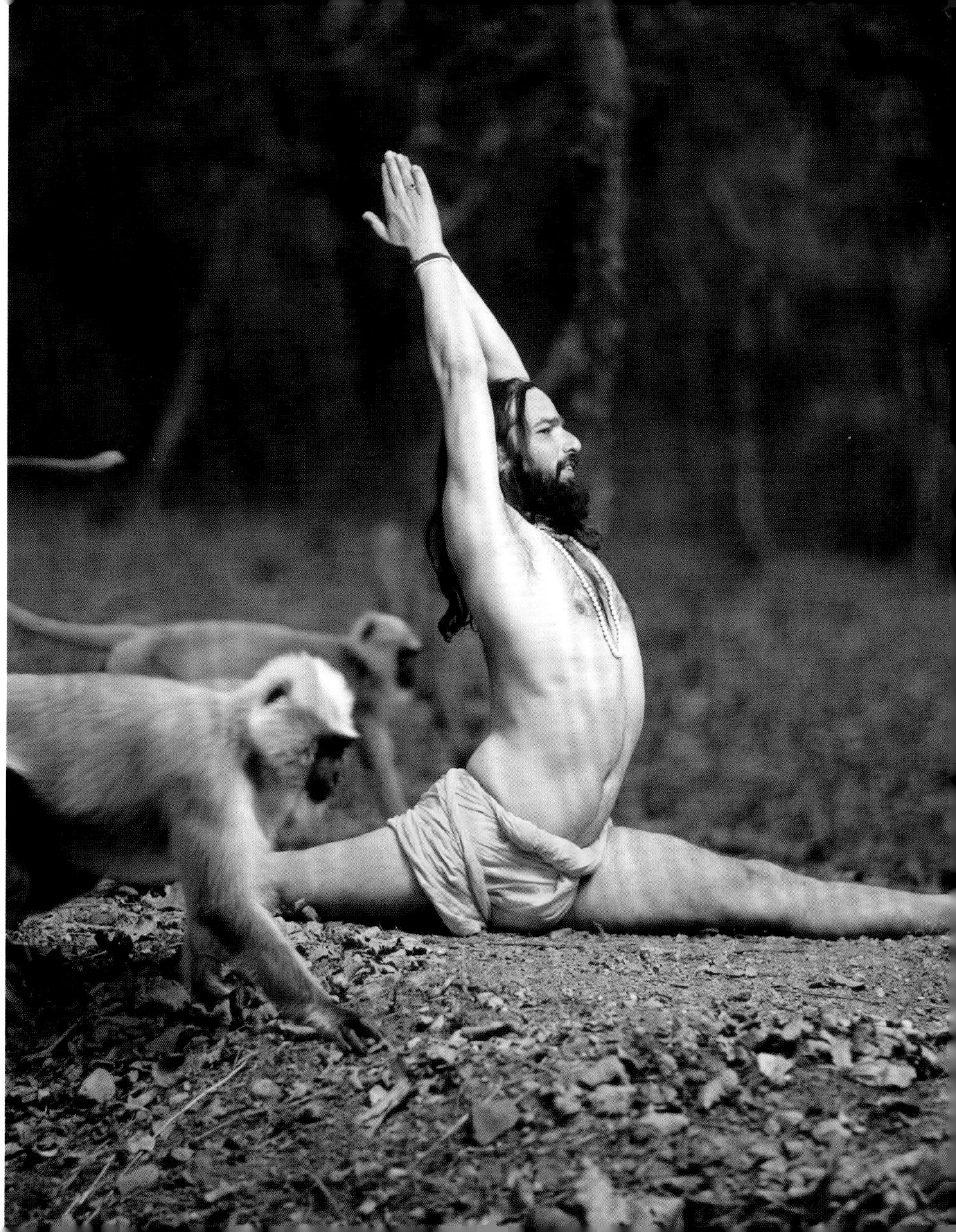

Sanskrit to English Translations

Sanskrit	Transliterated Sanskrit	English
अङ्ग	aṇga	body parts and organs
अङ्गुल	aṅgula	fingers
अङ्गुली (तर्जनी, मध्यमा, अनामिका, कनिष्ठिका), अङ्गुष्ठ	aṇgulī (tarjan, madhyamā, anāmikā, kaniṣthikā) aṅguṣṭha	fingers and toes (index, middle, ring, little), big toe
अधोपाद	adhopāda	feet, lower legs
अधोमुख	adhomukha	facing the ground
अन्तर्दृष्टि	antaṛdṛṣṭi	looking inside
अस्थि:	asthih	bones
मुखम्	mukham	face
उत्कफोणि	utkaphoṇi	elbows raised
उदर	udara	abdomen
हृदय:	hṛdayaḥ	heart
उरु	uru	thigh
कटि, श्रोणी	kaṭi, sroṇī	waist
कण्ठ:	kaṇth	throat
कपाल:	kāpāl	skull
कपोल:	kapolah	cheeks
कफोणि	kaphoṇi	elbow
कर	kara	hand
करतल	karatala	palm

Sanskrit	Transliterated Sanskrit	English
कर्ण	karṇa	ear, character from the Mahabarata
काख:, कुक्षि	kākhah, kukṣi	armpit
केश	keśa	hair
गर्भ	garbha	womb
गुल्फ	gulpha	ankle
गो	go	senses, cow
ग्रीवा	grīvā	neck
चक्र	cakra	wheel, spinning wheel, energy center
जटा	jaṭā	dreadlocks
जानु	jānu	knee
तिलक	tilaka	anointment of the third eye
त्वक् (त्वचा)	tvak (tvacā)	skin
दक्षिण	dakṣiṇa	South
दन्त:, दशन	dantah, daśana	teeth
दृष्टि	dṛṣṭi	gazing
देह, काय, शरीर	deha, kāya, sarīra	body
नख:	nakhah	nails
नाभ	nābha/nābhi	navel
नासिका	nāsikā	nose
नितम्ब	nitamba	buttocks, hips

Sanskrit	Transliterated Sanskrit	English
पाद	pāda	feet, legs, toes
पुच्छ	puccha	tail, feather
फुफ्फुस:	phuphphusah	lungs
पूर्व	pūrva	front, forward
पूर्वत:	pūrvatah	from the front
पृष्ठ	pṛṣṭha	back, behind
पृष्ठत:	pṛṣṭhatah	from the back
प्रपाद	prapāda	ball of the foot
बहिर्जानु	bahirjānu	outer edge of the knee
बहिर्दृष्टि	bahirdṛṣṭi	looking outside
बहिर्पाद	bahirpāda	outer edge of the feet
बहिर्पार्श्व	bahirpārśva	off to the side
बहिर्हस्त	bahirhasta	outer edge of the hands
बुद्धि, मनीषा, प्रज्ञा	buddhi, manīṣā, prajñā	intelligence
भुज	bhuja	arm
भ्रू:	bhrūh	eyebrows
मणि	maṇi	jewel
मन:	mana	mind
मस्तिष्कम्	mastiṣkam	brain
मुष्टि	muṣṭi	fist
मूल	mūla	root, source, foundation
मेरु	meru	spine, name of a sacred mountain
योनि, भग:	yoni, bhagah	species, vagina
रसना(जिह्वा)	rasanā, jihvā	tongue

Sanskrit	Transliterated Sanskrit	English
रोम:	romah	pores
ललाट, मस्तक	lalāṭa, mastaka	forehead
लिङ्गम्, शिश्न, मेढ्र:	liṅgam, siśna, meḍhrah	penis
वक्ष:	vakṣah	chest
वाम	vāma	left
शिखा	śikhā	top of the head, near the back
शिर	śira	head
शीर्ष	śīrṣa, randhra	crown of the head
सन्धि	sandhi	joints
समक्ष	samakṣa	front
समक्षत:	samakṣaṭah	from the front
समदृष्टि	samadṛṣti	steady gaze
सम्मुख	sammukha	facing forward, in front of
लघु आन्त्र	laghu āntra	small intestine
स्कन्ध	skandha	shoulder
दीर्घ आन्त्र	dhirgha āntra	large intestine
स्नायु:(नाडी)	snāyuh, naḍī	nerves
श्रोत्र	śrotra, karṇa	ear
हस्त	hasta	arm and hand
मणिबन्ध	maṇibandha	wrist
हनु	hanu	chin
नेत्रम्, लोचनम्	netram, locanam	eyes
नेत्रलोम	netraloma	eyelashes

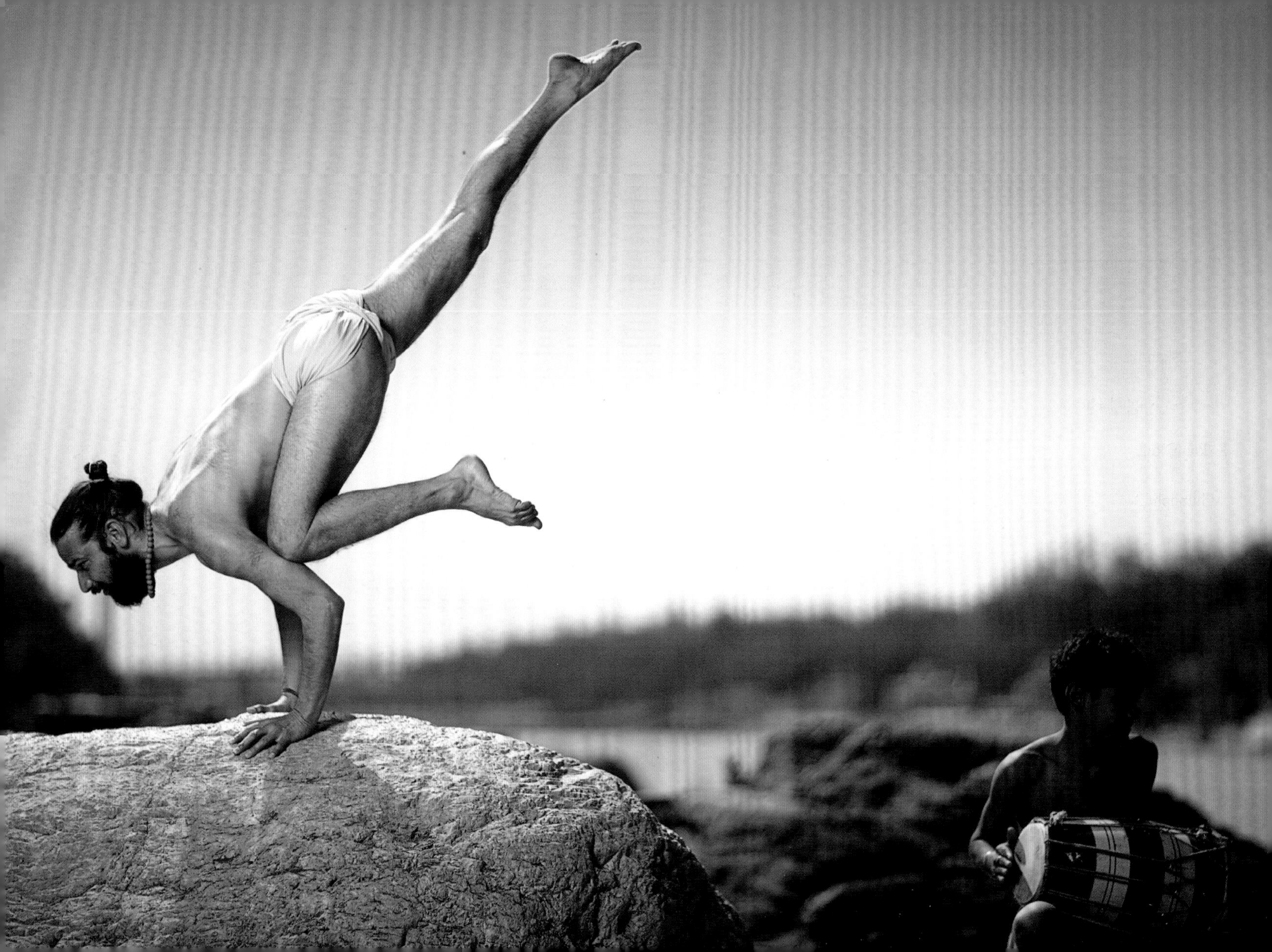

Sanskrit to English Diagram of the Body

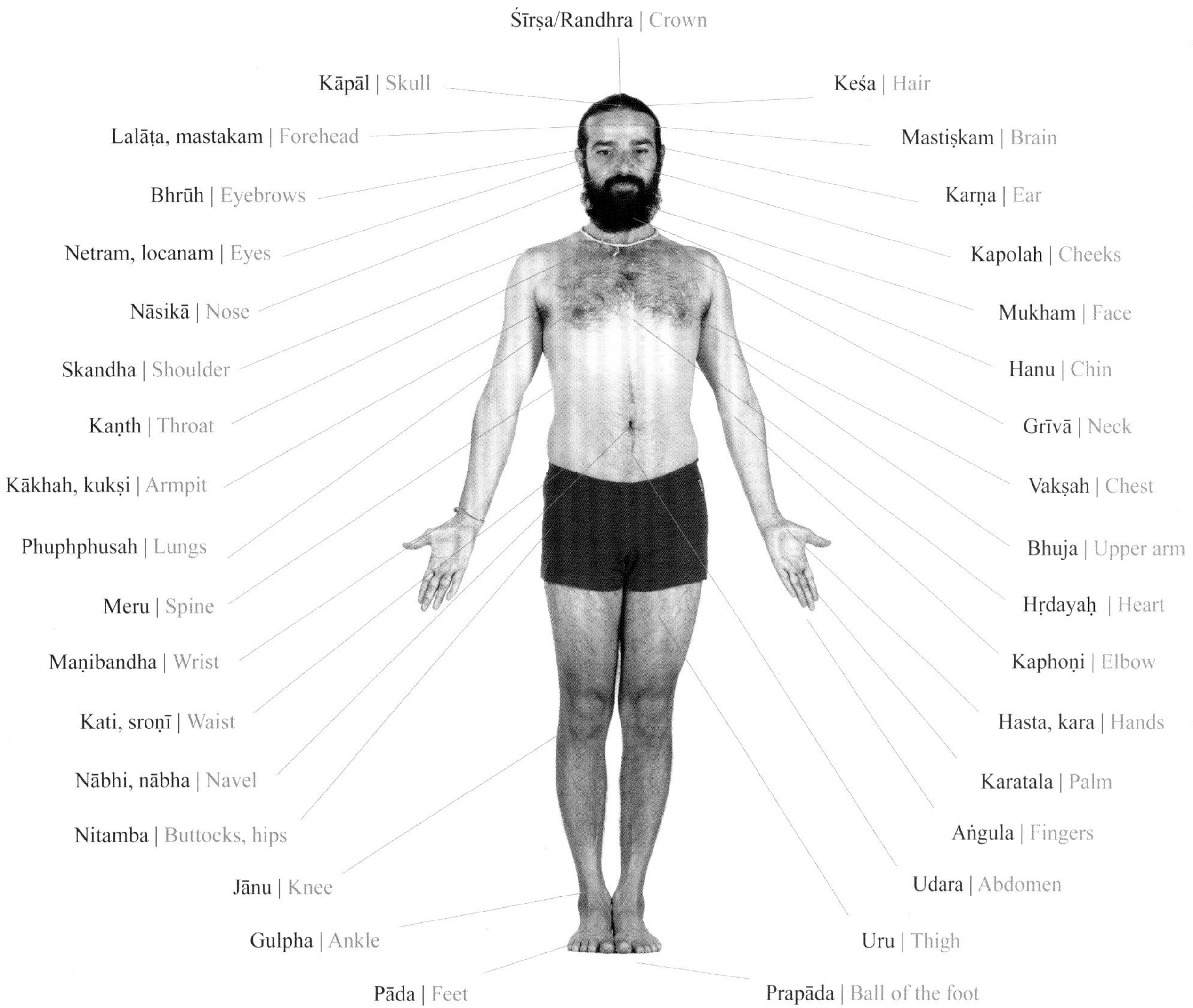

The Chakra System

The Hatha Yoga system was conceptualized primarily upon the energetic anatomy of the body, something easy to forget or overlook given the modern preoccupation with the physical. Hatha Yoga is rooted in Tantra, a complex system of philosophy and yogic practices that views the body as an important vehicle in the development of self-awareness. Ancient Hatha yogis saw the body as an interconnected energy system, with prana flowing through the nadis. There are said to be seventy-two thousand of these energy pathways in the body. The two key nadis are Ida, connected to the left nostril and the right hemisphere of the brain and characterized by a lunar, cooling, and restive energy, and Pingala, connected to the right nostril and the left hemisphere of the brain and characterized by a solar, heating, and active energy. As prana flows through the nadi system, the energy intersects at certain points in the body, known as chakras. Balancing these chakras is a major component of yoga.

The term Hatha breaks down into two root words: *ha*, meaning sun, and *tha*, meaning moon. This points to the primary focus of Hatha Yoga as an energetic practice in which we seek to balance the cosmic energies in the body. Maintaining this energy helps to raise our awareness, which in turn awakens Kundalini Shakti, or divine feminine energy, which is coiled at the base of the spine. One face of Shiva is Ardhanarishwara, who is depicted as both Shakti, the feminine divine (the left half of the body), and Shiva, the primordial masculine (the right half of the body). This representation is a beautiful and poetic metaphor for the union of polarities achieved through yoga. It is also said that while Shakti lives in the root as Kundalini, Shiva lives in the crown as consciousness. By working to enhance the flow of energy through the chakra system, we unite these two cosmic energies.

Balancing the chakras brings subtle physical, emotional, and mental benefits. A great deal of importance is placed on physical alignment, but yoga requires alignment on many other levels. In the *Yoga Sutras of Patanjali*, Patanjali says, "Sthiram sukham asanam," which means that yoga postures are characterized by both steadiness and ease. One translation of *sukham* is "deep contentment." I understand this to mean that yoga is the process and outcome of bringing intention, the physical body, the pranic body, the mental body, and the soul into alignment. This opens us up to the experience of Super Consciousness.

In this book, you will find the yantras, or geometric symbols of the chakras, above each posture. One pose can work to balance multiple chakras. Over time, you will intuitively understand and even experience each posture's effects on your chakra system. The guide on the following pages outlines the dominant energies and characteristics of each chakra. There are many wonderful books you can read to learn more about chakra energy, but most importantly, notice what you learn from your own practice.

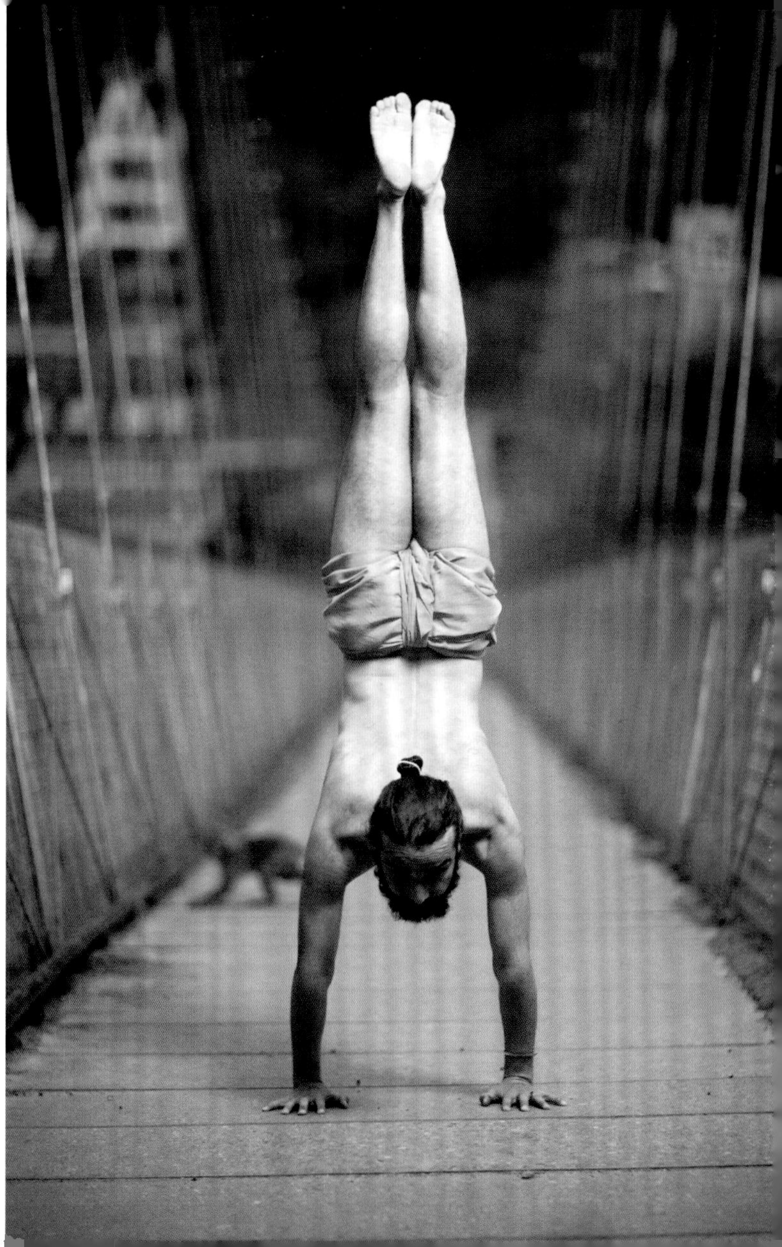

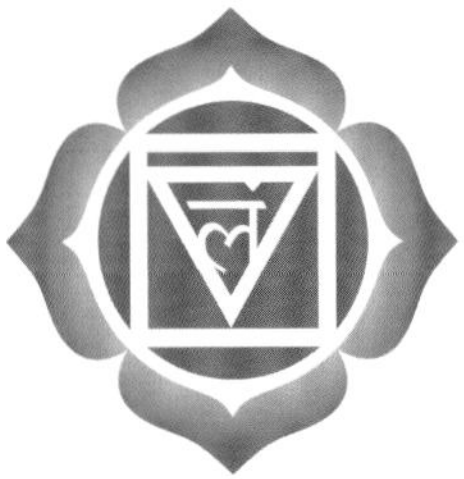

1
Muladhara Chakra
Root Chakra

Tattva (element): Earth
Bija (seed) mantra: LAM
Jnanendriya (sense): Smell

Associations: Groundedness; concentration; relationship to ancestors and biological family; relationship to food; sense of security, survival, and needs; health of the physical body, especially bonesand muscles

Related Asana: Standing and balancing poses; poses where the body has a lot of contact with the earth

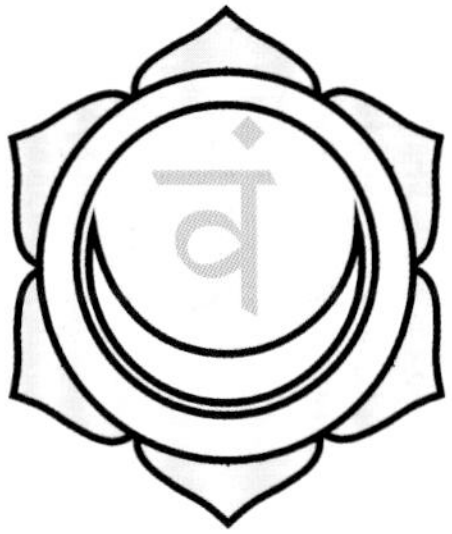

2
Swadhisthana Chakra
Sacral Chakra

Tattva: Water
Bija mantra: VAM
Jnanendriya: Taste

Associations: Circulation of blood and fluids, including hormones; ovaries and testes; sensuality; desire; wants; re-creation and renewal; creativity

Related Asana: Side-stretching poses; poses that compress the lower abdomen

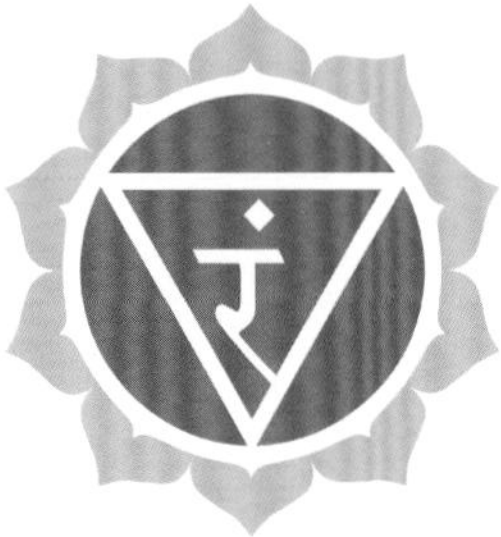

3
Manipura Chakra
Navel Chakra

Tattva: Fire
Bija mantra: RAM
Jnanendriya: Sight

Associations: Digestion; maintenance of body temperature, energy levels, and health of the physical body; motivation; ego, will, and confidence; vitality; anger, jealousy, anxiety, and fear; transforming, releasing, and letting go of negative emotions; adrenals; pancreas

Related Asana: Forward-bend poses; abdominal strengthening and twisting poses

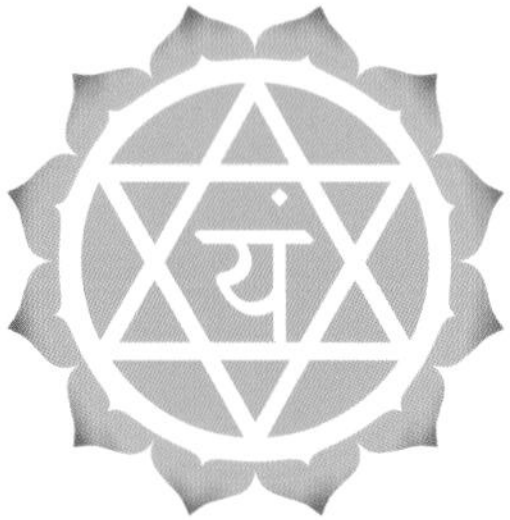

4
Anahata Chakra
Heart Chakra

Tattva: Air
Bija mantra: YAM
Jnanendriya: Touch

Associations: Giving and receiving unconditional love; compassion and loving; kindness; happiness without material objects; the mind and emotions; sharing; vulnerability and openness; heart issues on physical and emotional levels; devotion; deep contentment; relationship to the world; thymus gland

Related Asana: Heart-opening, chest-lifting, and backbending poses

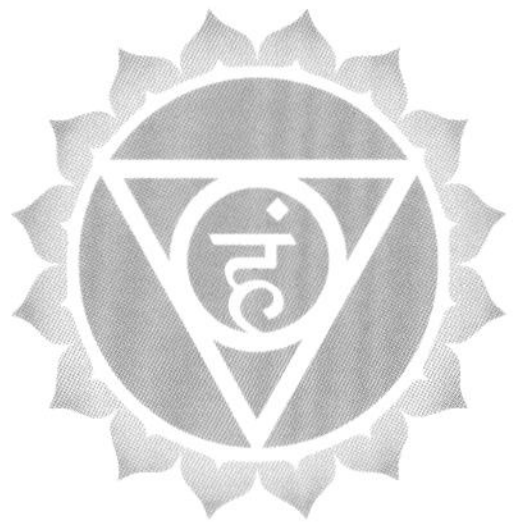

5
Vishuddha Chakra
Throat Chakra

Tattva: Ether
Bija mantra: HAM
Jnanendriya: Hearing

Associations: Sound, purification, vibration, and creative expression; self-expression and self-representation; working with blockages of the body and mind; sensitivity to sound; thyroid and parathyroid glands

Related Asana: Poses that constrict the throat; the release of emotion and tension by sounding and chanting

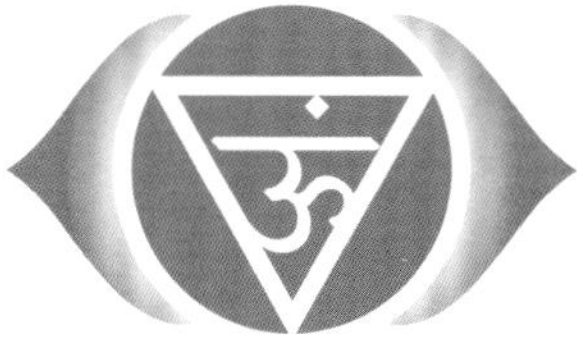

6
Ajna Chakra
Third-Eye Chakra

Tattva: Beyond the five elements
Bija mantra: OM
Jnanendriya: Subtle senses

Associations: Sattva Buddhi (intuitive center); concentration; conscious awareness; psychic center; knowing the past, present, and future; inner guidance and discriminating awareness; home of the pituitary (master) gland and the pineal gland

Related Asana: Balancing poses that improve concentration; inversions; meditation

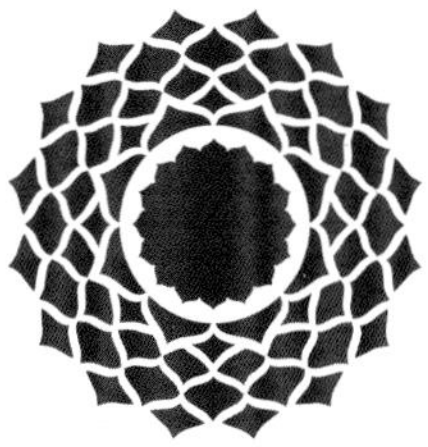

7
Sahasrara Chakra
Crown Chakra

Tattva: Beyond the five elements
Bija mantra: SOHUM
(union of the universe)
Jnanendriya: Subtle senses

Associations: Resting place of Shiva and Shakti (divine masculine and feminine energies); experience of union; point of connection to Brahma/Divinity/One-ness with the universe/Super Consciousness; experience of infinite expansion

Related Asana: Inversions; meditation

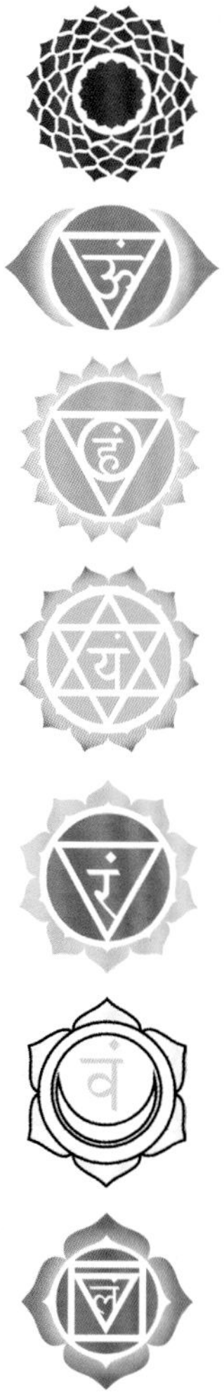

Standing

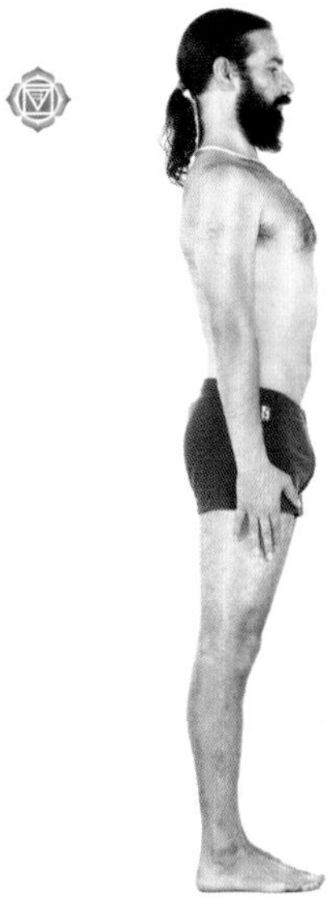

1
ताड आसन (सम स्थिति)
Tāḍa āsana (sama sthiti)
Palm tree pose (standing steady and even)

ताडासन (समस्थिति)
Tāḍāsana (samasthiti)

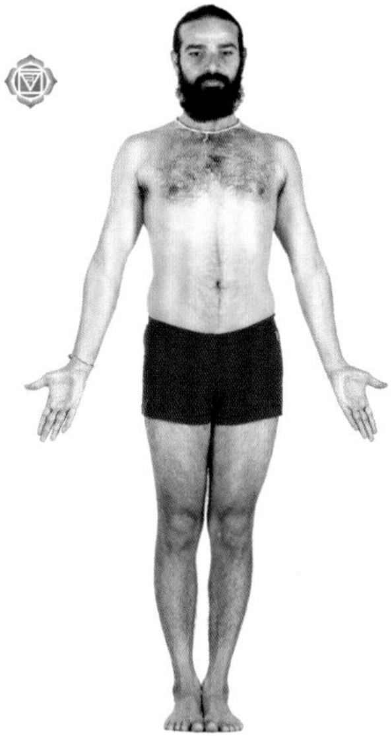

2
ताड आसन(सम स्थिति, हस्त बहिर्वृत्त)
Tāḍa āsana (sama sthiti, hasta bahirvṛtta)
Palm tree pose (standing steady, palms facing out)

ताडासन (समस्थिति, हस्तबहिर्वृत्त)
Tāḍāsana (samasthiti, hastabahirvṛtta)

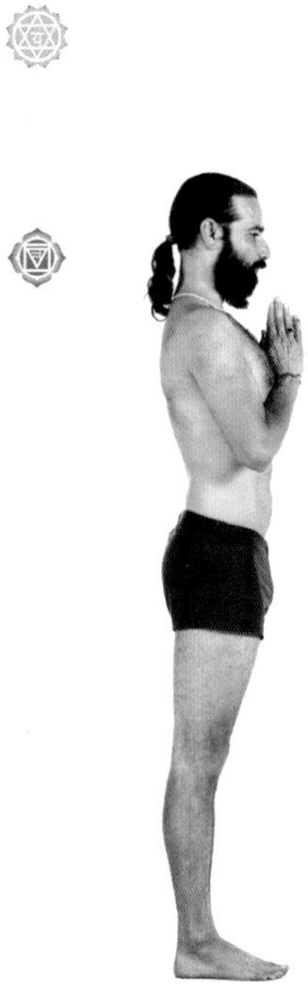

3
नमस्कार ताड आसन
Namaskāra tāḍa āsana
Prayer palm tree pose

नमस्कारताडासन
Namaskāratāḍāsana

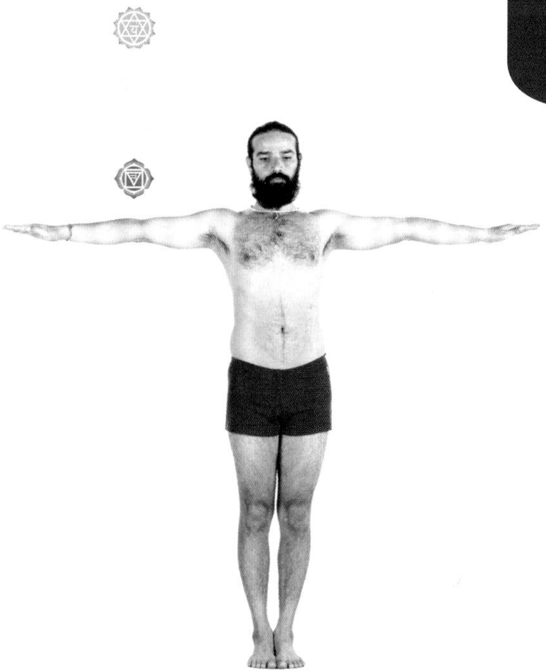

4
विराट हस्त ताड आसन
Tāḍa asana (virāṭa hasta)
Palm tree pose (hands extended wide)

ताडासन (विराटहस्त)
Tāḍasana (virātahasta)

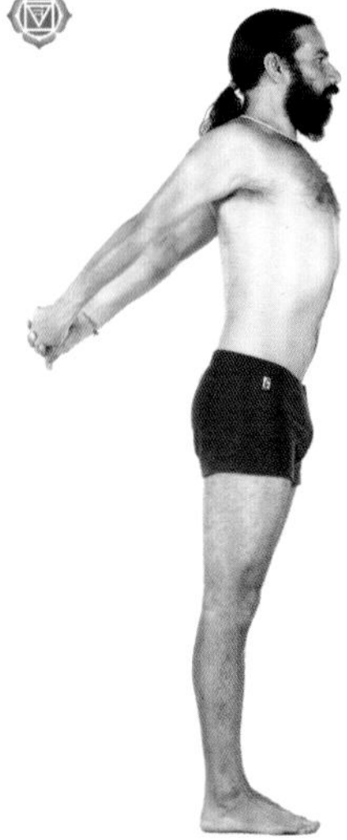

5
ताड आसन (पृष्ठ हस्त उत्तान)
Tāḍa āsana (pṛṣṭha hasta uttāna)
Palm tree pose (hands stretched behind)

ताडासन (पृष्ठहस्तोत्तान)
Tādāsana (pṛṣṭhahastottāna)

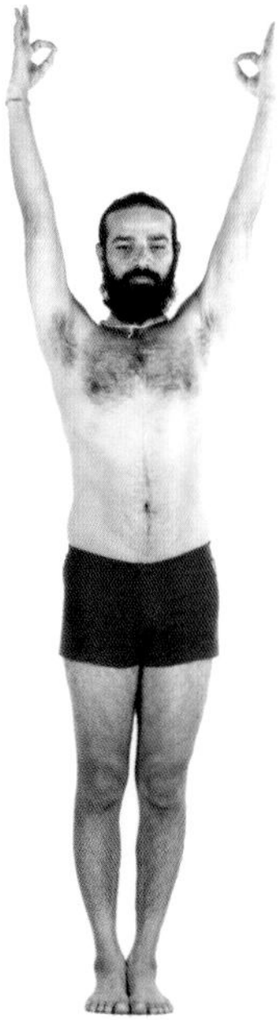

6
ताड आसन (ऊर्ध्व हस्त)
Tāḍa āsana (ūrdhva hasta)
Palm tree pose (arms overhead)

ताडासन (ऊर्ध्वहस्त)
Tāḍasana (ūrdhvahasta)

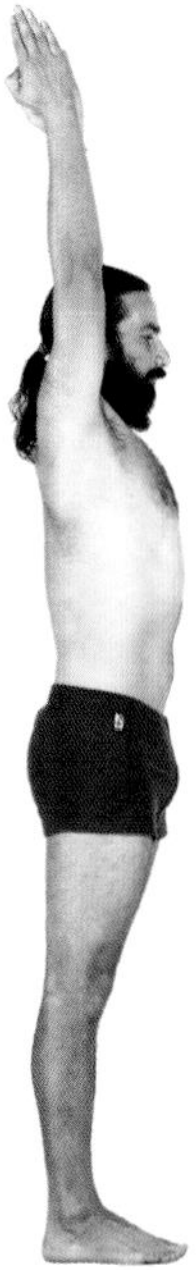

7
ताड आसन (ऊर्ध्व हस्त नमस्कार)
Tāḍa āsana (ūrdhva hasta namaskāra)
Palm tree pose (hands in prayer overhead)

ताडासन (ऊर्ध्वहस्तनमस्कार)
Tāḍāsana (ūrdhvahastanamaskāra)

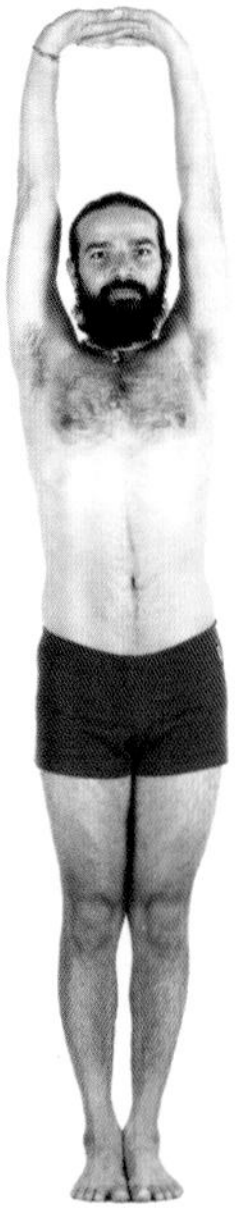

8
ताड आसन (ऊर्ध्व करतल)
Tāḍa āsana (ūrdhva karatala)
Palm tree pose (palms facing up)

ताडासन (ऊर्ध्वकरतल)
Tāḍāsana (ūrdhvakaratala)

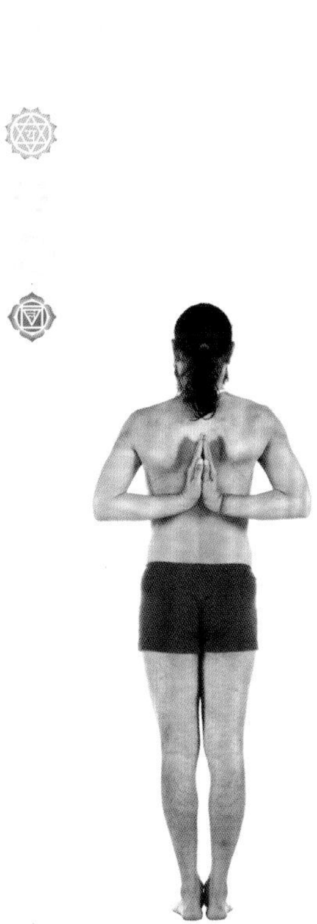

9
ताड आसन (पृष्ठ नमस्कार)
Tāḍa āsana (pṛṣṭha namaskāra)
Palm tree pose (hands in prayer behind)

ताडासन (पृष्ठनमस्कार)
Tāḍāsana (pṛṣṭhanamaskāra)

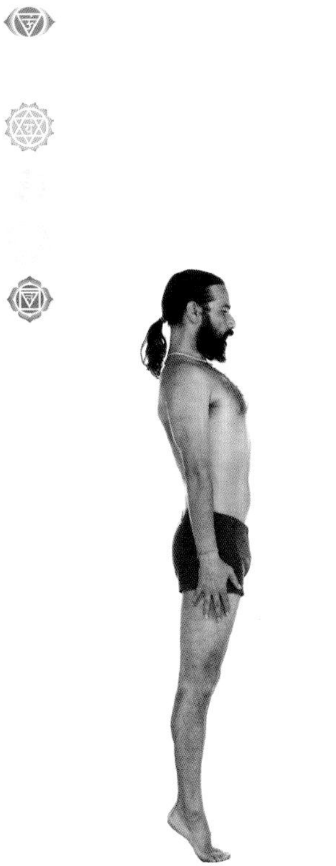

10
उत्तोलन ताड आसन
Uttolana tāḍa āsana
Balancing palm tree pose

उत्तोलनताडासन
Uttolanatāḍāsana

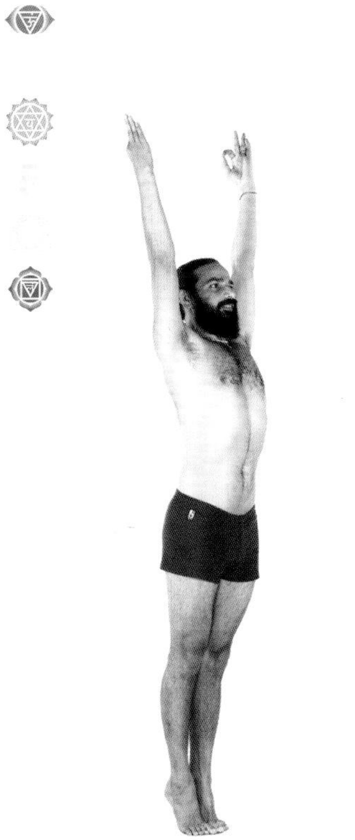

11
उत्तोलन ताड आसन (ऊर्ध्व हस्त)
Uttolana tāḍa āsana (ūrdhva hasta)
Balancing palm tree pose (arms overhead)

उत्तोलनताडासन (ऊर्ध्वहस्त)
Uttolanatāḍāsana (ūrdhvahasta)

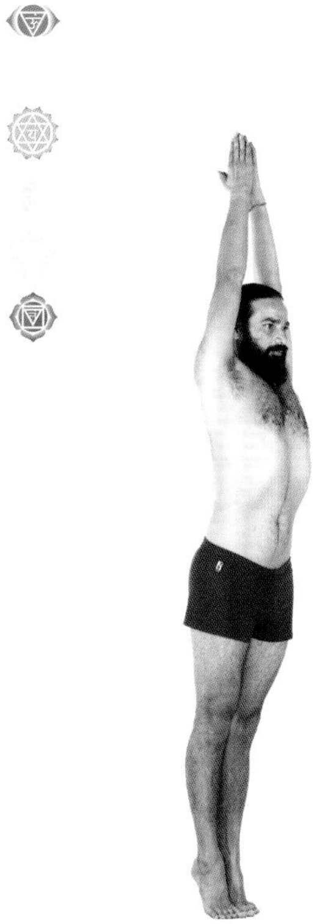

12
उत्तोलन ताड आसन (ऊर्ध्व हस्त नमस्कार)
Uttolana tāḍa āsana (ūrdhva hasta namaskāra)
Balancing palm tree pose
(arms overhead in prayer)

उत्तोलनताडासन (ऊर्ध्वहस्तनमस्कार)
Uttolanatāḍāsana (ūrdhvahastanamaskāra)

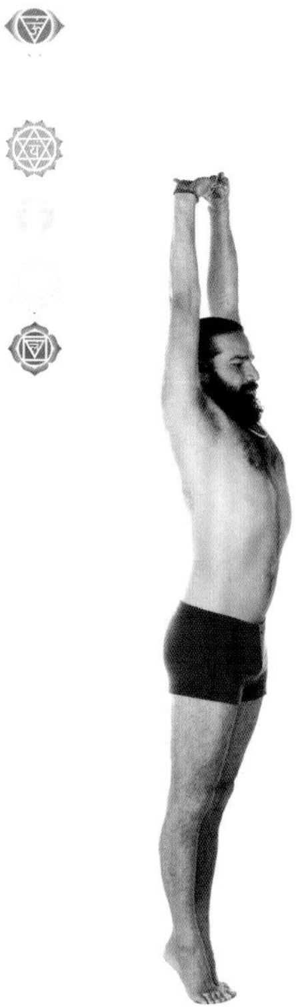

13
उत्तोलन ताड आसन (ऊर्ध्व करतल)
Uttolana tāḍa āsana (ūrdhva karatala)
Balancing palm tree pose (palms facing up)

उत्तोलनताडासन (ऊर्ध्वकरतल)
Uttolanatāḍāsana (ūrdhvakaratala)

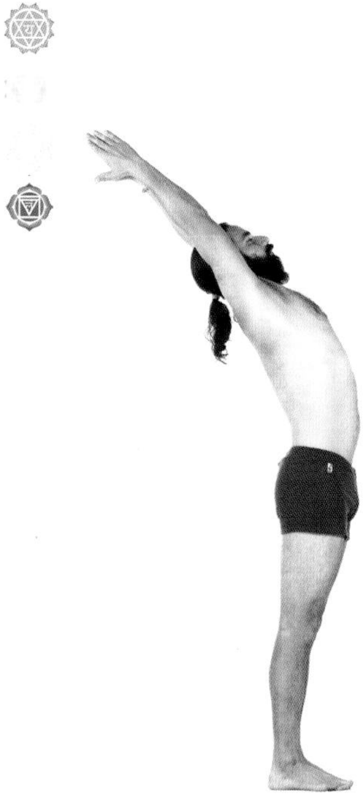

14
ऊर्ध्व हस्त उत्तान आसन
Ūrdhva hasta uttāna āsana
Overhead hands stretch pose

ऊर्ध्वहस्तोत्तानासन
Ūrdhvahastottānāsana

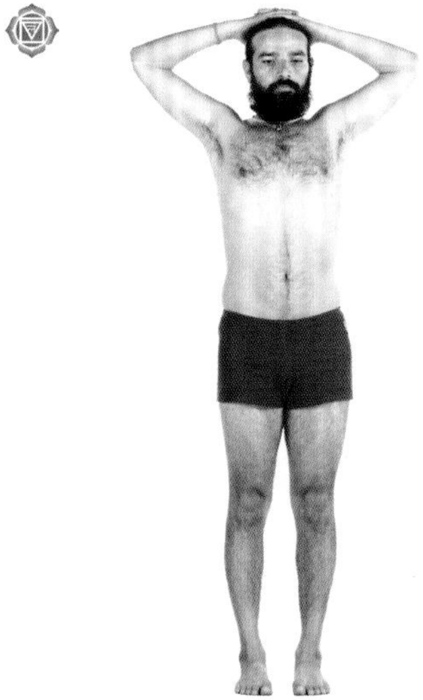

15
ताड आसन (शीर्ष हस्त)
Tāḍa āsana (śīrṣa hasta)
Palm tree pose (hands on head)

ताडासन (शीर्षहस्त)
Tāḍasana (śīrṣahasta)

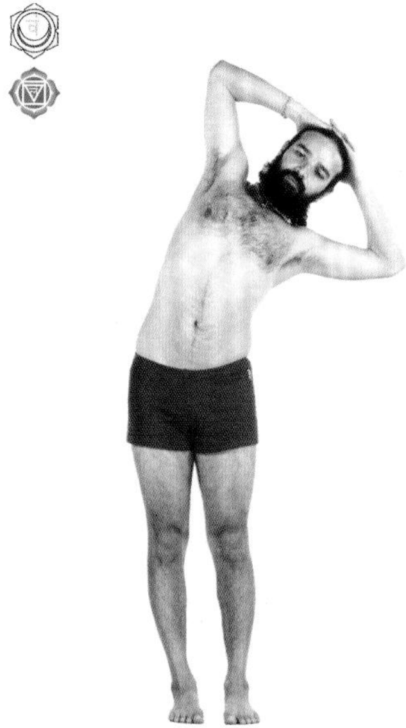

16
चन्द्र आसन (शीर्ष हस्त)
Candra āsana (śīrṣa hasta)
Moon pose (hands on head)

चन्द्रासन (शीर्षहस्त)
Candrāsana (śīrṣahasta)

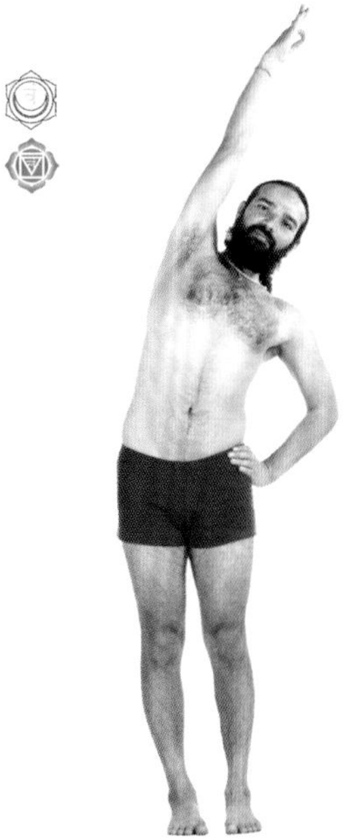

17
अर्ध चन्द्र आसन (एक कटि हस्त)
Ardha candra āsana (eka kati hasta)
Half moon pose (one hand on waist)

अर्धचन्द्रासन (एककटिहस्त)
Ardhacandrāsana (ekakatihasta)

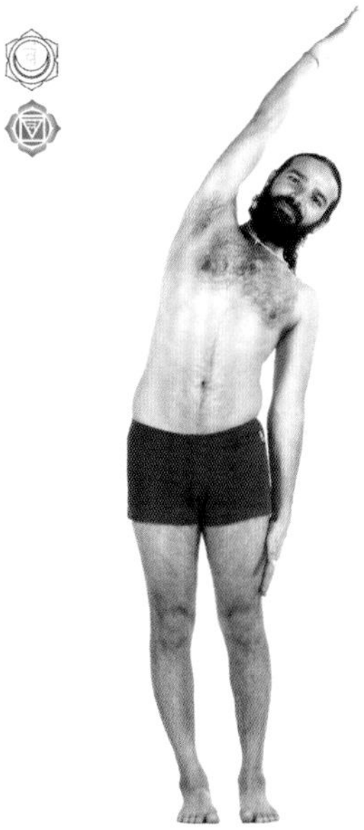

18
अर्ध चन्द्र आसन (एक हस्त उरु)
Ardha candra āsana (eka hasta uru)
Half moon pose (one hand on thigh)

अर्धचन्द्रासन (एकहस्तोरु)
Ardhacandrāsana (ekahastoru)

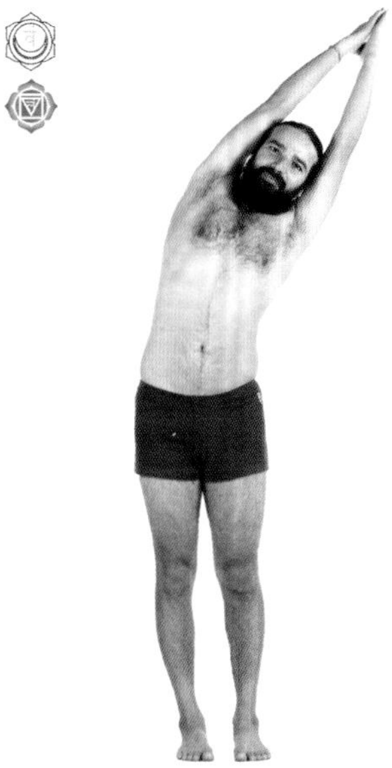

19
चन्द्र आसन (नमस्कार हस्त)
Candra āsana (namaskāra hasta)
Moon pose (prayer hands)

चन्द्रासन (नमस्कारहस्त)
Candrāsana (namaskārahasta)

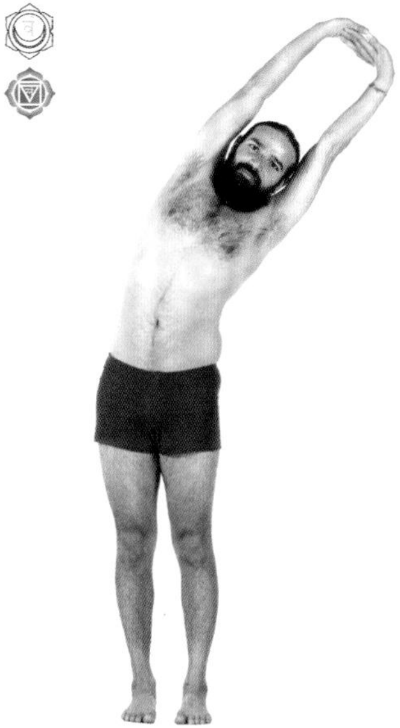

20
चन्द्र आसन (ऊर्ध्व करतल)
Candra āsana (ūrdhva karatala)
Moon pose (palms facing up)

चन्द्रासन (ऊर्ध्वकरतल)
Candrāsana (ūrdhvakaratala)

Balancing

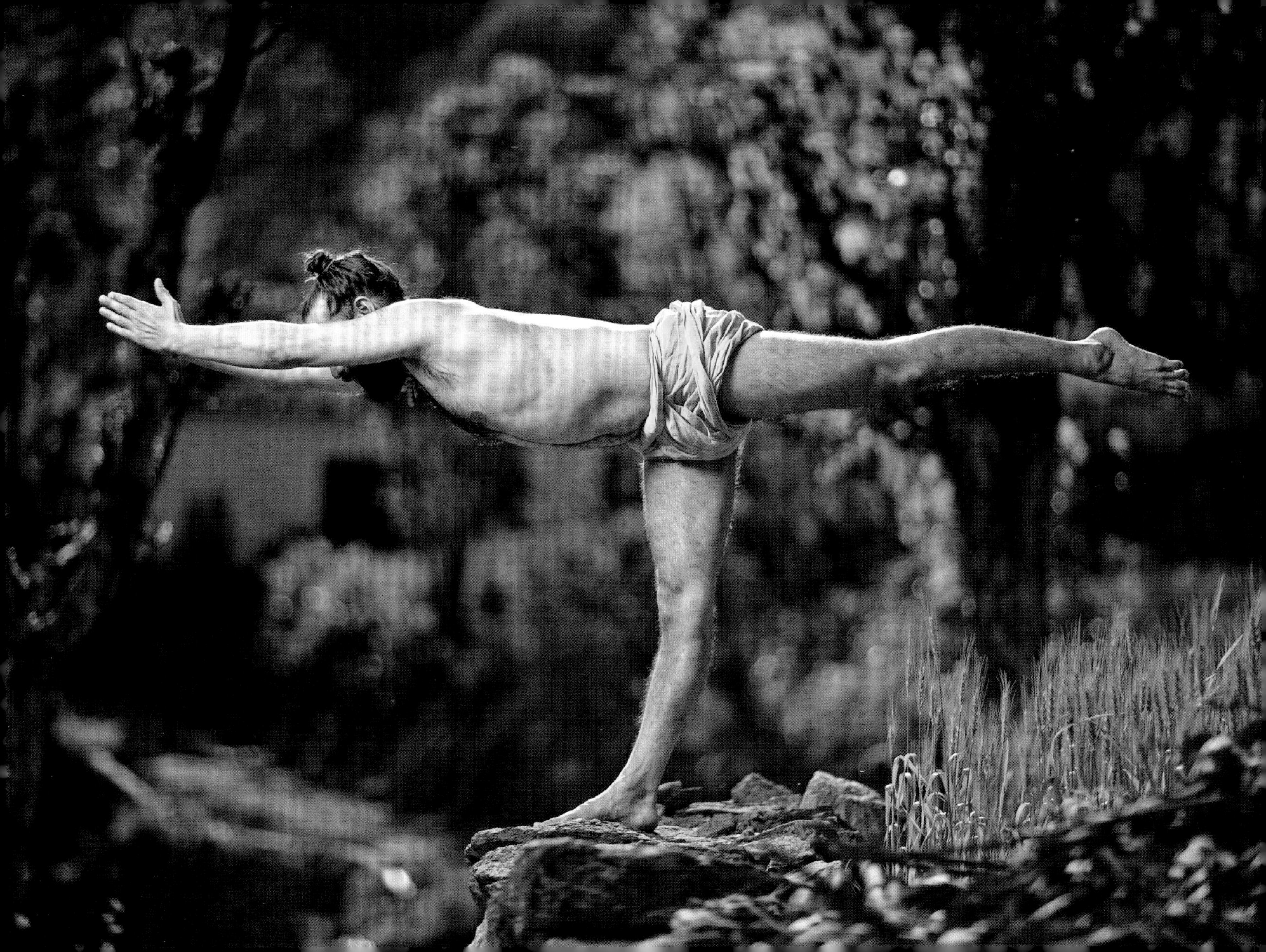

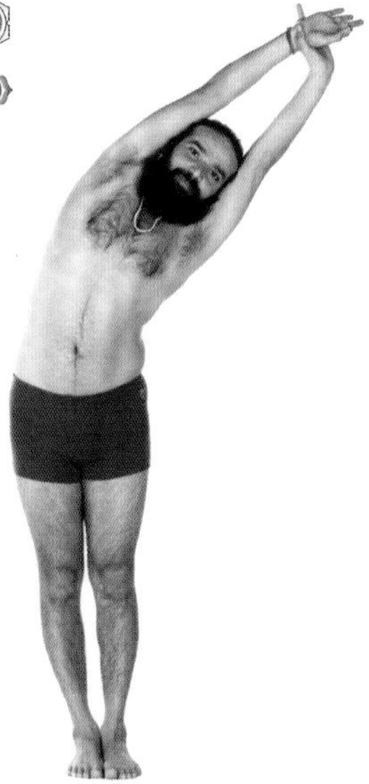

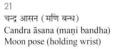

21
चन्द्र आसन (मणि बन्ध)
Candra āsana (maṇi bandha)
Moon pose (holding wrist)

चन्द्रासन (मणिबन्ध)
Candrāsana (maṇibandha)

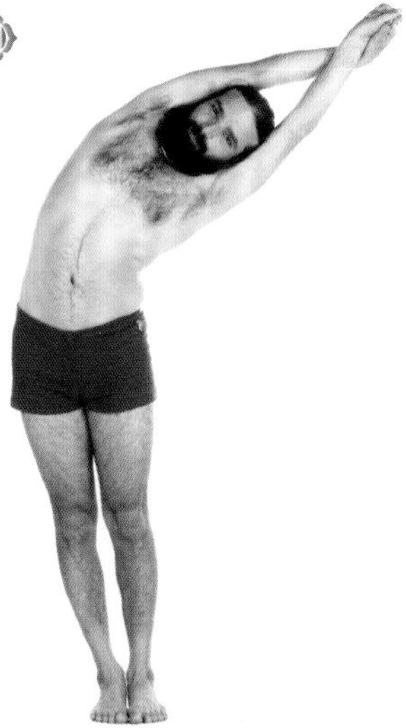

22
चन्द्र आसन (रज्जु हस्त)
Candra āsana (rajju hasta)
Moon pose (clasped hands)

चन्द्रासन (रज्जुहस्त)
Candrāsana (rajjuhasta)

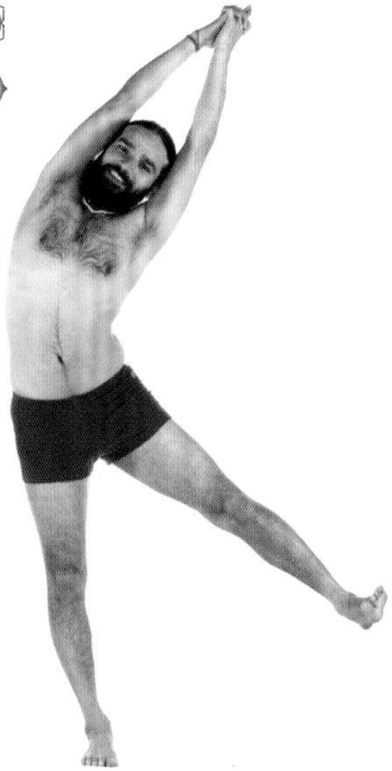

23
चन्द्र आसन (उत्तोलन एक पाद)
Candra āsana (uttolana eka pāda)
Moon pose (balancing on one foot)

चन्द्रासन (उत्तोलनैकपाद)
Candrāsana (uttolanaikapāda)

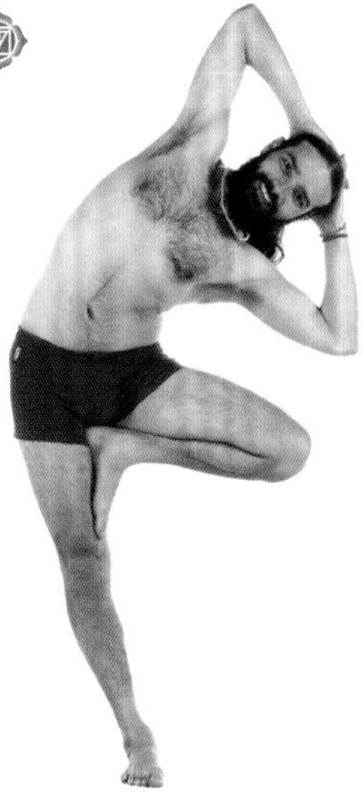

24
ध्रुव चन्द्र आसन (शीर्ष हस्त)
Dhruva candra āsana (śīrṣa hasta)
Fig tree moon pose (hands on head)

ध्रुवचन्द्रासन (शीर्षहस्त)
Dhruvacandrāsana (śīrṣahasta)

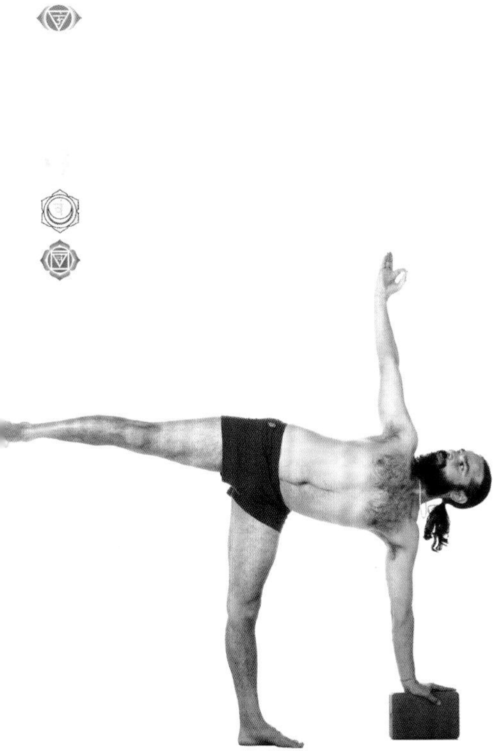

25
अर्ध चन्द्र कला आसन (सालम्ब हस्त)
Ardha candra kalā āsana (sālamba hasta)
Half moon phase pose (supported hand)

अर्धचन्द्रकलासन (सालम्बहस्त)
Ardhacandrakalāsana (sālambahasta)

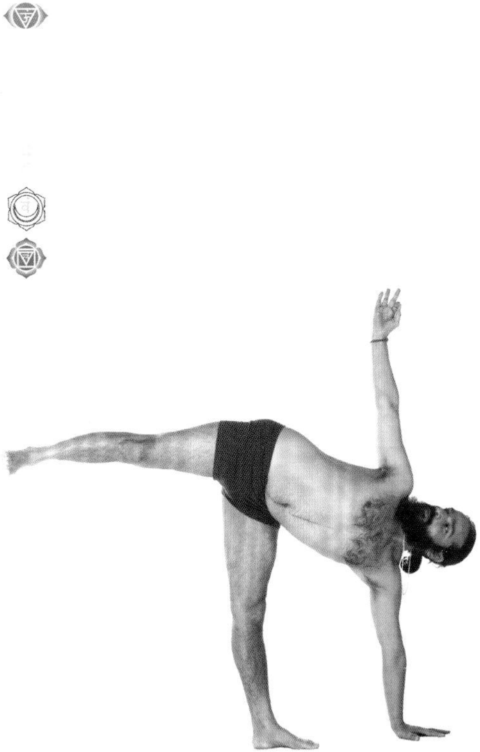

26
अर्ध चन्द्र कला आसन
Ardha candra kalā āsana
Half moon phase pose

अर्धचन्द्रकलासन
Ardhacandrakalāsana

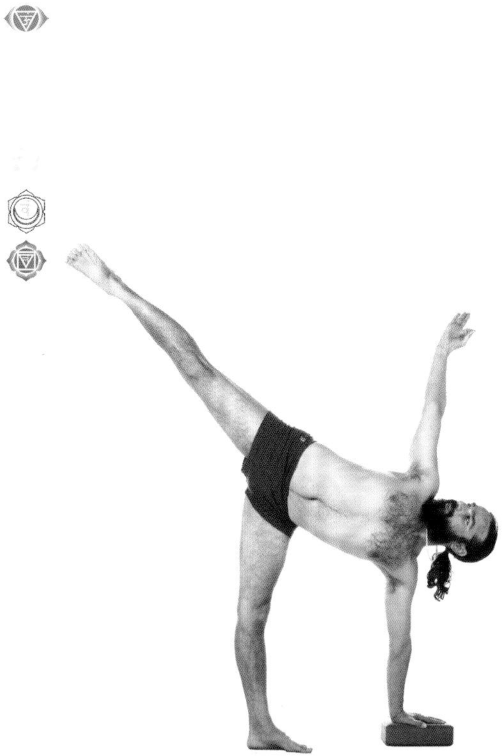

27
चन्द्र कला आसन (सालम्ब हस्त, व्योम पाद)
Candra kalā āsana (sālamba hasta, vyoma pāda)
Moon phase pose
(supported hand and externally rotated foot)

चन्द्रकलासन (सालम्बहस्त, व्योमपाद)
Candrakalāsana (sālambahasta, vyomapāda)

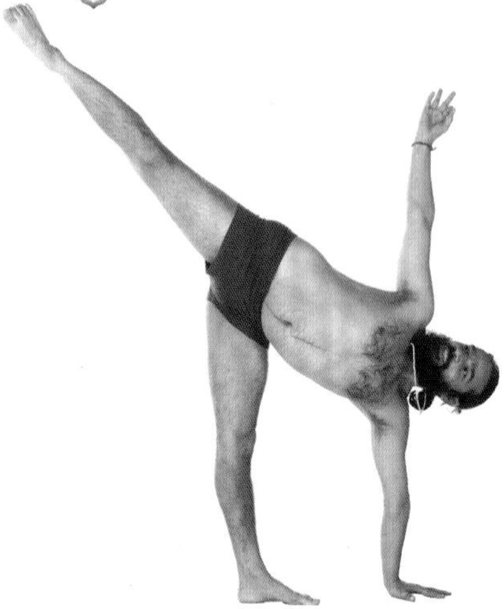

28
चन्द्र कला आसन
Candra kalā āsana
Moon phase pose

चन्द्रकलासन
Candrakalāsana

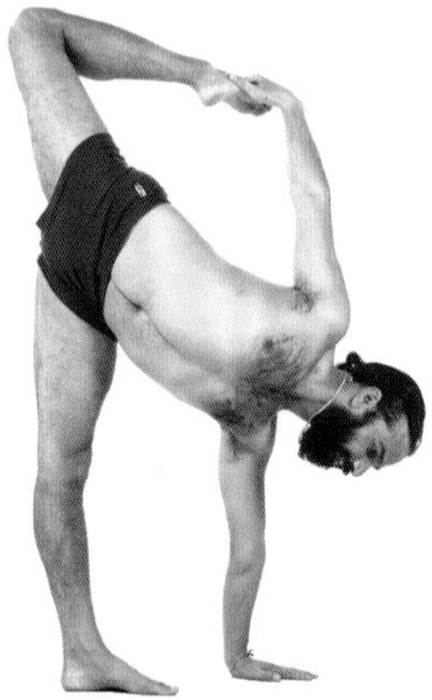

29
नृत्य चन्द्र कला आसन (अधो मुख)
Nṛtya candra kalā āsana (adho mukha)
Dancing moon phase pose (downward facing)

नृत्यचन्द्रकलासन (अधोमुख)
Nṛtyacandrakalāsana (adhomukha)

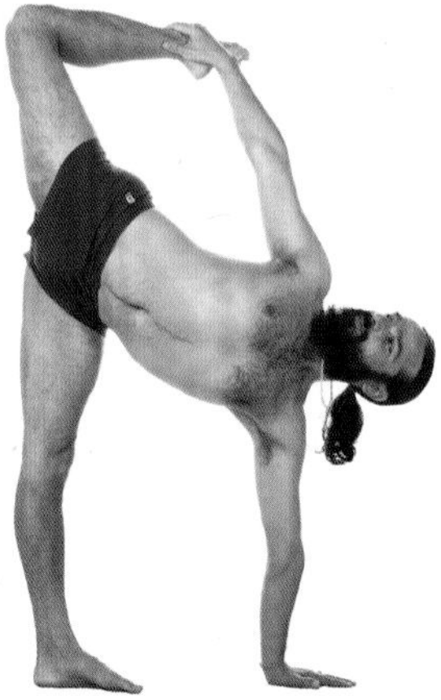

30
नृत्य चन्द्र कला आसन (ऊर्ध्व मुख)
Nṛtya candra kalā āsana (ūrdhva mukha)
Dancing moon phase pose (upward facing)

नृत्यचन्द्रकलासन(ऊर्ध्वमुख)
Nṛtyacandrakalāsana (ūrdhvamukha)

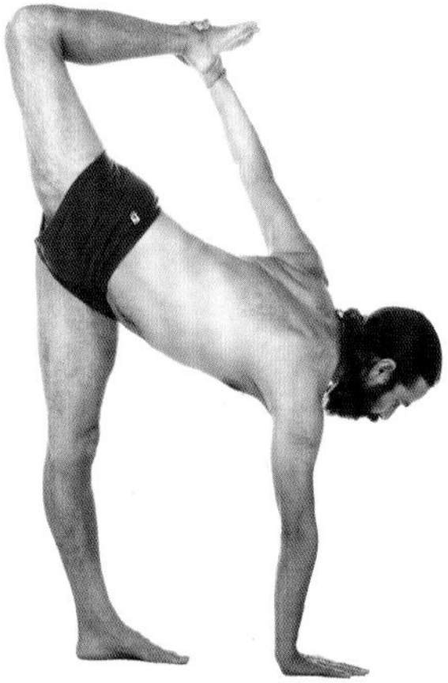

31
परिवृत्त नृत्य चन्द्र कला आसन (अधो मुख)
Parivṛtta nṛtya candra kalā āsana (adho mukha)
Twisted dancing moon phase pose
(downward facing)

परिवृत्तनृत्यचन्द्रकलासन (अधोमुख)
Parivṛttanṛtyacandrakalāsana (adhomukha)

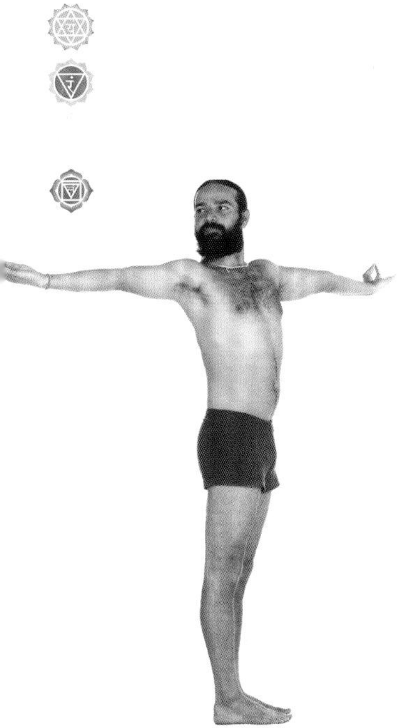

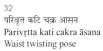

32
परिवृत्त कटि चक्र आसन
Parivṛtta kati cakra āsana
Waist twisting pose

परिवृत्तकटिचक्रासन
Parivṛttakaticakrāsana

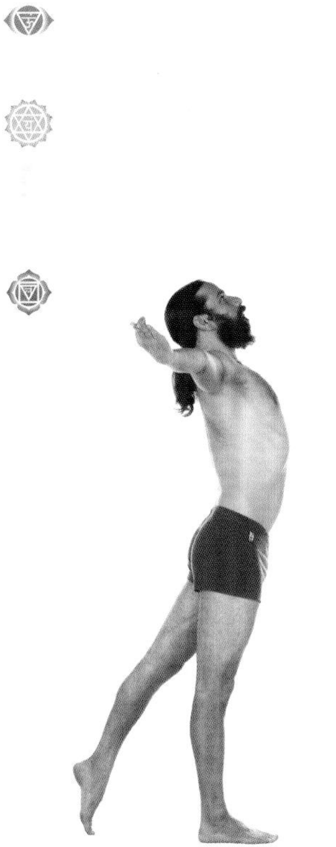

33
अप्सरा आसन (पृष्ठ पाद अङ्गुल भू)
Apsarā āsana (pṛṣṭha pāda aṅgula bhū)
Angel pose (back toes on the earth)

अप्सरासन (पृष्ठपादाङ्गुलभू)
Apsarāsana (pṛṣṭhapādāṅgulabhū)

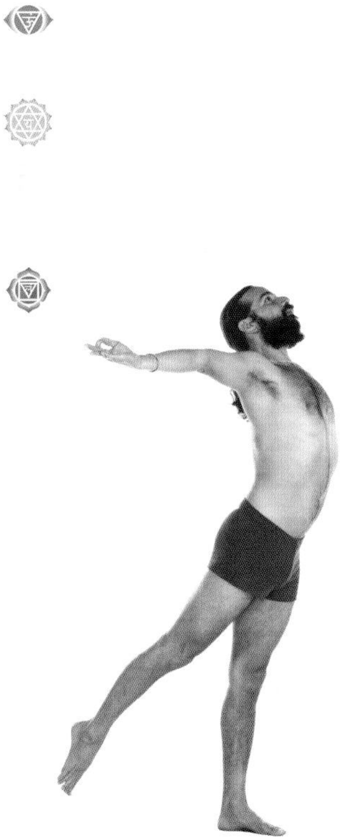

34
भद्र अप्सरा आसन
Bhadra apsarā āsana
Beautiful angel pose

भद्राप्सरासन
Bhadrāpsarāsana

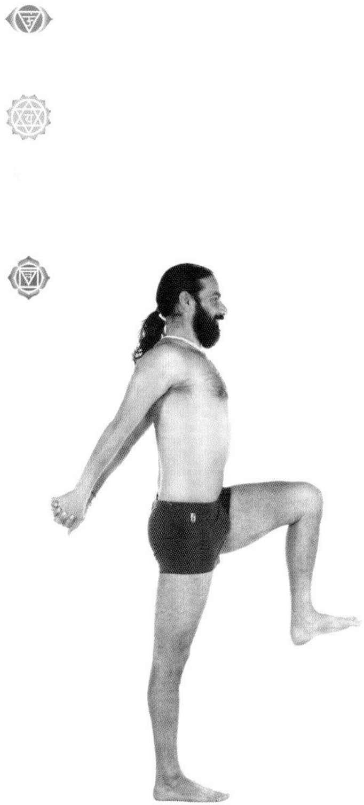

35
पवित्र आसन (पृष्ठ हस्त उत्तान)
Pavitra āsana (pṛṣṭha hasta uttāna)
Purity pose (hands stretched behind)

पवित्रासन (पृष्ठहस्तोत्तान)
Pavitrāsana (pṛṣṭhahastottāna)

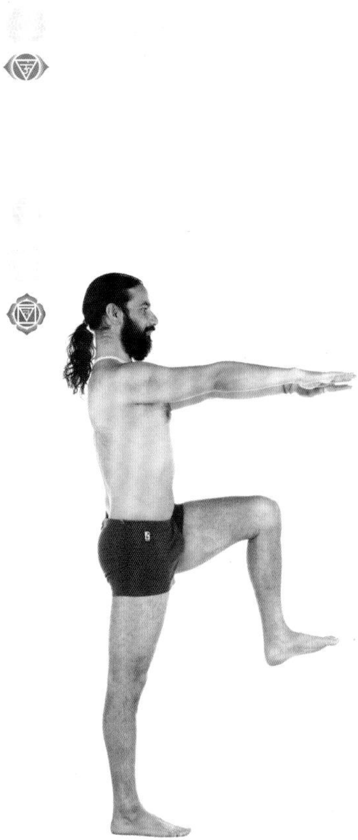

36
पवित्र आसन (समक्ष हस्त)
Pavitra āsana (samakṣa hasta)
Purity pose (hands in front)

पवित्रासन (समक्षहस्त)
Pavitrāsana (samakṣahasta)

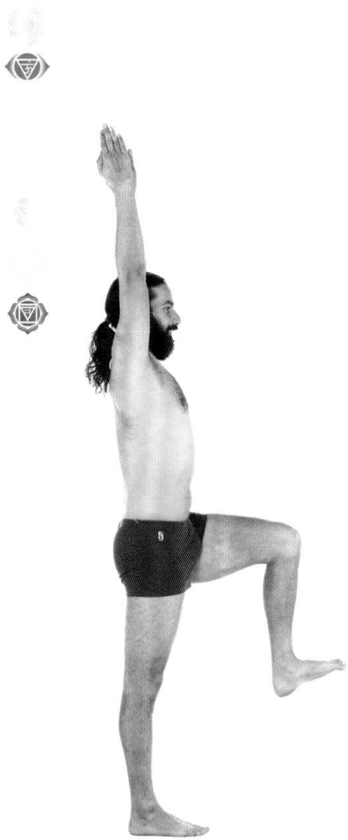

37
पवित्र आसन (ऊर्ध्व हस्त)
Pavitra āsana (ūrdhva hasta)
Purity pose (hands overhead)

पवित्रासन (ऊर्ध्वहस्त)
Pavitrāsana (ūrdhvahasta)

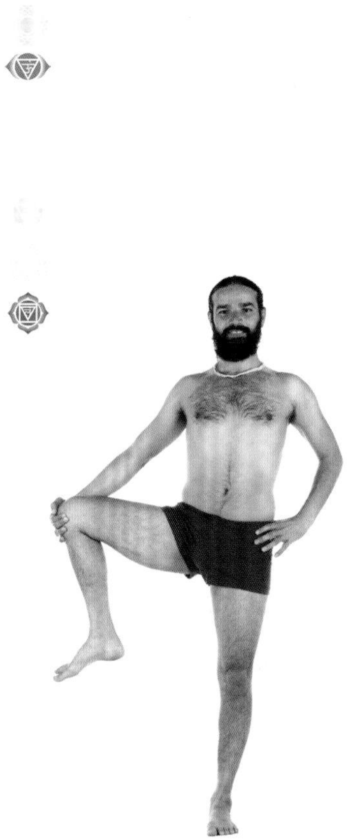

38
पवित्र आसन (पार्श्व कटि जानु हस्त)
Pavitra āsana (pārśva kati jānu hasta)
Purity pose (hand on waist and knee open to the side)

पवित्रासन (पार्श्वकटिजानुहस्त)
Pavitrāsana (pārśvakatijānuhasta)

Your true nature is blissful, joyful, playful, and fearless.

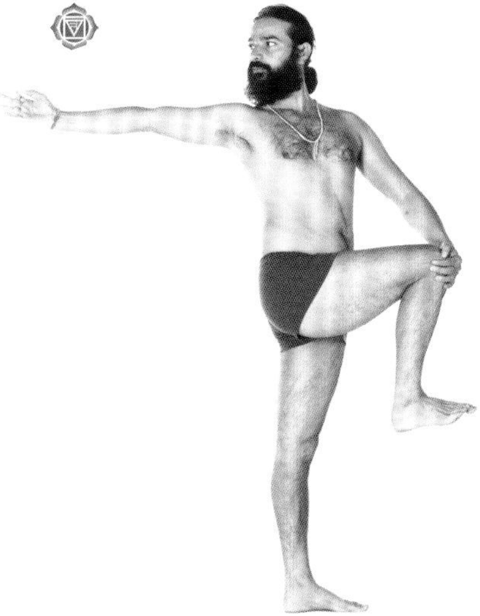

39
परिवृत्त पवित्र आसन (एक जानु हस्त)
Parivṛtta pavitra āsana (eka jānu hasta)
Twisted purity pose (one hand on knee)

परिवृत्तपवित्रासन (एकजानुहस्त)
Parivṛttapavitrāsana (ekajānuhasta)

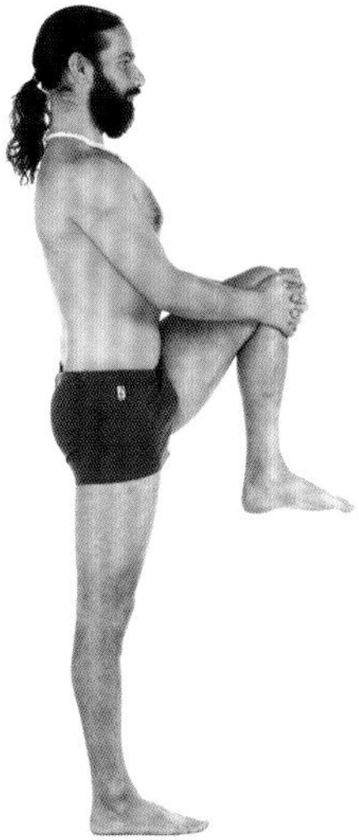

40
पवित्र आसन (जानु बद्ध)
Pavitra āsana (jānu baddha)
Purity pose (holding knee)

पवित्रासन (जानुबद्ध)
Pavitrāsana (jānubaddha)

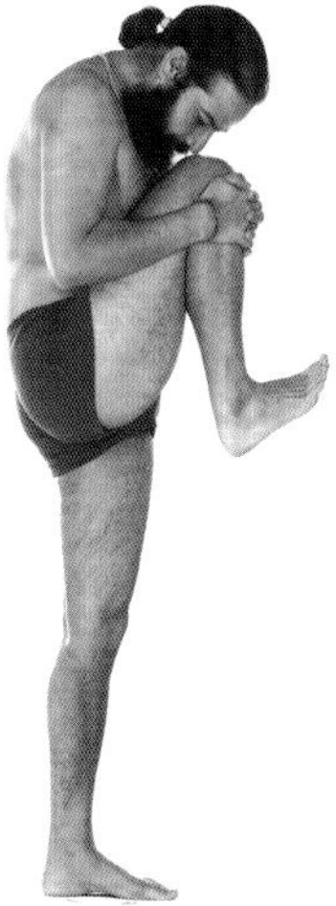

41
पवित्र आसन (जानु शिर)
Pavitra āsana (jānu śira)
Purity pose (head to knee)

पवित्रासन (जानुशिर)
Pavitrāsana (jānuśira)

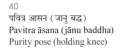

*Yoga is not a workout;
it is a journey inward.*

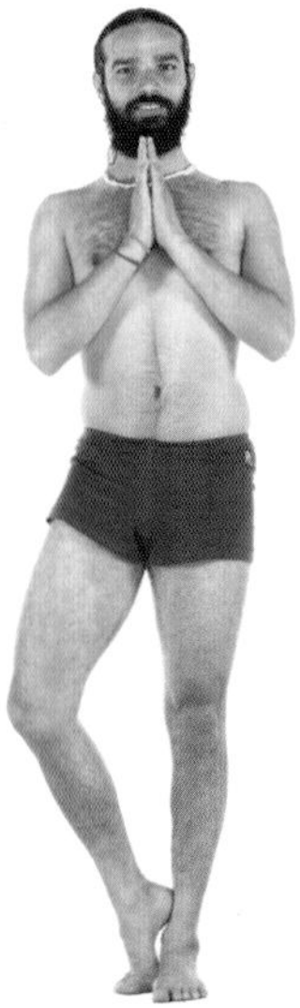

42
ध्रुव आसन (प्रपदिक)
Dhruva āsana (prapadika)
Fig tree pose (ball of toes on the earth)

ध्रुवासन(प्रपदिक)
Dhruvāsana (prapadika)

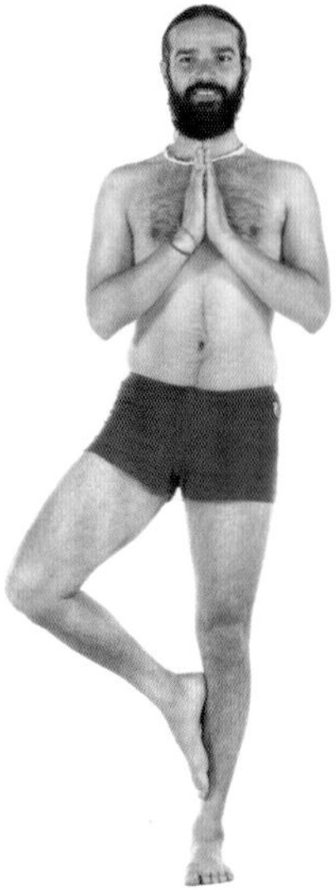

43
ध्रुव आसन (गुल्फ पाद)
Dhruva āsana (gulpha pāda)
Fig tree pose (foot on ankle)

ध्रुवासन (गुल्फपाद)
Dhruvāsana (gulphapāda)

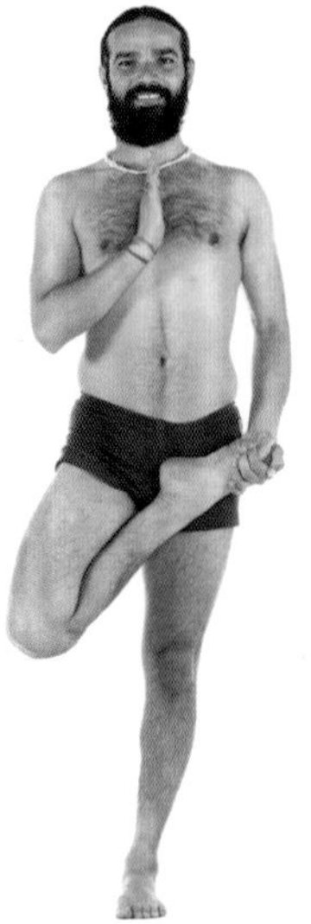

44
अर्ध पद्म ध्रुव आसन (एक हस्त नमस्कार)
Ardha padma dhruva āsana
(eka hasta namaskāra)
Half lotus fig tree pose
(one hand in prayer)

अर्धपद्मध्रुवासन (एकहस्तनमस्कार)
Ardhapadmadhruvāsana (ekahastanamaskāra)

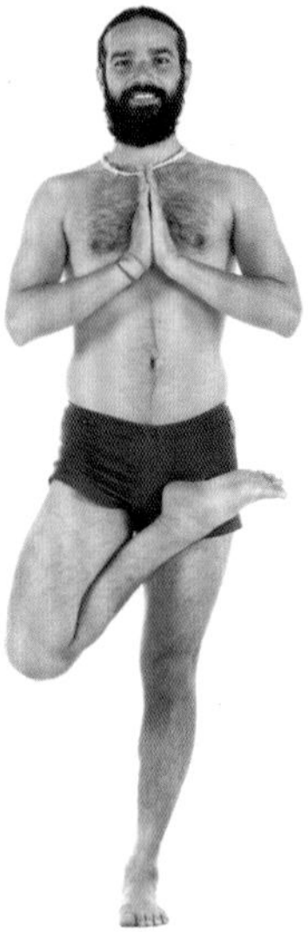

45
अर्ध पद्म ध्रुव आसन (नमस्कार हस्त)
Ardha padma dhruva āsana (namaskāra hasta)
Half lotus fig tree pose (hands in prayer)

अर्धपद्मध्रुवासन (नमस्कारहस्त)
Ardhapadmadhruvāsana (namaskārahasta)

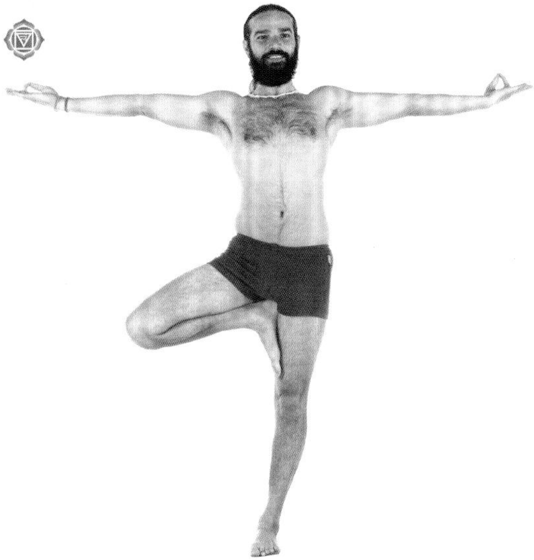

46
ध्रुव आसन (विराट हस्त)
Dhruva āsana (virāṭa hasta)
Fig tree pose (hands extended wide)

ध्रुवासन (विराटहस्त)
Dhruvāsana (virātahasta)

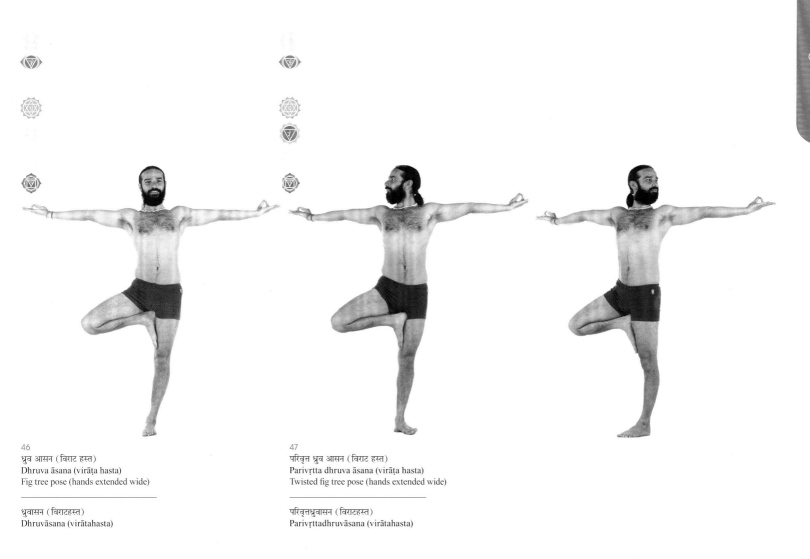

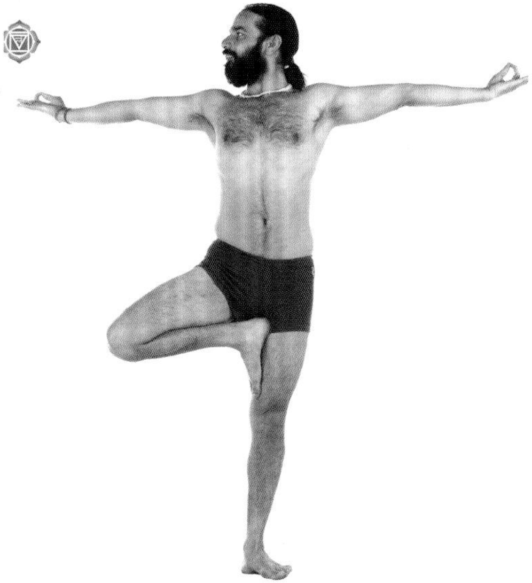

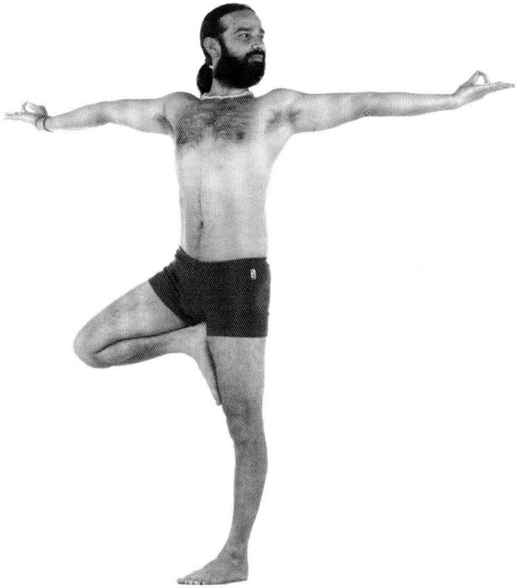

47
परिवृत्त ध्रुव आसन (विराट हस्त)
Parivṛtta dhruva āsana (virāṭa hasta)
Twisted fig tree pose (hands extended wide)

परिवृत्तध्रुवासन (विराटहस्त)
Parivṛttadhruvāsana (virātahasta)

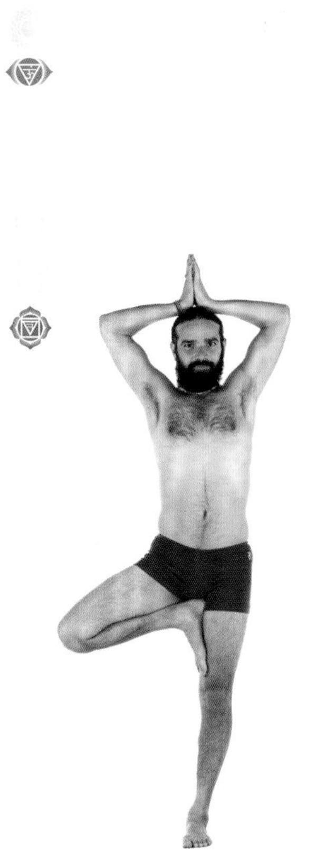

48
ध्रुव आसन (शिखा नमस्कार)
Dhruva āsana (śikhā namaskāra)
Fig tree pose (hands in prayer on the head)

ध्रुवासन (शिखानमस्कार)
Dhruvāsana (śikhānamaskāra)

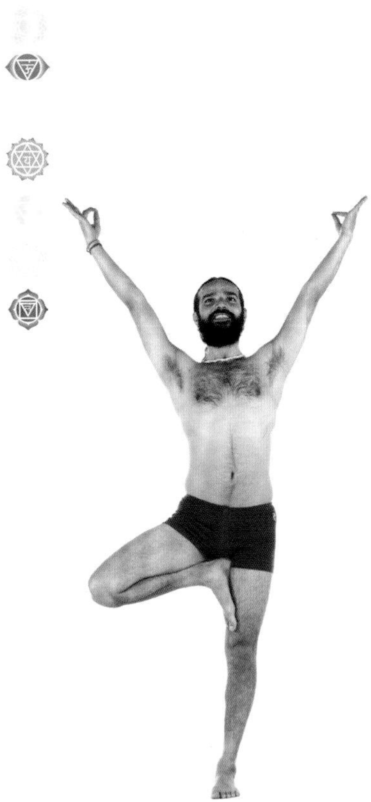

49
आनन्द ध्रुव आसन
Ānanda dhruva āsana
Blissful fig tree pose

आनन्दध्रुवासन
Ānandadhruvāsana

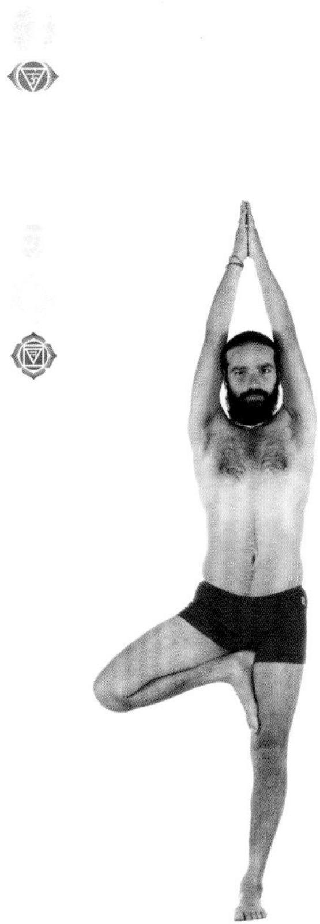

50
ध्रुव आसन
Dhruva āsana
Fig tree pose

ध्रुवासन
Dhruvāsana

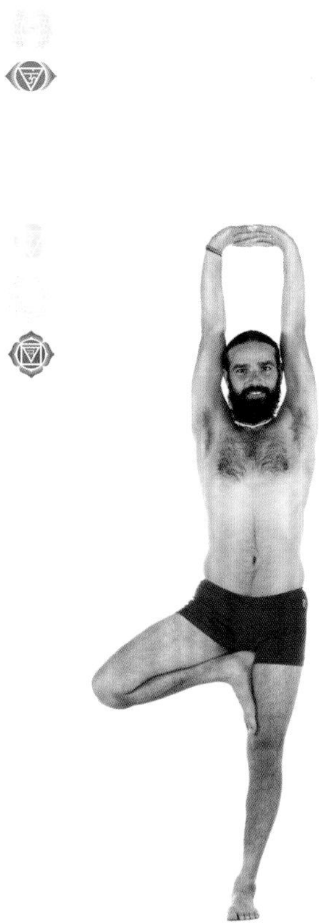

51
ध्रुव आसन (ऊर्ध्व करतल)
Dhruva āsana (ūrdhva karatala)
Fig tree pose (palms facing up)

ध्रुवासन (ऊर्ध्वकरतल)
Dhruvāsana (ūrdhvakaratala)

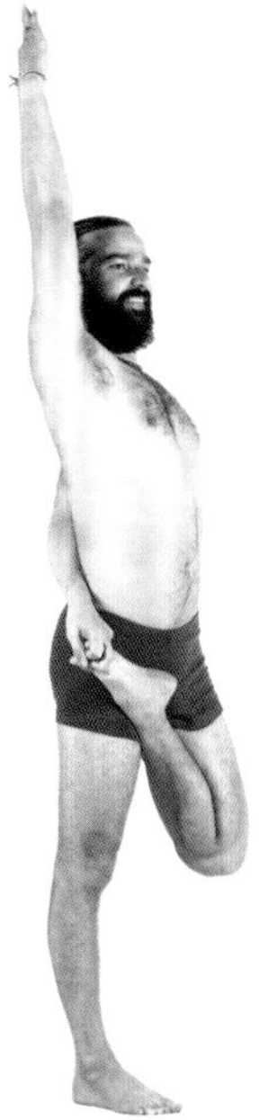

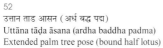

52
उत्तान ताड आसन (अर्ध बद्ध पद्म)
Uttāna tāḍa āsana (ardha baddha padma)
Extended palm tree pose (bound half lotus)

उत्तानताडासन (अर्धबद्धपद्म)
Uttānatāḍāsana (ardhabaddhapadma)

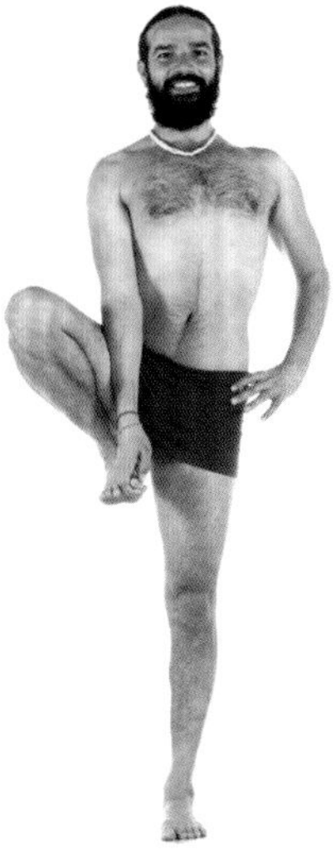

53
उत्थित हस्त पाद अङ्गुष्ठ आसन (आरम्भ अवस्था)
Utthita hasta pāda aṅguṣṭha āsana (ārambha avasthā)
Standing hand to big toe pose (starting position)

उत्थितहस्तपादाङ्गुष्ठासन (आरम्भावस्था)
Utthitahastapādāṅguṣṭhāsana (ārambhāvasthā)

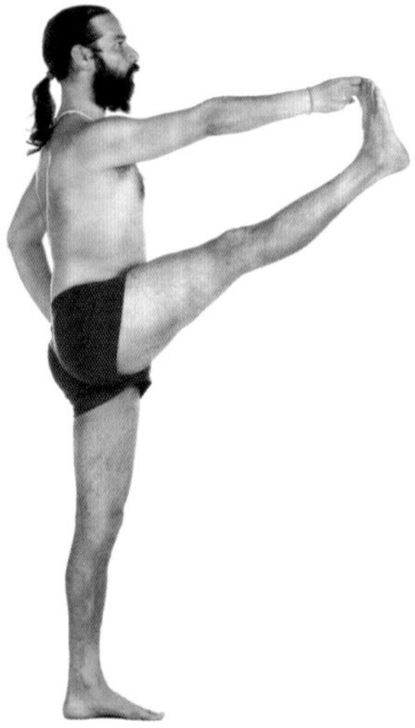

54
उत्थित हस्त पाद अङ्गुष्ठ आसन
Utthita hasta pāda āṅguṣṭha āsana
Standing hand to big toe pose

उत्थितहस्तपादाङ्गुष्ठासन
Utthitahastapādāṅguṣṭhāsana

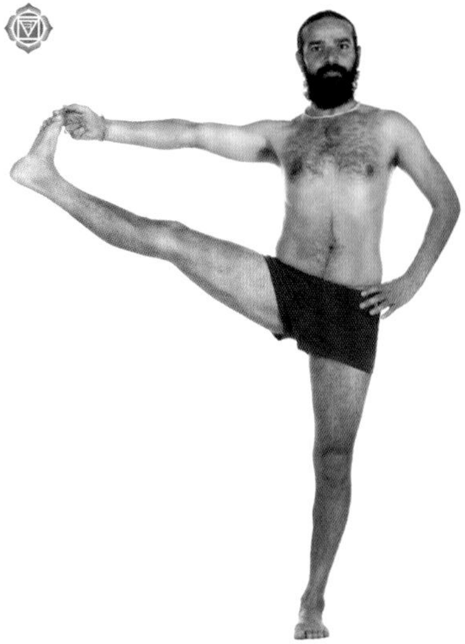

55
उत्थित हस्त पाद अङ्गुष्ठ आसन (पार्श्व)
Utthita hasta pāda āṅguṣṭha āsana (pārśva)
Standing hand to big toe pose (open to the side)

उत्थितहस्तपादाङ्गुष्ठासन (पार्श्व)
Utthitahastapādāṅguṣṭhāsana (pārśva)

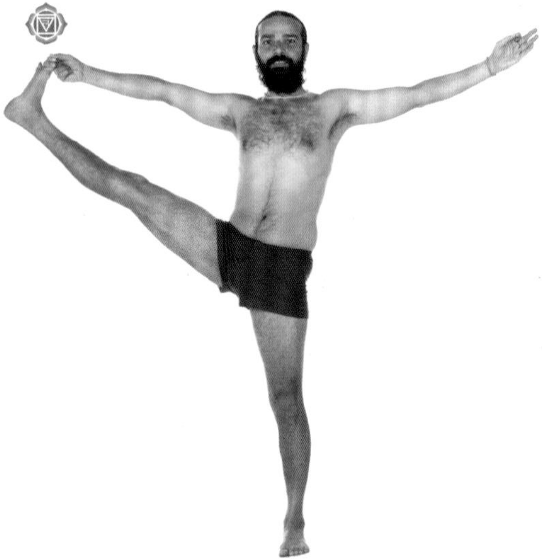

56
उत्थित पार्श्व हस्त पाद अङ्गुष्ठ आसन (पार्श्व, विराट हस्त)
Utthita hasta pāda āṅguṣṭha āsana (pārśva, virāṭa hasta)
Standing hand to big toe pose (open to the side, hand extended)

उत्थितहस्तपादाङ्गुष्ठासन (पार्श्व,विराटहस्त)
Utthitahastapādāṅguṣṭhāsana (pārśva, virāṭahasta)

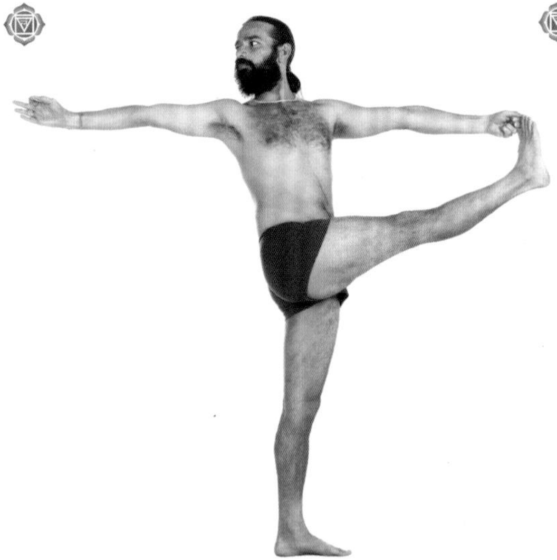

57
उत्थित परिवृत्त हस्त पाद अङ्गुष्ठ आसन (विराट हस्त)
Utthita parivṛtta hasta pāda aṅguṣṭha āsana (virāṭa hasta)
Standing twisted hand to big toe pose (hand extended)

उत्थितपरिवृत्तहस्तपादाङ्गुष्ठासन (विराटहस्त)
Utthitaparivṛttahastapādāṅguṣṭhāsana (virāṭahasta)

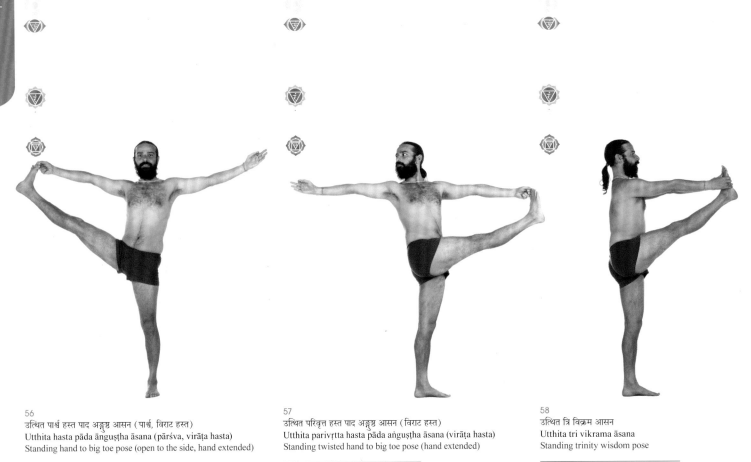

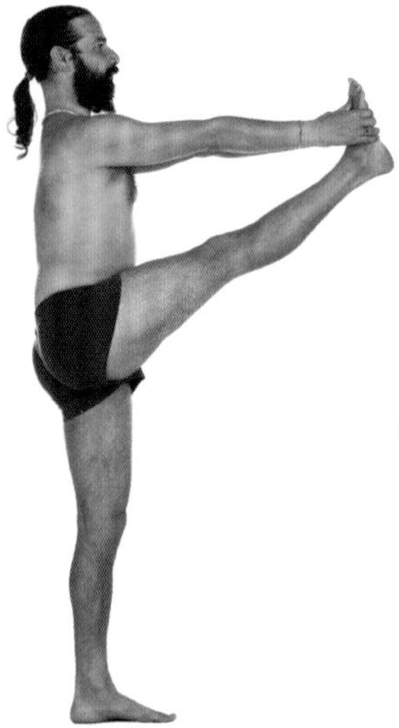

58
उत्थित त्रि विक्रम आसन
Utthita tri vikrama āsana
Standing trinity wisdom pose

उत्थितत्रिविक्रमासन
Utthitatrivikramāsana

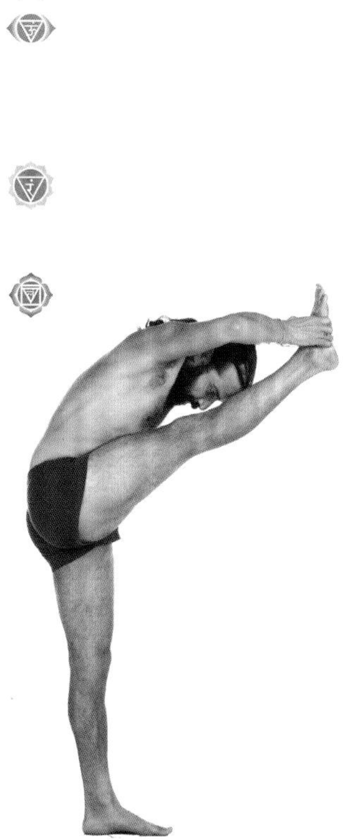

59
उत्थित त्रि विक्रम आसन (जानु शिर)
Utthita tri vikrama āsana (jānu śira)
Standing trinity wisdom pose (head to knee)

उत्थितत्रिविक्रमासन (जानुशिर)
Utthitatrivikramāsana (jānuśira)

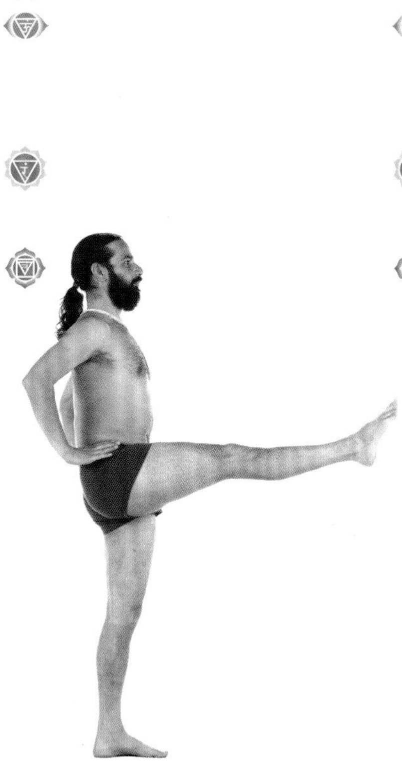

60
उत्थित एक पाद दण्ड आसन (कटि हस्त)
Utthita eka pāda daṇḍa āsana (kati hasta)
Standing one leg stick pose (hands on waist)

उत्थितैकपाददण्डासन (कटिहस्त)
Utthitaikapādaṇḍaḍāsana (katihasta)

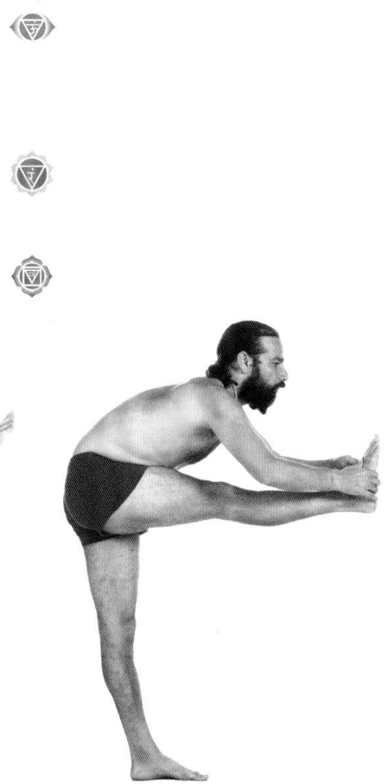

61
उत्थित एक पाद जानु शिर आसन (पूर्व मुख)
Utthita eka pāda jānu śira āsana (pūrva mukha)
Standing one leg head to knee pose (facing forward)

उत्थितैकपादजानुशिरासन (पूर्वमुख)
Utthitaikapādajānuśirāsana (pūrvamukha)

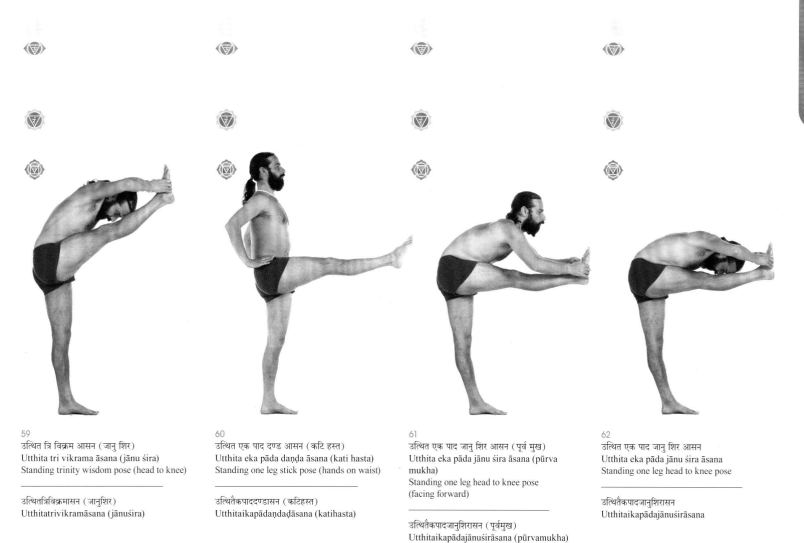

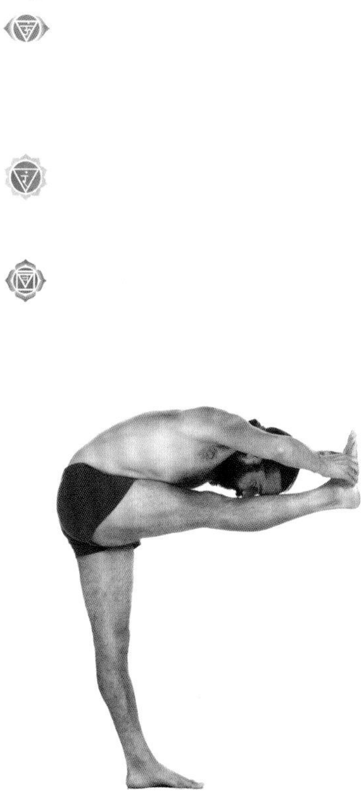

62
उत्थित एक पाद जानु शिर आसन
Utthita eka pāda jānu śira āsana
Standing one leg head to knee pose

उत्थितैकपादजानुशिरासन
Utthitaikapādajānuśirāsana

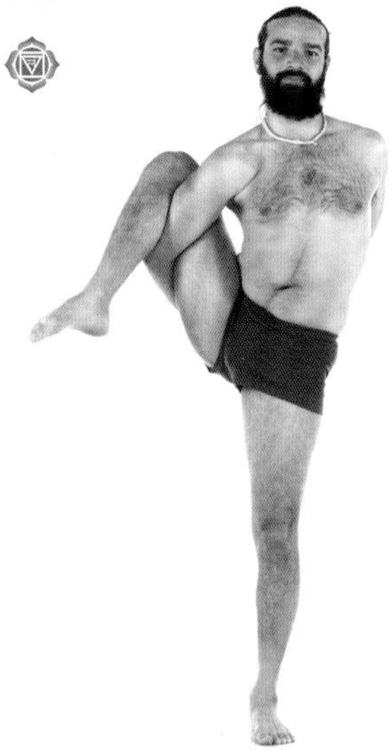

63
पार्श्व त्रि विक्रम आसन (रज्जु हस्त,आरम्भ अवस्था)
Pārśva tri vikrama āsana (rajju hasta, ārambha avasthā)
Side trinity wisdom pose (bound hands, starting position)

पार्श्वत्रिविक्रमासन (रज्जुहस्त, आरम्भावस्था)
Pārśvatrivikramāsana (rajjuhasta, ārambhāvasthā)

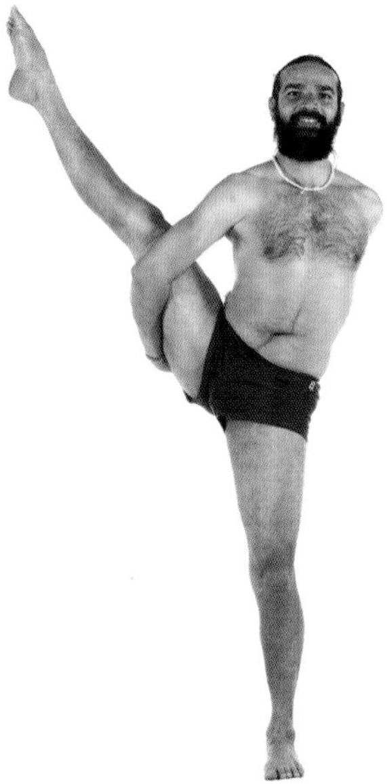

64
पूर्ण पार्श्व त्रि विक्रम आसन (रज्जु हस्त)
Pūrṇa pārśva tri vikrama āsana (rajju hasta)
Side full trinity wisdom pose (bound hands)

पूर्णपार्श्वत्रिविक्रमासन (रज्जुहस्त)
Pūrṇapārśvatrivikramāsana (rajjuhasta)

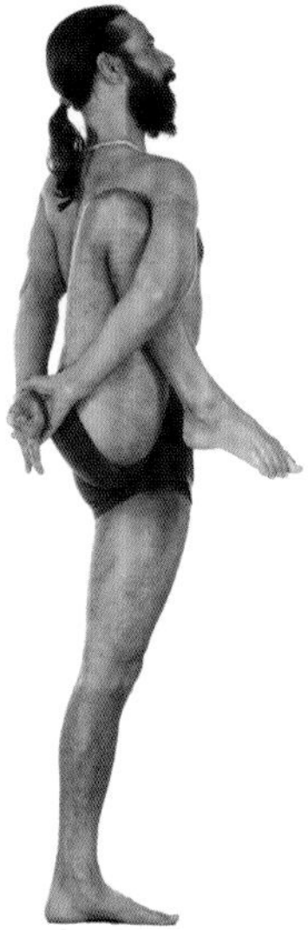

65
जटायु आसन
Jaṭāyu āsana
Vulture pose

जटायुासन
Jaṭāyuāsana

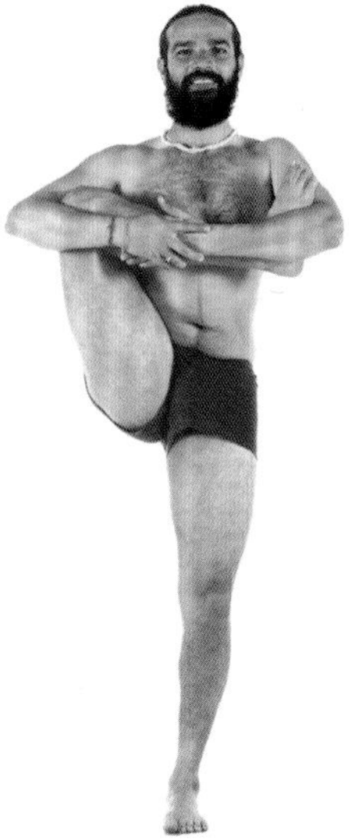

66
उत्थितशिशु वात्सल्य आसन
Utthita śīṣu vātsalya āsana
Standing baby cradling pose

उत्थितशिशुवात्सल्यासन
Utthitaśīṣuvātsalyāsana

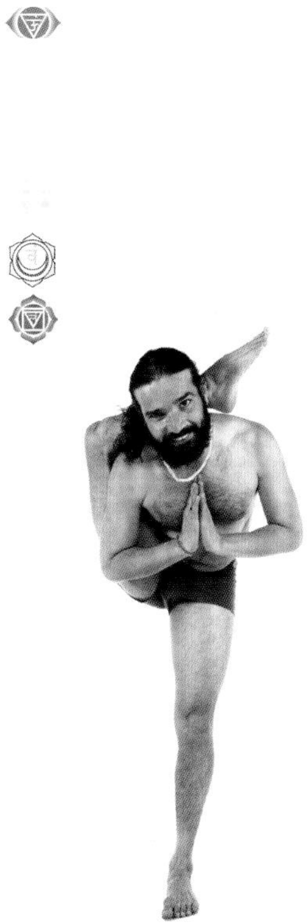

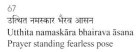

67
उत्थित नमस्कार भैरव आसन
Utthita namaskāra bhairava āsana
Prayer standing fearless pose

उत्थितनमस्कारभैरवासन
Utthitanamaskārabhairavāsana

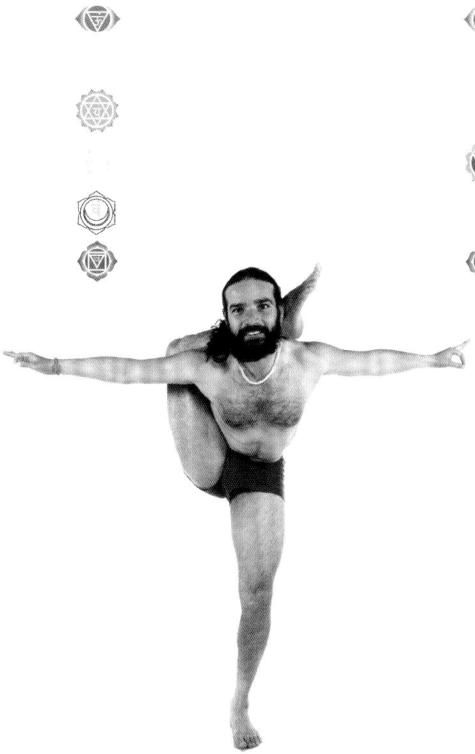

68
उत्थित भैरव आसन (विराट हस्त)
Utthita bhairava āsana (virāṭa hasta)
Standing fearless pose (hands extended wide)

उत्थितभैरवासन (विराटहस्त)
Utthitabhairavāsana (virāṭahasta)

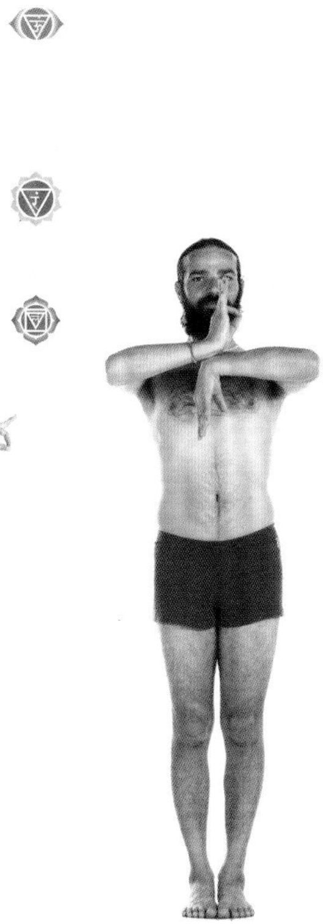

69
नट राज आसन (आरम्भ अवस्था)
Naṭa rāja āsana (ārambha avasthā)
Lord of the Dance pose (starting position)

नटराजासन(आरम्भावस्था)
Naṭarājāsana (ārambhavasthā)

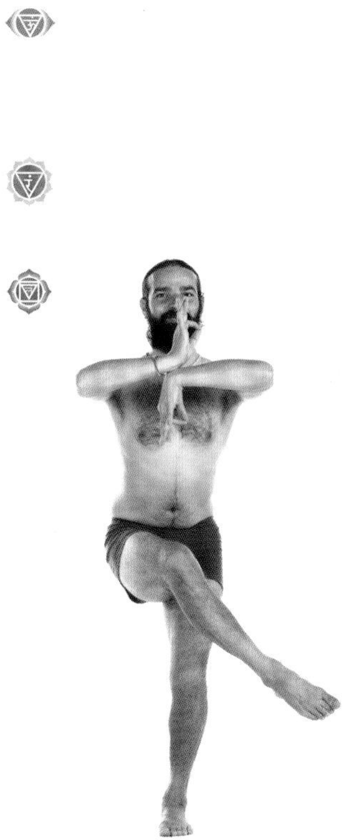

70
शाम्भवी नट राज आसन
Śāmbhavī naṭa rāja āsana
Shiva-Shakti Lord of the Dance pose

शाम्भवीनटराजासन
Śāmbhavīnaṭarājāsana

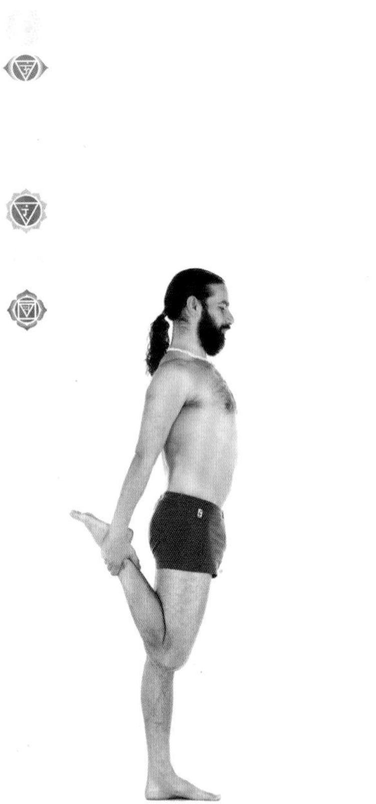

71
मृदुल नट राज आसन (आरम्भ अवस्था)
Mṛdula nata rāja āsana (ārambha avasthā)
Happy Lord of the Dance pose (starting position)

मृदुलनटराजासन (आरम्भावस्था)
Mṛdulanatarājāsana (ārambhāvasthā)

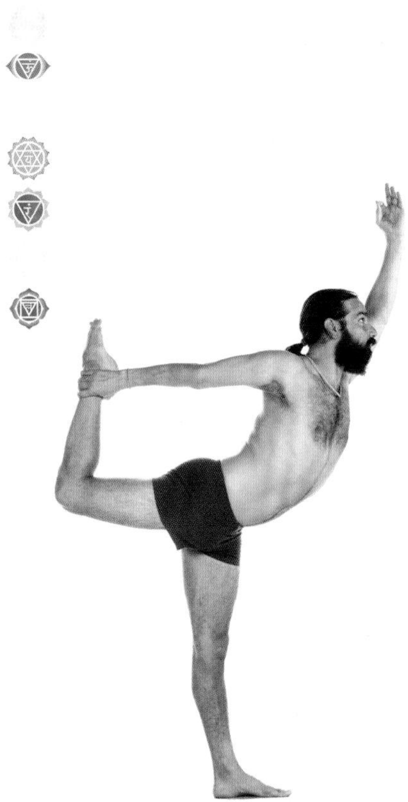

72
नट राज आसन (बहिः गुल्फ हस्त)
Naṭa rāja āsana (bahiḥ gulpha hasta)
Lord of the Dance pose (hand outside ankle)

नटराजासन (बहिर्गुल्फहस्त)
Naṭarājāsana (bahirgulphahasta)

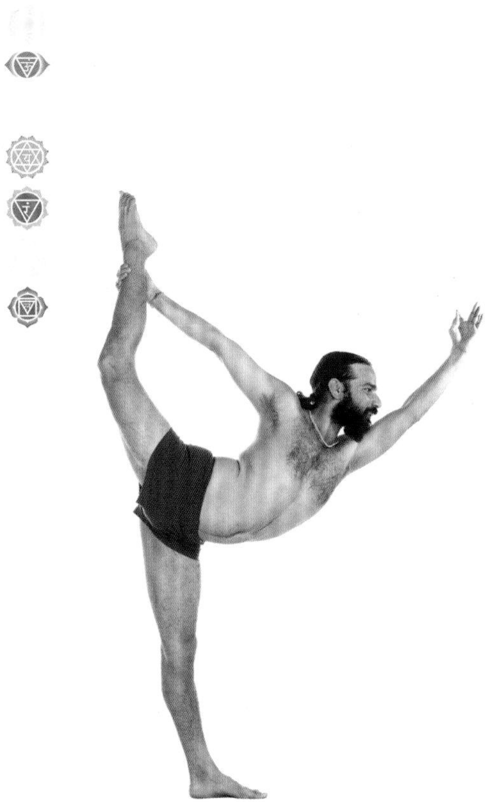

73
नट राज आसन (अन्तः गुल्फ हस्त)
Naṭa rāja āsana (antar gulpha hasta)
Lord of the Dance pose (hand inside ankle)

नटराजासन (अन्तर्गुल्फहस्त)
Naṭarājāsana (antargulphahasta)

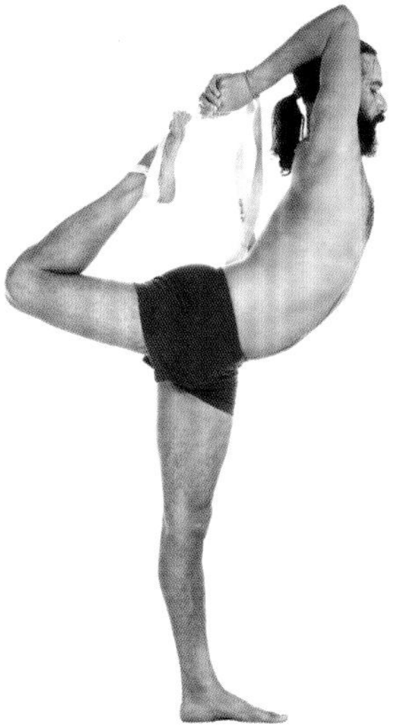

74
नट राज आसन (सरज्जु)
Nata rāja āsana (sarajju)
Lord of the Dance pose (supported by strap)

नटराजासन (सरज्जु)
Natarājāsana (sarajju)

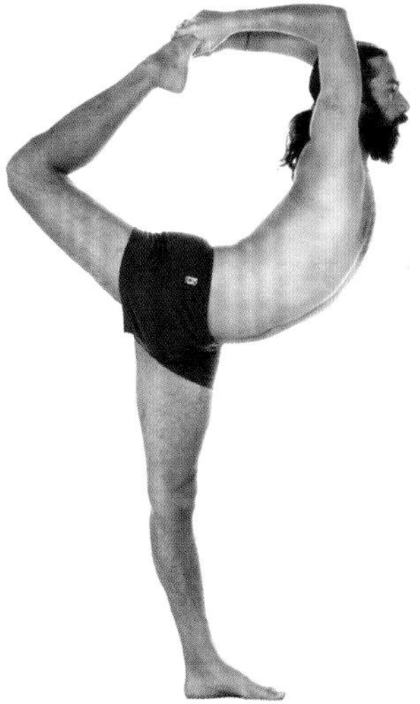

75
नट राज आसन (द्वि हस्त पाद)
Nata rāja āsana (dvi hasta pāda)
Lord of the Dance pose (two hands on foot)

नटराजासन (द्विहस्तपाद)
Natarājāsana (dvihastapāda)

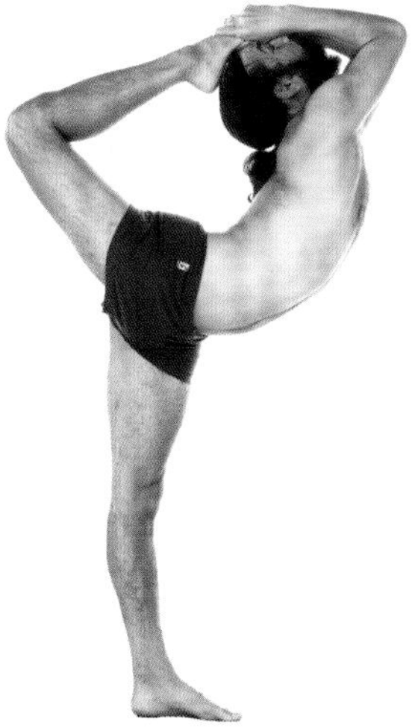

76
पूर्ण नट राज आसन
Pūrṇa nata rāja āsana
Full Lord of the Dance pose

पूर्णनटराजासन
Pūrṇanatarājāsana

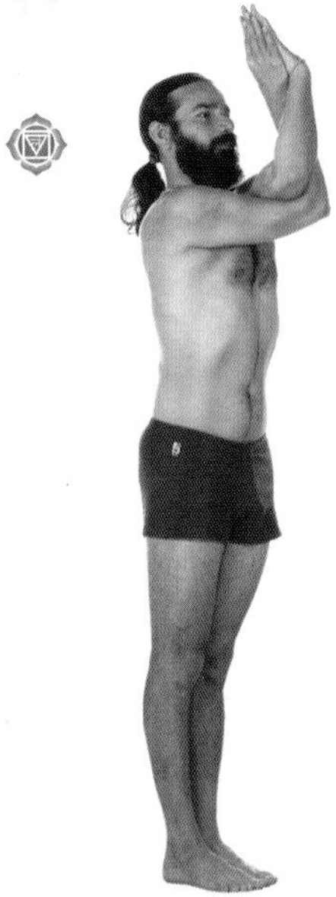

77
गरुड आसन (आरम्भ अवस्था)
Garuḍa āsana (ārambha avasthā)
Eagle pose (starting position)

गरुडासन (आरम्भावस्था)
Garuḍāsana (ārambhavasthā)

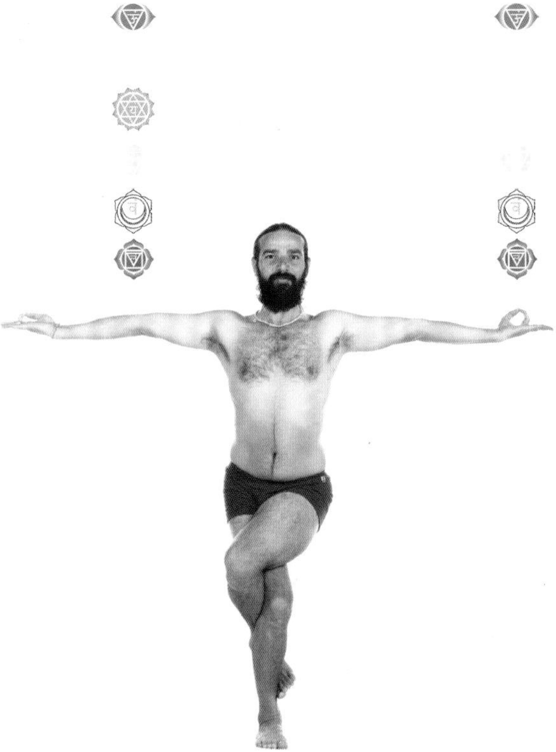

78
गरुड आसन (विराट हस्त)
Garuḍa āsana (virāṭa hasta)
Eagle pose (hands extended wide)

गरुडासन (विराटहस्त)
Garuḍāsana (virātahasta)

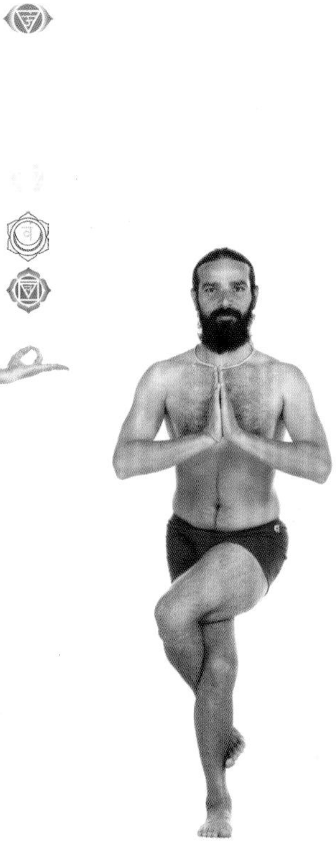

79
नमस्कार गरुडासन
Namaskāra garuḍa āsana
Prayer eagle pose

नमस्कारगरुडासन
Namaskāragaruḍāsana

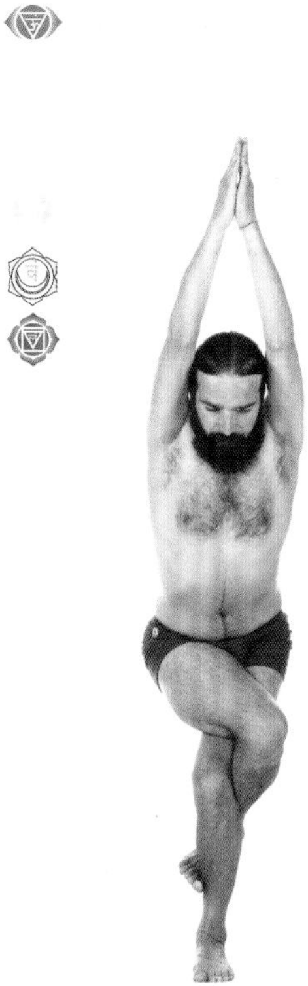

80
गरुड आसन (ऊर्ध्व हस्त नमस्कार)
Garuḍa āsana (ūrdhva hasta namaskāra)
Eagle pose (hands in prayer overhead)

गरुडासन (ऊर्ध्वहस्तनमस्कार)
Garuḍāsana (ūrdhvahastanamaskāra)

Life is enthusiasm and excitement!

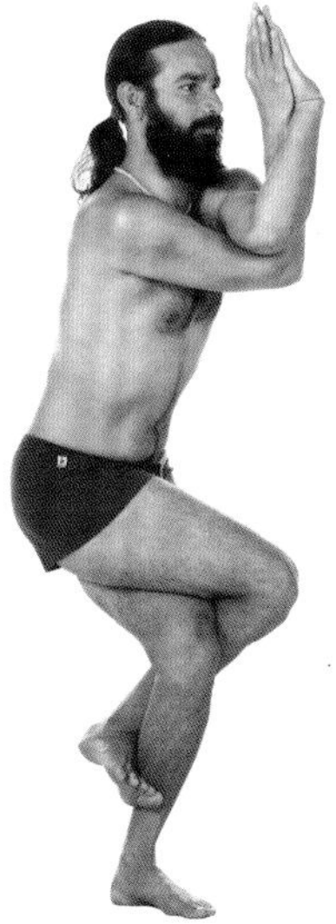

81
गरुड आसन
Garuḍa āsana
Eagle pose

गरुडासन
Garuḍāsana

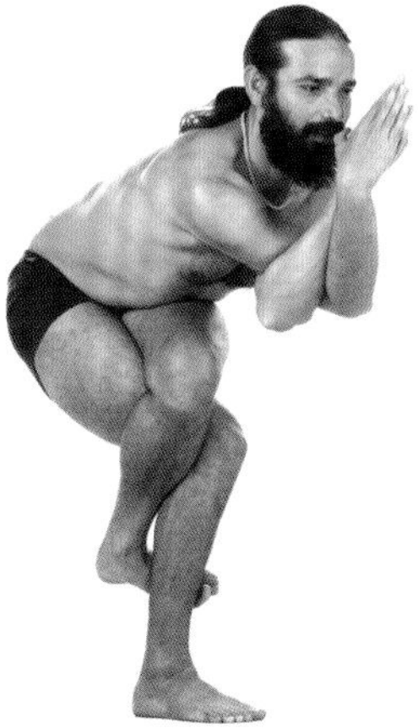

82
विनत गरुड आसन
Vinata garuḍa āsana
Humble eagle pose

विनतगरुडासन
Vinatagaruḍāsana

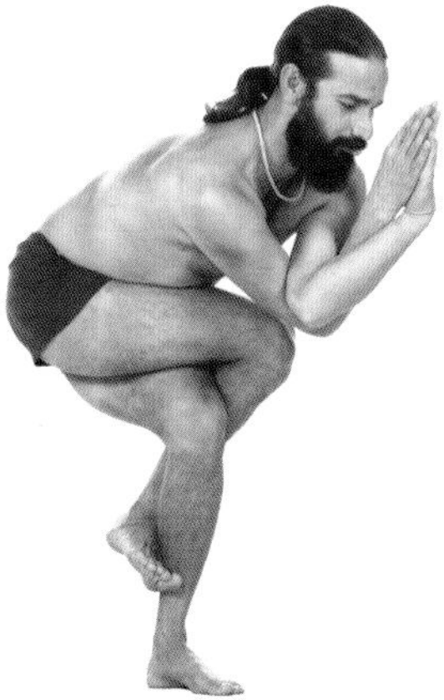

83
गरुड आसन (कफोणि जानु)
Garuḍa āsana (kaphoṇi jānu)
Eagle pose (elbow to knee)

गरुडासन (कफोणिजानु)
Garuḍāsana (kaphoṇijānu)

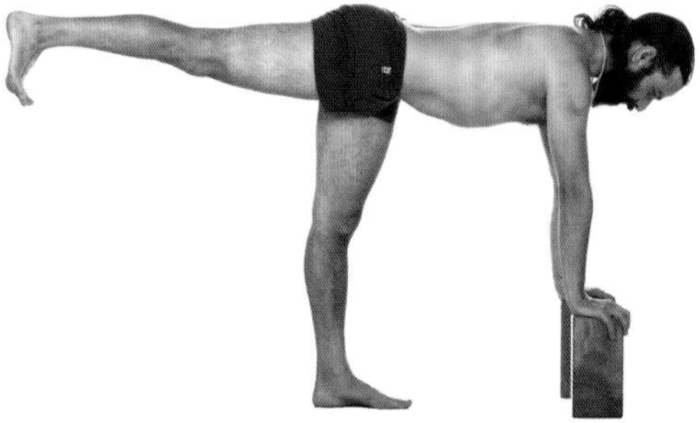

84
उत्तोलन एक पाद आसन (सालम्ब हस्त)
Uttolana eka pāda āsana (sālamba hasta)
Balancing one leg pose (supported hands)

उत्तोलनैकपादासन (सालम्बहस्त)
Uttolanaikapādāsana (sālambahasta)

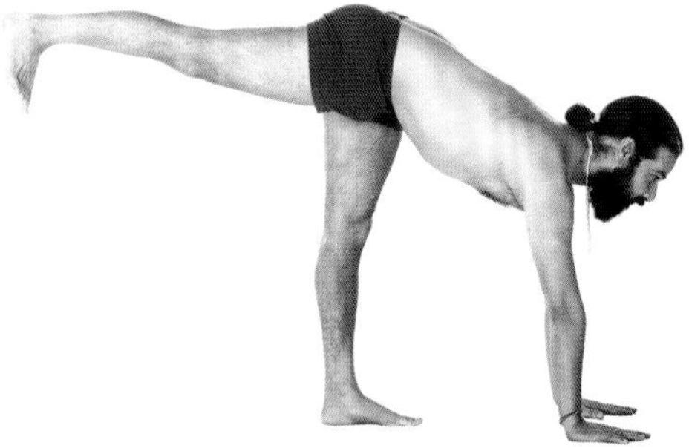

85
उत्तोलन एक पाद आसन (हस्त भू)
Uttolana eka pāda āsana (hasta bhū)
Balancing one leg pose (hands on the earth)

उत्तोलनैकपादासन (हस्तभू)
Uttolanaikapādāsana (hastabhū)

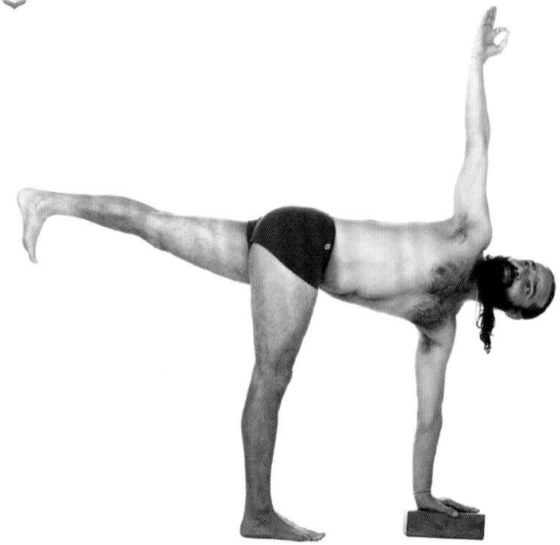

86
परिवृत्त उत्तोलन एक पाद आसन (सालम्ब हस्त)
Parivṛtta uttolana eka pāda āsana (sālamba hasta)
Twisted balancing one leg pose (supported hand)

परिवृत्तोत्तोलनैकपादासन (सालम्बहस्त)
Parivṛttottolanaikapādāsana (sālambahasta)

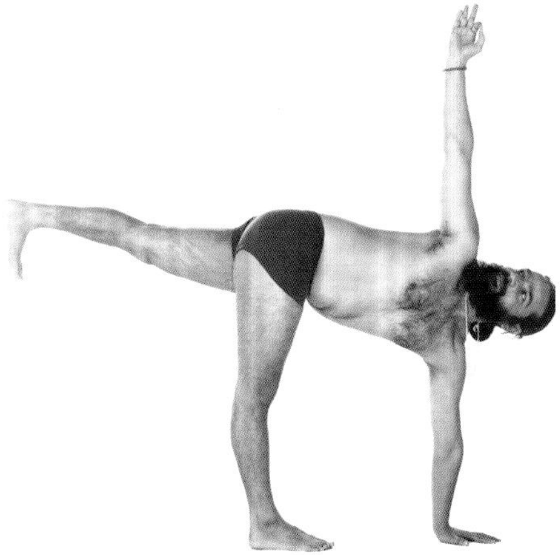

87
परिवृत्त उत्तोलन एक पाद आसन (हस्त भू)
Parivṛtta uttolana eka pāda āsana (hasta bhū)
Twisted balancing one leg pose (hand on the earth)

परिवृत्तोत्तोलनैकपादासन (हस्तभू)
Parivṛttottolanaikapādāsana (hastabhū)

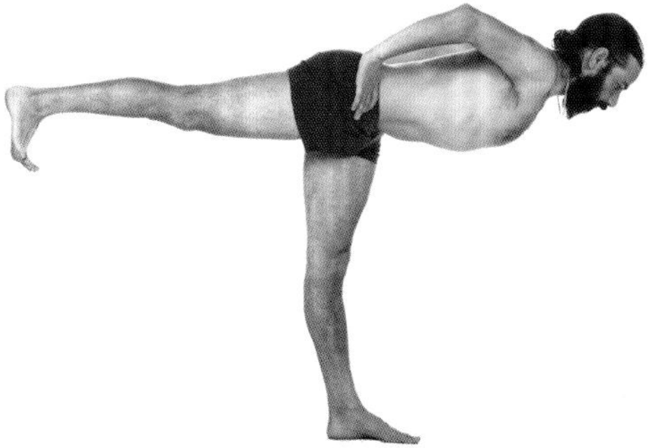

88
उत्तोलन एक पाद आसन (कटि हस्त)
Uttolana eka pāda āsana (kaṭi hasta)
Balancing one leg pose (hands on waist)

उत्तोलनैकपादासन (कटिहस्त)
Uttolanaikapādāsana (kaṭihasta)

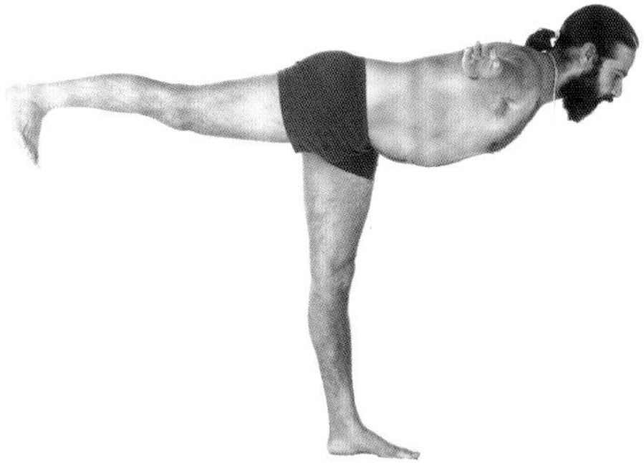

89
उत्तोलन एक पाद आसन (विराट हस्त)
Uttolana eka pāda āsana (virāṭa hasta)
Balancing one leg pose (hands extended wide)

उत्तोलनैकपादासन (विराटहस्त)
Uttolanaikapādāsana (virātahasta)

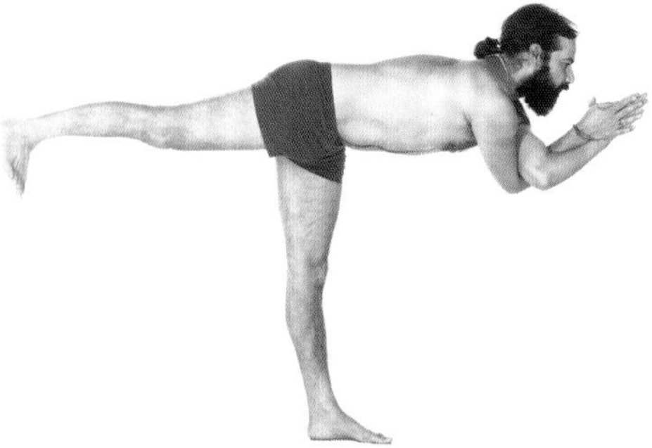

90
उत्तोलन एक पाद आसन (गरुड हस्त)
Uttolana eka pāda āsana (garuḍa hasta)
Balancing one leg pose (eagle hands)

उत्तोलनैकपादासन (गरुडहस्त)
Uttolanaikapādāsana (garuḍahasta)

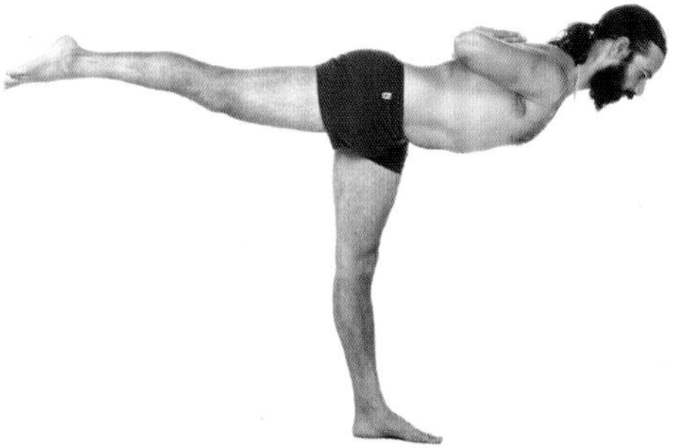

91
उत्तोलन एक पाद आसन (पृष्ठ नमस्कार)
Uttolana eka pāda āsana (pṛṣṭha namaskāra)
Balancing one leg pose (hands in prayer behind)

उत्तोलनैकपादासन (पृष्ठनमस्कार)
Uttolanaikapādāsana (pṛṣṭhanamaskāra)

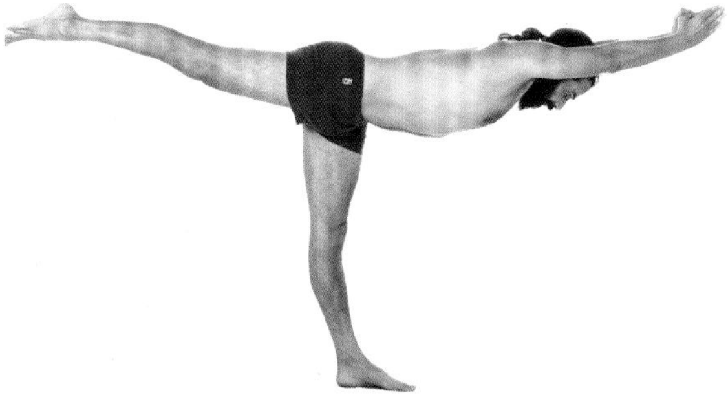

92
पूर्ण उत्तोलन एक पाद आसन
Pūrṇa uttolana eka pāda āsana
Full balancing one leg pose

पूर्णोत्तोलनैकपादासन
Pūrṇottolanaikapādāsana

Moving Toward the Earth

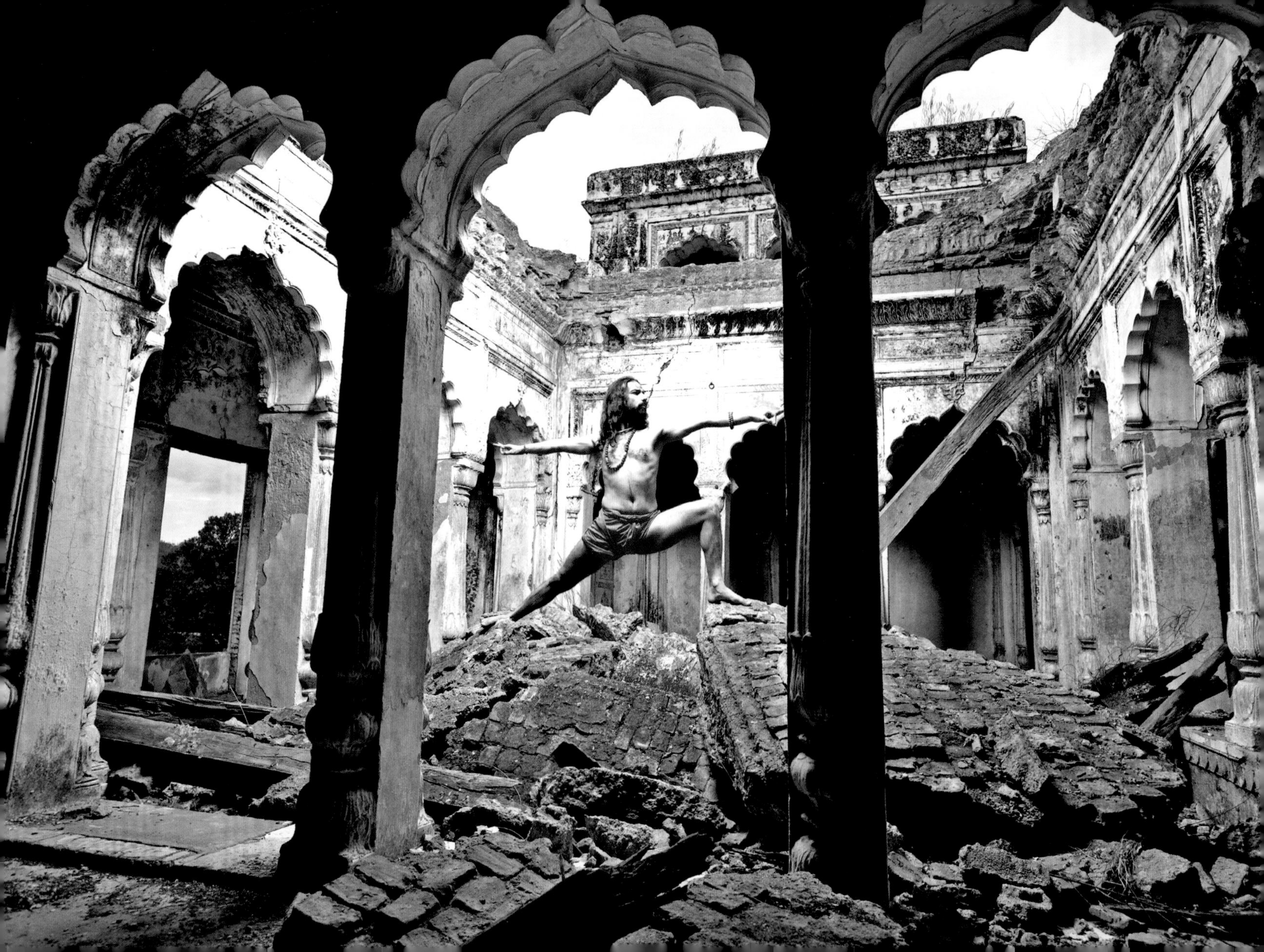

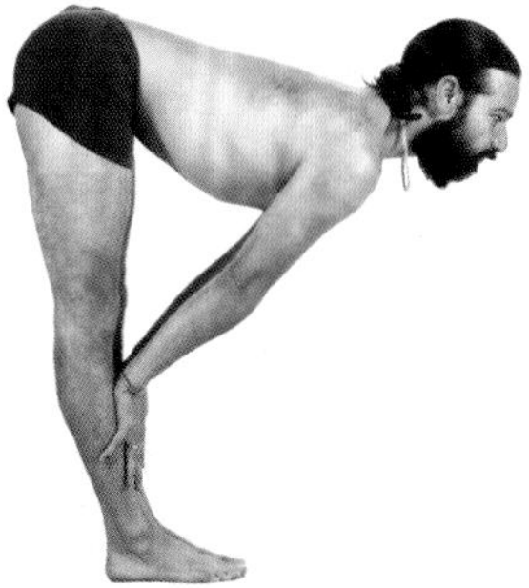

93
अर्ध पृष्ठ उत्तान आसन (पूर्व मुख)
Ardha pṛṣṭha uttāna āsana (pūrva mukha)
Half back stretch pose (facing forward)

अर्धपृष्ठोत्तानासन (पूर्वमुख)
Ardhapṛṣṭhottānāsana (pūrvamukha)

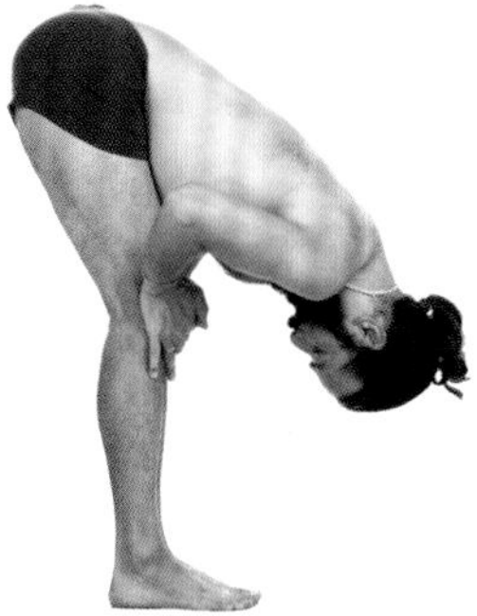

94
पृष्ठ उत्तान आसन (करतल जानु)
Pṛṣṭha uttāna āsana (karatala jānu)
Back stretch pose (palms on knee)

पृष्ठोत्तानासन (करतलजानु)
Pṛṣṭhottānāsana (karatalajānu)

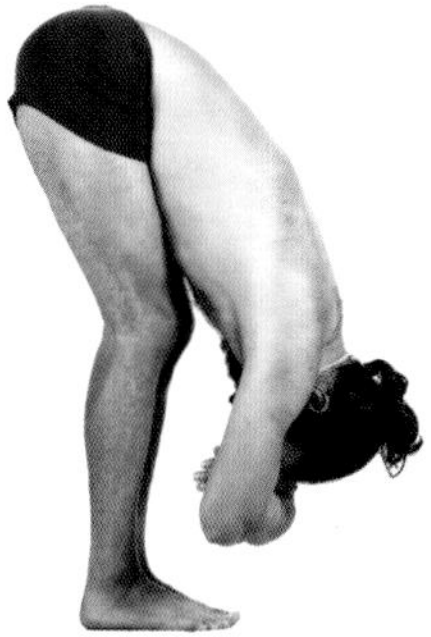

95
पृष्ठ उत्तान आसन (बद्ध कफोणि)
Pṛṣṭha uttāna āsana (baddha kaphoṇi)
Back stretch pose (elbows bound)

पृष्ठोत्तानासन (बद्धकफोणि)
Pṛṣṭhottānāsana (baddhakaphoṇi)

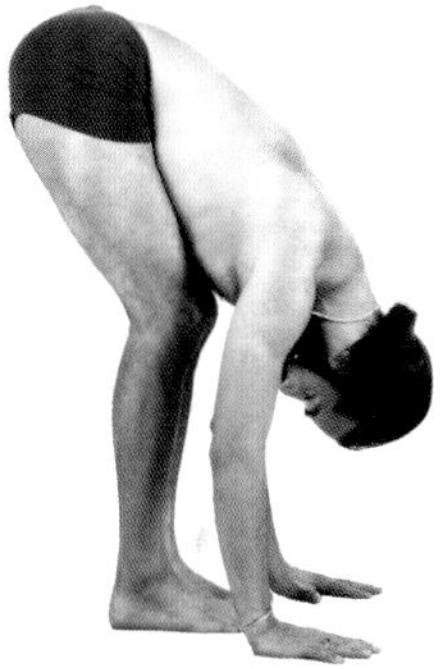

96
पृष्ठ उत्तान आसन (हस्त भू)
Pṛṣṭha uttāna āsana (hasta bhū)
Back stretch pose (hands on the earth, knees bent)

पृष्ठोत्तानासन (हस्तभू)
Pṛṣṭhottānāsana (hastabhū)

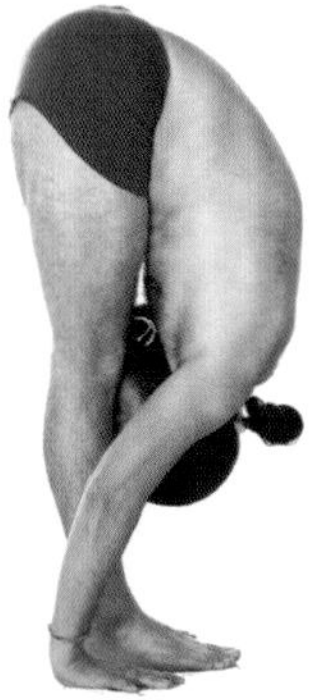

97
पृष्ठ उत्तान आसन (हस्त भू)
Pṛṣṭha uttāna āsana (hasta bhū)
Back stretch pose (hands on the earth)

पृष्ठोत्तानासन (हस्तभू)
Pṛṣṭhottānāsana (hastabhū)

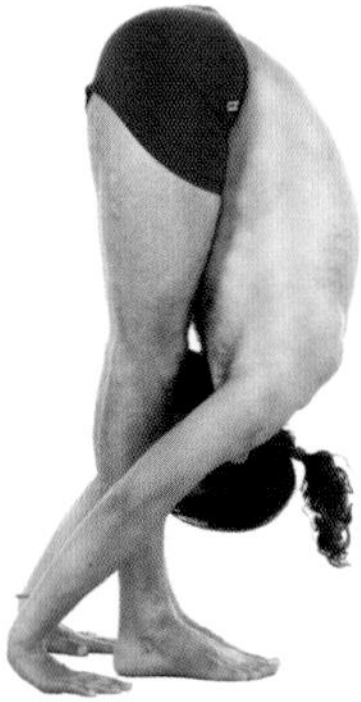

98
पृष्ठ उत्तान आसन (पृष्ठ हस्त भू)
Pṛṣṭha uttāna āsana (pṛṣṭha hasta bhū)
Back stretch pose (hands on the earth behind)

पृष्ठोत्तानासन (पृष्ठहस्तभू)
Pṛṣṭhottānāsana (pṛṣṭhahastabhū)

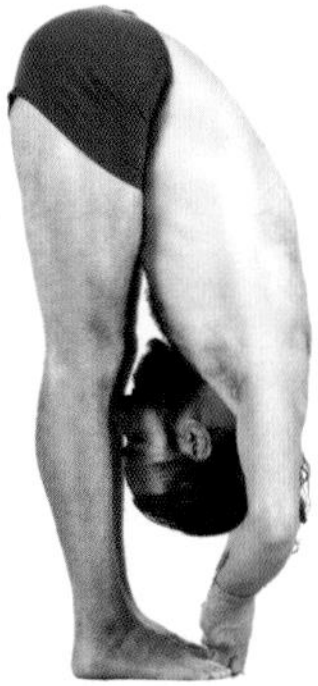

99
पृष्ठ उत्तान आसन (पाद अङ्गुष्ठ)
Pṛṣṭha uttāna āsana (pāda aṅguṣṭha)
Back stretch pose (holding big toes)

पृष्ठोत्तानासन (पादाङ्गुष्ठ)
Pṛṣṭhottānāsana (pādāṅguṣṭha)

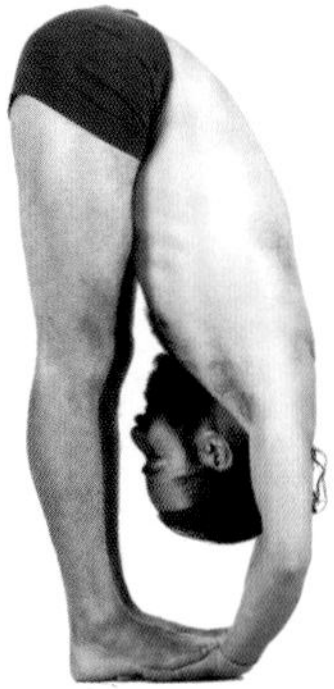

100
पृष्ठ उत्तान आसन (पाद हस्त)
Pṛṣṭha uttāna āsana (pāda hasta)
Back stretch pose (hands under feet)

पृष्ठोत्तानासन (पादहस्त)
Pṛṣṭhottānāsana (pādāhasta)

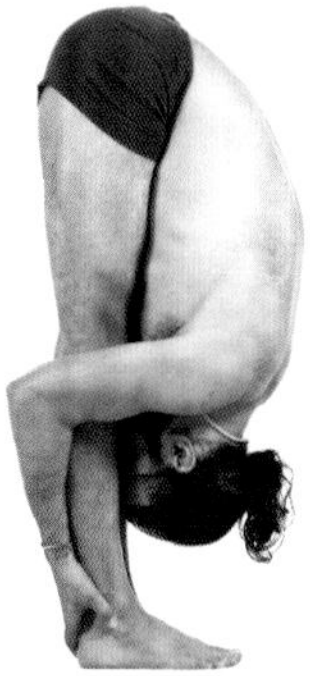

101
पृष्ठ उत्तान आसन (गुल्फ बद्ध)
Pṛṣṭha uttāna āsana (gulpha baddha)
Back stretch pose (holding ankles)

पृष्ठोत्तानासन (गुल्फबद्ध)
Pṛṣṭhottānāsana (gulphabaddha)

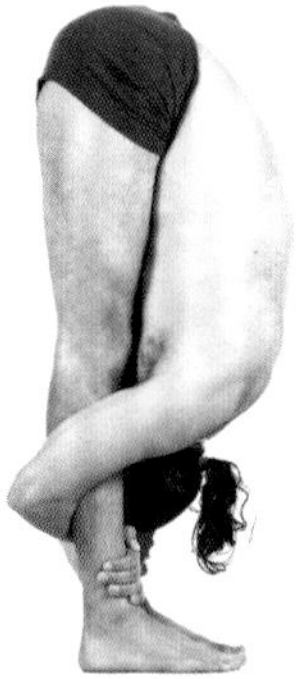

102
पृष्ठ उत्तान आसन (विपरीत गुल्फ बद्ध)
Pṛṣṭha uttāna āsana (viparīta gulpha baddha)
Back stretch pose (hands holding opposite ankles)

पृष्ठोत्तानासन (विपरीतगुल्फबद्ध)
Pṛṣṭhottānāsana (viparītagulphabaddha)

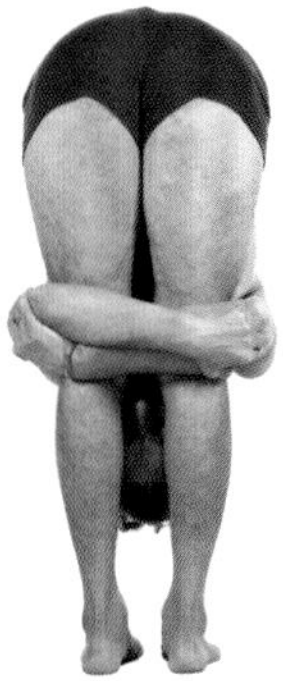

103
पृष्ठ उत्तान आसन (पृष्ठ पाद रज्जु हस्त)
Pṛṣṭha uttāna āsana (pṛṣṭha pāda rajju hasta)
Back stretch pose (elbows clasped behind legs)

पृष्ठोत्तानासन (पृष्ठपादरज्जुहस्त)
Pṛṣṭhottānāsana (pṛṣṭhapādarajjuhasta)

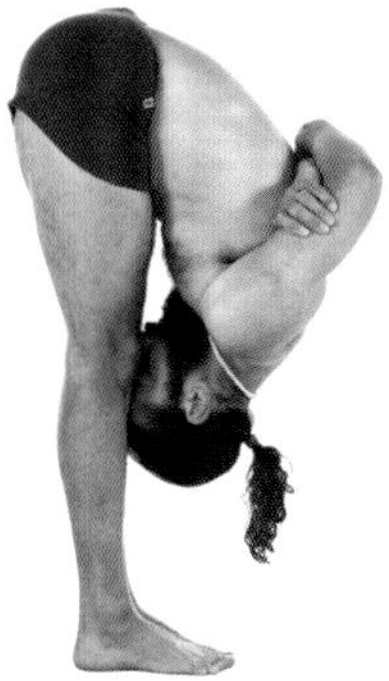

104
पृष्ठ उत्तान आसन (पृष्ठ कफोणि बद्ध)
Pṛṣṭha uttāna āsana (pṛṣṭha kaphoṇi baddha)
Back stretch pose (holding elbows behind the back)

पृष्ठोत्तानासन (पृष्ठकफोणिबद्ध)
Pṛṣṭhottānāsana (pṛṣṭhakaphoṇibaddha)

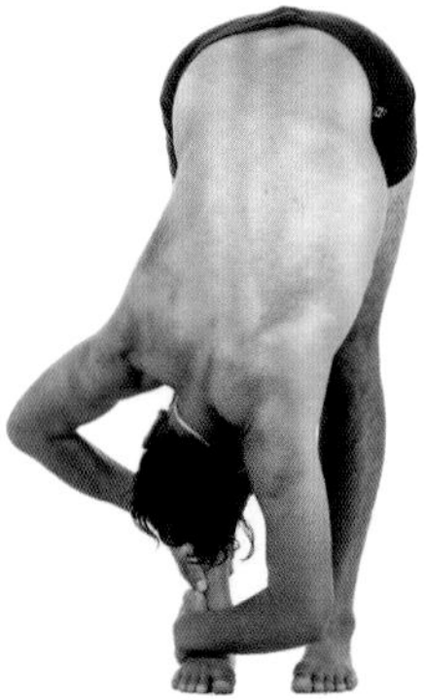

105
पृष्ठ उत्तान आसन (पार्श्व एक पाद)
Pṛṣṭtha uttāna āsana (pārśva eka pāda)
Back stretch pose (holding one leg)

पृष्ठोत्तानासन (पार्श्वैकपाद)
Pṛṣṭthottānāsana (pārśvaikapāda)

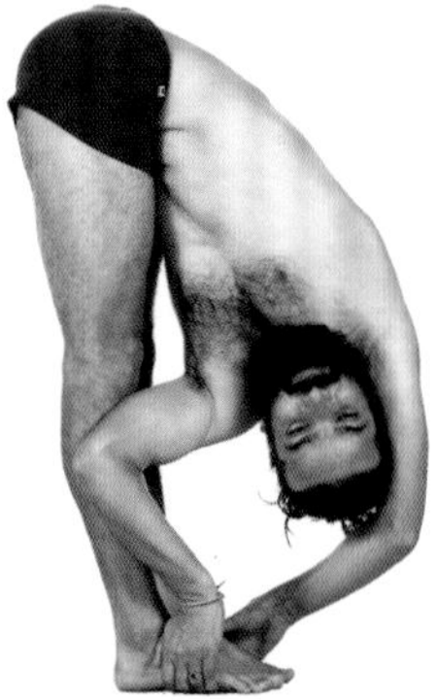

106
परिवृत्त पृष्ठ उत्तान आसन
Parivṛtta pṛṣṭha uttāna āsana
Twisted back stretch pose

परिवृत्तपृष्ठोत्तानासन
Parivṛttapṛṣṭhottānāsana

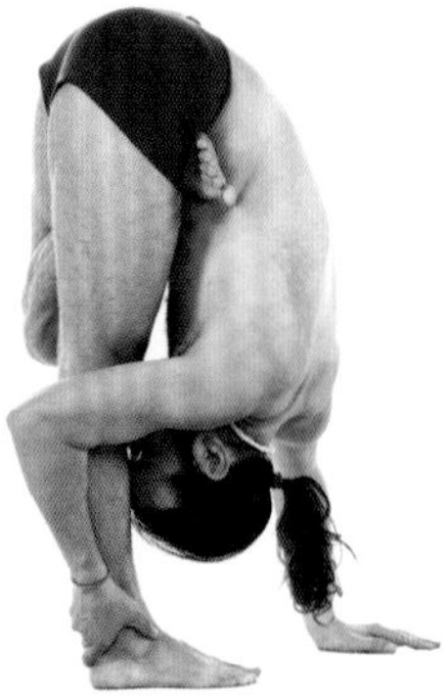

107
पृष्ठ उत्तान आसन (अर्ध पद्म पाद)
Pṛṣṭha uttāna āsana (ardha padma pāda)
Back stretch pose (half lotus foot)

पृष्ठोत्तानासन (अर्धपद्मपाद)
Pṛṣṭhottānāsana (ardhapadmapāda)

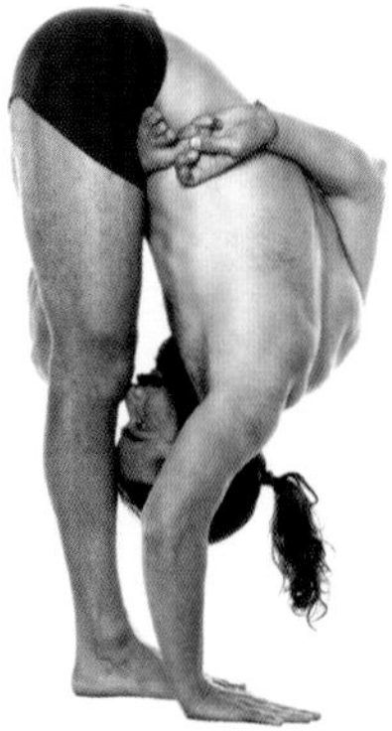

108
पृष्ठ उत्तान आसन (अर्ध बद्ध पद्म)
Pṛṣṭha uttāna āsana (ardha baddha padma)
Back stretch pose (bound half lotus)

पृष्ठोत्तानासन (अर्धबद्धपद्म)
Pṛṣṭhottānāsana (ardhabaddhapadma)

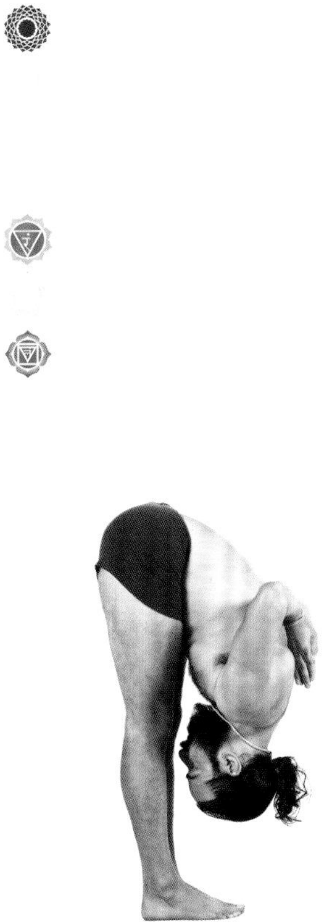

109
पृष्ठ उत्तान आसन (पृष्ठ नमस्कार)
Pṛṣṭha uttāna āsana (pṛṣṭha namaskāra)
Back stretch pose (hands in prayer behind)

पृष्ठोत्तानासन (पृष्ठनमस्कार)
Pṛṣṭhottānāsana (pṛṣṭhanamaskāra)

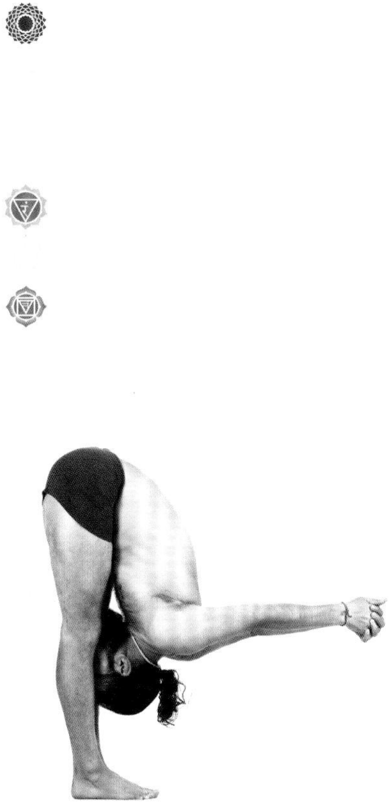

110
पृष्ठ उत्तान आसन (पृष्ठ हस्त उत्तान)
Pṛṣṭha uttāna āsana (pṛṣṭha hasta uttāna)
Back stretch pose (hands stretched behind)

पृष्ठोत्तानासन (पृष्ठहस्तोत्तान)
Pṛṣṭhottānāsana (pṛṣṭhahastottāna)

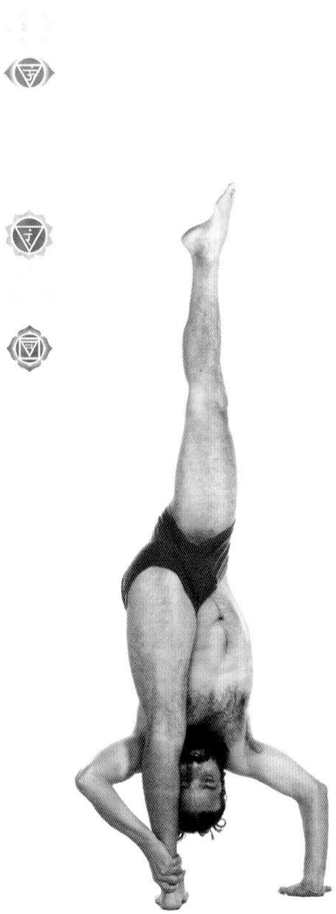

111
पृष्ठ उत्तान आसन (ऊर्ध्व एक पाद)
Pṛṣṭha uttāna āsana (ūrdhva eka pāda)
Back stretch pose (one leg overhead)

पृष्ठोत्तानासन (ऊर्ध्वैकपाद)
Pṛṣṭhottānāsana (ūrdhvaikapāda)

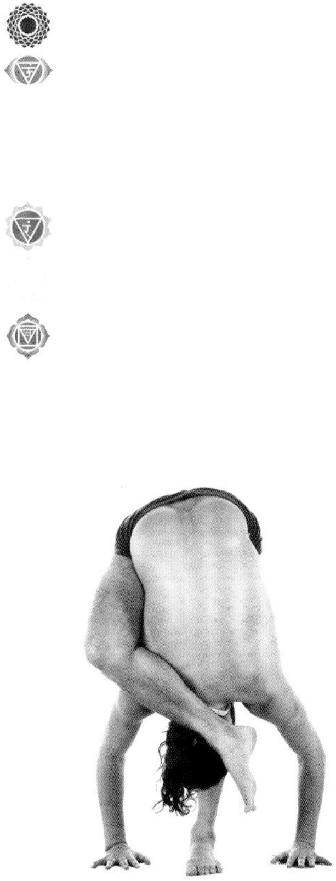

112
भैरव पृष्ठ उत्तान आसन
Bhairava pṛṣṭha uttāna āsana
Fearless back stretch pose

भैरवपृष्ठोत्तानासन
Bhairavapṛṣṭhottānāsana

Yoga is transformation.

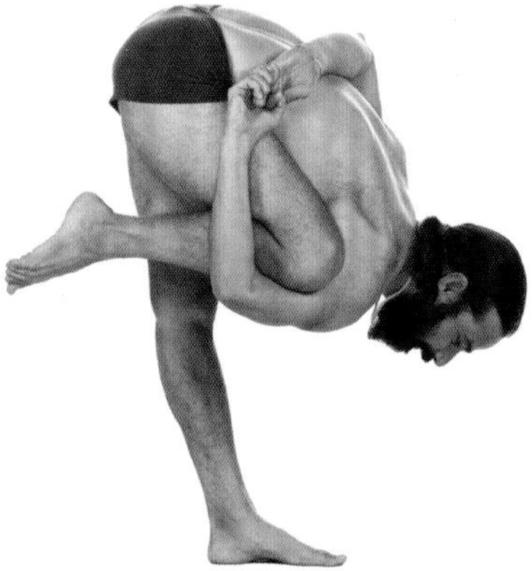

113
जटायु पृष्ठ उत्तान आसन
Jatāyu pṛṣṭha uttāna āsana
Vulture back stretch pose

जटायुपृष्ठोत्तानासन
Jatāyupṛṣṭhottānāsana

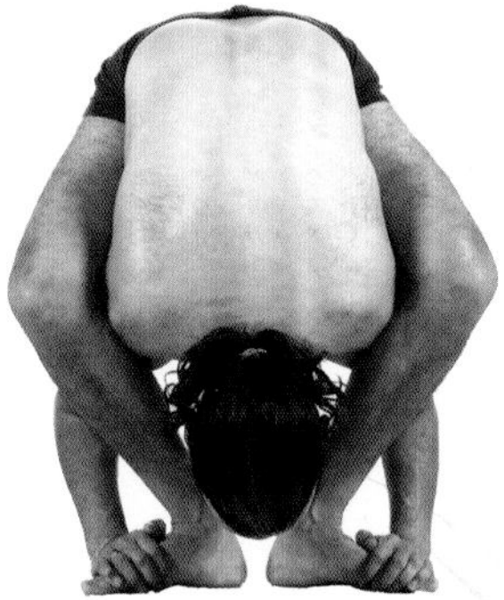

114
शिर पाद उत्तान आसन (बद्ध हस्त पाद)
Śira pāda uttāna āsana (baddha hasta pāda)
Head to feet stretch pose (hands holding feet)

शिरपादोत्तानासन (बद्धहस्तपाद)
Śirapādottānāsana (baddhahastapāda)

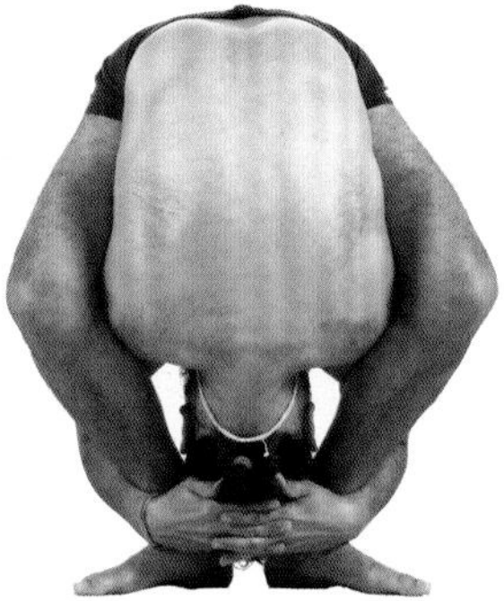

115
शिर पाद उत्तान आसन (बद्ध हस्त शिर)
Śira pāda uttāna āsana (baddha hasta śira)
Head to feet stretch pose (hands bound to head)

शिरपादोत्तानासन (बद्धहस्तशिर)
Śirapādottānāsana (baddhahastaśira)

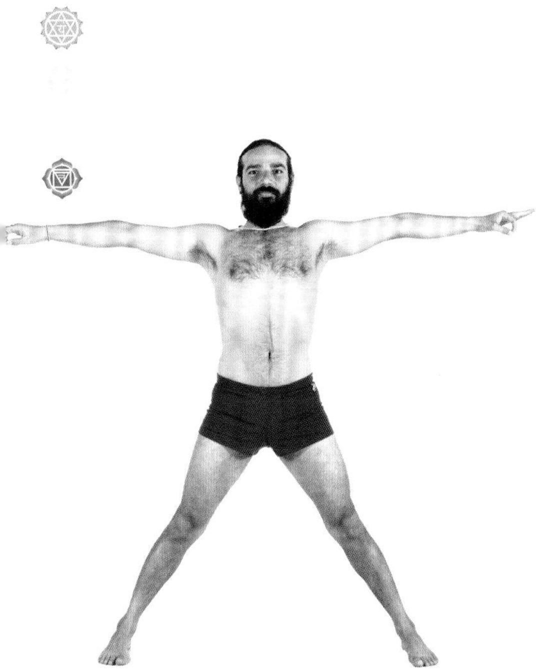

116
प्रसरित पाद आसन (विराट हस्त)
Prasarita pāda āsana (virāṭa hasta)
Wide-leg pose (extended arms)

प्रसरितपादासन (विराटहस्त)
Prasaritapādāsana (virāṭahasta)

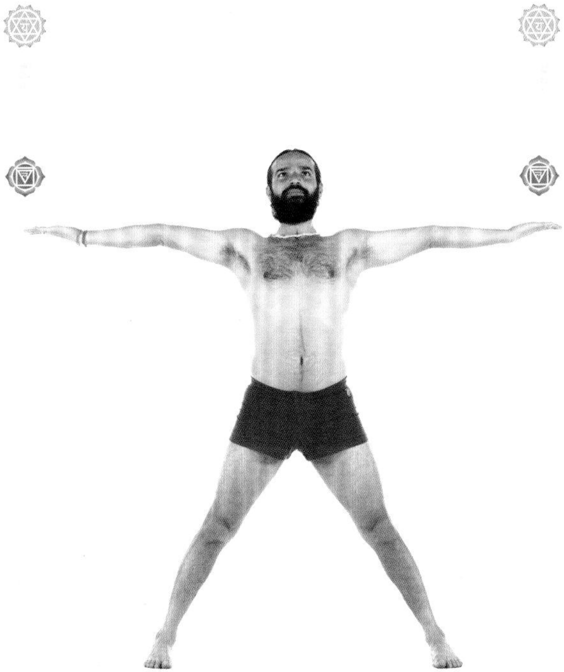

117
प्रसरित पाद आसन (विराट हस्त, ऊर्ध्व करतल)
Prasarita pāda āsana (virāṭa hasta, ūrdhva karatala)
Wide-leg pose (extended arms, palm facing up)

प्रसरितपादासन (विराटहस्त,ऊर्ध्वकरतल)
Prasaritapādāsana (virāṭahasta, ūrdhvakaratala)

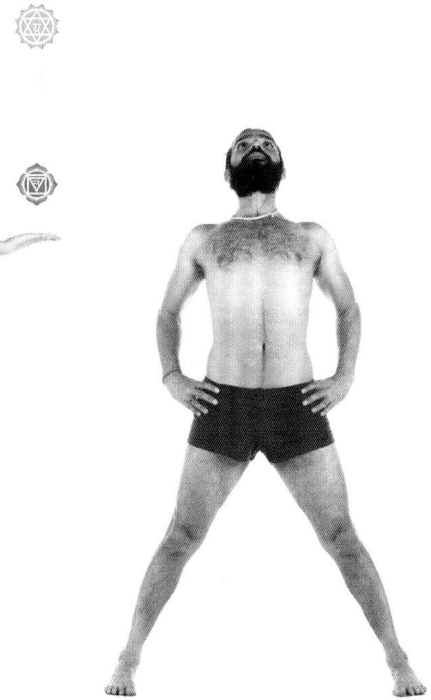

118
प्रसरित पाद आसन (कटि हस्त, ऊर्ध्व मुख)
Prasarita pāda āsana (kaṭi hasta, ūrdhva mukha)
Wide-leg pose (hands on waist, upward facing)

प्रसरितपादासन (कटिहस्त, ऊर्ध्वमुख)
Prasaritapādāsan (kaṭihasta, ūrdhvamukha)

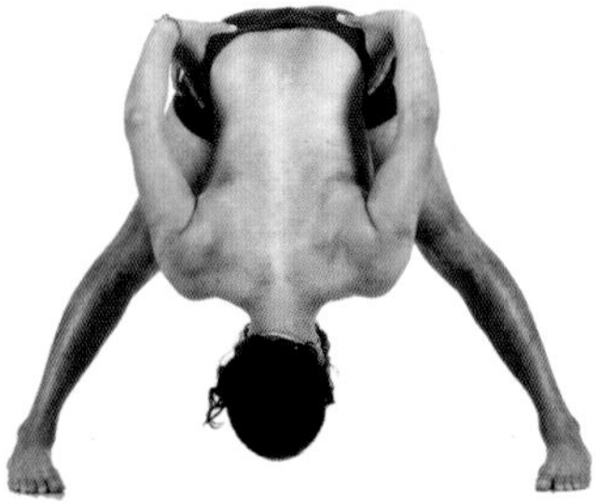

119
प्रसरित पाद उत्तान आसन (कटि हस्त)
Prasarita pāda uttāna āsana (kati hasta)
Wide-leg forward stretch pose (hands on waist)

प्रसरितपादोत्तानासन (कटिहस्त)
Prasaritapādottānāsana (katihasta)

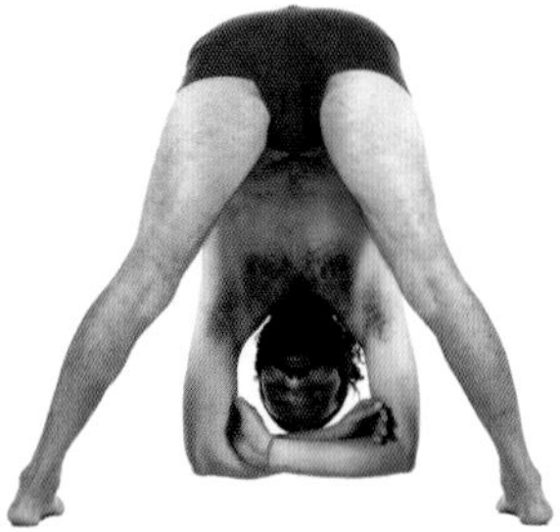

120
प्रसरित पाद उत्तान आसन (बद्ध कफोणि)
Prasarita pāda uttāna āsana (baddha kaphoṇi)
Wide-leg forward stretch pose (clasped elbows)

प्रसरितपादोत्तानासन (बद्धकफोणि)
Prasaritapādottānāsana (baddhakaphoṇi)

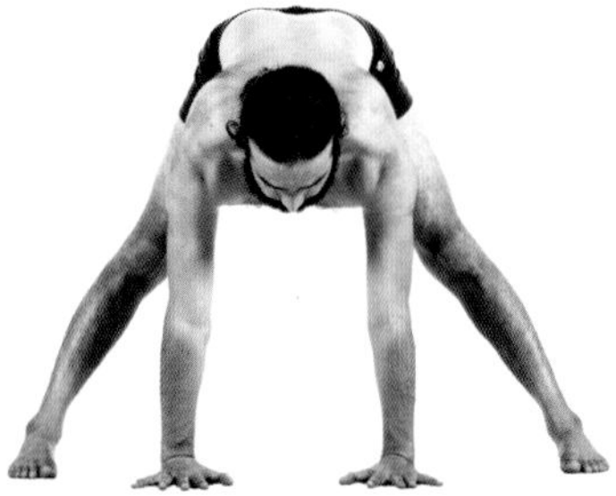

121
प्रसरित पाद उत्तान आसन (हस्त भू पूर्व मुख)
Prasarita pāda uttāna āsana
(hasta bhū pūrva mukha)
Wide-leg forward stretch pose
(hands on the earth facing forward)

प्रसरितपादोत्तानासन (हस्तभूपूर्वमुख)
Prasaritapādottānāsana (hastabhūpūrvamukha)

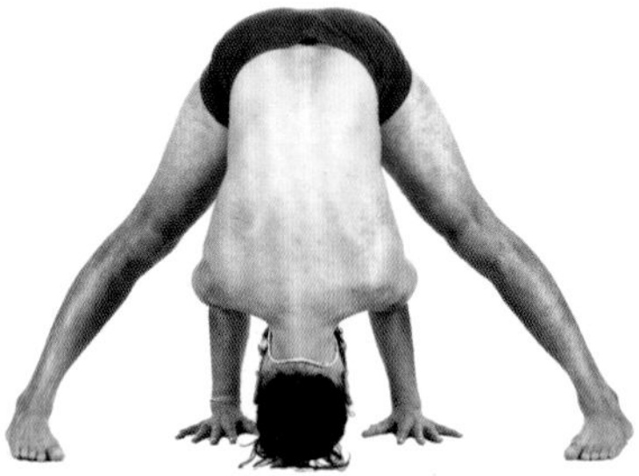

122
प्रसरित पाद उत्तान आसन (हस्त भू)
Prasarita pāda uttāna āsana (hasta bhū)
Wide-leg forward stretch pose (hands on the earth)

प्रसरितपादोत्तानासन (हस्तभू)
Prasaritapādottānāsana (hastabhū)

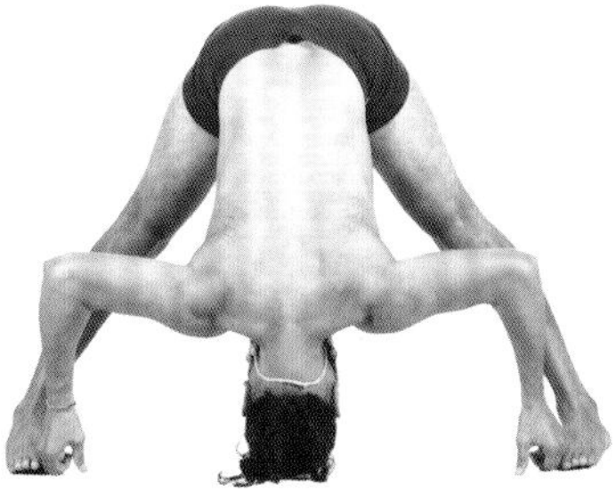

123
प्रसरित पाद उत्तान आसन (बद्ध पाद अङ्गुष्ठ)
Prasarita pāda uttāna āsana
(baddha pāda aṅguṣṭha)
Wide-leg forward stretch pose (holding big toes)

प्रसरितपादोत्तानासन (बद्धपादाङ्गुष्ठ)
Prasaritapādottānāsana
(baddhapādāṅguṣṭha)

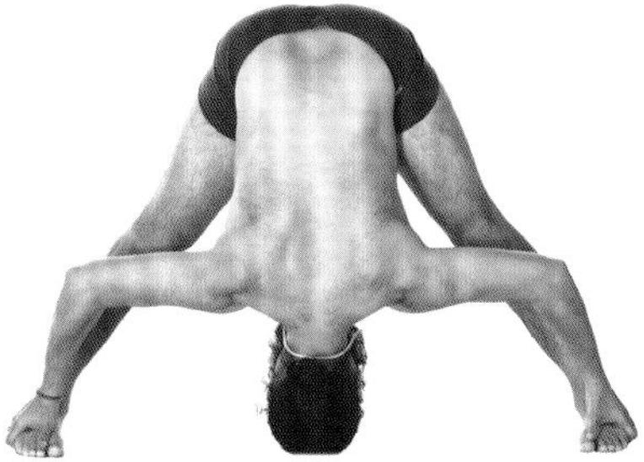

124
प्रसरित पाद उत्तान आसन (बद्ध बहिर्पाद)
Prasarita pāda uttāna āsana
(baddha bahirpāda)
Wide-leg forward stretch pose
(holding outside of the feet)

प्रसरितपादोत्तानासन (बद्धबहिर्पाद)
Prasaritapādottānāsana (baddhabahirpāda)

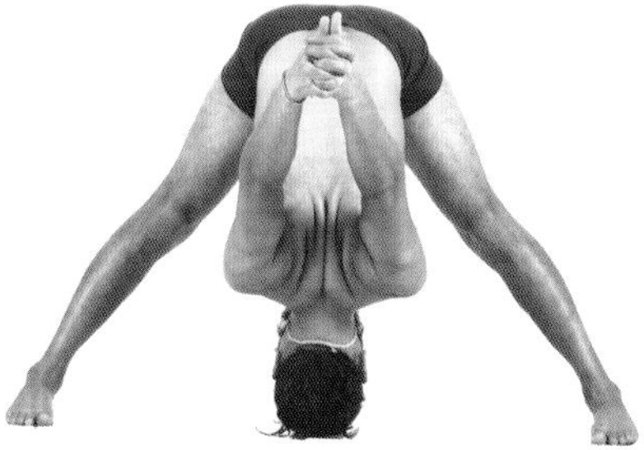

125
प्रसरित पाद उत्तान आसन (पृष्ठ हस्त उत्तान)
Prasarita pāda uttāna āsana
(pṛṣṭha hasta uttāna)
Wide-leg forward stretch pose
(hands extended behind)

प्रसरितपादोत्तानासन (पृष्ठहस्तोत्तान)
Prasaritapādottānāsana (pṛṣṭhahastottāna)

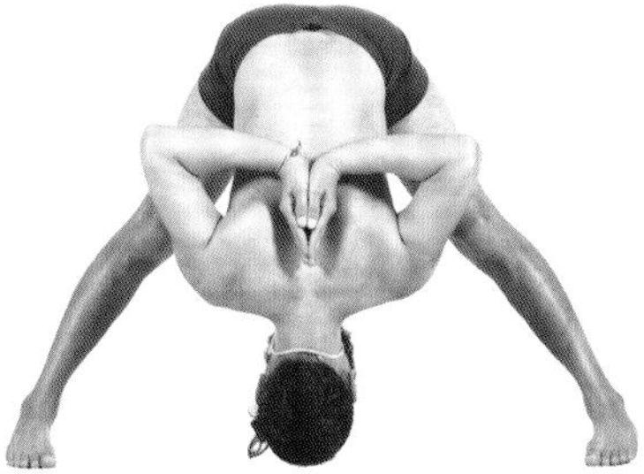

126
प्रसरित पाद उत्तान आसन (पृष्ठ नमस्कार)
Prasarita pāda uttāna āsana
(pṛṣṭha namaskāra)
Wide-leg forward stretch pose
(hands behind in prayer)

प्रसरितपादोत्तानासन (पृष्ठनमस्कार)
Prasaritapādottānāsana (pṛṣṭhanamaskāra)

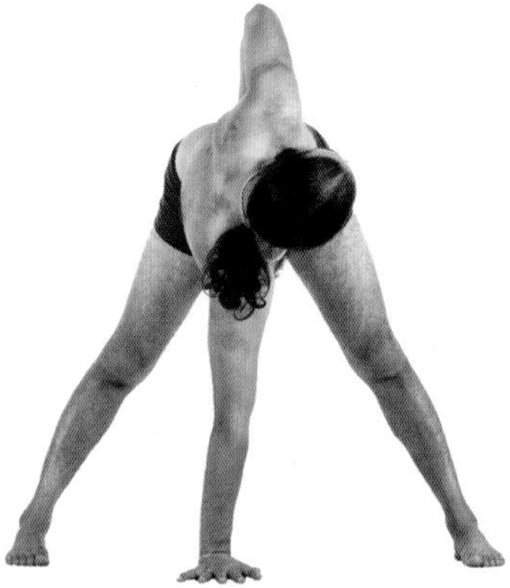

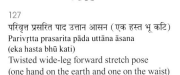

127
परिवृत्त प्रसरित पाद उत्तान आसन (एक हस्त भू कटि)
Parivṛtta prasarita pāda uttāna āsana
(eka hasta bhū kati)
Twisted wide-leg forward stretch pose
(one hand on the earth and one on the waist)

परिवृत्तप्रसरितपादोत्तानासन (एकहस्तभूकटि)
Parivṛttaprasaritapādottānāsana (ekahastabhūkati)

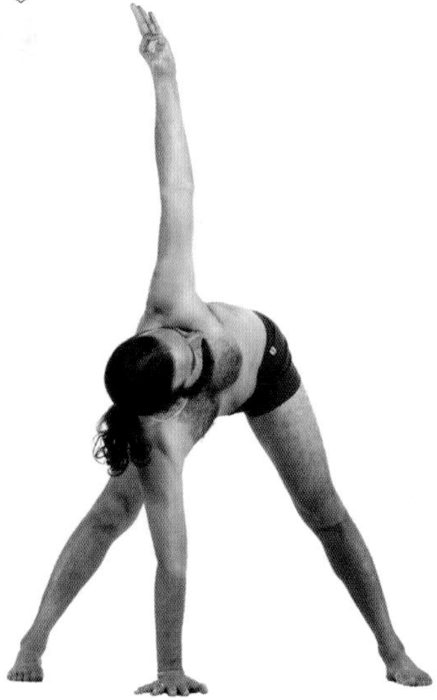

128
परिवृत्त प्रसरित पाद उत्तान आसन (विराट हस्त भू)
Parivṛtta prasarita pāda uttāna āsana
(virāṭa hasta bhū)
Twisted wide-leg forward stretch pose
(one hand on the earth and one extended)

परिवृत्तप्रसरितपादोत्तानासन (विराटहस्तभू)
Parivṛttaprasaritapādottānāsana (virāṭahastabhū)

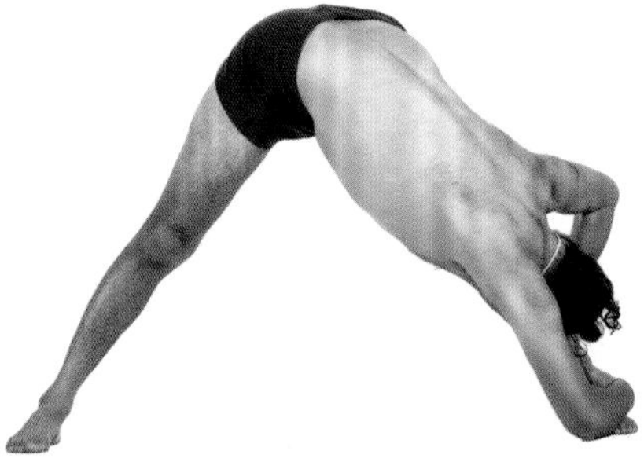

129
पार्श्व प्रसरित पाद उत्तान आसन (गुल्फ बद्ध)
Pārśva prasarita pāda uttāna āsana
(gulpha baddha)
Wide-leg forward side stretch pose
(holding ankle)

पार्श्वप्रसरितपादोत्तानासन (गुल्फबद्ध)
Pārśvaprasaritapādottānāsana
(gulphabaddha)

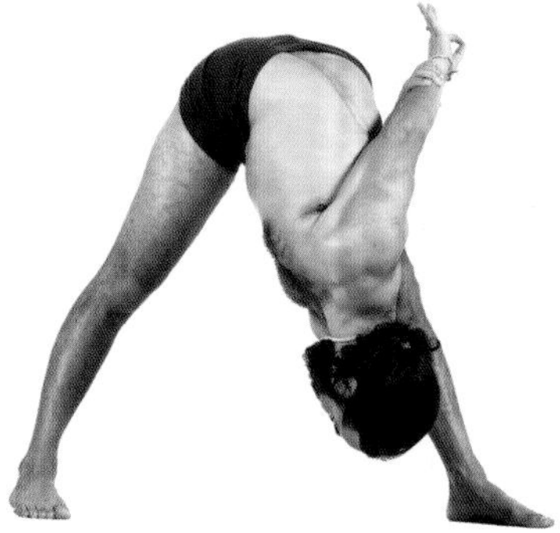

130
प्रसरित पाद उत्तान आसन (पार्श्व पाद हस्त बद्ध)
Prasarita pāda uttāna āsana
(pārśva pāda hasta baddha)
Wide-leg forward stretch pose
(hands clasped around leg)

प्रसरितपादोत्तानासन (पार्श्वपादहस्तबद्ध)
Prasaritapādottānāsana
(pārśvapādahastabaddha)

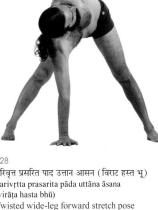

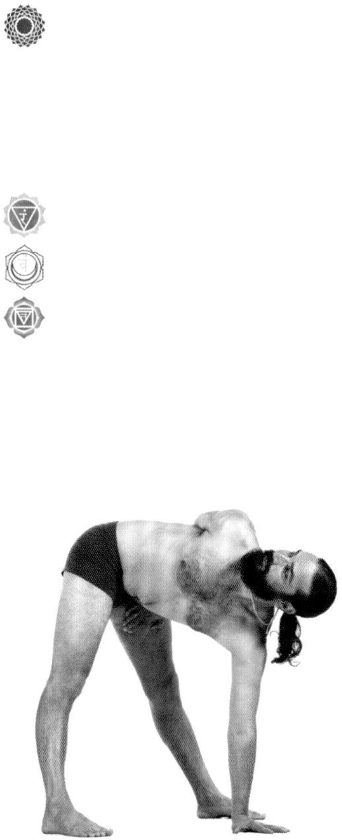

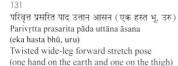

131
परिवृत्त प्रसरित पाद उत्तान आसन (एक हस्त भू, उरु)
Parivṛtta prasarita pāda uttāna āsana
(eka hasta bhū, uru)
Twisted wide-leg forward stretch pose
(one hand on the earth and one on the thigh)

परिवृत्तप्रसरितपादोत्तानासन (एकहस्तभू, उरु)
Parivṛttaprasaritapādottānāsana
(ekahastabhū, uru)

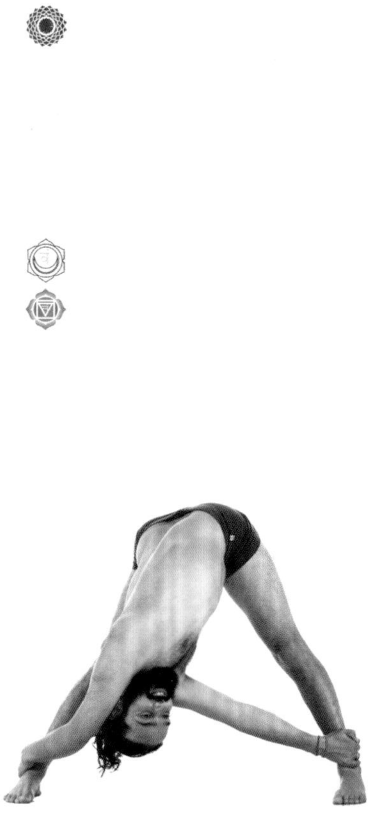

132
परिवृत्त प्रसरित पाद उत्तान आसन (विपरीत गुल्फ बद्ध)
Parivṛtta prasarita pāda uttāna āsana
(viparīta gulpha baddha)
Twisted wide-leg forward stretch pose
(holding opposite ankles)

परिवृत्तप्रसरितपादोत्तानासन (विपरीतगुल्फबद्ध)
Parivṛttaprasaritapādottānāsana
(viparītagulphabaddha)

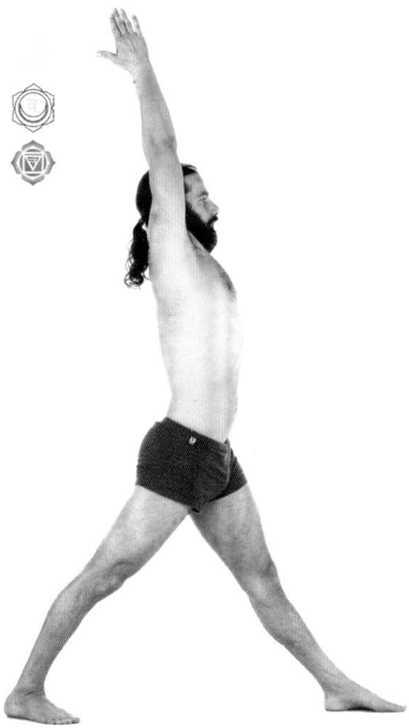

133
पार्श्व उत्तान आसन (ऊर्ध्व हस्त आरम्भ अवस्था)
Pārśva uttāna āsana
(ūrdhva hasta, ārambhā avasthā)
Side stretch pose
(hands overhead, starting position)

पार्श्वोत्तानासन (ऊर्ध्वहस्तारम्भावस्था)
Pārśvottānāsana (ūrdhvahasta, ārambhāvasthā)

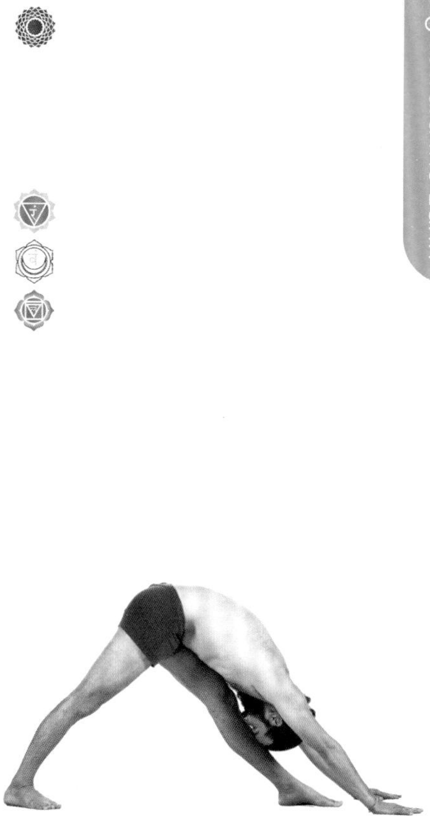

134
पार्श्व उत्तान आसन (हस्त भू)
Pārśva uttāna āsana (hasta bhū)
Side stretch pose (hands on the earth)

पार्श्वोत्तानासन (हस्तभू)
Pārśvottānāsana (hastabhū)

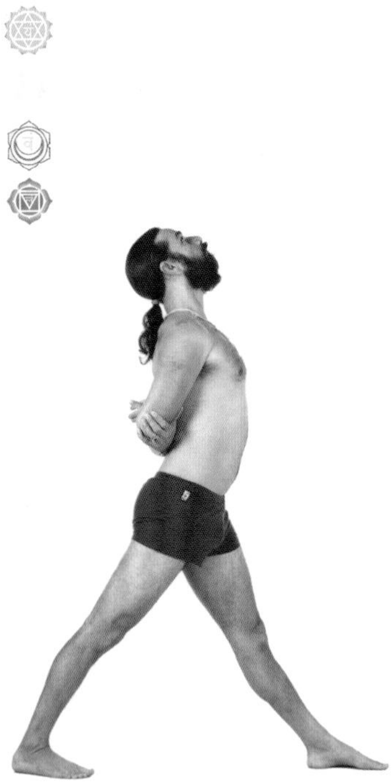

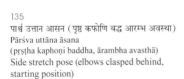

135
पार्श्व उत्तान आसन (पृष्ठ कफोणि बद्ध आरम्भ अवस्था)
Pārśva uttāna āsana
(pṛṣṭha kaphoṇi baddha, ārambha avasthā)
Side stretch pose (elbows clasped behind, starting position)

पार्श्वोत्तानासन (पृष्ठकफोणिबद्धारम्भावस्था)
Pārśvottānāsana (pṛṣṭhakaphoṇibaddhārambhāvasthā)

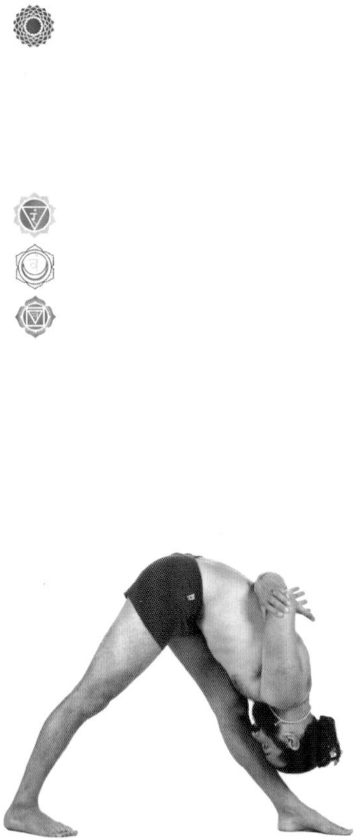

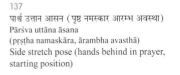

136
पार्श्व उत्तान आसन (पृष्ठ कफोणि बद्ध)
Pārśva uttāna āsana (pṛṣṭha kaphoṇi baddha)
Side stretch pose (elbows clasped behind)

पार्श्वोत्तानासन (पृष्ठकफोणिबद्ध)
Pārśvottānāsana (pṛṣṭhakaphoṇibaddha)

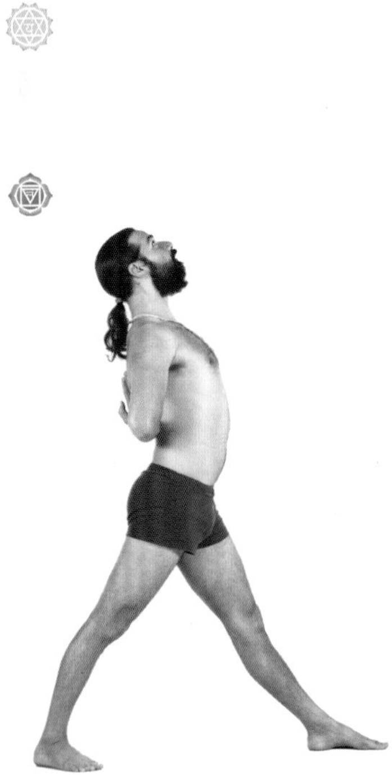

137
पार्श्व उत्तान आसन (पृष्ठ नमस्कार आरम्भ अवस्था)
Pārśva uttāna āsana
(pṛṣṭha namaskāra, ārambha avasthā)
Side stretch pose (hands behind in prayer, starting position)

पार्श्वोत्तानासन (पृष्ठनमस्कारारम्भावस्था)
Pārśvottānāsana (pṛṣṭhanamaskārārambhāvasthā)

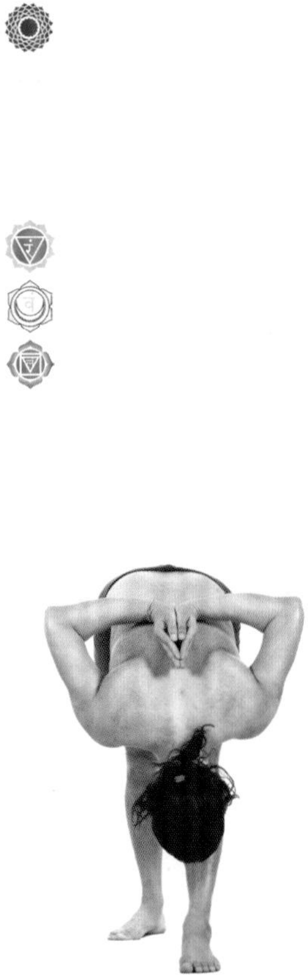

138
पार्श्व उत्तान आसन (पृष्ठ नमस्कार)
Pārśva uttāna āsana (pṛṣṭha namaskāra)
Side stretch pose (hands behind in prayer)

पार्श्वोत्तानासन (पृष्ठनमस्कार)
Pārśvottānāsana (pṛṣṭhanamaskāra)

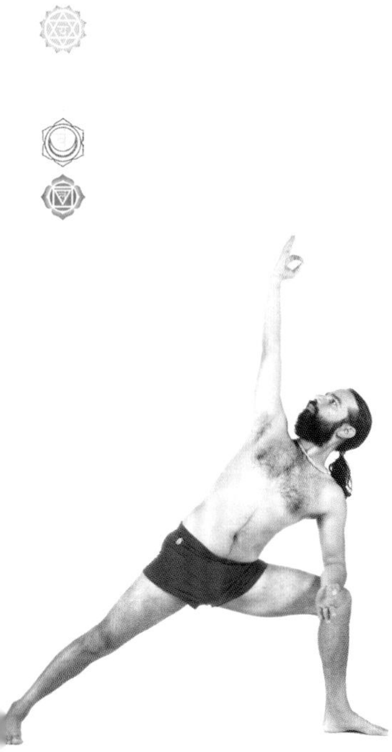

139
अर्ध पार्श्व कोण आसन
Ardha pārśva koṇa āsana
Half side angle pose

अर्धपार्श्वकोणासन
Ardhapārśvakoṇāsana

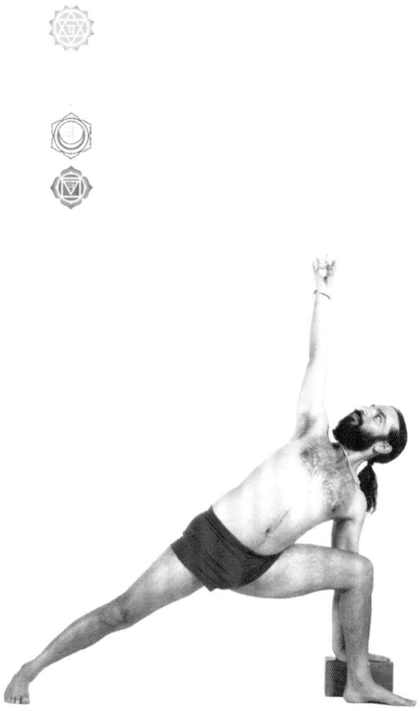

140
पार्श्व कोण आसन (सालम्ब बहिर्हस्त)
Pārśva koṇa āsana (sālamba bahirhasta)
Side angle pose (supported hand on the outside)

पार्श्वकोणासन (सालम्बबहिर्हस्त)
Pārśvakoṇāsana (sālambabahirhasta)

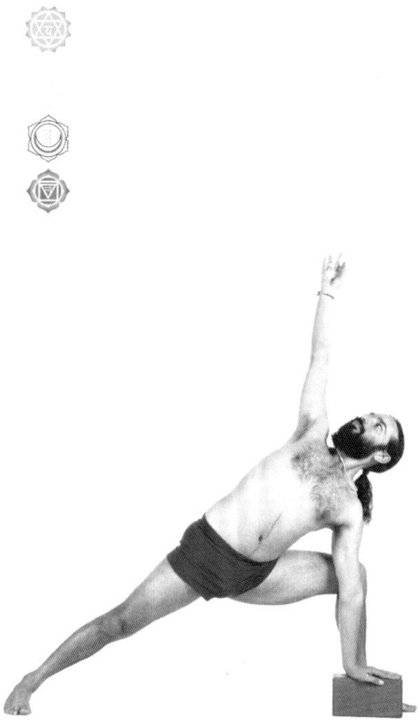

141
पार्श्व कोण आसन (सालम्ब अन्तर्हस्त)
Pārśva koṇa āsana (sālamba antarhasta)
Side angle pose (supported hand on the inside)

पार्श्वकोणासन (सालम्बान्तर्हस्त)
Pārśvakoṇāsana (sālambantarhasta)

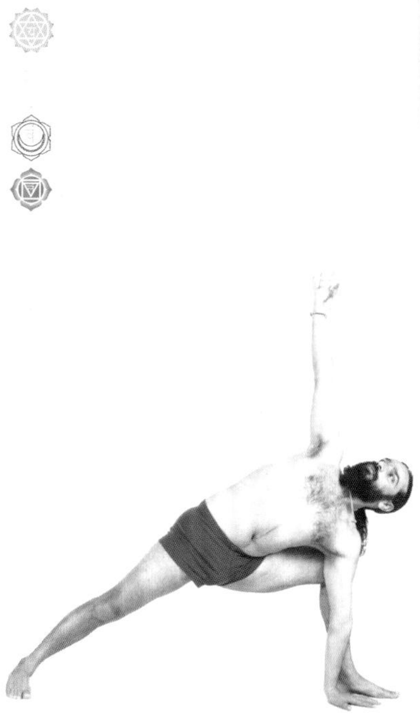

142
पार्श्व कोण आसन (अन्तर्हस्त)
Pārśva koṇa āsana (antarhasta)
Side angle pose (hand on the inside)

पार्श्वकोणासन (अन्तर्हस्त)
Pārśvakoṇāsana (antarhasta)

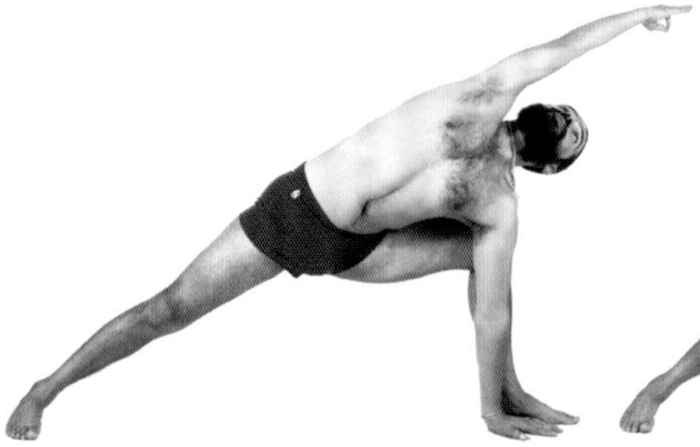

143
पूर्ण पार्श्व कोण आसन (अन्तर्हस्त)
Pūrṇa pārśva koṇa āsana (antarhasta)
Full side angle pose (hand on the inside)

पूर्णपार्श्वकोणासन (अन्तर्हस्त)
Pūrṇapārśvakoṇāsana (antarhasta)

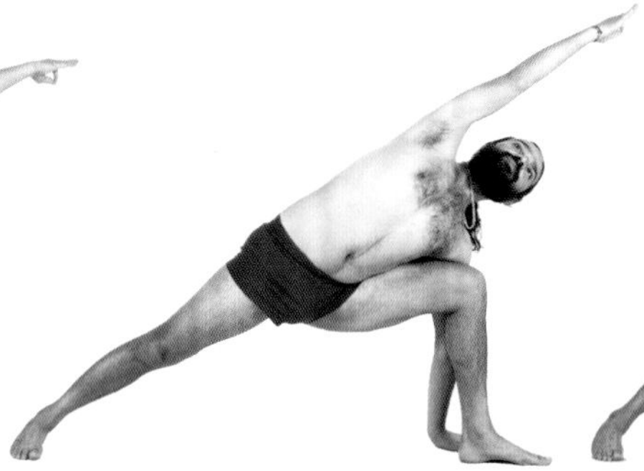

144
पूर्ण पार्श्व कोण आसन (बहिर्हस्त)
Pūrṇa pārśva koṇa āsana (bahirhasta)
Full side angle pose (hand on the outside)

पूर्णपार्श्वकोणासन (बहिर्हस्त)
Pūrṇapārśvakoṇāsana (bahirhasta)

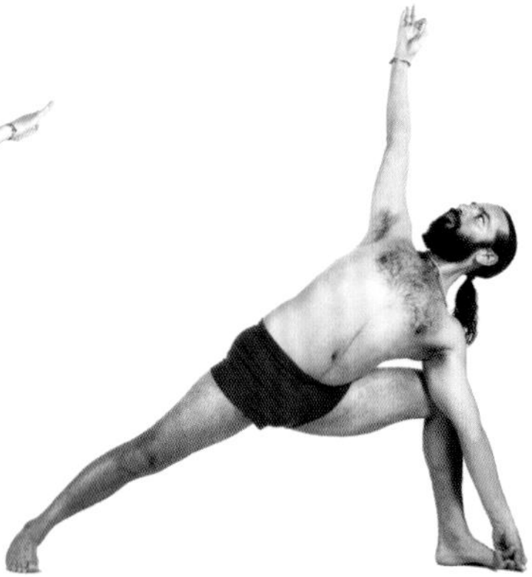

145
पार्श्व कोण आसन (बद्ध पाद अङ्गुष्ठ)
Pārśva koṇa āsana (baddha pāda aṅguṣṭha)
Side angle pose (holding big toe)

पार्श्वकोणासन (बद्धपादाङ्गुष्ठ)
Pārśvakoṇāsana (baddhapādāṅguṣṭha)

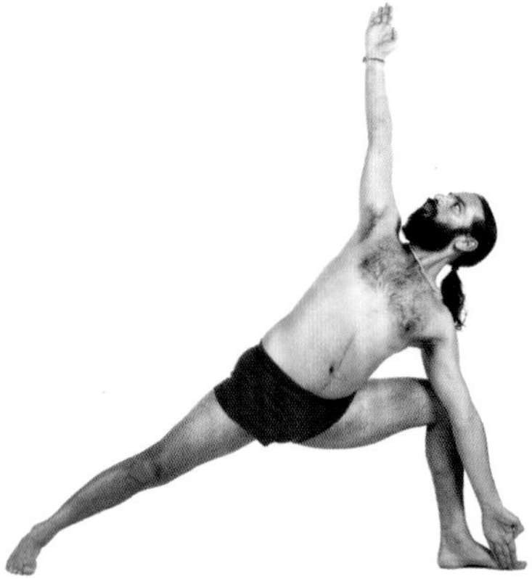

146
पार्श्व कोण आसन
Pārśva koṇa āsana
Side angle pose

पार्श्वकोणासन
Pārśvakoṇāsana

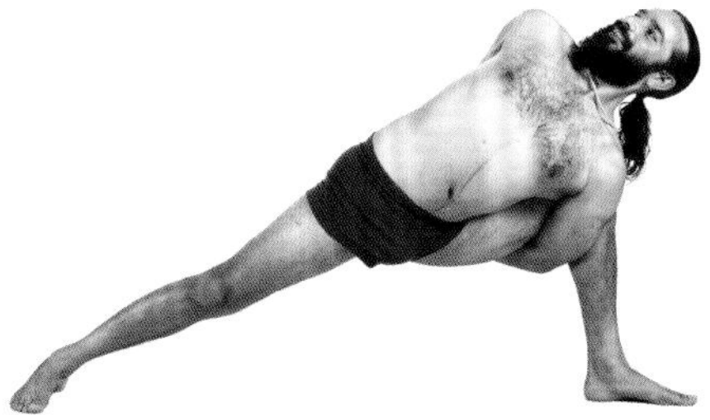

147
पार्श्व कोण आसन (उरु रज्जु हस्त)
Pārśva koṇa āsana (uru rajju hasta)
Side angle pose (hands bound around thigh)

पार्श्वकोणासन (उरुरज्जुहस्त)
Pārśvakoṇāsana (ururajjuhasta)

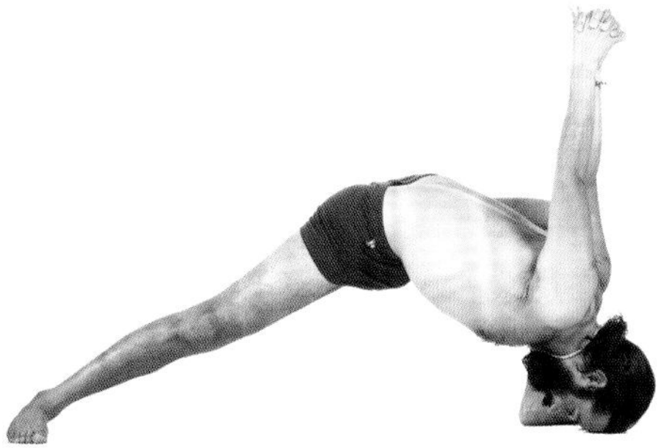

148
शीर्ष पाद अङ्गुष्ठ पार्श्व कोण आसन
Śirṣa pāda aṅguṣṭha pārśva koṇa āsana
Head to big toe side angle pose

शीर्षपादाङ्गुष्ठपार्श्वकोणासन
Śirṣapādāṅguṣṭhapārśvakoṇāsana

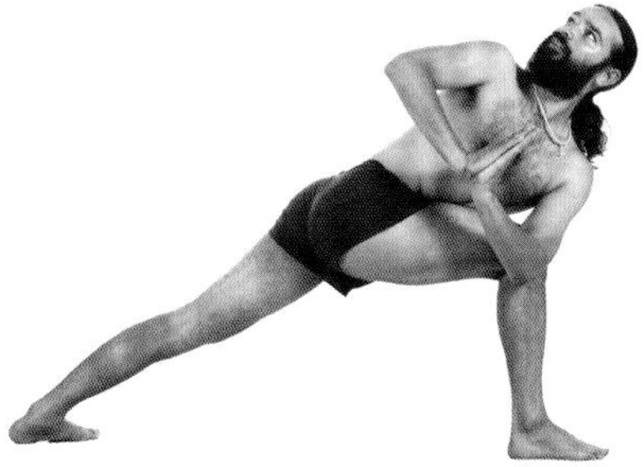

149
परिवृत्त पार्श्व कोण आसन (नमस्कार हस्त)
Parivṛtta pārśva koṇa āsana (namaskāra hasta)
Twisted side angle pose (hands in prayer)

परिवृत्तपार्श्वकोणासन (नमस्कारहस्त)
Parivṛttapārśvakoṇāsana (namaskārahasta)

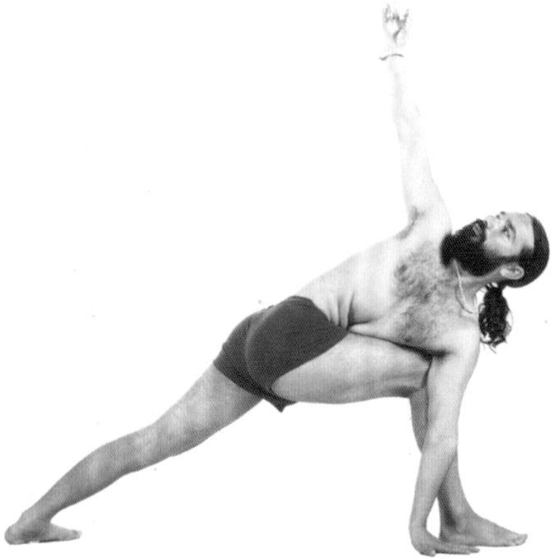

150
परिवृत्त पार्श्व कोण आसन
Parivṛtta pārśva koṇa āsana
Twisted side angle pose

परिवृत्तपार्श्वकोणासन
Parivṛttapārśvakoṇāsana

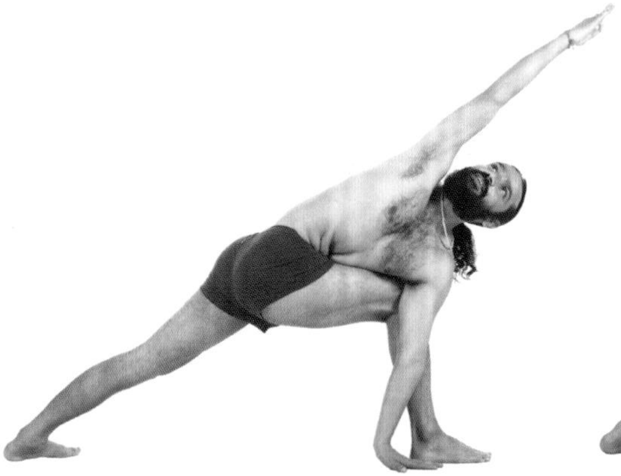

151
परिवृत्त पूर्ण पार्श्व कोण आसन
Parivṛtta pūrṇa pārśva koṇa āsana
Fully twisted side angle pose

परिवृत्तपूर्णपार्श्वकोणासन
Parivṛttapūrṇapārśvakoṇāsana

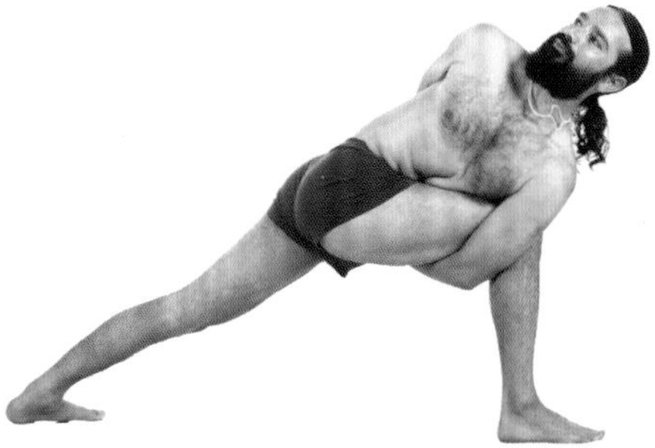

152
परिवृत्त पार्श्व कोण आसन (रज्जु हस्त)
Parivṛtta pārśva koṇa āsana (rajju hasta)
Twisted side angle pose (bound arms)

परिवृत्तपार्श्वकोणासन (रज्जुहस्त)
Parivṛttapārśvakoṇāsana (rajjuhasta)

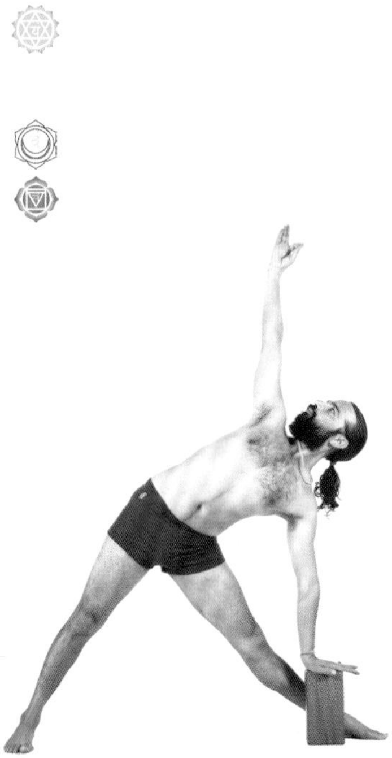

153
त्रिकोण आसन (सालम्ब अन्तर्हस्त)
Trikoṇa āsana (sālamba antarhasta)
Triangle pose (supported hand on the inside)

त्रिकोणासन (सालम्ब अन्तर्हस्त)
Trikoṇāsana (sālamba antarhasta)

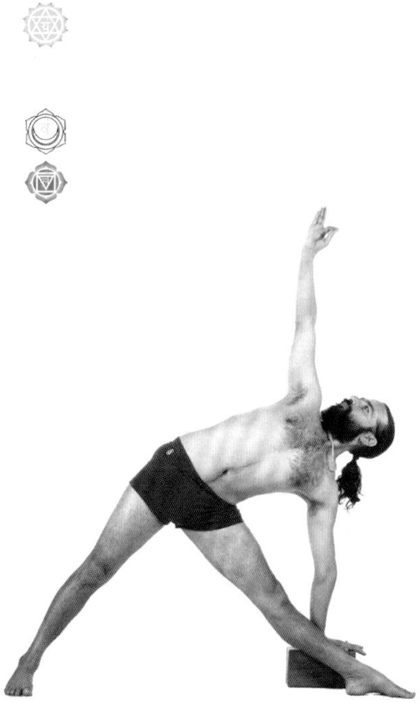

154
त्रिकोण आसन (सालम्ब बहिर्हस्त)
Trikoṇa āsana (sālamba bahirhasta)
Triangle pose (supported hand on the outside)

त्रिकोणासन (सालम्ब बहिर्हस्त)
Trikoṇāsana (sālambabahirhasta)

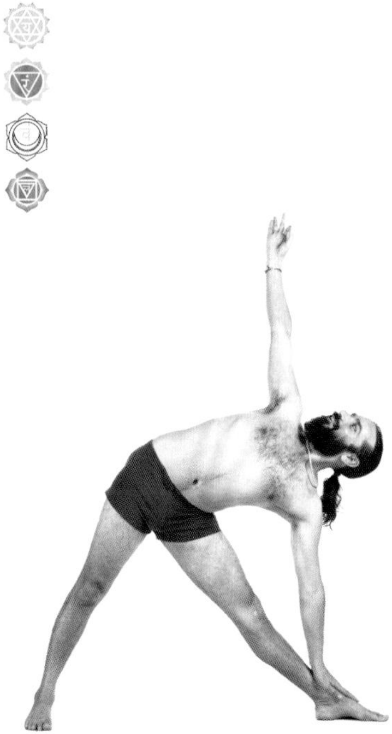

155
त्रिकोण आसन (पाद हस्त)
Trikoṇa āsana (pāda hasta)
Triangle pose (hand on foot)

त्रिकोणासन (पादहस्त)
Trikoṇāsana (pādahasta)

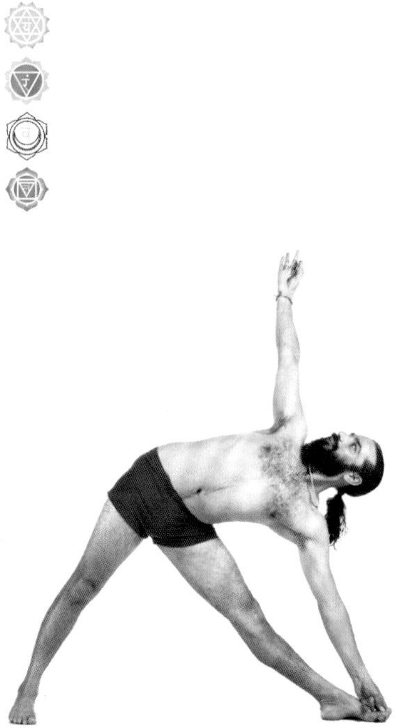

156
त्रिकोण आसन (बद्ध पाद अङ्गुष्ठ)
Trikoṇa āsana (baddha pāda aṅguṣṭha)
Triangle pose (holding big toe)

त्रिकोणासन (बद्धपादाङ्गुष्ठ)
Trikoṇāsana (baddhapādāṅguṣṭha)

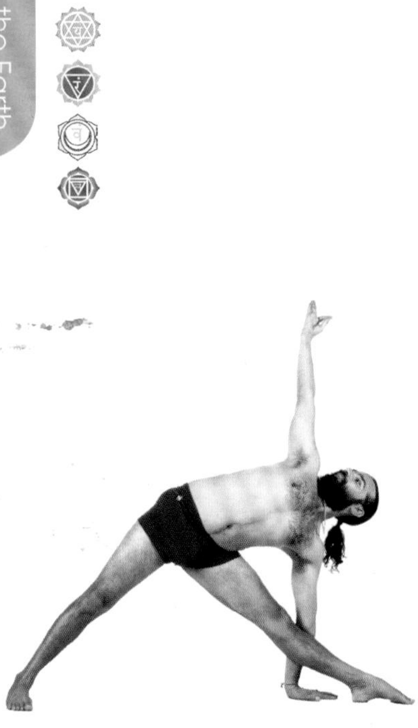

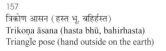

157
त्रिकोण आसन (हस्त भू, बहिर्हस्त)
Trikoṇa āsana (hasta bhū, bahirhasta)
Triangle pose (hand outside on the earth)

त्रिकोणासन (हस्तभू,बहिर्हस्त)
Trikoṇāsana (hastabhū, bahirhasta)

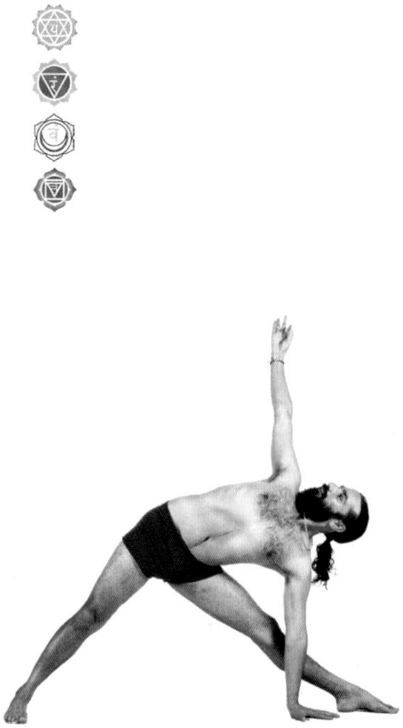

158
त्रिकोण आसन (हस्त भू, अन्तर्हस्त)
Trikoṇa āsana (hasta bhū, antarhasta)
Triangle pose (hand inside on the earth)

त्रिकोणासन (हस्तभू,अन्तर्हस्त)
Trikoṇāsana (hastabhū, antarhasta)

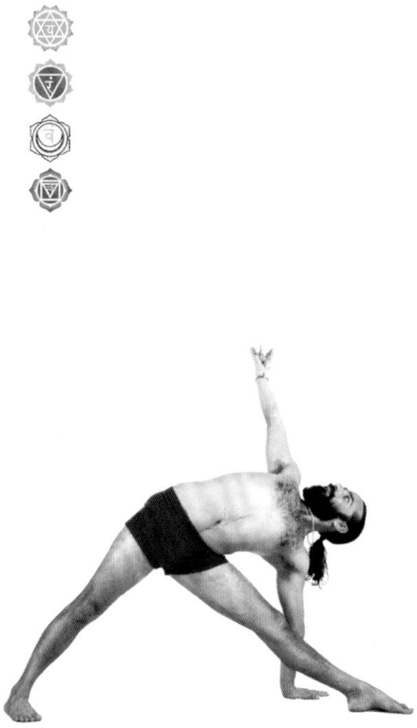

159
त्रिकोण आसन (हस्त भू, बहिर्हस्त परिवृत्तबहिः)
Trikoṇa āsana (hasta bhū, bahirhasta parivṛtta bahiḥ)
Triangle pose (hand outside on the earth, twisting open)

त्रिकोणासन (हस्तभू, बहिर्हस्तपरिवृत्तबहिः)
Trikoṇāsana (hastabhū, bahirhastaparivṛttabahiḥ)

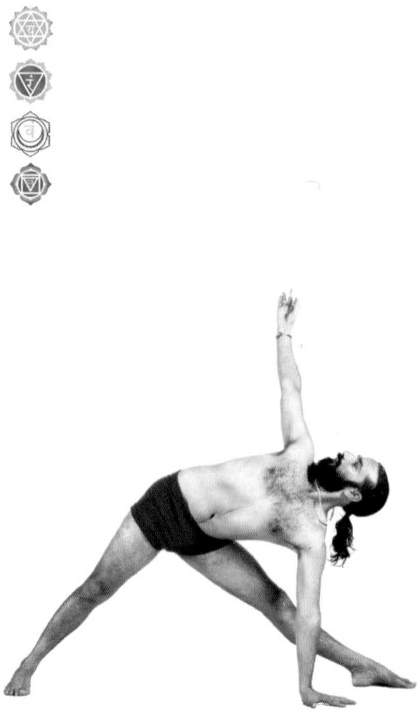

160
त्रिकोण आसन (हस्त भू, अन्तर्हस्त परिवृत्तबहिः)
Trikoṇa āsana (hasta bhū, antarhasta parivṛtta bahiḥ)
Triangle pose (hand inside on the earth, twisting open)

त्रिकोणासन (हस्तभू, अन्तर्हस्तपरिवृत्तबहिः)
Trikoṇāsana (hastabhū, antarhastaparivṛttabahiḥ)

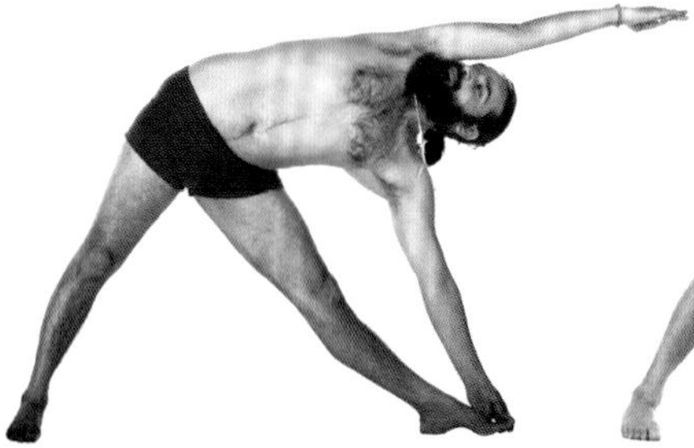

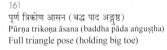

161
पूर्ण त्रिकोण आसन (बद्ध पाद अङ्गुष्ठ)
Pūrṇa trikoṇa āsana (baddha pāda aṅguṣṭha)
Full triangle pose (holding big toe)

पूर्णत्रिकोणासन (बद्धपादाङ्गुष्ठ)
Pūrṇatrikoṇāsana (baddhapādaṅguṣṭha)

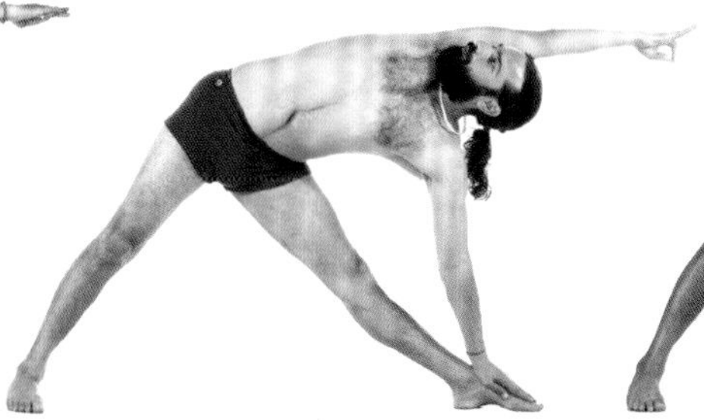

162
पूर्ण त्रिकोण आसन (पाद हस्त)
Pūrṇa trikoṇa āsana (pāda hasta)
Full triangle pose (hand on foot)

पूर्णत्रिकोणासन (पादहस्त)
Pūrṇatrikoṇāsana (pādahasta)

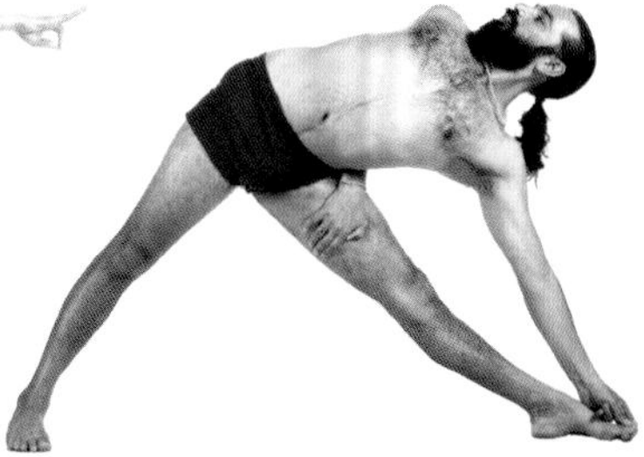

163
त्रिकोण आसन (बद्ध पाद अङ्गुष्ठ, उरु हस्त)
Trikoṇa āsana (baddha pāda aṅguṣṭha, uru hasta)
Triangle pose (holding big toe, hand on thigh)

त्रिकोणासन (बद्धपादाङ्गुष्ठ, उरुहस्त)
Trikoṇāsana (baddhapādāṅguṣṭha, uruhasta)

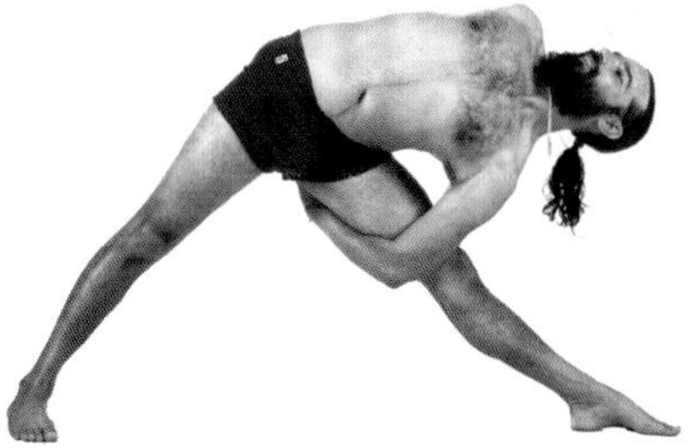

164
विक त्रिकोण आसन (उरु बद्ध, रज्जु हस्त)
Vika trikoṇa āsana (uru baddha, rajju hasta)
Challenging triangle pose (hands bound around thigh)

विकत्रिकोणासन (उरुबद्ध, रज्जुहस्त)
Vikatrikoṇāsana (urubaddha, rajjuhasta)

Before learning something new, practice what you already know.

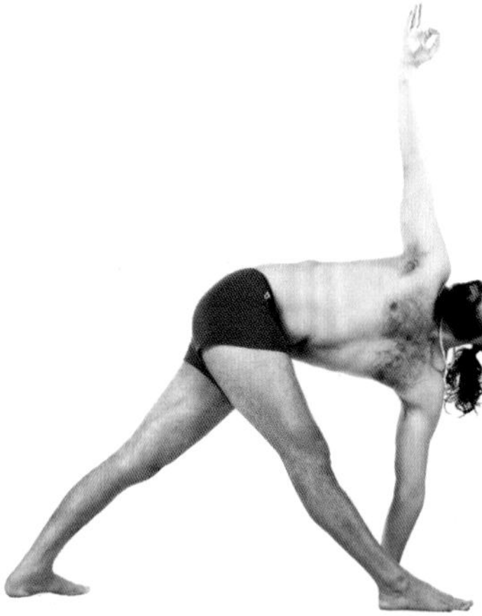

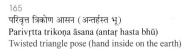

165
परिवृत्त त्रिकोण आसन (अन्तर्हस्त भू)
Parivṛtta trikoṇa āsana (antaṛ hasta bhū)
Twisted triangle pose (hand inside on the earth)

परिवृत्तत्रिकोणासन (अन्तर्हस्तभू)
Parivṛttatrikoṇāsana (antaṛhastabhū)

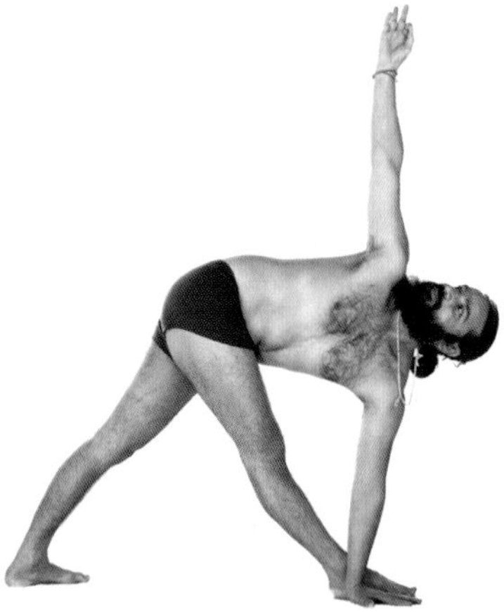

166
परिवृत्त त्रिकोण आसन (बहिर्हस्त भू)
Parivṛtta trikoṇa āsana (bahir hasta bhū)
Twisted triangle pose (hand outside on the earth)

परिवृत्तत्रिकोणासन (बहिर्हस्तभू)
Parivṛttatrikoṇāsana (bahirhastabhū)

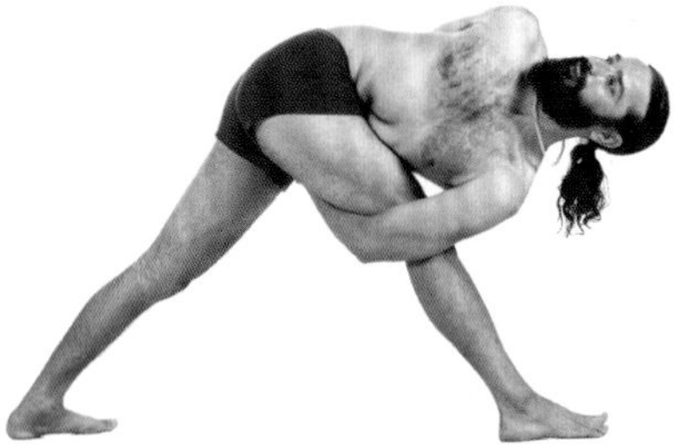

167
परिवृत्त विकटत्रिकोण आसन (रज्जु हस्त)
Parivṛtta vikaṭa trikoṇa āsana (rajju hasta)
Challenging twisted triangle pose (hands bound)

परिवृत्तविकटत्रिकोणासन (रज्जुहस्त)
Parivṛttavikaṭatrikoṇāsana (rajjuhasta)

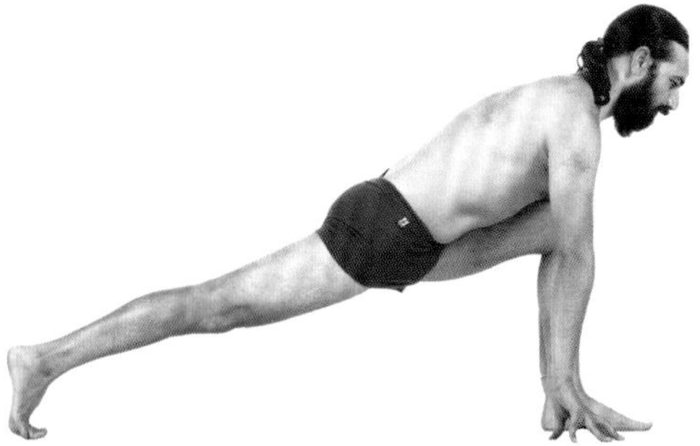

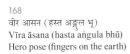

168
वीर आसन (हस्त अङ्गुल भू)
Vīra āsana (hasta aṅgula bhū)
Hero pose (fingers on the earth)

वीरासन (हस्ताङ्गुलभू)
Vīrāsana (hastāṅgulabhū)

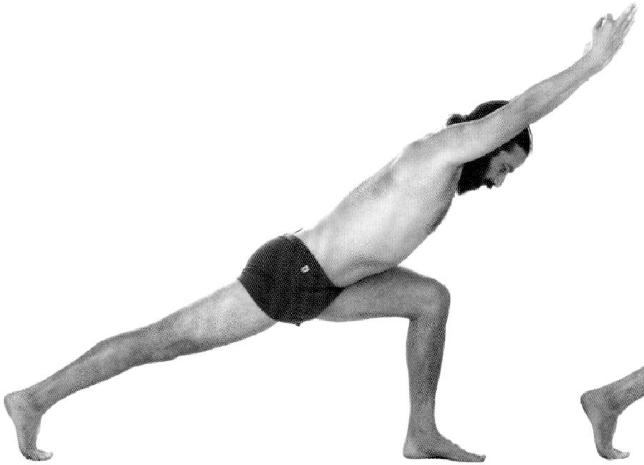

169
क्षितिज वीर आसन (अधोमुख)
Kṣitija vīra āsana (adhomukha)
Horizon hero pose (downward facing)

क्षितिजवीरासन (अधोमुख)
Kṣitijavīrāsana (adhomukha)

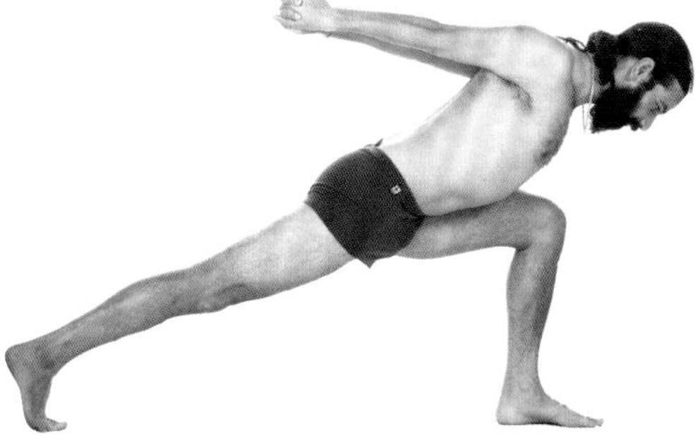

170
क्षितिज वीर आसन (पृष्ठ हस्त उत्तान)
Kṣitija vīra āsana (pṛṣṭha hasta uttāna)
Horizon hero pose (hands stretched behind)

क्षितिजवीरासन (पृष्ठहस्तोत्तान)
Kṣitijavīrāsana (pṛṣṭhahastottāna)

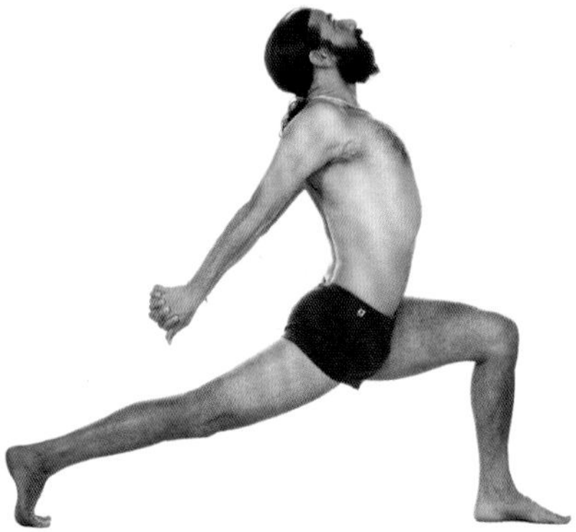

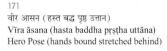

171
वीर आसन (हस्त बद्ध पृष्ठ उत्तान)
Vīra āsana (hasta baddha pṛṣṭha uttāna)
Hero Pose (hands bound stretched behind)

वीरासन (हस्तबद्धपृष्ठोत्तान)
Vīrāsana (hastabaddhapṛṣṭhottāna)

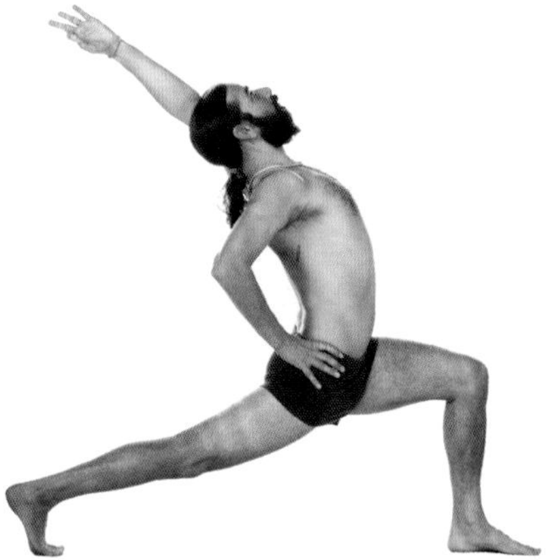

172
वीर आसन (एक कटि हस्त)
Vīra āsana (eka kaṭi hasta)
Hero pose (one hand on waist)

वीरासन (एककटिहस्त)
Vīrāsana (ekakaṭihasta)

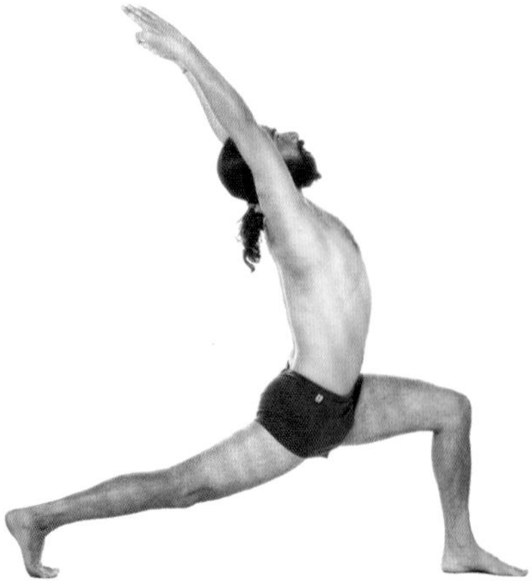

173
वीर आसन (ज्ञान मुद्रा)
Vīra āsana (jñāna mudrā)
Hero pose (hands in jñāna mudrā)

वीरासन (ज्ञानमुद्रा)
Vīrāsana (jñanamudrā)

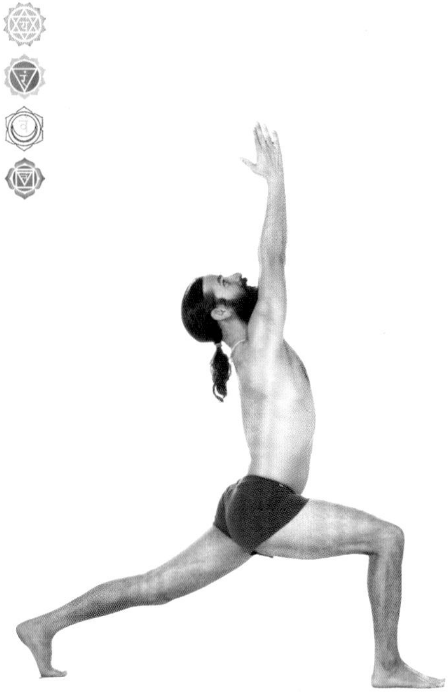

174
वीर आसन
Vīra āsana
Hero pose

वीरासन
Vīrāsana

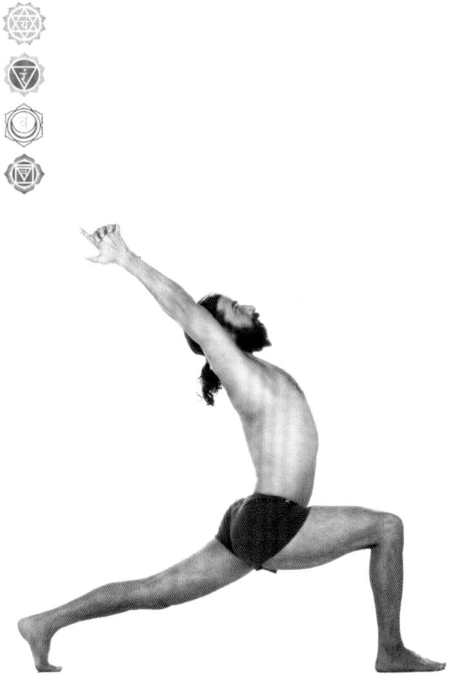

175
वीर आसन (आकाश तर्जनी मुद्रा)
Vīra āsana (ākāśa tarjanī mudrā)
Hero pose (pointing index fingers to the sky)

वीरासन (आकाशतर्जनीमुद्रा)
Vīrāsana (ākāśatarjanīmudrā)

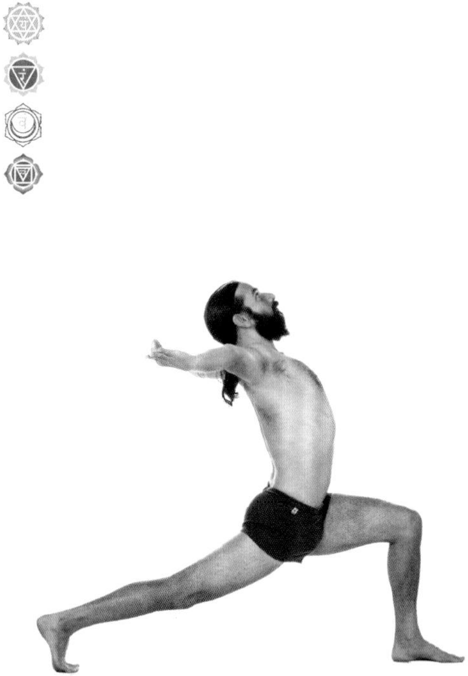

176
वीर आसन (विराट हस्त ज्ञान मुद्रा)
Vīra āsana (virāṭa hasta jñāna mudrā)
Hero pose (arms extended wide hands in jñāna mudrā)

वीरासन (विराटहस्तज्ञानमुद्रा)
Vīrāsana (virāṭahastajñānamudrā)

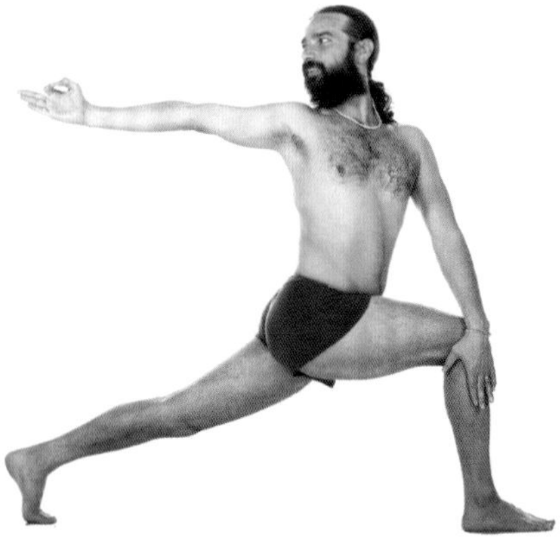

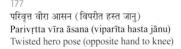

177
परिवृत्त वीरा आसन (विपरीत हस्त जानु)
Parivṛtta vīra āsana (viparīta hasta jānu)
Twisted hero pose (opposite hand to knee)

परिवृत्तवीरासन (विपरीतहस्तजानु)
Parivṛttavīrāsana (viparītahastajānu)

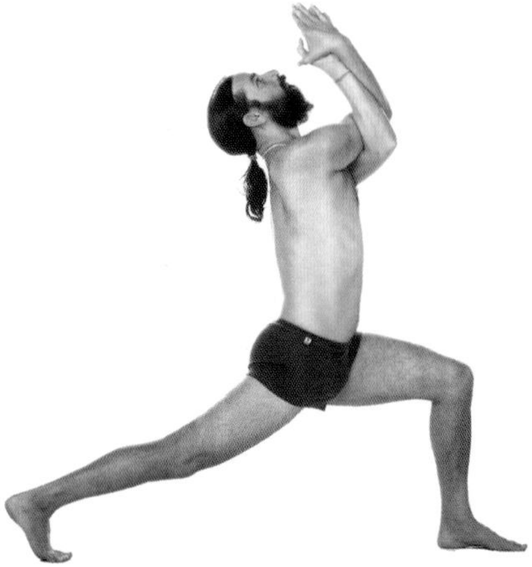

178
वीर आसन (गरुड हस्त)
Vīra āsana (garuḍa hasta)
Hero pose (eagle arms)

वीरासन (गरुडहस्त)
Vīrāsana (garuḍahasta)

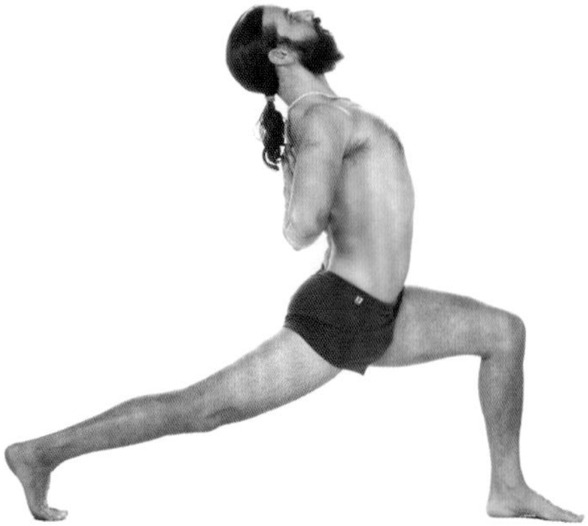

179
वीर आसन (पृष्ठ नमस्कार)
Vīra āsana (pṛṣṭha namaskāra)
Hero pose (hands behind in prayer)

वीरासन (पृष्ठनमस्कार)
Vīrāsana (pṛṣṭhanamaskāra)

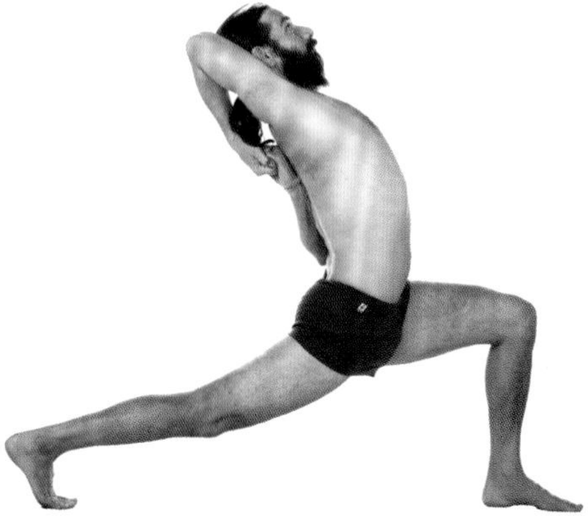

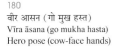

180
वीर आसन (गो मुख हस्त)
Vīra āsana (go mukha hasta)
Hero pose (cow-face hands)

वीरासन (गोमुखहस्त)
Vīrāsana (gomukhahasta)

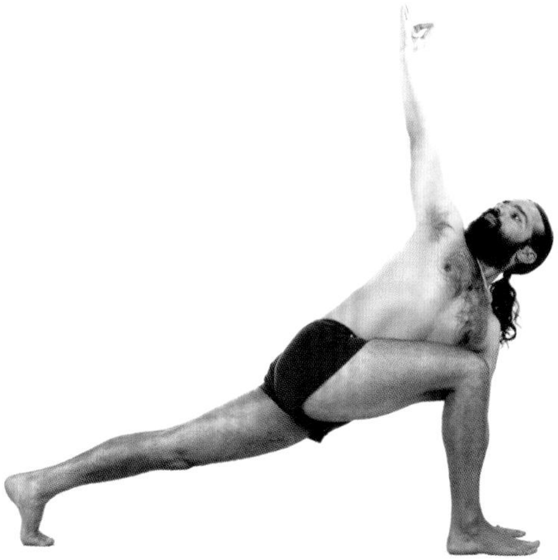

181
परिवृत्त वीर आसन (अन्तर्हस्त, विराट हस्त)
Parivṛtta vīra āsana (antarhasta, virāṭa hasta)
Twisted hero pose (hand inside, arms extended)

परिवृत्तवीरासन (अन्तर्हस्त, विराटहस्त)
Parivṛttavīrāsana (antarhasta, virātahasta)

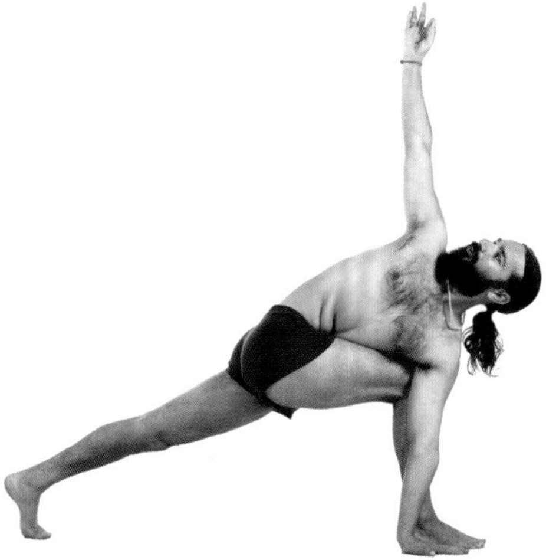

182
परिवृत्त वीर आसन (बहिर्हस्त, विराट हस्त)
Parivṛtta vīra āsana (bahirhasta, virāṭa hasta)
Twisted hero pose (hands outside, arms extended)

परिवृत्तवीरासन (बहिर्हस्त, विराटहस्त)
Parivṛttavīrarāsana (bahirhasta, virātahasta)

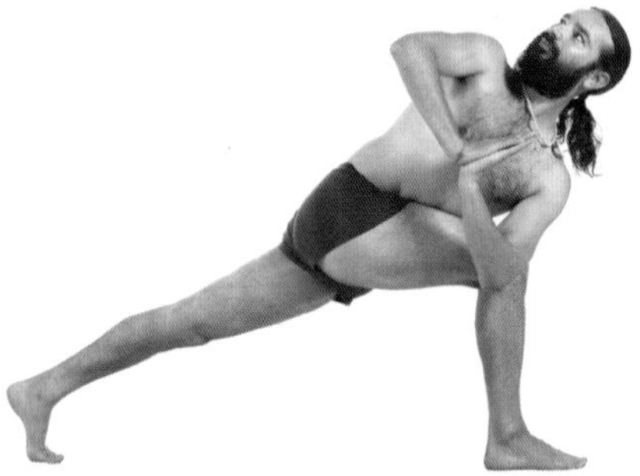

183
परिवृत्त नमस्कार वीर आसन
Parivṛtta namaskāra vīra āsana
Praying twisted hero pose

परिवृत्तनमस्कारवीरासन
Parivṛttanamaskāravīrāsana

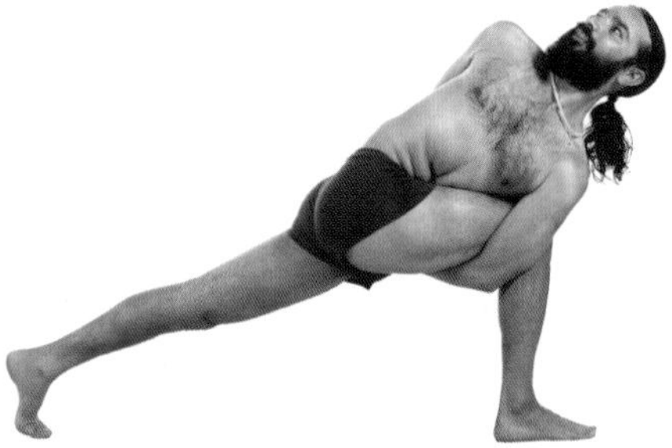

184
परिवृत्त वीर आसन (रज्जु हस्त)
Parivṛtta vīra āsana (rajju hasta)
Twisted hero pose (bound hands)

परिवृत्तवीरासन (रज्जुहस्त)
Parivṛttavīrāsana (rajjuhasta)

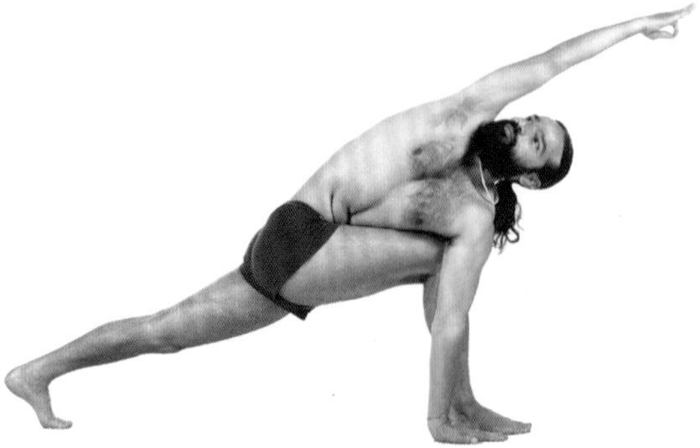

185
परिवृत्त पूर्ण वीर आसन (बहिर्हस्त भू)
Parivṛtta pūrṇa vīra āsana (bahirhasta bhū)
Fully twisted hero pose (hand on the earth, outside foot)

परिवृत्तपूर्णवीरासन (बहिर्हस्तभू)
Parivṛttapūrṇavīrāsana (bahirhastabhū)

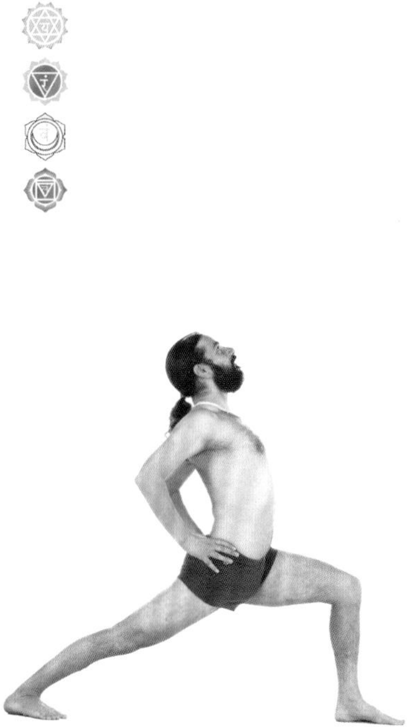

186
वीर भद्र आसन (कटि हस्त)
Vīra bhadra āsana (kati hasta)
Beautiful warrior pose (hands on waist)

वीरभद्रासन (कटिहस्त)
Vīrabhadrāsana (kaṭihasta)

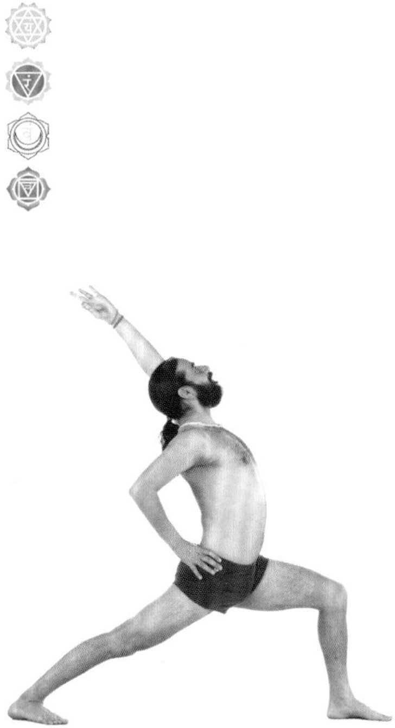

187
वीर भद्र आसन (एक कटि हस्त)
Vīra bhadra āsana (eka kati hasta)
Beautiful warrior pose (one hand on waist)

वीरभद्रासन (एककटिहस्त)
Vīrabhadrāsana (ekakaṭihasta)

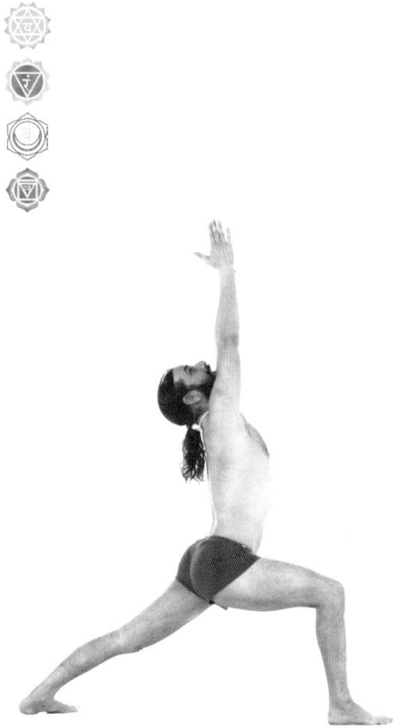

188
वीर भद्र आसन (ऊर्ध्व नमस्कार)
Vīra bhadra āsana (ūrdhva namaskāra)
Beautiful warrior pose (hands overhead in prayer)

वीरभद्रासन (ऊर्ध्वनमस्कार)
Vīrabhadrāsana (ūrdhvanamaskāra)

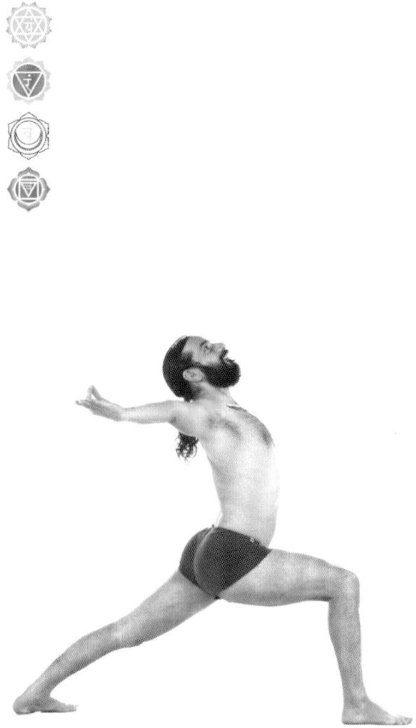

189
वीर भद्र आसन (विराट हस्त)
Vīra bhadra āsana (virāṭa hasta)
Beautiful warrior pose (hands extended wide)

वीरभद्रासन (विराटहस्त)
Vīrabhadrāsana (virāṭahasta)

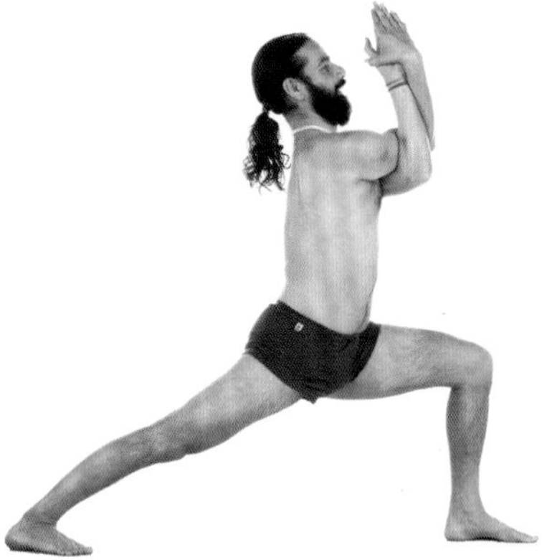

190
वीर भद्र आसन (गरुड हस्त)
Vīra bhadra āsana (garuḍa hasta)
Beautiful warrior pose (eagle arms)

वीरभद्रासन (गरुडहस्त)
Vīrabhadrāsana (garuḍahasta)

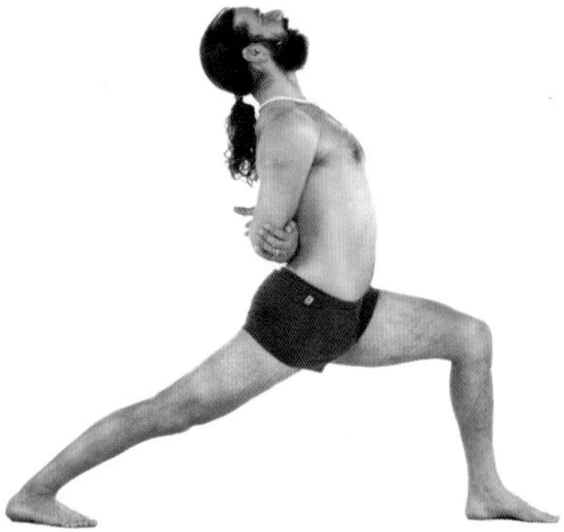

191
वीर भद्र आसन (पृष्ठ कफोणि बद्ध)
Vīra bhadra āsana (pṛṣṭha kaphoṇi baddha)
Beautiful warrior pose (elbows bound behind)

वीरभद्रासन (पृष्ठकफोणिबद्ध)
Vīrabhadrāsana (pṛṣṭhakaphoṇibaddha)

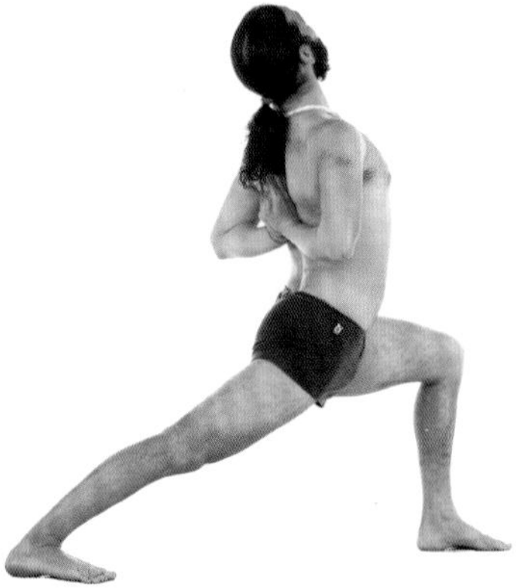

192
वीर भद्र आसन (पृष्ठ नमस्कार)
Vīra bhadra āsana (pṛṣṭha namaskāra)
Beautiful warrior pose (hands behind in prayer)

वीरभद्रासन (पृष्ठनमस्कार)
Vīrabhadrāsana (pṛṣṭhanamaskāra)

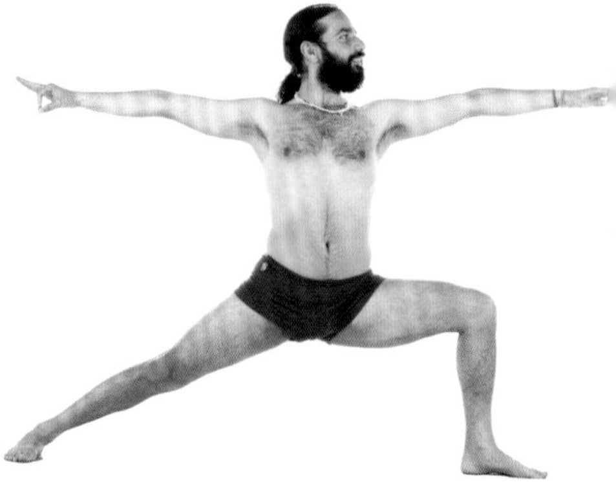

193
महा वीर भद्र आसन (ज्ञान मुद्रा)
Mahā vīra bhadra āsana (jñāna mudrā)
Great beautiful warrior pose (hands in jñāna mudrā)

महावीरभद्रासन (ज्ञानमुद्रा)
Mahāvīrabhadrāsana (jñānamudrā)

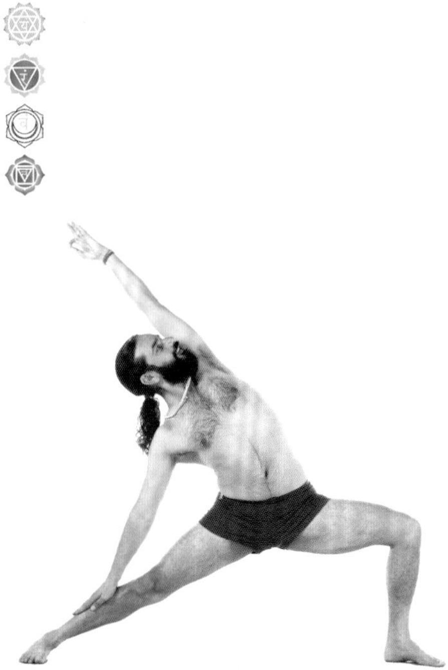

194
नृत्त महा वीर भद्र आसन (ऊर्ध्व मुख)
Nṛtya mahā vīra bhadra āsana (ūrdhva mukha)
Dancing great beautiful warrior pose (facing upward)

नृत्तमहावीरभद्रासन (ऊर्ध्वमुख)
Nṛtyamahāvīrabhadrāsana (ūrdhvamukha)

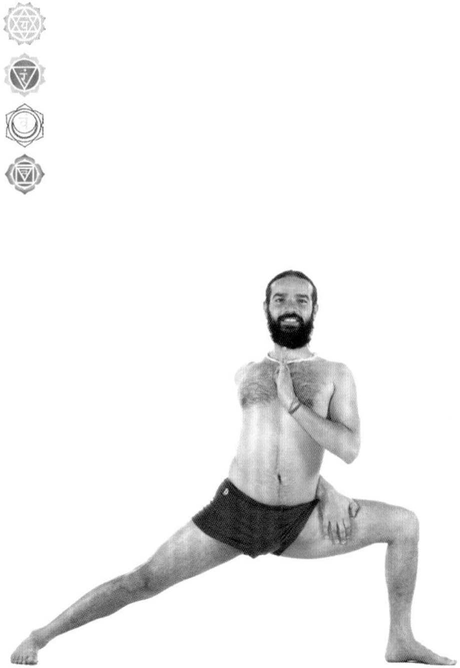

195
महा वीर भद्र आसन (उरु हस्त, ज्ञान मुद्रा)
Mahā vīra bhadra āsana (uru hasta, jñāna mudrā)
Great beautiful warrior pose (hand on thigh, hand in jñāna mudrā)

महावीरभद्रासन (उरुहस्त, ज्ञानमुद्रा)
Mahāvīrabhadrāsana (uruhasta, jñānamudrā)

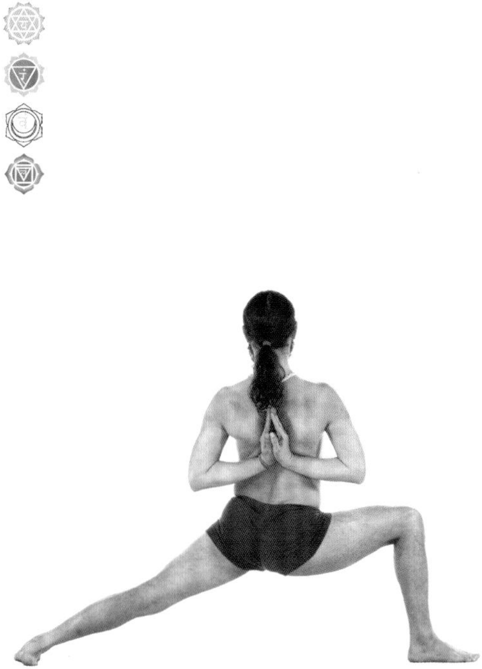

196
महा वीर भद्र आसन (पृष्ठ नमस्कार)
Mahā vīra bhadra āsana (pṛṣṭha namaskāra)
Great beautiful warrior pose (hands behind in prayer)

महावीरभद्रासन (पृष्ठनमस्कार)
Mahāvīrabhadrāsana (pṛṣṭhanamaskāra)

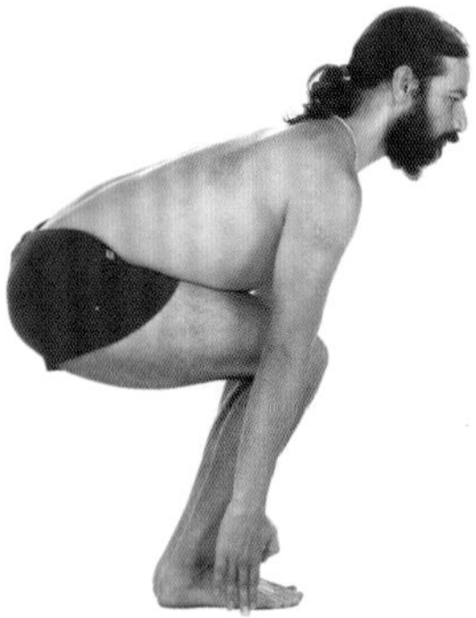

197
उत्कट आसन (हस्त अङ्गुल भू)
Utkaṭa āsana (hasta aṅgula bhū)
Strong pose (fingers on the earth)

उत्कटासन (हस्ताङ्गुलभू)
Utkaṭāsana (hastāṅgulabhū)

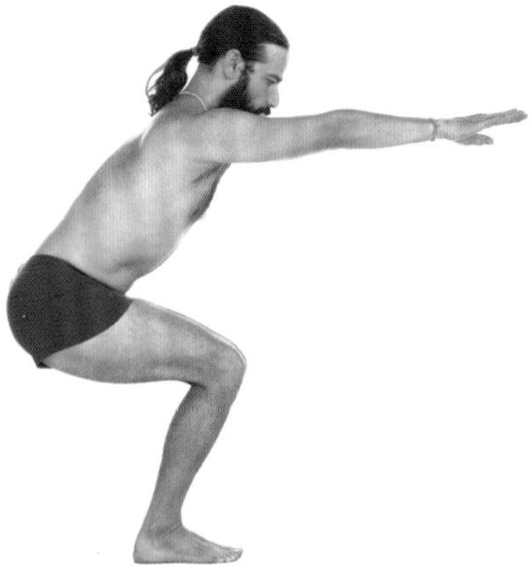

198
उत्कट आसन (समक्ष हस्त)
Utkaṭa āsana (samakṣa hasta)
Strong pose (hands facing forward)

उत्कटासन (समक्षहस्त)
Utkaṭāsana (samakṣahasta)

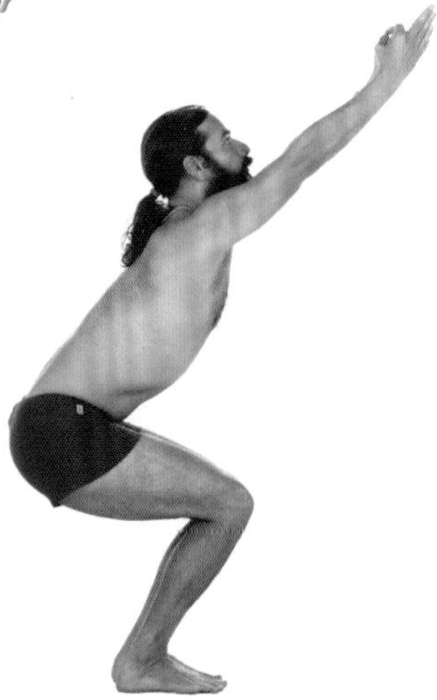

199
उत्कट आसन (ज्ञान मुद्रा)
Utkaṭa āsana (jñāna mudrā)
Strong pose (hands in jñāna mudrā)

उत्कटासन (ज्ञानमुद्रा)
Utkaṭāsana (jñānamudrā)

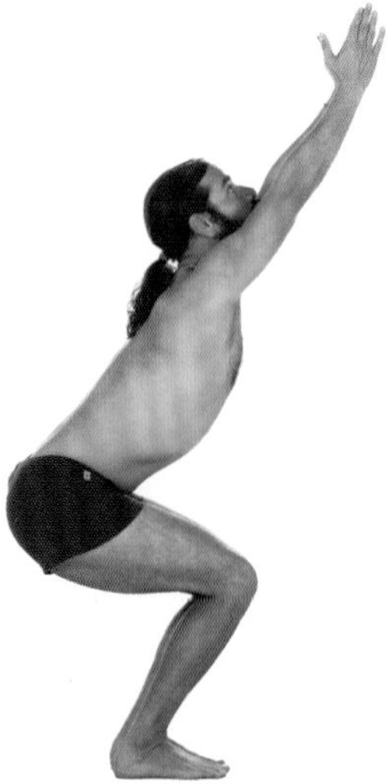

200
उत्कट आसन
Utkaṭa āsana
Strong pose

उत्कटासन
Utkaṭāsana

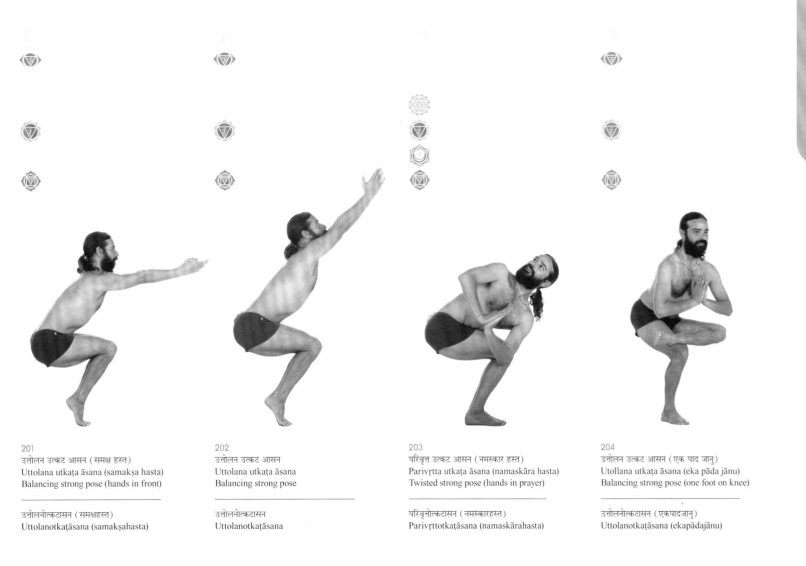

201
उत्तोलन उत्कट आसन (समक्ष हस्त)
Uttolana utkaṭa āsana (samakṣa hasta)
Balancing strong pose (hands in front)

उत्तोलनोत्कटासन (समक्षहस्त)
Uttolanotkaṭāsana (samakṣahasta)

202
उत्तोलन उत्कट आसन
Uttolana utkaṭa āsana
Balancing strong pose

उत्तोलनोत्कटासन
Uttolanotkaṭāsana

203
परिवृत्त उत्कट आसन (नमस्कार हस्त)
Parivṛtta utkaṭa āsana (namaskāra hasta)
Twisted strong pose (hands in prayer)

परिवृत्तोत्कटासन (नमस्कारहस्त)
Parivṛttotkaṭāsana (namaskārahasta)

204
उत्तोलन उत्कट आसन (एक पाद जानु)
Utollana utkaṭa āsana (eka pāda jānu)
Balancing strong pose (one foot on knee)

उत्तोलनोत्कटासन (एकपादजानु)
Uttolanotkaṭāsana (ekapādajānu)

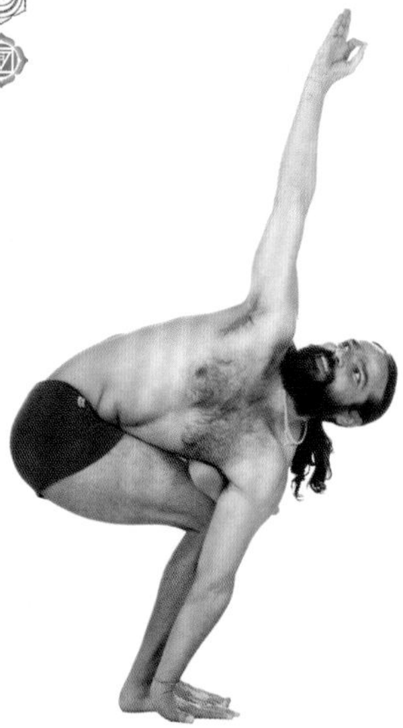

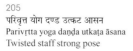

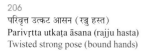

205
परिवृत्त योग दण्ड उत्कट आसन
Parivṛtta yoga daṇḍa utkaṭa āsana
Twisted staff strong pose

परिवृत्तयोगदण्डोत्कटासन
Parivṛttayogadaṇḍotkaṭāsana

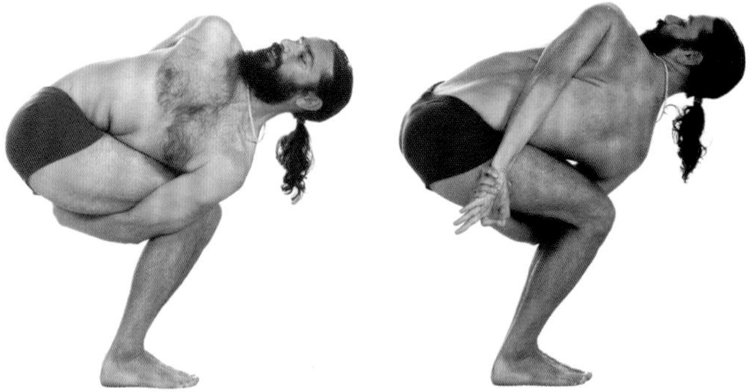

206
परिवृत्त उत्कट आसन (रज्जु हस्त)
Parivṛtta utkaṭa āsana (rajju hasta)
Twisted strong pose (bound hands)

परिवृत्तोत्कटासन (रज्जुहस्त)
Parivṛttotkaṭāsana (rajjuhasta)

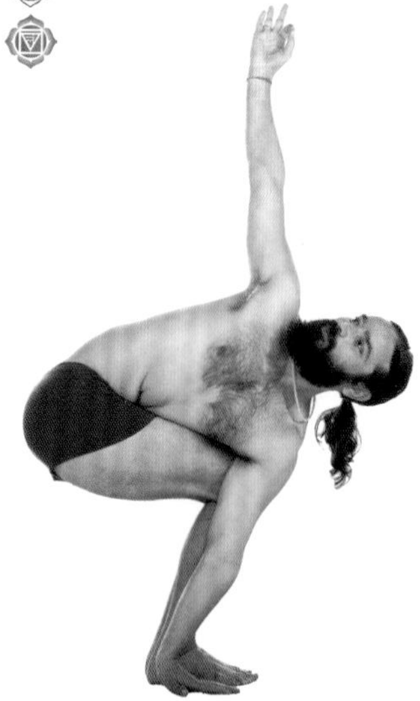

207
परिवृत्त उत्कट आसन (विराट हस्त भू)
Parivṛtta utkaṭa āsana (virāṭa hasta bhū)
Twisted strong pose (extended hand on the earth)

परिवृत्तोत्कटासन (विराटहस्तभू)
Parivṛttotkaṭāsana (virāṭahastabhū)

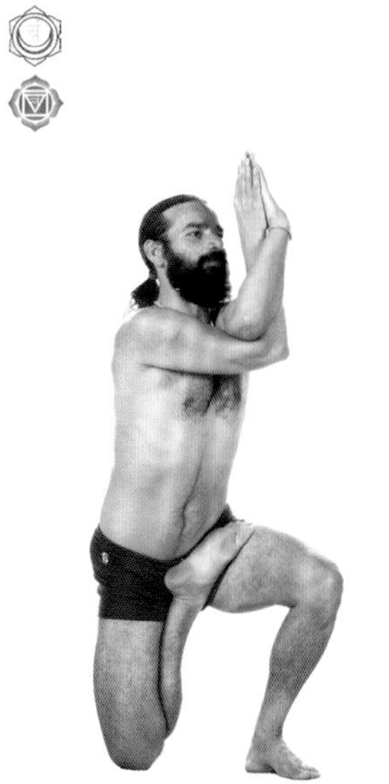

208
वातायन आसन (गरुड हस्त)
Vātāyana āsana (garuḍa hasta)
Window pose (eagle hands)

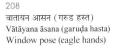

वातायनासन (गरुडहस्त)
Vātāyanāsana (garuḍahasta)

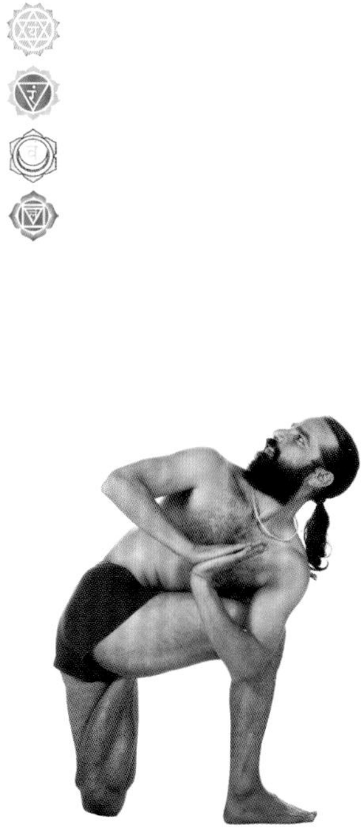

209
परिवृत्त वातायनासन (नमस्कार हस्त)
Parivṛtta vātāyana āsana (namaskāra hasta)
Twisted window pose (hands in prayer)

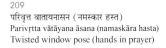

परिवृत्तवातायनासन (नमस्कारहस्त)
Parivṛttavātāyanāsana (namaskārahasta)

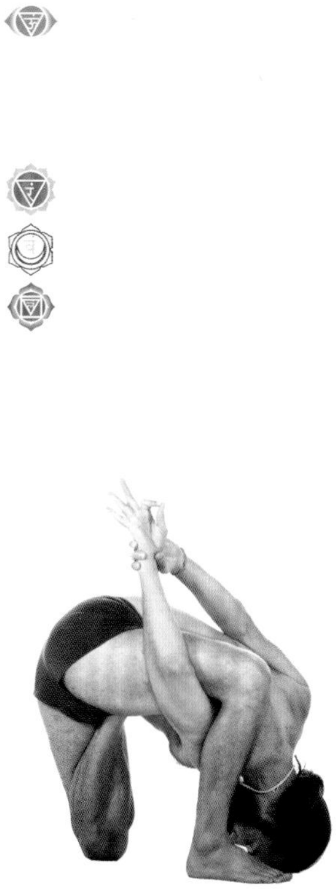

210
वातायन आसन (ललाट भू,रज्जु हस्त)
Vātāyana āsana (lalāṭa bhū, rajju hasta)
Window pose (forehead on the earth, bound hands)

वातायनासन (ललाटभू, रज्जुहस्त)
Vātāyanāsana (lalāṭabhū, rajjuhasta)

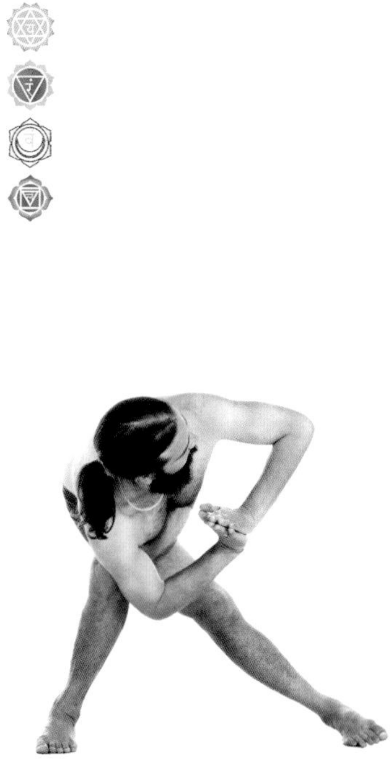

211
निरङ्कार नमस्कार आसन
Niraṅkāra namaskāra āsana
Formless prayer pose

निरङ्कारनमस्कारासन
Niraṅkāranamaskārāsana

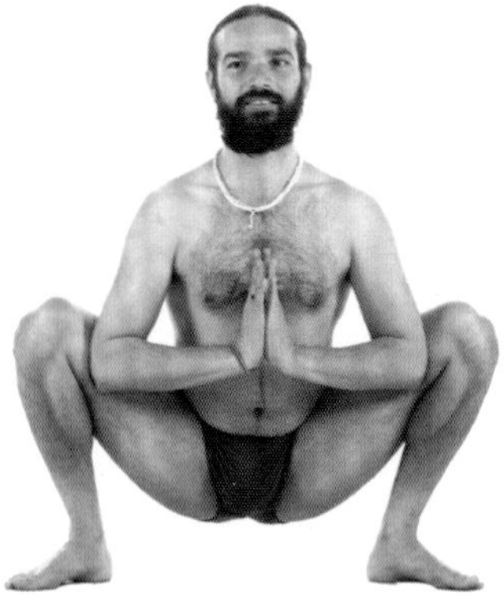

212
भू मङ्गला देवी आसन (नमस्कार)
Bhū maṅgalā devī āsana (namaskāra)
Goddess of Auspiciousness pose (hands in prayer)

भूमङ्गलादेवीासन (नमस्कार)
Bhūmaṅgalādevīāsana (namaskāra)

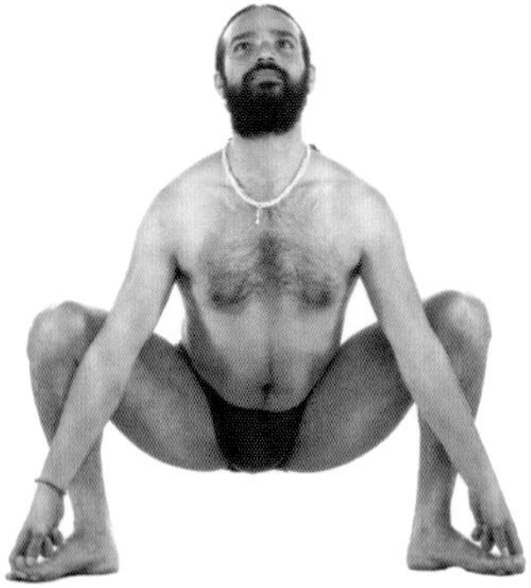

213
भू मङ्गला देवी आसन
Bhū maṅgalā devī āsana
Goddess of Auspiciousness pose

भूमङ्गलादेवीासन
Bhūmaṅgalādevīāsana

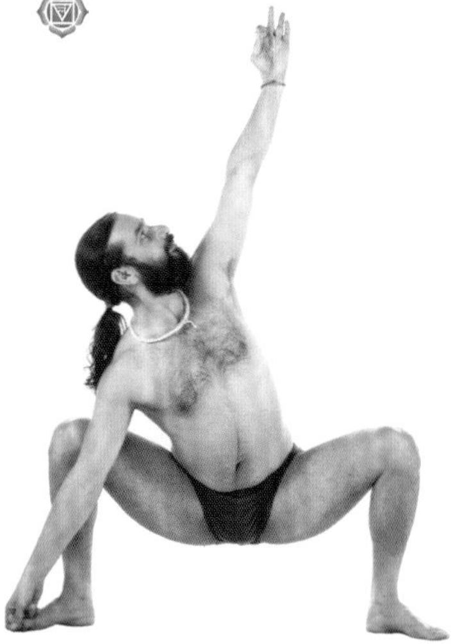

214
धात्री देवी आसन
Dhātri devī āsana
Goddess of Giving pose

धात्रीदेवीासन
Dhātridevīāsana

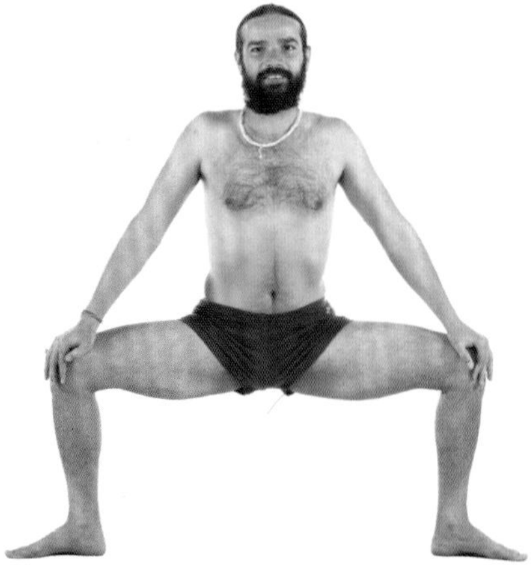

215
देवी शैल पुत्री आसन
Devī śaila putrī āsana
Daughter of the Mountain Goddess pose

देवीशैलपुत्रीासन
Devīśailaputrīāsana

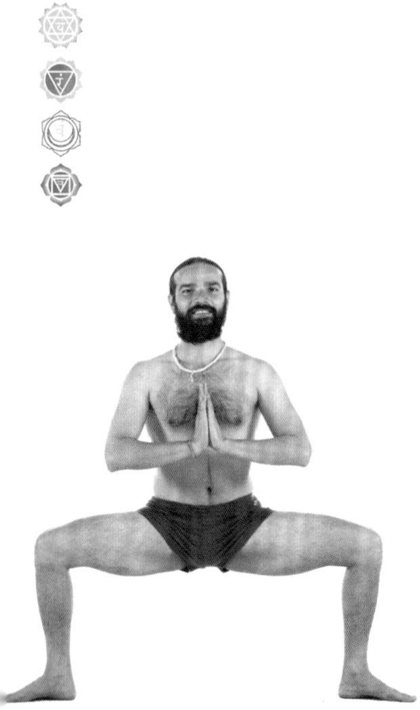

216
देवी ब्रह्म चारिणी आसन (नमस्कार)
Devī brahma cāriṇī āsana (namaskāra)
Austere Goddess pose (hands in prayer)

देवीब्रह्मचारिण्यासन (नमस्कार)
Devībrahmacāriṇyāsana (namaskāra)

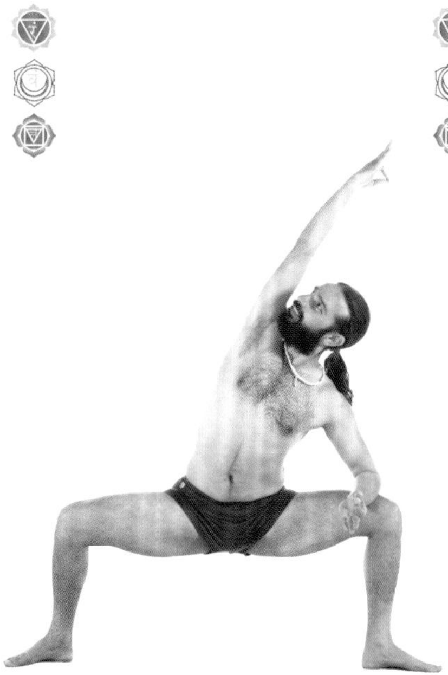

217
देवी चन्द्र घण्टा आसन
Devī candra ghaṇṭā āsana
Bell of the Moon Goddess pose

देवीचन्द्रघण्टासन
Devīcandraghaṇṭāsana

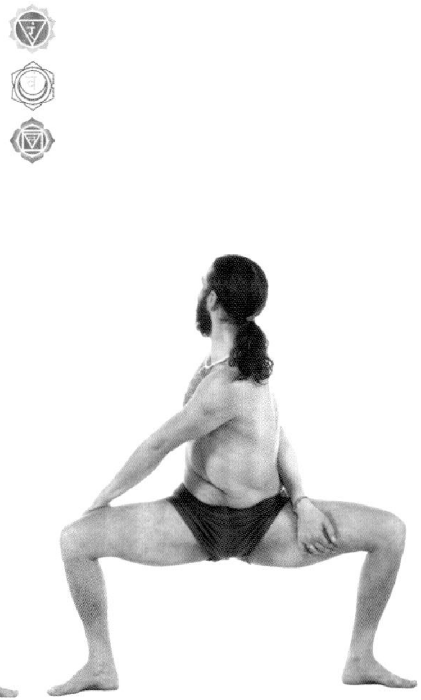

218
देवी कुण्डलिनी आसन
Devī kuṇḍalinī āsana
Goddess of Serpent power pose

देवीकुण्डलिन्यासन
Devīkuṇḍalinyāsana

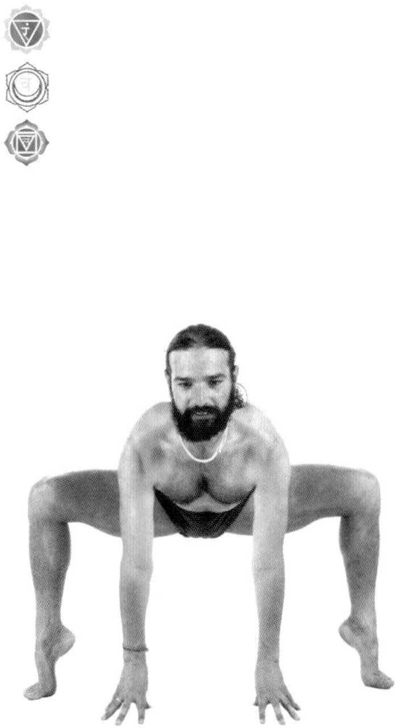

219
उत्तोलन भू देवी आसन
Utollana bhū devī āsana
Balancing Earth Goddess pose

उत्तोलनभूदेवीसन
Utollanabhūdevīāsana

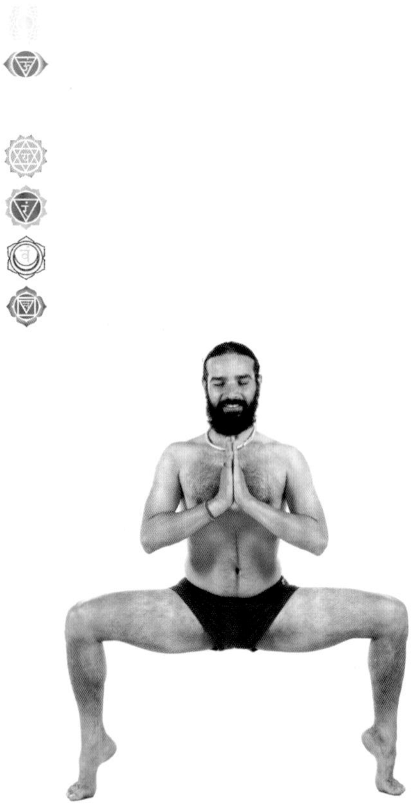

220
उत्तोलन भू देवी आसन (नमस्कार)
Utollana bhū devi āsana (namaskāra)
Balancing Earth Goddess pose (hands in prayer)

उत्तोलनभूदेवीासन (नमस्कार)
Utollanabhūdeviāsana (namaskāra)

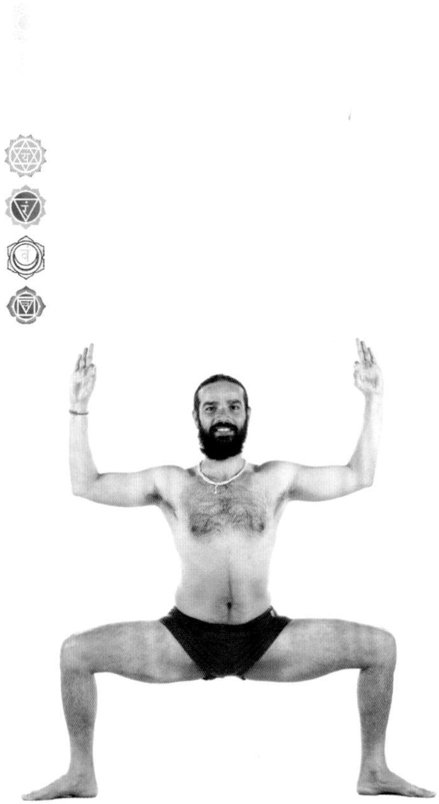

221
देवी भैरवी आसन
Devī bhairavī āsana
Fearless Goddess pose

देवीभैरवीासन
Devībhairavīāsana

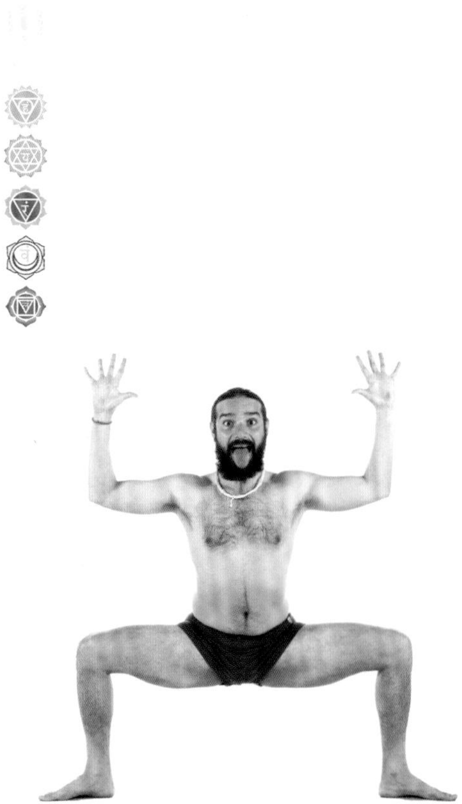

222
देवी काली आसन
Devī kālī āsana
Goddess of Time pose

देवीकालीासन
Devīkālīāsana

Every moment is full and complete.

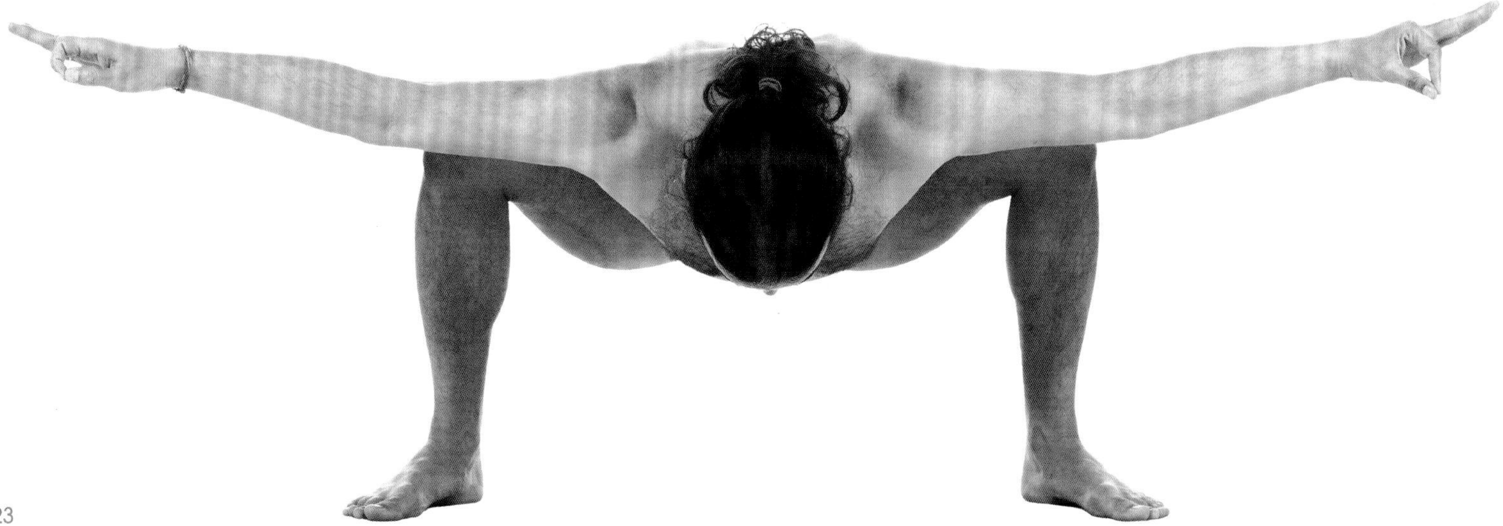

223
शक्ति कामाक्षी देवी आसन
Śakti kāmākṣī devī āsana
Goddess of Beauty and Divine Power pose

शक्तिकामाक्षीदेवीासन
Śaktikāmākṣīdevīāsana

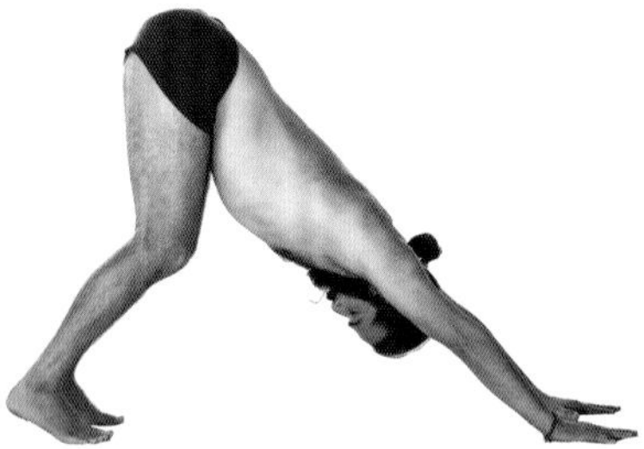

224
अर्ध पर्वत आसन
Ardha parvata āsana
Half mountain pose

अर्धपर्वतासन
Ardhaparvatāsana

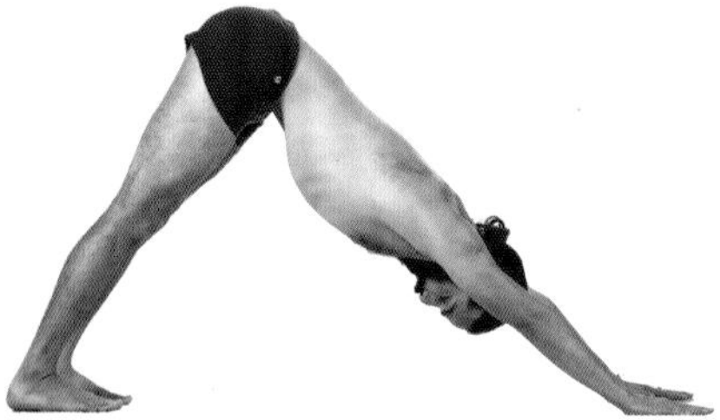

225
पर्वत आसन
Parvata āsana
Mountain pose

पर्वतासन
Parvatāsana

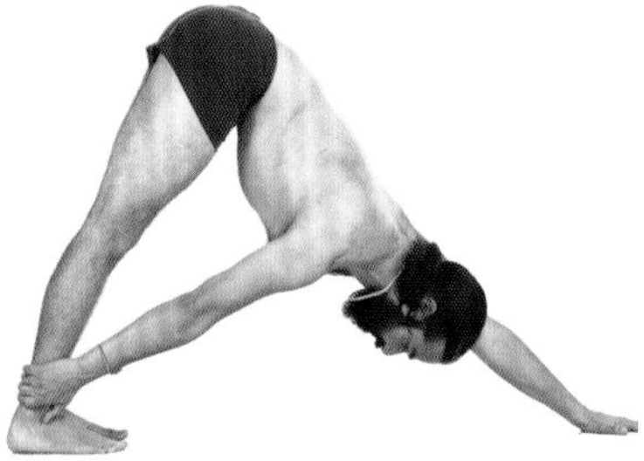

226
पर्वत आसन (एक हस्त पाद बद्ध)
Parvata āsana (eka hasta pāda baddha)
Mountain pose (holding one ankle)

पर्वतासन (एकहस्तपादबद्ध)
Parvatāsana (ekahastapādabaddha)

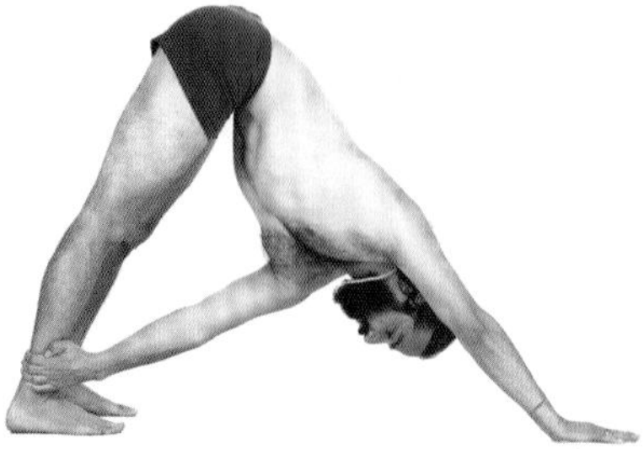

227
पर्वत आसन (विपरीत एक हस्त पाद बद्ध)
Parvata āsana (viparīta eka pāda hasta baddha)
Mountain pose (one hand holding opposite ankle)

पर्वतासन (विपरीतैकपादहस्तबद्ध)
Parvatāsana (viparītaikapādahastabaddha)

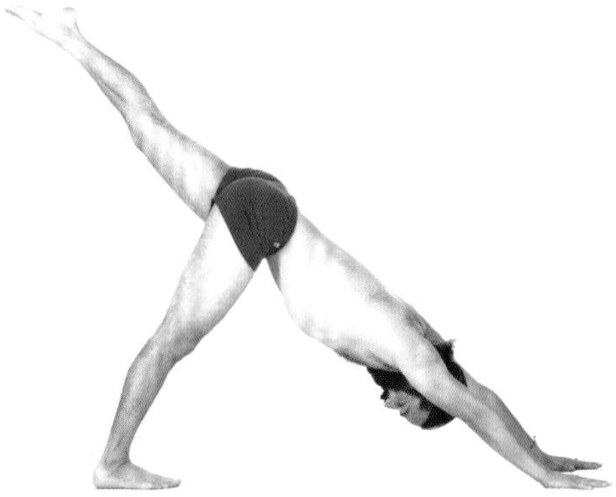

228
पर्वत आसन (ऊर्ध्व एक पाद)
Parvata āsana (ūrdhva eka pāda)
Mountain pose (one leg raised)

पर्वतासन (ऊर्ध्वैकपाद)
Parvatāsana (ūrdhvaikapāda)

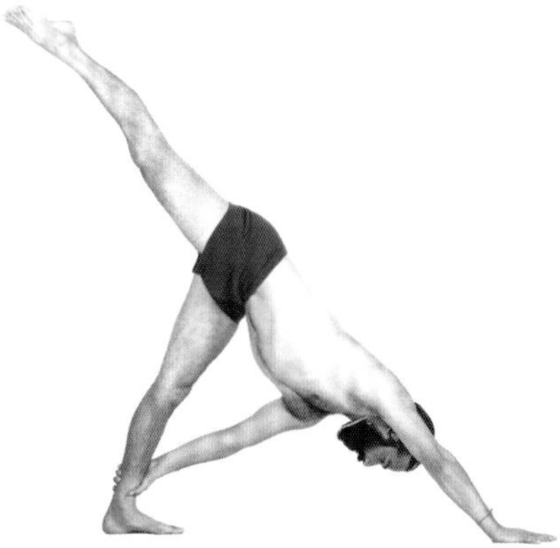

229
पर्वत आसन (एक हस्त पाद बद्ध, ऊर्ध्व एक पाद)
Parvata āsana (hasta pāda baddha, ūrdhva eka pāda)
Mountain pose (one leg raised, holding one ankle)

पर्वतासन (हस्तपादबद्ध, ऊर्ध्वैकपाद)
Parvatāsana (hastapādabaddha, ūrdhvaikapāda)

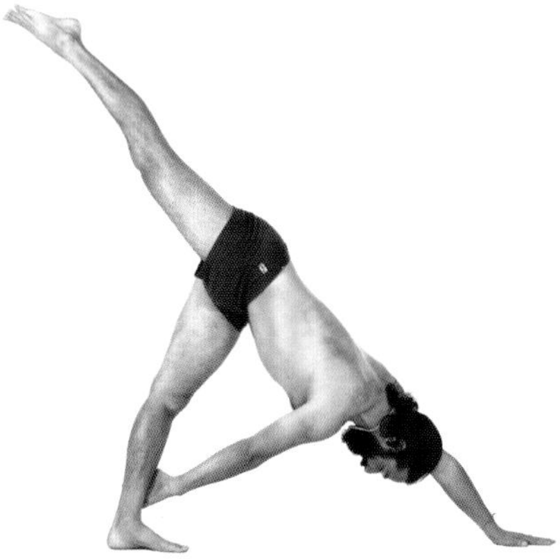

230
पर्वत आसन (विपरीत एक हस्त पाद बद्ध, ऊर्ध्व एक पाद)
Parvata āsana (viparīta eka hasta pāda baddha, ūrdhva eka pāda)
Mountain pose (holding opposite ankle, one leg raised)

पर्वतासन (विपरीतहस्तपादबद्ध, ऊर्ध्वैकपाद)
Parvatāsana (viparītaikahastapādabaddha, ūrdhvaikapāda)

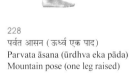

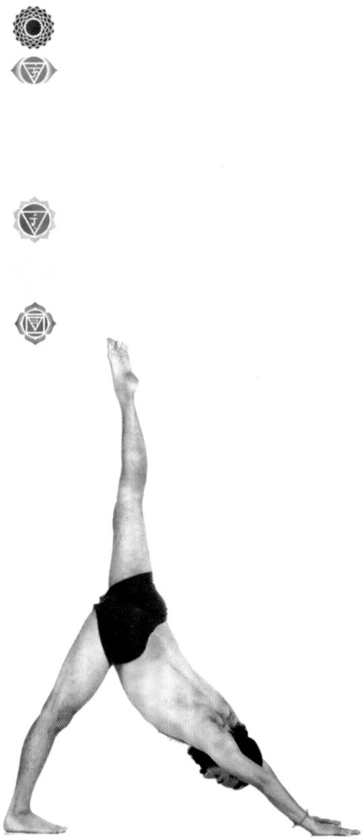

231
पर्वत आसन (ऊर्ध्व एक पाद, बहिर्वृत्त)
Parvata āsana (ūrdhva eka pāda, bahirvṛtta)
Mountain pose (one leg raised, turned out)

पर्वतासन (ऊर्ध्वैकपाद, बहिर्वृत्त)
Parvatāsana (ūrdhvaikapāda, bahirvṛtta)

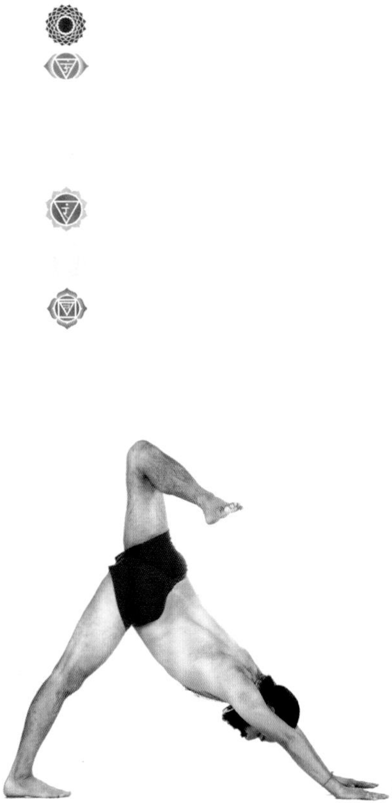

232
पर्वत आसन (एक पाद वृश्चिक)
Parvata āsana (eka pāda vṛścika)
Mountain pose (one leg in scorpion)

पर्वतासन (एकपादवृश्चिक)
Parvatāsana (ekapādavṛścika)

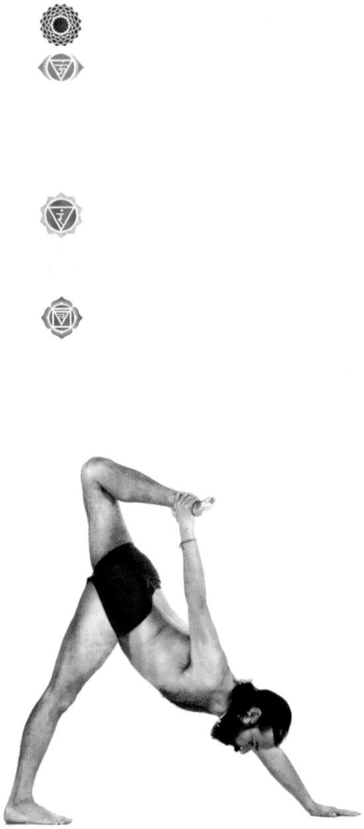

233
वृश्चिक पर्वत आसन (विकट)
Vṛścika parvata āsana (vikaṭa)
Scorpion mountain pose (challenging variation)

वृश्चिकपर्वतासन (विकट)
Vṛścikaparvatāsana (vikata)

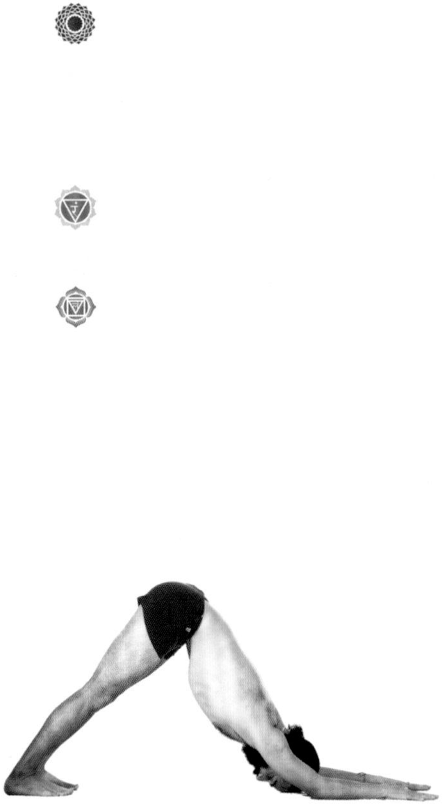

234
पर्वत आसन (कफोणि भू)
Parvata āsana (kaphoṇi bhū)
Mountain pose (elbows on the earth)

पर्वतासन (कफोणिभू)
Parvatāsana (kaphonibhū)

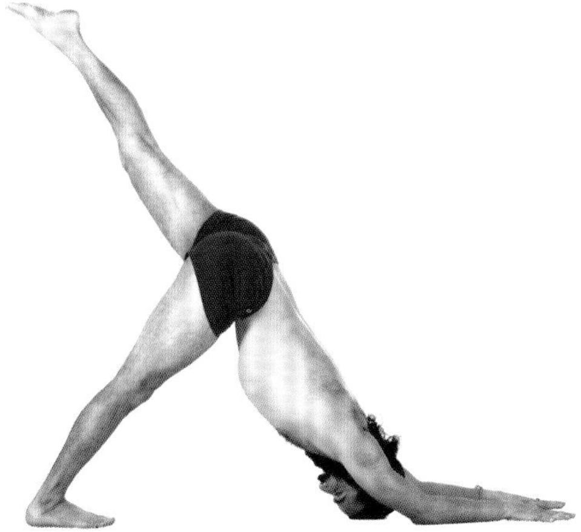

235
पर्वत आसन (कफोणि भू, ऊर्ध्व एक पाद)
Parvata āsana (kaphoṇi bhū, ūrdhva eka pāda)
Mountain pose (elbows on the earth, one leg raised)

पर्वतासन (कफोणिभू, ऊर्ध्वैकपाद)
Parvatāsana (kaphoṇibhū, ūrdhvaikapāda)

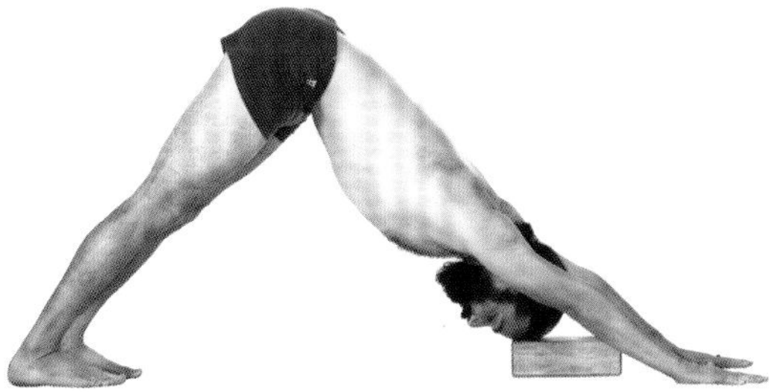

236
अधोमुख श्वान आसन (सालम्ब)
Adhomukha śvāna āsana (sālamba)
Downward facing dog (supported)

अधोमुखश्वानासन (सालम्ब)
Adhomukhaśvānāsana (sālamba)

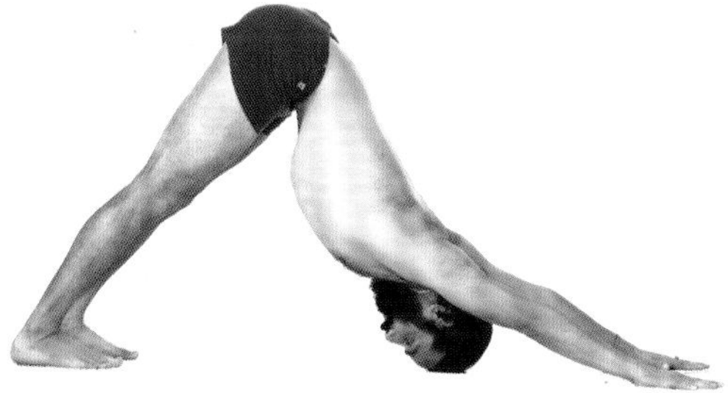

237
अधोमुख श्वान आसन
Adhomukha śvāna āsana
Downward facing dog

अधोमुखश्वानासन
Adhomukhaśvānāsana

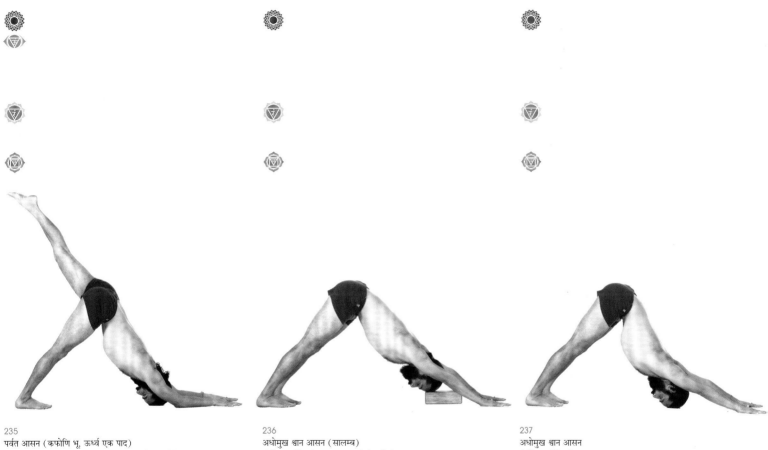

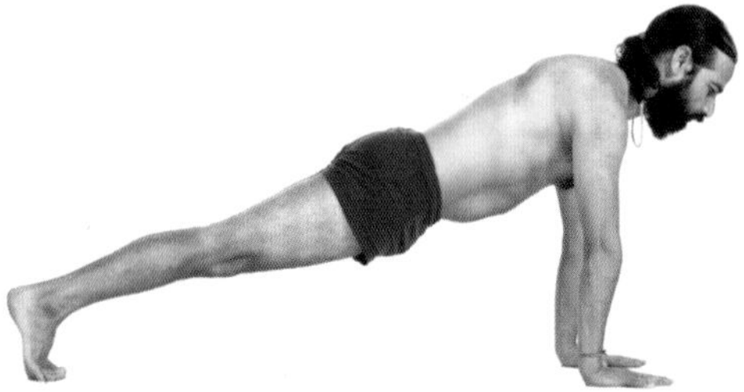

238
चतुः अङ्ग दण्ड आसन
Catuḥ aṅga daṇḍa āsana
Four limb staff pose

चतुरङ्गदण्डासन
Caturaṅgadaṇḍāsana

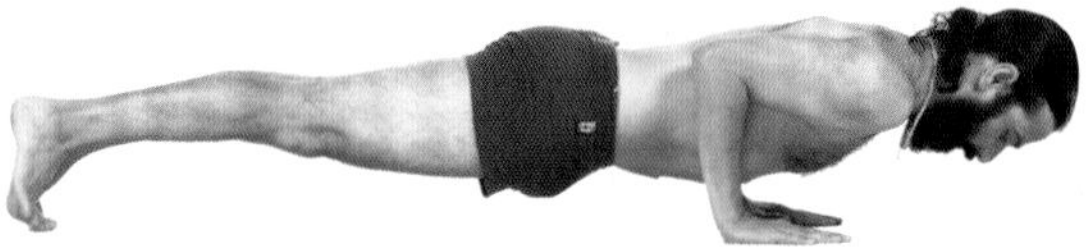

239
चतुः अङ्ग भू दण्ड आसन
Catuḥ aṅga bhū daṇḍa āsana
Four limb earth staff pose

चतुरङ्गभूदण्डासन
Caturaṅgabhūdaṇḍāsana

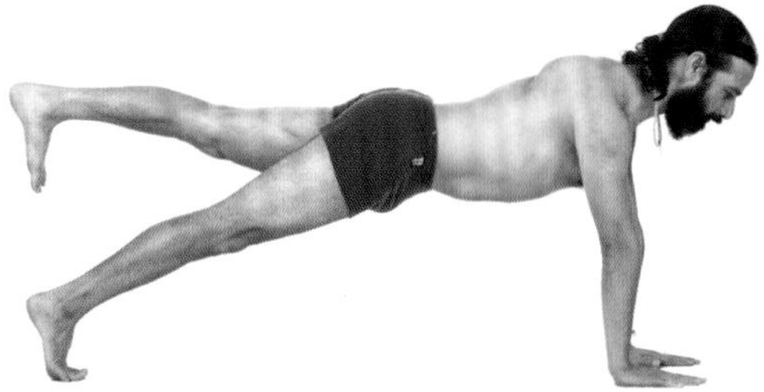

240
त्रि अङ्ग दण्ड आसन
Tri aṅga daṇḍa āsana
Three limb staff pose

त्रयङ्गदण्डासन
Trayaṅgadaṇḍāsana

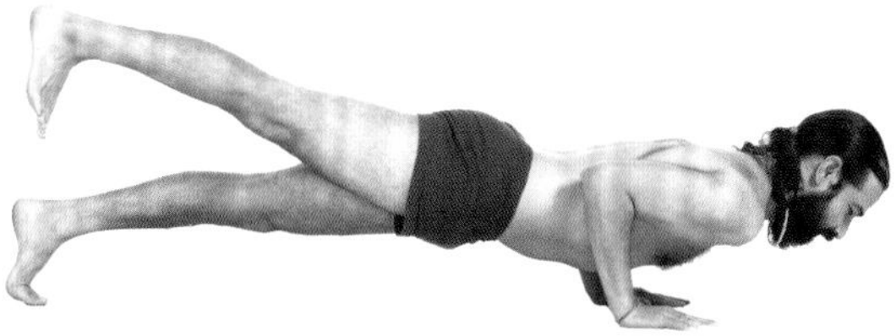

241
त्रि अङ्ग भू दण्ड आसन
Tri aṅga bhū daṇḍa āsana
Three limb earth staff pose

त्रयङ्गभूदण्डासन
Trayaṅgabhūdaṇḍāsana

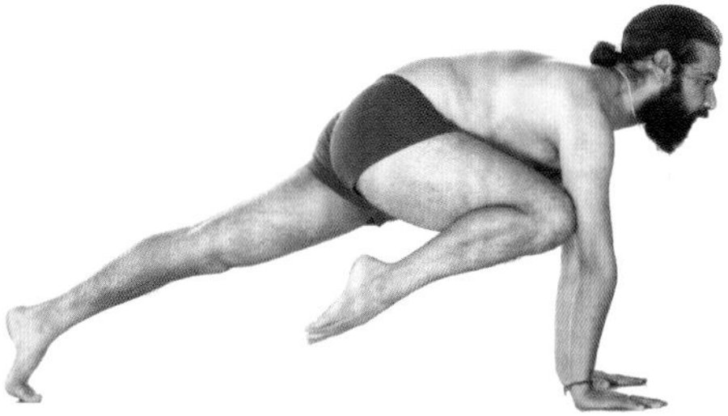

242
चतुः अङ्ग दण्ड आसन (जानु कफोणि)
Catuḥ aṅga daṇḍa āsana (jānu kaphoṇi)
Four limb staff pose (knee to elbow)

चतुरङ्गदण्डासन (जानुकफोणि)
Caturaṅgadaṇḍāsana (jānukaphoṇi)

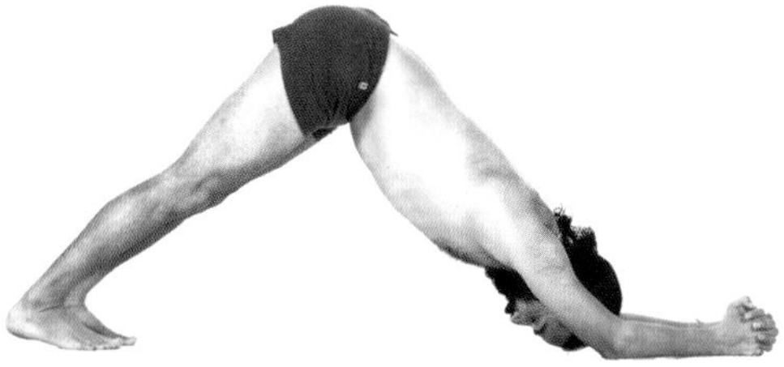

243
पर्वत आसन (कफोणि भू, बद्ध अङ्गुल)
Parvata āsana (kaphoṇi bhū, baddha aṅgula)
Mountain pose (elbows on the earth, clasped fingers)

पर्वतासन (कफोणिभू, बद्धाङ्गुल)
Parvatāsana (kaphoṇibhū, baddhaṅgula)

Every obstacle in life is an opportunity for growth.

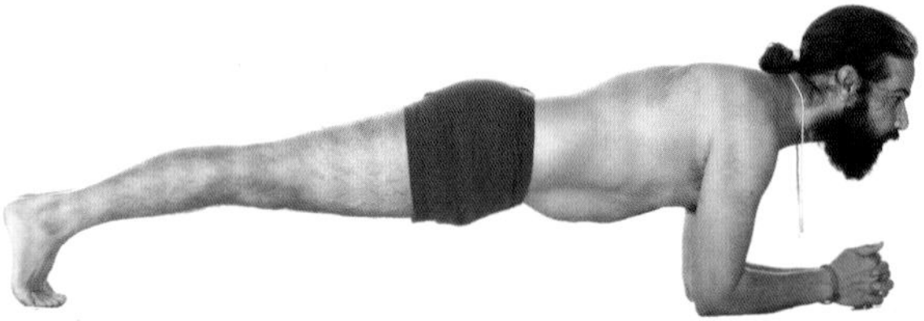

244
चतु: अङ्ग दण्ड आसन (कफोणि भू बद्ध अङ्गुल)
Catuḥ aṅga daṇḍa āsana (kaphoṇi bhū baddha aṅgula)
Four limb staff pose (elbows on the earth, bound fingers)

चतुरङ्गदण्डासन (कफोणिभूबद्धाङ्गुल)
Caturaṅgadaṇḍāsana (kaphoṇibhūbaddhāṅgula)

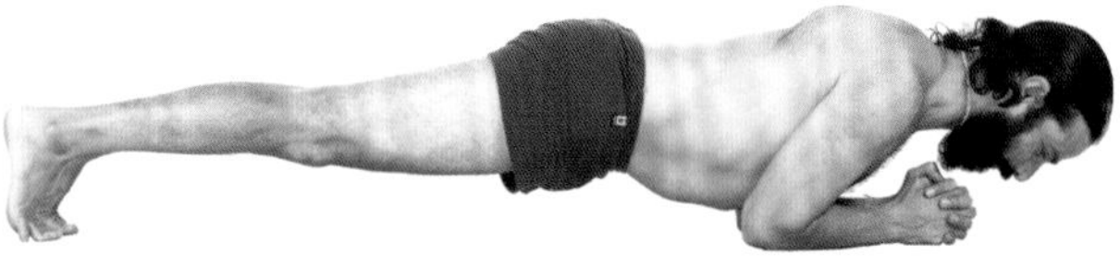

245
चतु: अङ्ग भू दण्ड आसन (कफोणि भू बद्ध अङ्गुल)
Catuḥ aṅga bhū daṇḍa āsana (kaphoṇi bhū baddha aṅgula)
Four limb earth staff pose (elbows on the earth, bound fingers)

चतुरङ्गभूदण्डासन (कफोणिभूबद्धाङ्गुल)
Caturaṅgabhūdaṇḍāsana (kaphoṇibhūbaddhāṅgula)

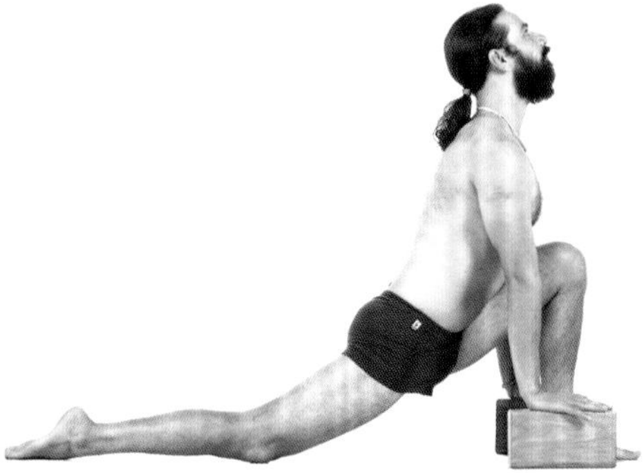

246
चेतक आसन (सालम्ब)
Cetaka āsana (sālamba)
Horse pose (supported)

चेतकासन (शालम्ब)
Cetakāsana (sālamba)

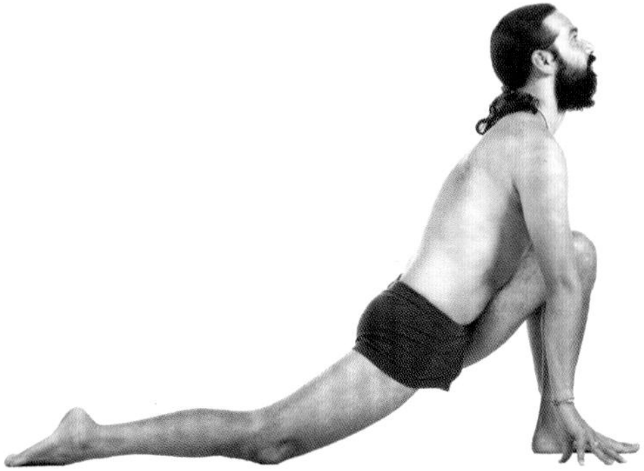

247
चेतक आसन (हस्त अङ्गुल भू)
Cetaka āsana (hasta aṅgula bhū)
Horse pose (fingers on the earth)

चेतकासन (हस्ताङ्गुलभू)
Cetakāsana (hastāṅgulabhū)

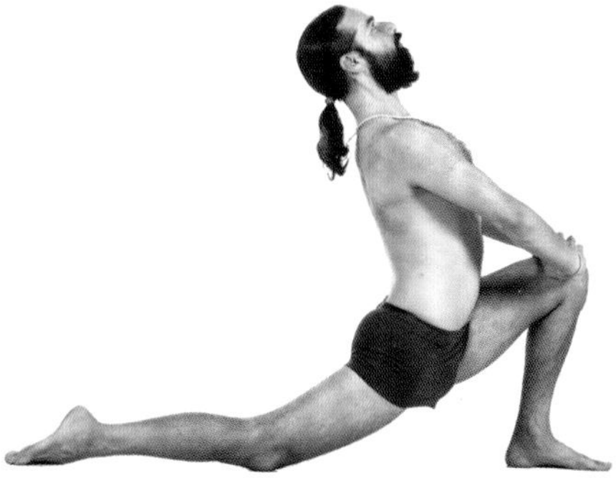

248
चेतक आसन (जानु हस्त)
Cetaka āsana (jānu hasta)
Horse pose (hands on knee)

चेतकासन (जानुहस्त)
Cetakāsana (jānuhasta)

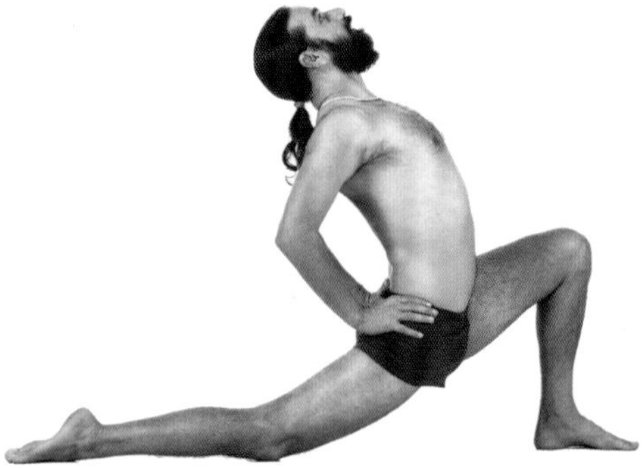

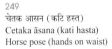

249
चेतक आसन (कटि हस्त)
Cetaka āsana (kati hasta)
Horse pose (hands on waist)

चेतकासन (कटिहस्त)
Cetakāsana (katihasta)

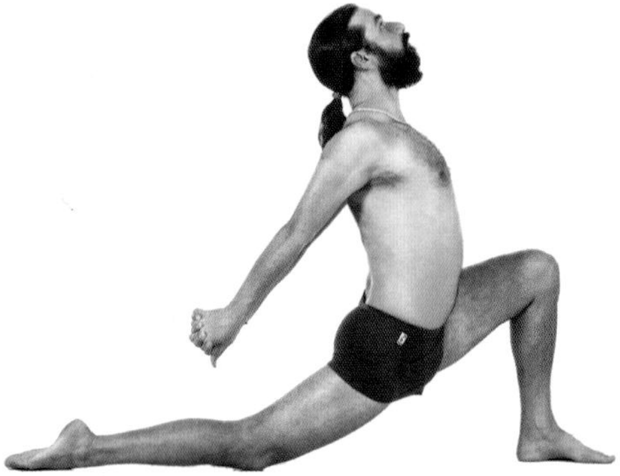

250
चेतक आसन (पृष्ठ हस्त उत्तान)
Cetaka āsana (pṛṣṭha hasta uttāna)
Horse pose (hands stretched behind)

चेतकासन (पृष्ठहस्तोत्तान)
Cetakāsana (pṛṣṭhahastottāna)

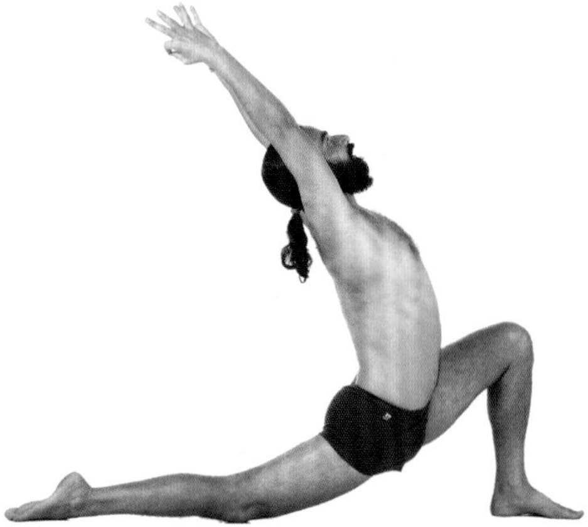

251
चेतक आसन
Cetaka āsana
Horse pose

चेतकासन
Cetakāsana

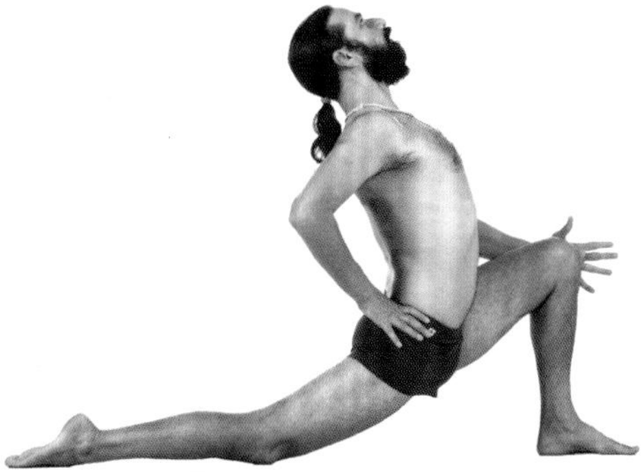

252
चेतक आसन (जानु कटि हस्त)
Cetaka āsana (jānu kati hasta)
Horse pose (hands on knee and waist)

चेतकासन (जानुकटिहस्त)
Cetakāsana (jānukatihasta)

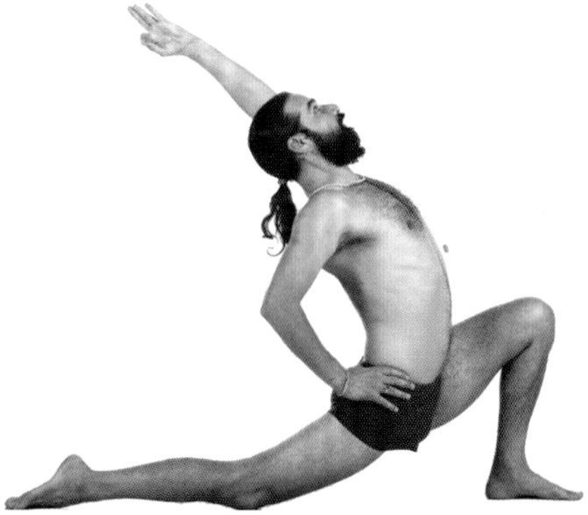

253
चेतक आसन (एक हस्त ऊर्ध्व कटि)
Cetaka āsana (eka hasta ūrdhva kati)
Horse pose (one hand on waist, one hand overhead)

चेतकासन (एकहस्तोर्ध्वकटि)
Cetakāsana (ekahastordhvakati)

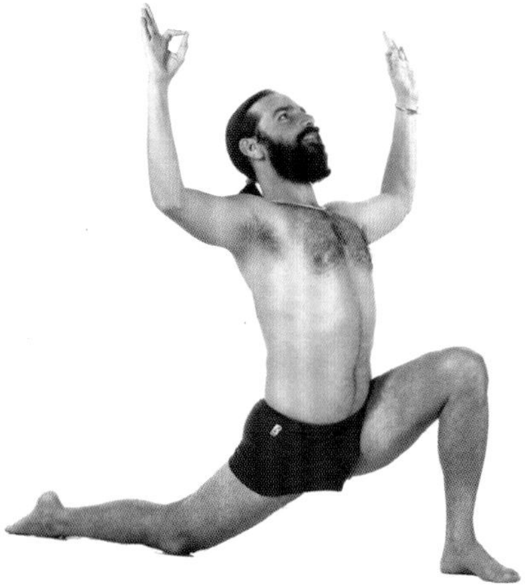

254
चेतक आसन (देवी हस्त)
Cetaka āsana (devī hasta)
Horse pose (goddess arms)

चेतकासन (देवीहस्त)
Cetakāsana (devīhasta)

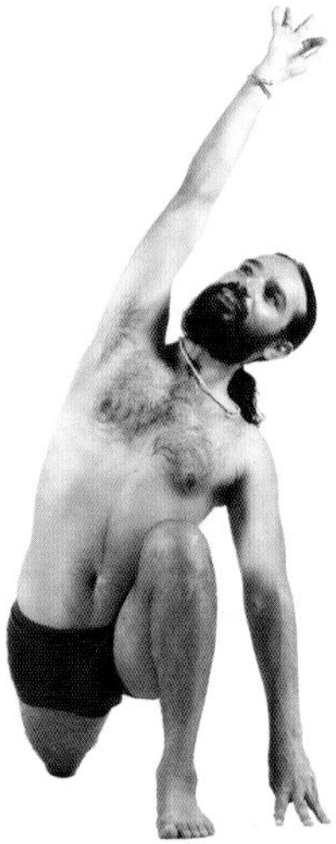

255
पार्श्व चेतक आसन (एक हस्त अङ्गुल भू)
Pārśva cetaka āsana (eka hasta aṅgula bhū)
Side horse pose (one hand on the earth)

पार्श्वचेतकासन (एकहस्ताङ्गुलभू)
Pārśvacetakāsana (ekahastaṅgulabhū)

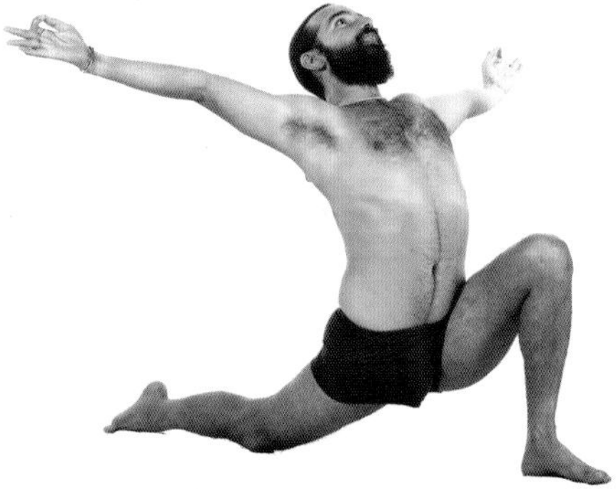

256
चेतक आसन (विराट हस्त)
Cetaka āsana (virāṭa hasta)
Horse pose (arms extended wide)

चेतकासन (विराटहस्त)
Cetakāsana (virāṭahasta)

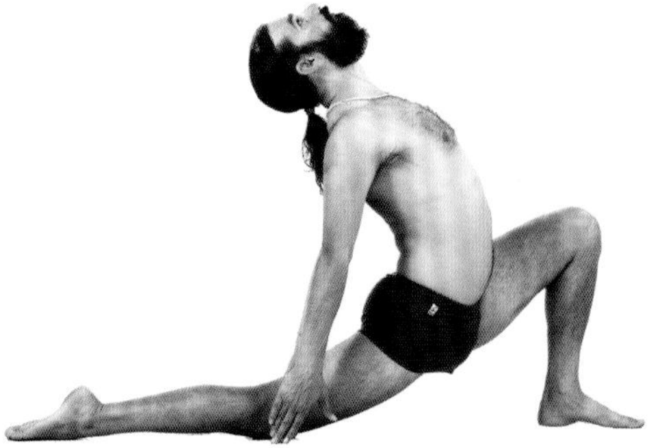

257
चेतक आसन (पृष्ठ अङ्गुल भू)
Cetaka āsana (pṛṣṭha aṅgula bhū)
Horse pose (fingers on the earth behind)

चेतकासन (पृष्ठाङ्गुलभू)
Cetakāsana (pṛṣṭhaṅgulabhū)

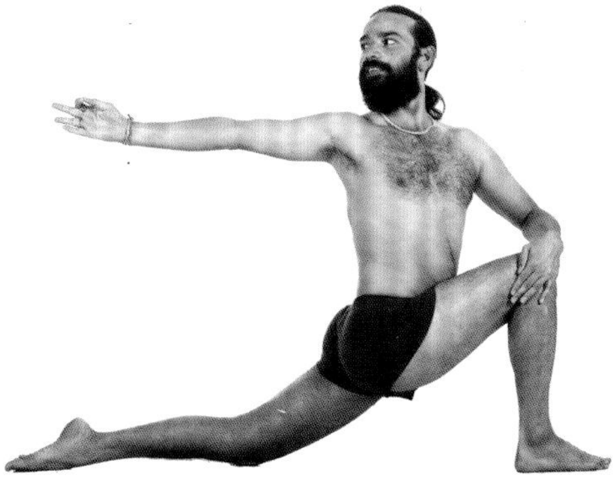

258
परिवृत्त चेतक आसन (विपरीत हस्त जानु)
Parivṛtta cetaka āsana (viparīta hasta jānu)
Twisted horse pose (opposite hand on knee)

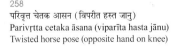

परिवृत्तचेतकासन (विपरीतहस्तजानु)
Parivṛttacetakāsana (viparītahastajānu)

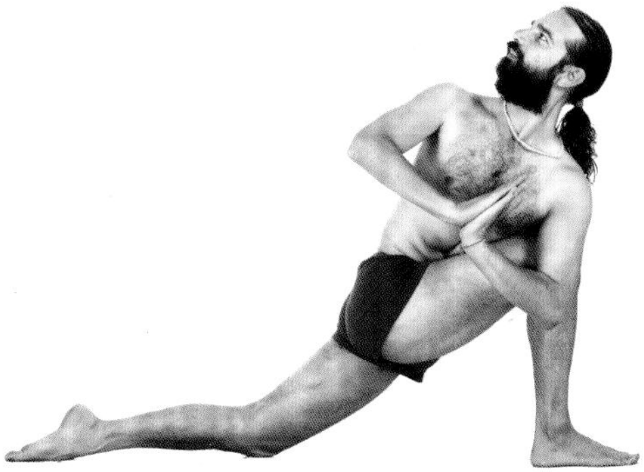

259
परिवृत्त चेतक आसन (नमस्कार हस्त)
Parivṛtta cetaka āsana (namaskāra hasta)
Twisted horse pose (hands in prayer)

परिवृत्तचेतकासन (नमस्कारहस्त)
Parivṛttacetakāsana (namaskārahasta)

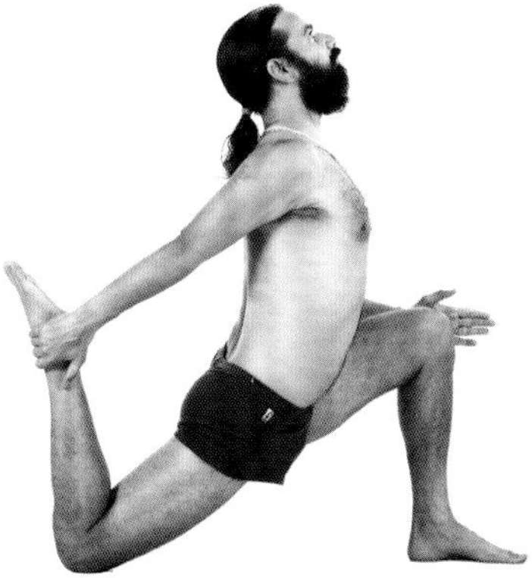

260
धनुः चेतक आसन (एक हस्त जानु)
Dhanuḥ cetaka āsana (eka hasta jānu)
Bow horse pose (one hand on knee)

धनुश्चेतकासन (एकहस्तजानु)
Dhanuścetakāsana (ekahastajānu)

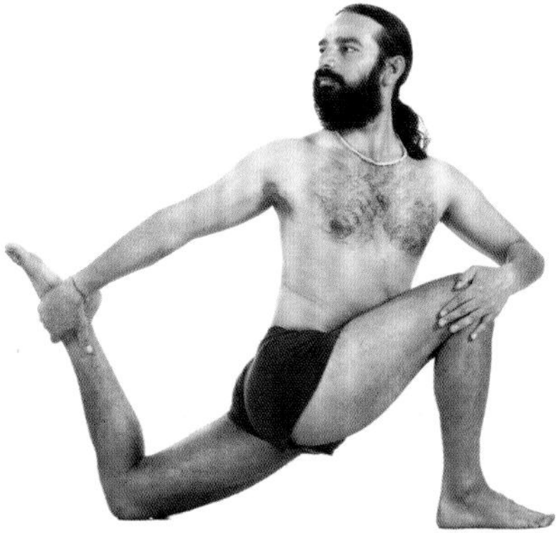

261
परिवृत्त धनुःचेतक आसन (विपरीत हस्त जानु)
Parivṛtta dhanuḥ cetaka āsana (viparīta hasta jānu)
Twisted bow horse pose (hand on opposite knee)

परिवृत्तधनुश्चेतकासन (विपरीतहस्तजानु)
Parivṛttadhanuścetakāsana (viparītahastajānu)

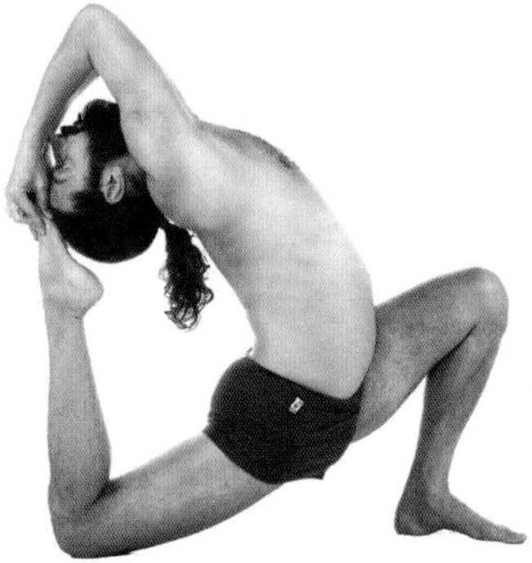

262
चेतक कपोत आसन (पाद ललाट)
Cetaka kapota āsana (pāda lalāṭa)
Pigeon horse pose (foot to forehead)

चेतककपोतासन (पादललाट)
Cetakakapotāsana (pādalalāṭa)

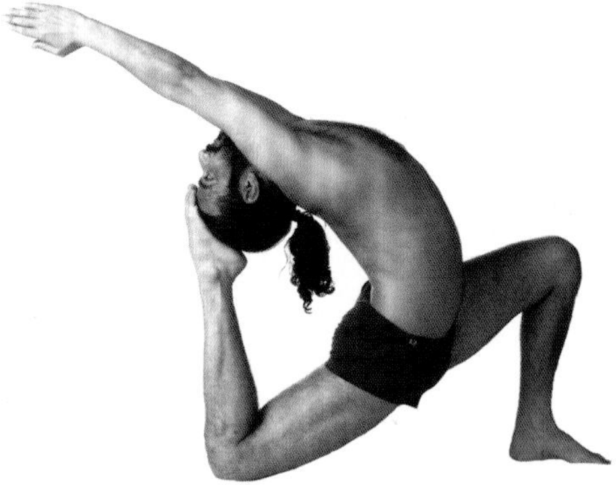

263
चेतक कपोत आसन (पादललाट,हस्त उत्तान)
Cetaka kapota āsana (pāda lalāṭa, hasta uttāna)
Pigeon horse pose (foot to forehead, extended arms)

चेतककपोतासन (पादललाट,हस्तोत्तान)
Cetakakapotāsana (pādalalāṭa, hastottāna)

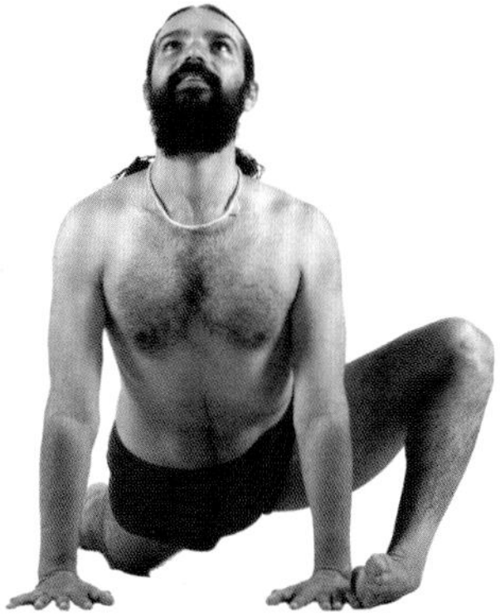

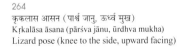

264
कृकलास आसन (पार्श्व जानु, ऊर्ध्व मुख)
Kṛkalāsa āsana (pārśva jānu, ūrdhva mukha)
Lizard pose (knee to the side, upward facing)

कृकलासासन (पार्श्वजानु, ऊर्ध्वमुख)
Kṛkalāsāsana (pārśvajānu, ūrdhvamukha)

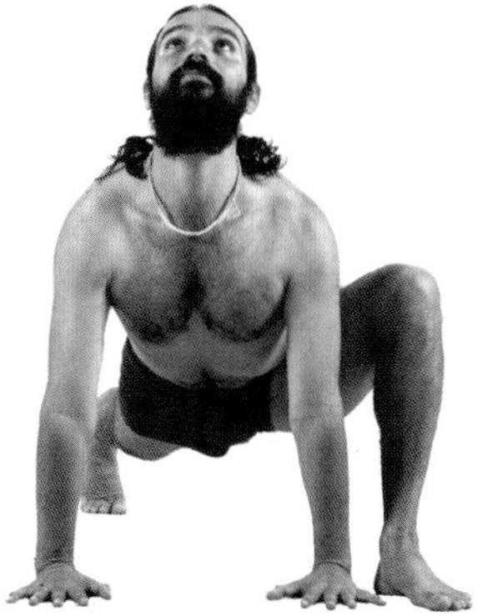

265
कृकलास आसन (ऊर्ध्व मुख)
Kṛkalāsa āsana (ūrdhva mukha)
Lizard pose (upward facing)

कृकलासासन (ऊर्ध्वमुख)
Kṛkalāsāsana (ūrdhvamukha)

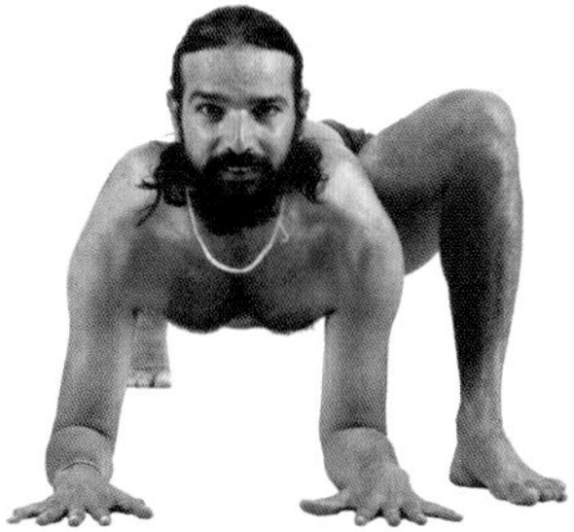

266
कृकलास आसन (कफोणि भू)
Kṛkalāsa āsana (kaphoṇi bhū)
Lizard pose (elbows on the earth)

कृकलासासन (कफोणिभू)
Kṛkalāsāsana (kaphoṇibhū)

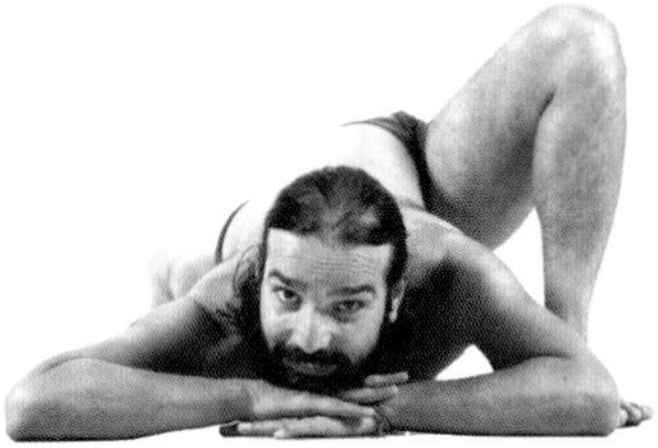

267
पूर्ण कृकलास आसन
Pūrṇa kṛkalāsa āsana
Full lizard pose

पूर्णकृकलासासन
Pūrṇakṛkalāsāsana

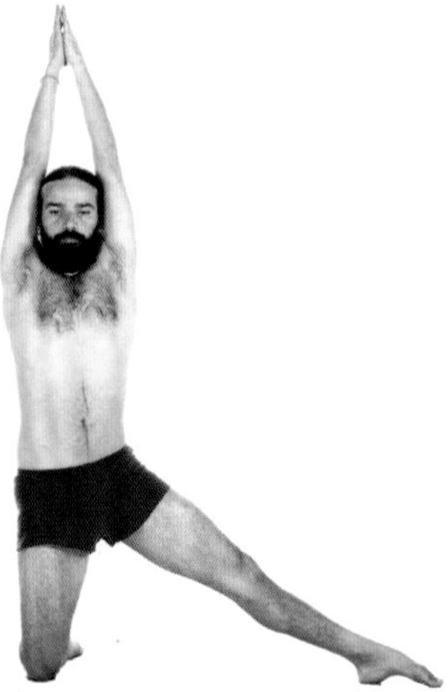

268
नमस्कार परिघ आसन
Namaskāra parigha āsana
Prayer gate pose

नमस्कारपरिघासन
Namaskāraparighāsana

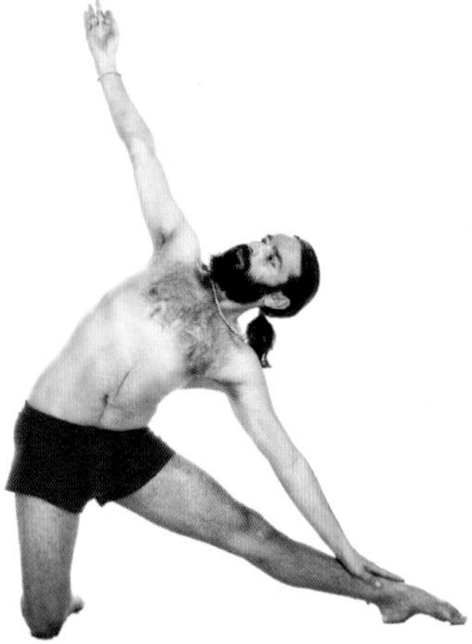

269
चन्द्र परिघ आसन (विराट हस्त)
Candra parigha āsana (virāṭa hasta)
Moon gate pose (hands extended wide)

चन्द्रपरिघासन (विराटहस्त)
Candraparighāsana (virāṭahasta)

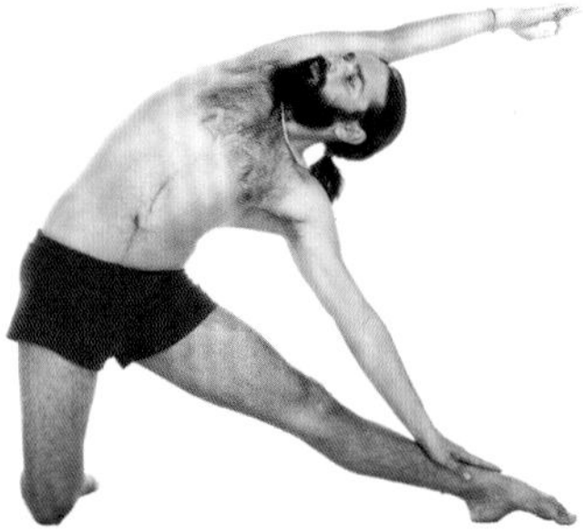

270
कोण परिघ आसन
Koṇa parigha āsana
Angled gate pose

कोणपरिघासन
Koṇaparighāsana

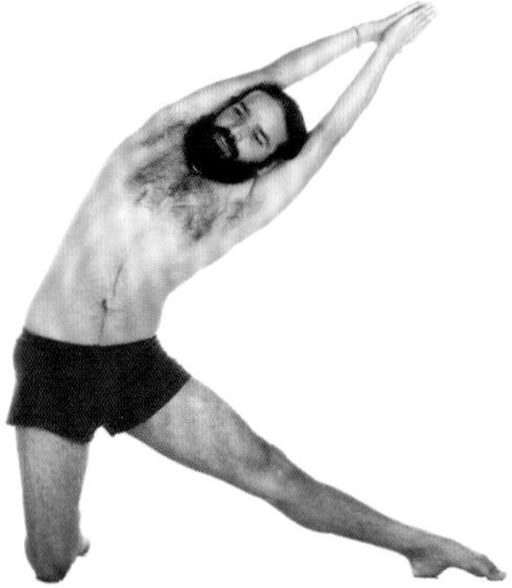

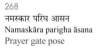

271
नमस्कार चन्द्र परिघ आसन
Namaskāra candra parigha āsana
Prayer moon gate pose

नमस्कारचन्द्रपरिघासन
Namaskāracandraparighāsana

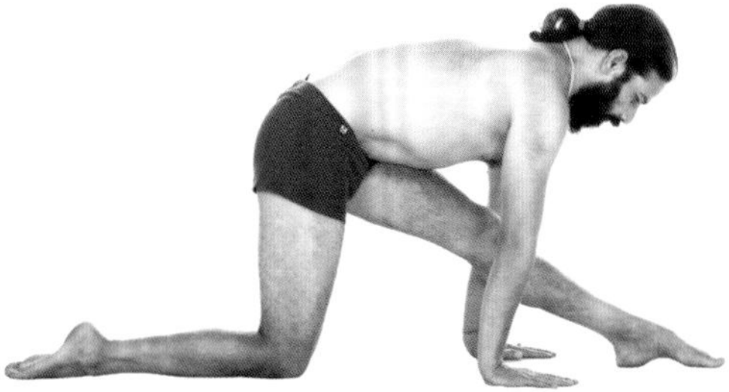

272
परिघ आसन (हस्त भू समक्ष)
Parigha āsana (hasta bhū samakṣa)
Gate pose (hands on the earth in front)

परिघासन (हस्तभूसमक्ष)
Parighāsana (hastabhūsamakṣa)

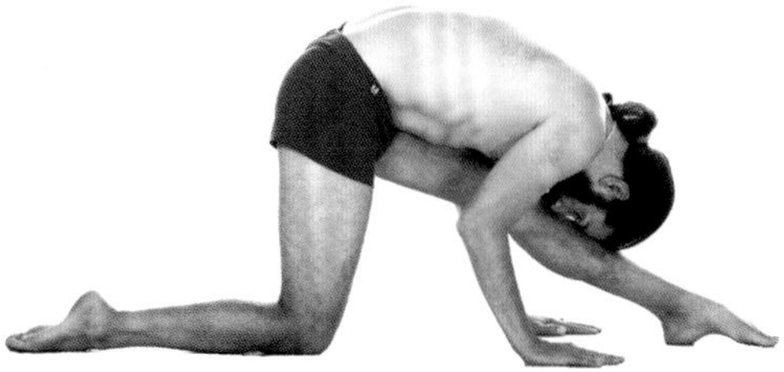

273
जानु शिर परिघ आसन (हस्त भू समक्ष)
Jānu śira parigha āsana (hasta bhū samakṣa)
Head to knee gate pose (hands on the earth in front)

जानुशिरपरिघासन (हस्तभूसमक्ष)
Jānuśiraparighāsana (hastabhūsamakṣa)

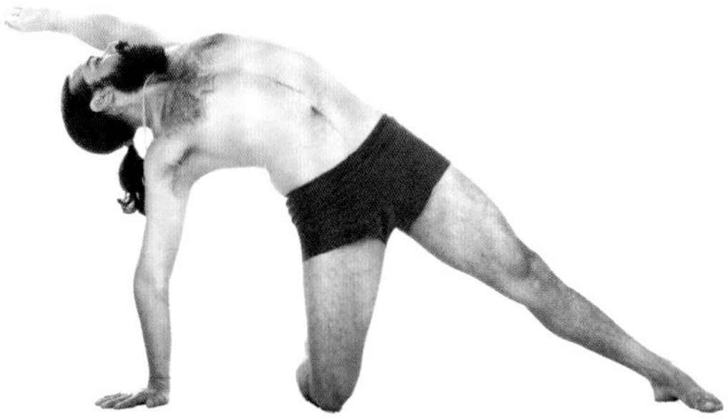

274
अप्सरा परिघ आसन (एक हस्त भू)
Apsarā parigha āsana (eka hasta bhū)
Angel gate pose (one hand on the earth)

अप्सरापरिघासन (एकहस्तभू)
Apsarāparighāsana (ekahastabhū)

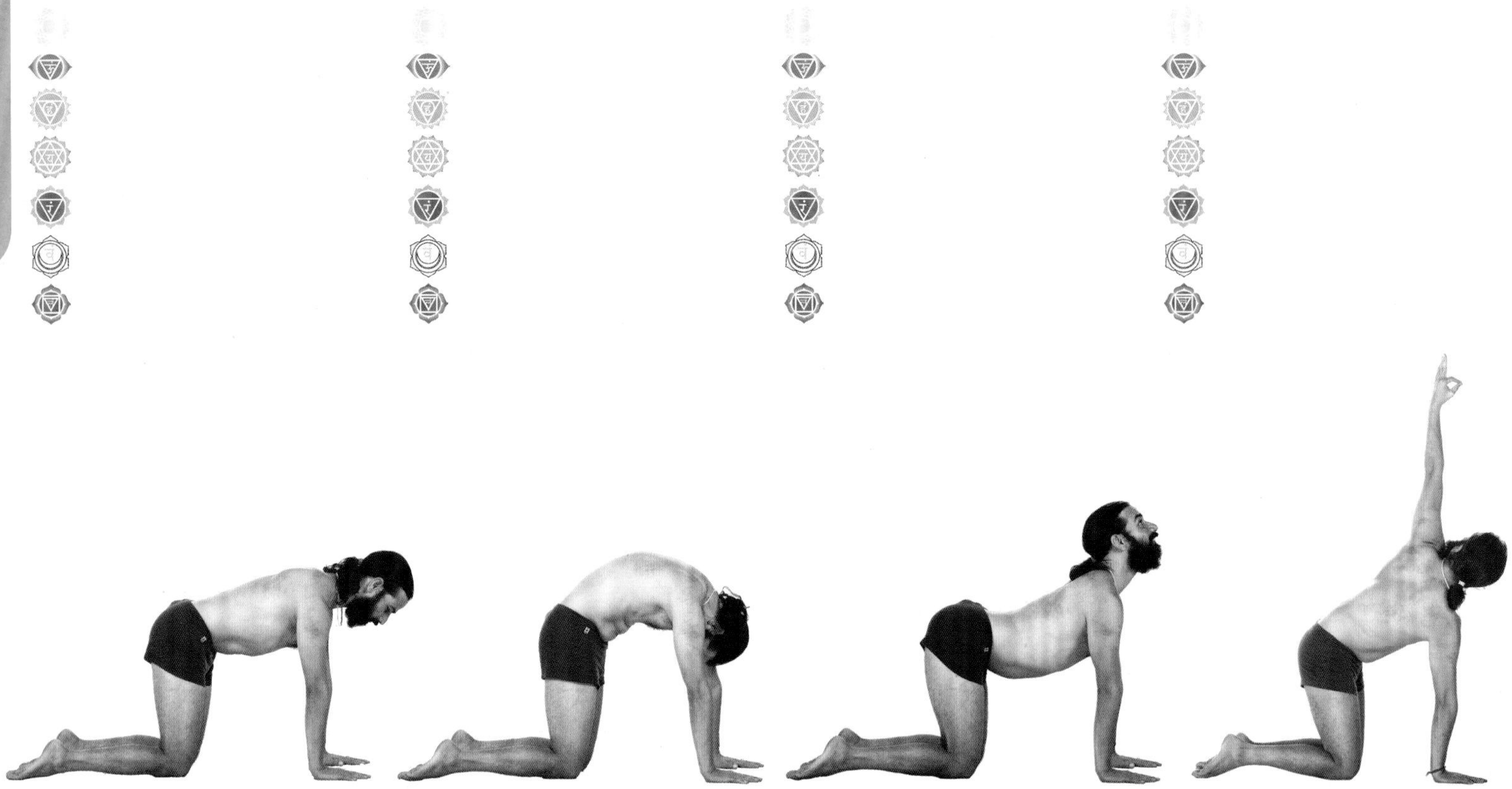

275
फलकम् आसन (मार्जारी आरम्भ अवस्था)
Phalakaṃ āsana (mārjārī ārambha avasthā)
Table pose (cat starting position)

फलकमासन (मार्जार्यारम्भावस्था)
Phalakamāsana (mārjāryārambhavasthā)

276
अधो मुख मार्जारी आसन
Adho mukha mārjārī āsana
Downward facing cat pose

अधोमुखमार्जार्यासन
Adhomukhamārjāryāsana

277
ऊर्ध्व मुख मार्जारी आसन
Ūrdhva mukha mārjārī āsana
Upward facing cat pose

ऊर्ध्वमुखमार्जार्यासन
Ūrdhvamukhamārjāryāsana

278
परिवृत्त मार्जारी आसन (विराट हस्त)
Parivṛtta mārjāri āsana (virāṭa hasta)
Twisted cat pose (arms extended wide)

परिवृत्तमार्जारासन (विराटहस्त)
Parivṛttamārjārāsana (virāṭahasta)

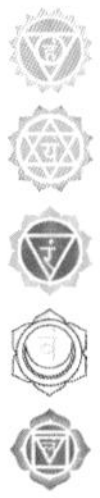

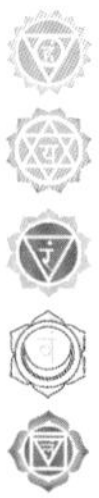

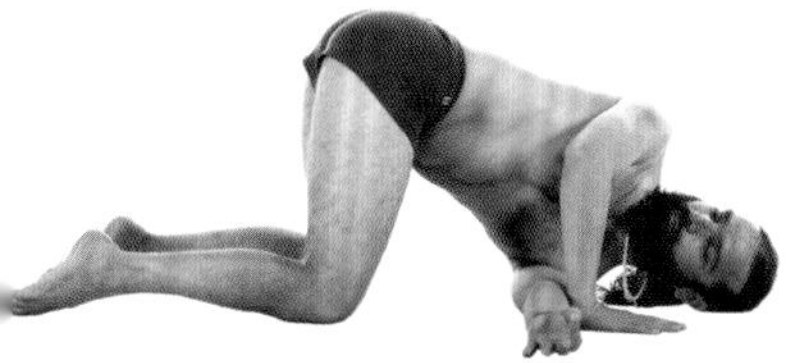

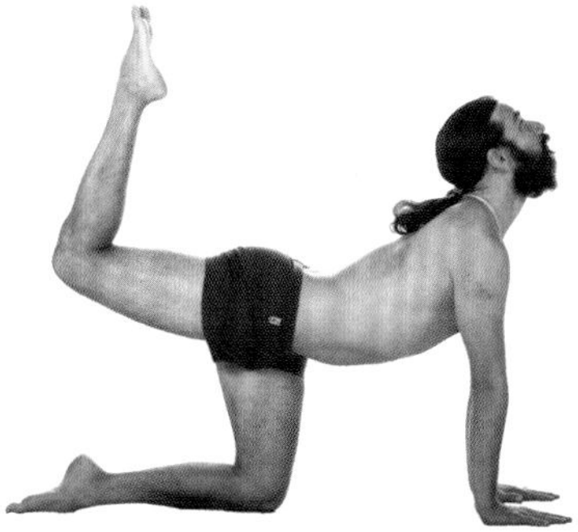

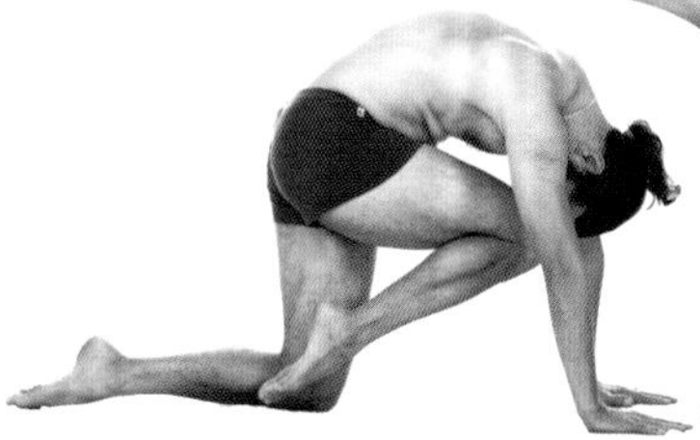

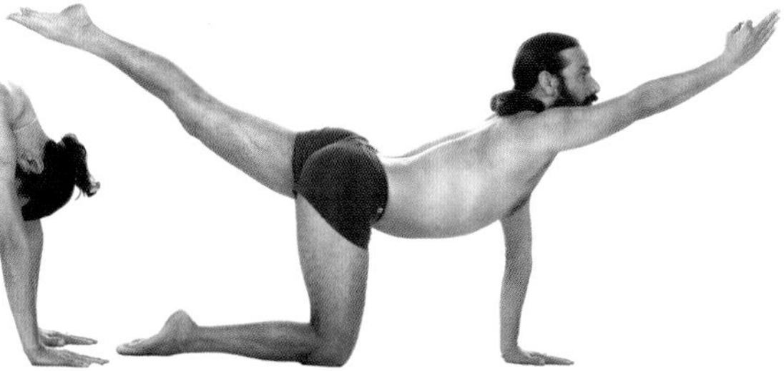

279
परिवृत्त मार्जार आसन (स्कन्ध भू)
Parivṛtta mārjāra āsana (skandha bhū)
Twisted cat pose (shoulder on the earth)

परिवृत्तमार्जारासन(स्कन्धभू)
Parivṛttamārjārāsana (skandhabhū)

280
शार्दूल आसन (ऊर्ध्व मुख)
Śārdūla āsana (ūrdhva mukha)
Tiger pose (upward facing)

शार्दूलासन (ऊर्ध्वमुख)
Śārdūlāsana (ūrdhvamukha)

281
शार्दूल आसन (जानुललाट)
Śārdūla āsana (jānu lalāṭa)
Tiger pose (knee to forehead)

शार्दूलासन (जानुललाट)
Śārdūlāsana (jānulalāṭa)

282
उत्तोलन शार्दूल आसन
Uttolana śārdūla āsana
Balancing tiger pose

उत्तोलनशार्दूलासन
Uttolanaśārdūlāsana

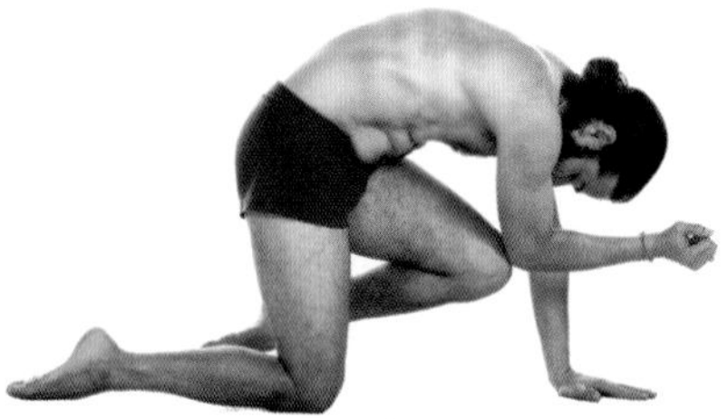

283
उत्तोलन शार्दूल आसन (विपरीत जानु कफोणि)
Uttolana śārdūla āsana (viparīta jānu kaphoṇi)
Balancing tiger pose (opposite knee to elbow)

उत्तोलनशार्दूलासन (विपरीतजानुकफोणि)
Uttolanaśārdūlāsana (viparītajānukaphoṇi)

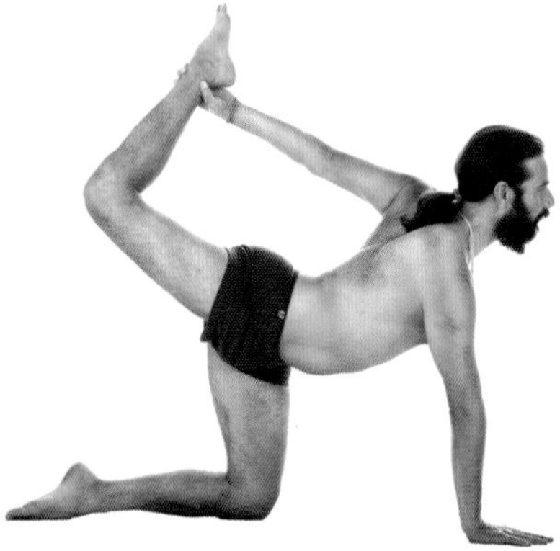

284
धनुः शार्दूल आसन (विपरीत एक हस्त)
Dhanuḥ śārdūla āsana (viparīta eka hasta)
Bowed tiger pose (opposite hand to leg)

धनुर्शार्दूलासन (विपरीतैकहस्त)
Dhanurśārdūlāsana (viparītaikahasta)

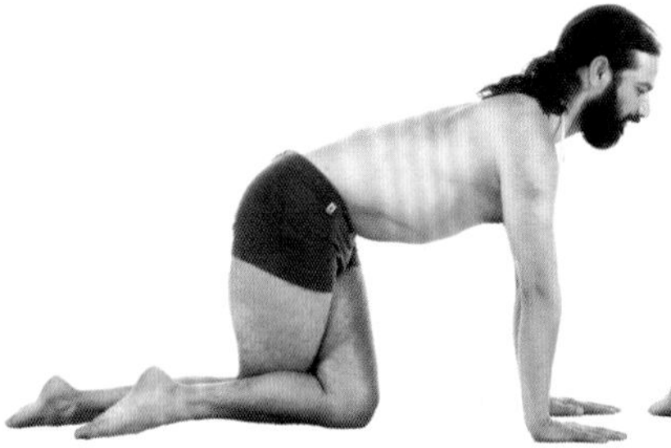

285
गरुड पाद फलकम् आसन
Garuḍa pāda phalakaṃ āsana
Eagle leg table pose

गरुडपादफलकमासन
Garuḍapādaphalakamāsana

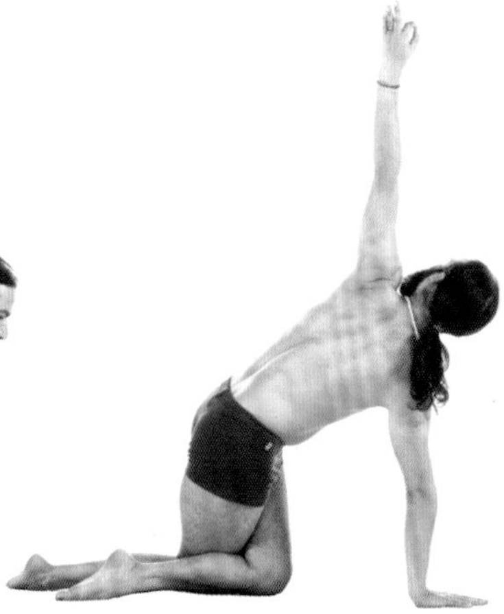

286
परिवृत्त गरुड पाद फलकम् आसन (विराट हस्त)
Parivṛtta garuḍa pāda phalakaṃ āsana (virāṭa hasta)
Twisted eagle leg table pose (arms extended wide)

परिवृत्तगरुडपादफलकमासन (विराटहस्त)
Parivṛttagaruḍapādaphalakamāsana (virāṭahasta)

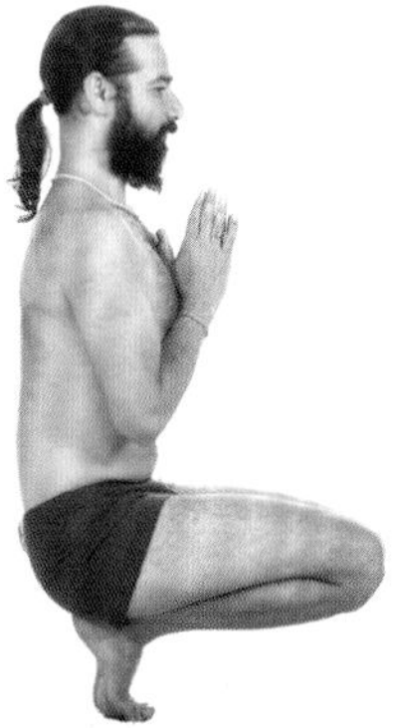

287
उत्तोलन पाद अङ्गुष्ठ आसन (नमस्कार)
Uttolana pāda aṅguṣṭha āsana (namaskāra)
Balancing toes pose (hands in prayer)

उत्तोलनपादाङ्गुष्ठासन (नमस्कार)
Uttolanapādāṅguṣṭhāsana (namaskāra)

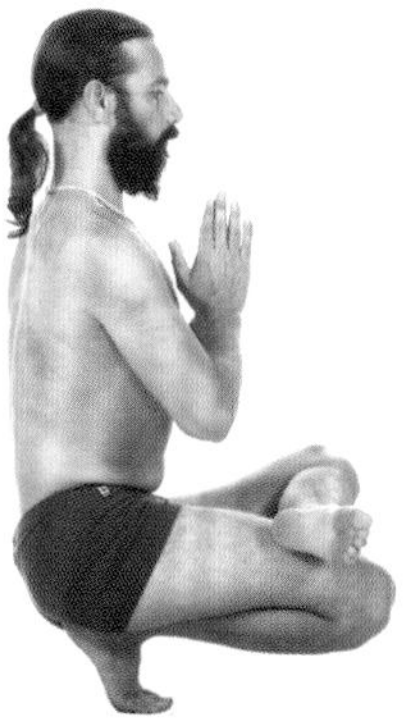

288
उत्तोलन एक पाद अङ्गुष्ठ आसन (नमस्कार)
Uttolana eka pāda aṅguṣṭha āsana (namaskāra)
Balancing one leg on toes pose (hands in prayer)

उत्तोलनैकपादाङ्गुष्ठासन (नमस्कार)
Uttolanaikapādāṅguṣṭhāsana (namaskāra)

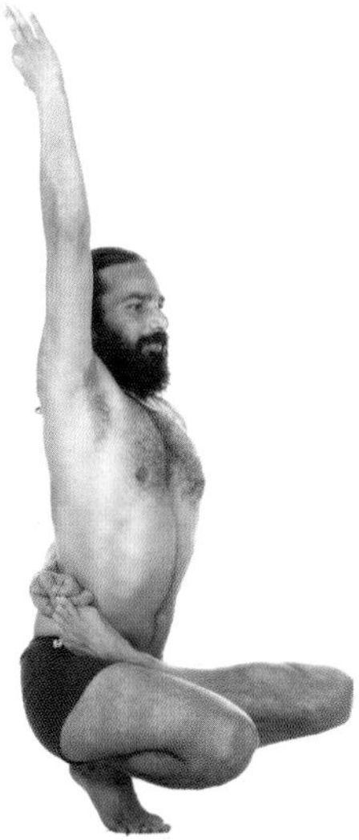

289
उत्तोलन एक पाद अङ्गुष्ठ आसन (अर्ध बद्ध पद्म, एक ऊर्ध्व हस्त)
Uttolana eka pāda aṅguṣṭha āsana (ardha baddha padma, eka ūrdhva hasta)
Balancing one leg on toes pose (bound half lotus, one arm overhead)

उत्तोलनैकपादाङ्गुष्ठासन (अर्धबद्धपद्म, एकोर्ध्वहस्त)
Uttolanaikapādāṅguṣṭhāsana (ardhabaddhapadma, ekordhvahasta)

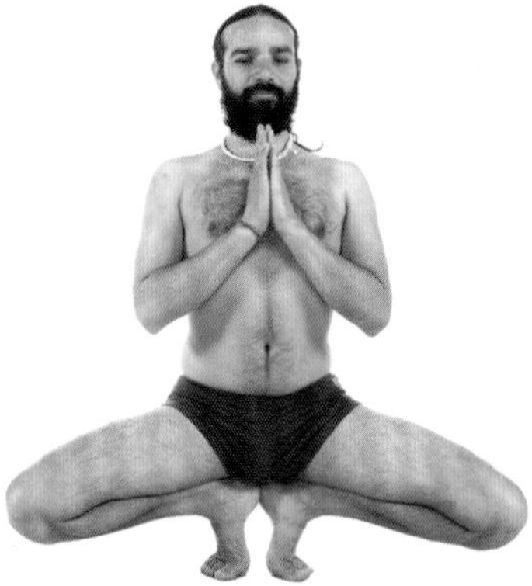

290
उत्तोलन पाद अङ्गुष्ठ आसन (प्रसरित जानु, हृदय नमस्कार)
Uttolana pāda aṅguṣṭha āsana
(prasarita jānu, hṛdayaḥ namaskāra)
Balancing toes pose (wide knees, hands in prayer)

उत्तोलनपादाङ्गुष्ठासन (प्रसरितजानु, हृदयनमस्कार)
Uttolanapādāṅguṣṭhāsana (prasaritajānu, hṛdayanamaskāra)

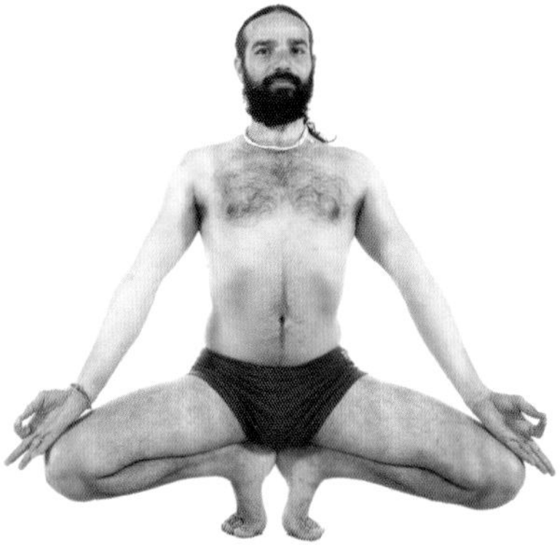

291
उत्तोलन पाद अङ्गुष्ठ आसन (प्रसरित जानु)
Uttolana pāda aṅguṣṭha āsana (prasarita jānu)
Balancing toes pose (wide knees)

उत्तोलनपादाङ्गुष्ठासन (प्रसरितजानु)
Uttolanapādāṅguṣṭhāsana (prasaritajānu)

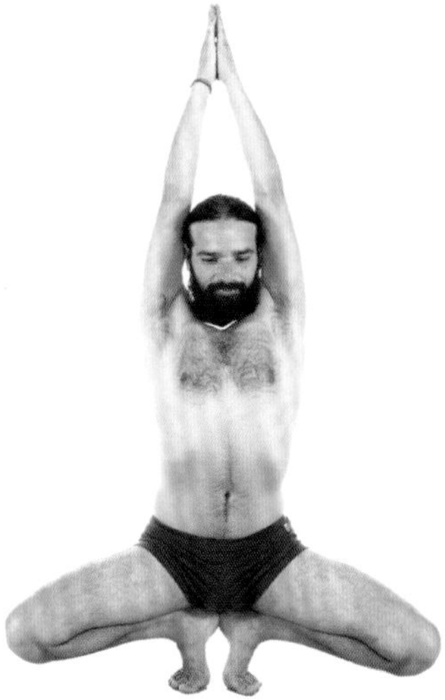

292
उत्तोलन पाद अङ्गुष्ठ आसन (प्रसरितजानु, ऊर्ध्व हस्त नमस्कार)
Uttolana pāda aṅguṣṭha āsana (prasarita jānu, ūrdhva hasta namaskā
Balancing toes pose (wide-knees, hands overhead in prayer)

उत्तोलनपादाङ्गुष्ठासन (प्रसरितजानु, ऊर्ध्वहस्तनमस्कार)
Uttolanapādāṅguṣṭhāsana (prasaritajānu, ūrdhvahastanamaskāra)

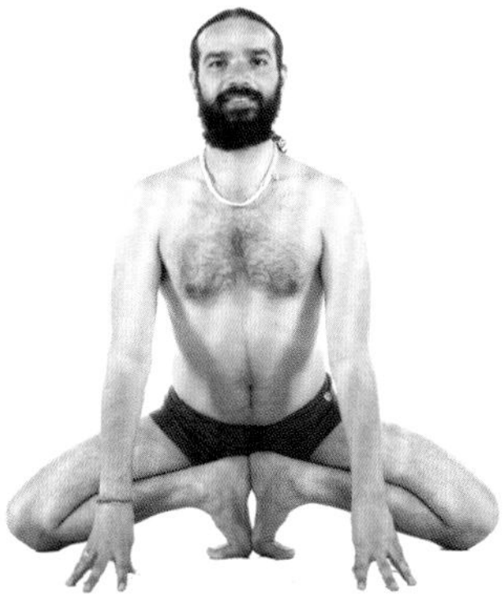

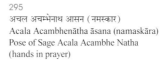

293
योनि मुद्रा आसन (हस्त अङ्गुल भू)
Yoni mudrā āsana (hasta aṅgula bhū)
Source of life pose (fingers on the earth)

योनिमुद्रासन (हस्ताङ्गुलभू)
Yonimudrāsana (hastāṅgulabhū)

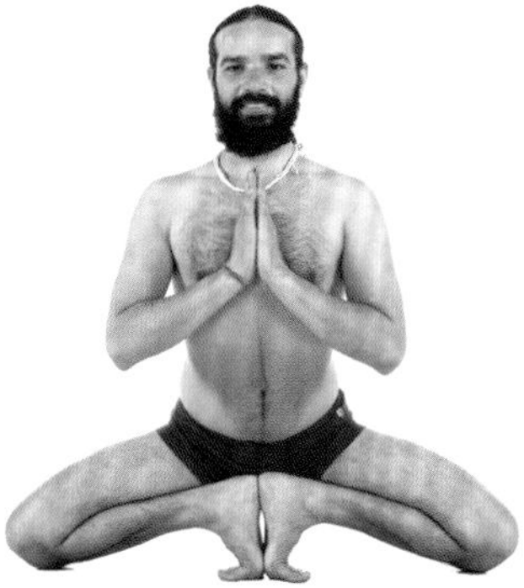

294
नमस्कार योनि मुद्रा आसन
Namaskāra yoni mudrā āsana
Prayer source of life pose

नमस्कारयोनिमुद्रासन
Namaskārayonimudrāsana

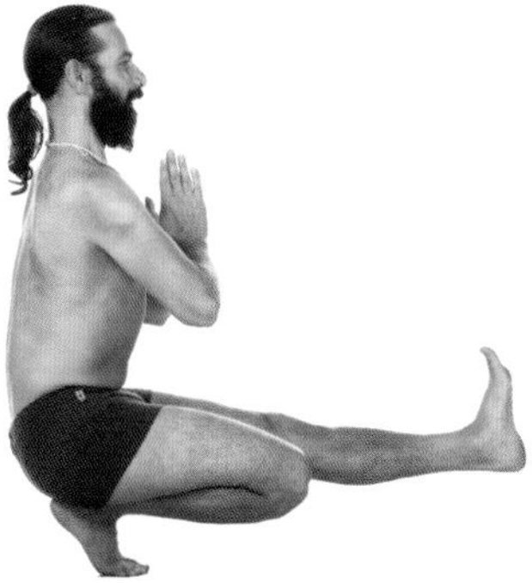

295
अचल अचम्भेनाथ आसन (नमस्कार)
Acala Acambhenātha āsana (namaskāra)
Pose of Sage Acala Acambhe Natha
(hands in prayer)

अचल अचम्भेनाथासन (नमस्कार)
Acalaacambhenāthāsana (namaskāra)

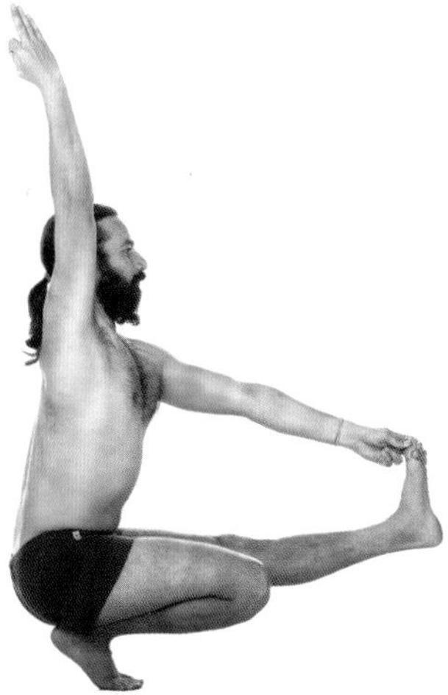

296
अचल अचम्भेनाथ आसन
Acala Acambhenātha āsana
Pose of Sage Acala Acambhe Natha

अचल अचम्भेनाथासन
Acalaacambhenātha āsana

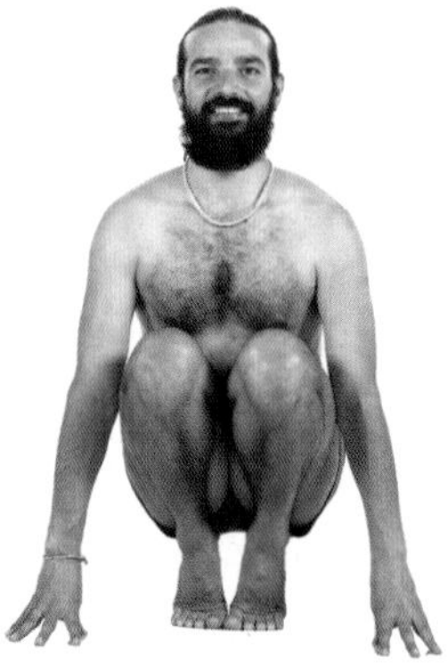

297
उत्तोलन काग आसन (हस्त अङ्गुल भू)
Uttolana kāga āsana (hasta aṅgula bhū)
Balancing crow pose (fingers on the earth)

उत्तोलनकागासन (हस्ताङ्गुलभू)
Uttolanakāgāsana (hastāṅgulabhū)

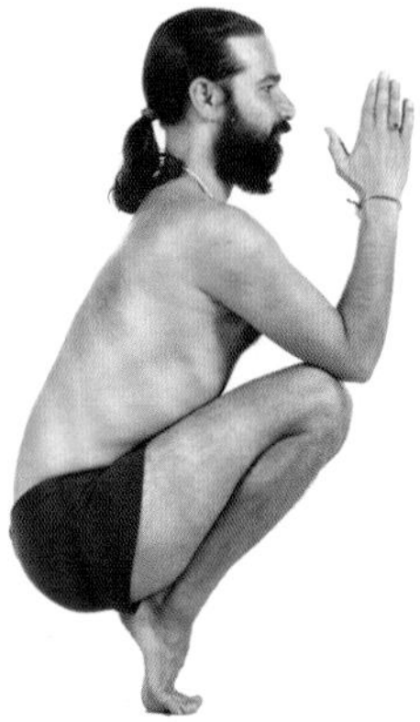

298
उत्तोलन नमस्कार काग आसन
Uttolana namaskāra kāga āsana
Balancing praying crow pose

उत्तोलननमस्कारकागासन
Uttolananamaskārakāgāsana

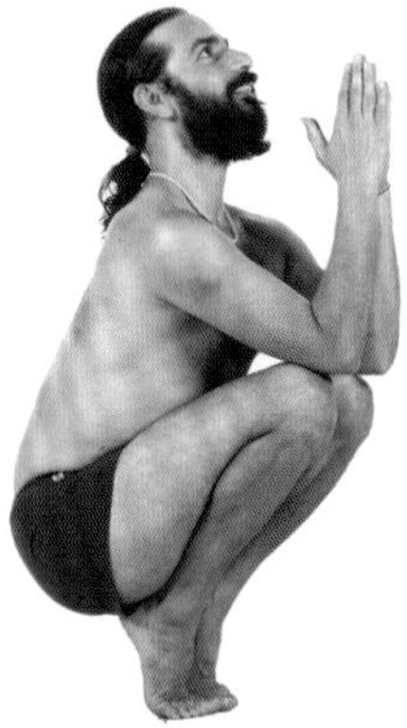

299
उत्तोलन नमस्कार काग आसन (ऊर्ध्व दृष्टि)
Uttolana namaskāra kāga āsana (ūrdhva dṛṣṭi)
Balancing praying crow pose (gazing upward)

उत्तोलननमस्कारकागासन (ऊर्ध्वदृष्टि)
Uttolananamaskārakāgāsana (ūrdhvadṛṣṭi)

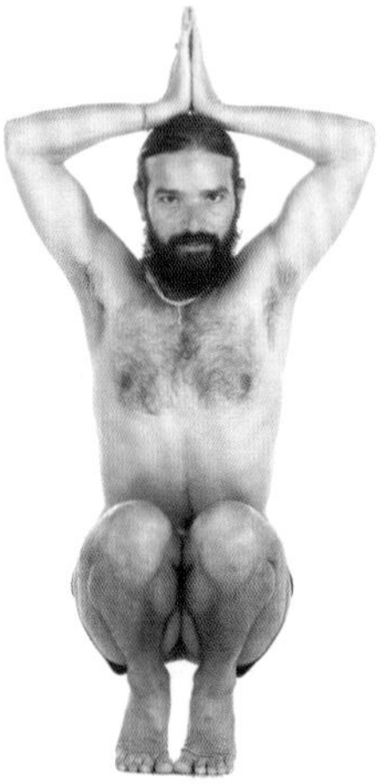

300
उत्तोलन काग आसन (शीर्ष नमस्कार)
Uttolana kāga āsana (śīrṣa namaskāra)
Balancing crow pose (hands in prayer on top of the head)

उत्तोलनकागासन (शीर्षनमस्कार)
Uttolanakāgāsana (śīrṣanamaskāra)

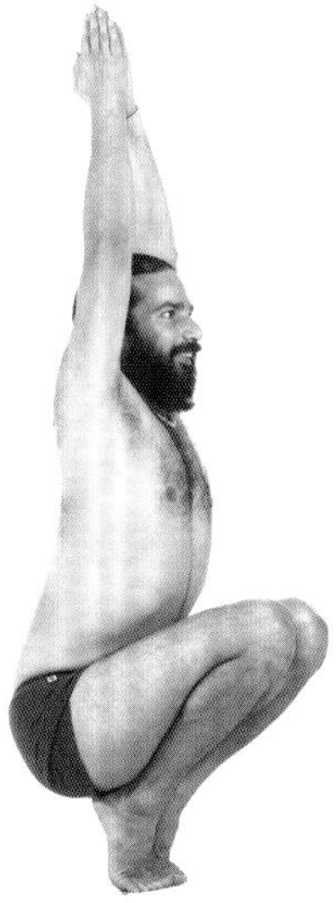

301
उत्तोलन काग आसन (ऊर्ध्व हस्त)
Uttolana kāga āsana (ūrdhva hasta)
Balancing crow pose (hands overhead)

उत्तोलनकागासन (ऊर्ध्वहस्त)
Uttolanakāgāsana (ūrdhvahasta)

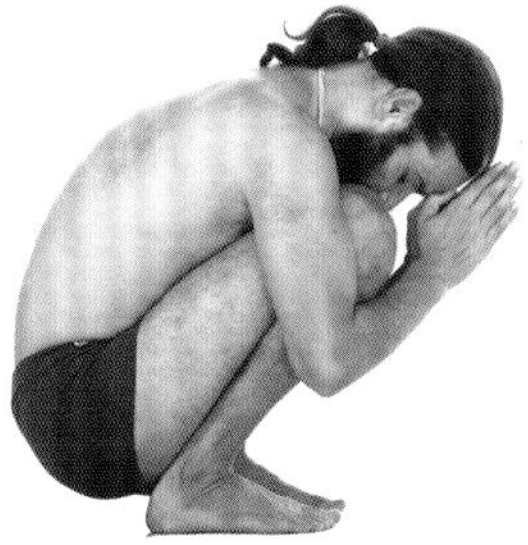

302
नमस्कार काग आसन
Namaskāra kāga āsana
Praying crow pose

नमस्कारकागासन
Namaskārakāgāsana

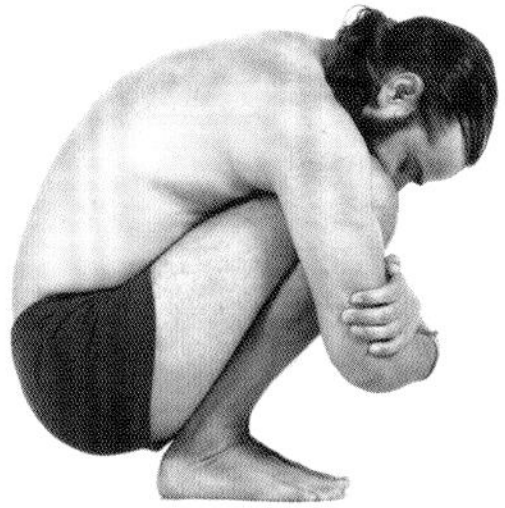

303
काग आसन (जानु बद्ध)
Kāga āsana (jānu baddha)
Crow pose (bound knees)

कागासन (जानुबद्ध)
Kāgāsana (jānubaddha)

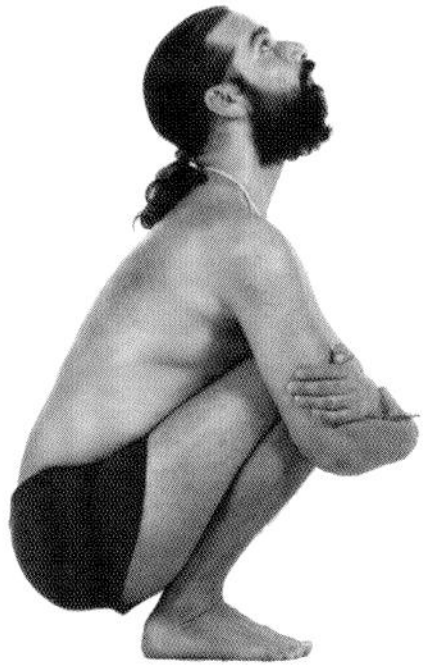

304
काग आसन (जानु बद्ध ,ऊर्ध्व दृष्टि)
Kāga āsana (jānu baddha, ūrdhva dṛṣṭi)
Crow pose (bound knees, gazing upward)

कागासन (जानुबद्ध ,ऊर्ध्वदृष्टि)
Kāgāsana (jānubaddha, ūrdhvadṛṣṭi)

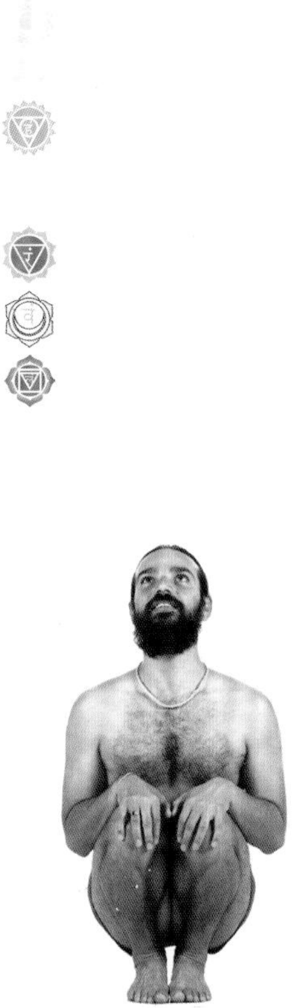

305
काग आसन (ऊर्ध्वदृष्टि)
Kāga āsana (ūrdhva dṛṣṭi)
Crow pose (gazing upward)

काागासन (ऊर्ध्वदृष्टि)
Kāgāsana (ūrdhvadṛṣṭi)

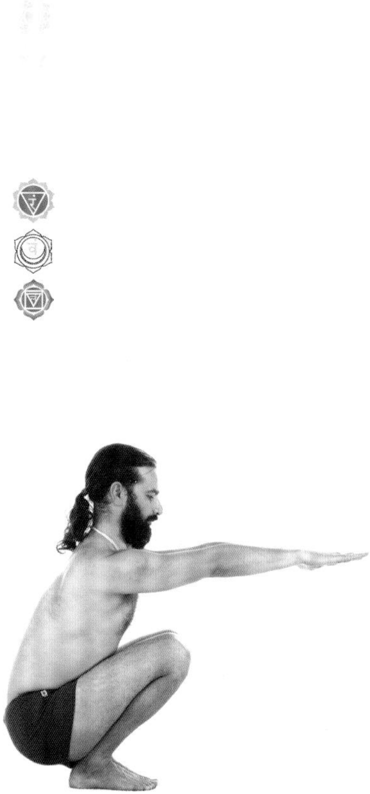

306
काग आसन (समक्ष हस्त)
Kāga āsana (samakṣa hasta)
Crow pose (hands extended in front)

कागासन (समक्षहस्त)
Kāgāsana (samakṣahasta)

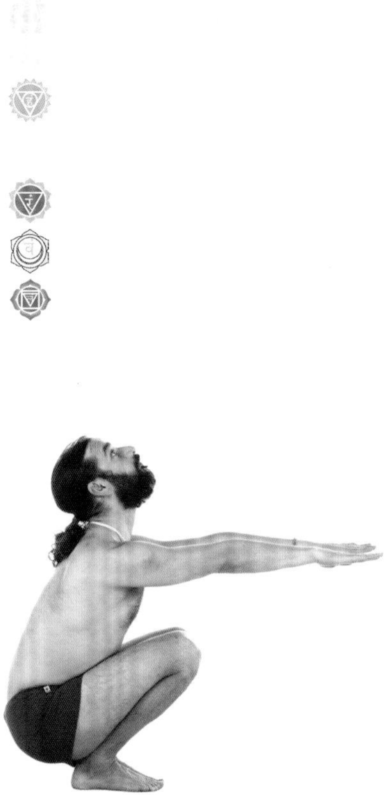

307
काग आसन (समक्ष हस्त, ऊर्ध्व दृष्टि)
Samakṣa hasta kāga āsana (ūrdhva dṛṣṭi)
Crow pose (hands extended in front, gazing upward)

कागासन (समक्षहस्त, ऊर्ध्वदृष्टि)
Samakṣahastakāgāsana (ūrdhvadṛṣṭi)

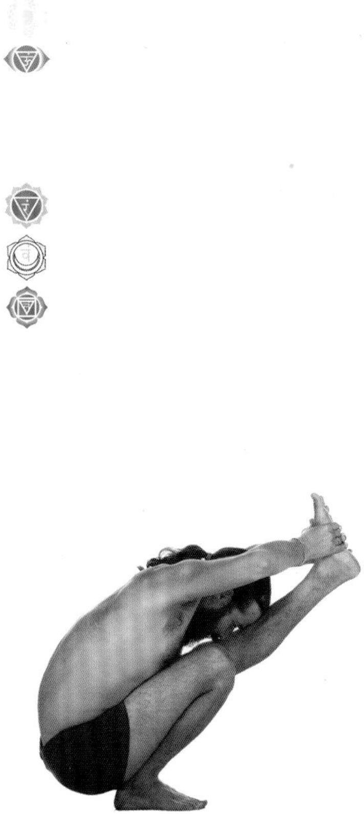

308
जानु शिर काग आसन (क्षितिज पाद)
Jānuśira kāga āsana (kṣitija pāda)
Head to knee crow pose (leg extended to horizon)

जानुशिरकागासन (क्षितिजपाद)
Jānuśirakāgāsana (kṣitijapāda)

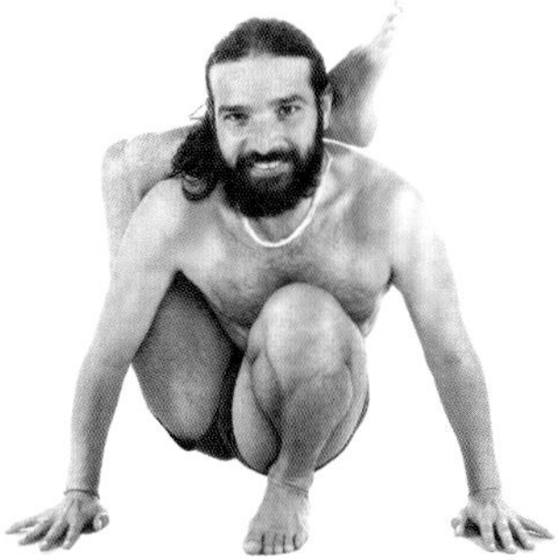

309
भैरव काग आसन
Bhairava kāga āsana
Fearless crow pose

भैरवकागासन
Bhairavakāgāsana

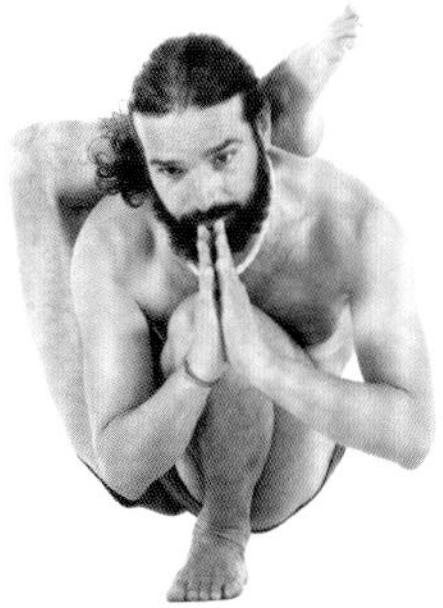

310
नमस्कार भैरव काग आसन
Namaskāra bhairava kāga āsana
Fearless praying crow pose

नमस्कारभैरवकागासन
Namaskārabhairavakāgāsana

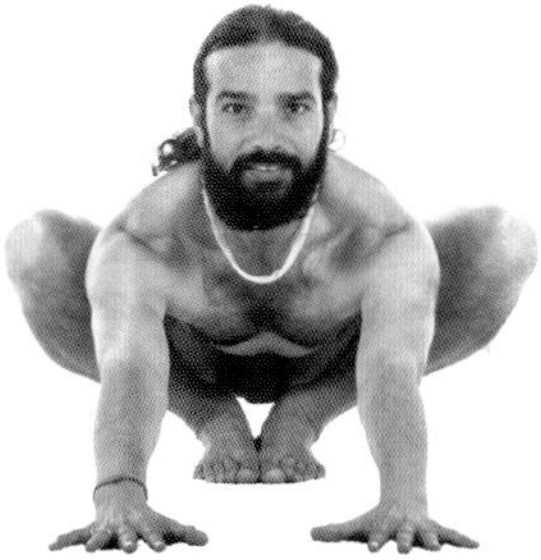

311
काग आसन (भू नमन ,समक्ष दृष्टि)
Kāga āsana (bhū namana, samakṣa dṛṣṭi)
Crow pose (bowing to the earth, gazing forward)

कागासन (भूनमन, समक्षदृष्टि)
Kāgāsana (bhūnamana, samakṣadṛṣṭi)

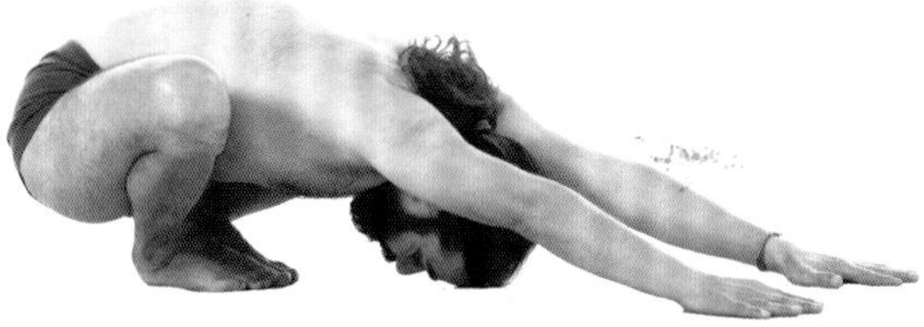

312
काग आसन (भू नमन)
Kāga āsana (bhū namana)
Crow pose (bowing to the earth)

कागासन (भूनमन)
Kāgāsana (bhūnamana)

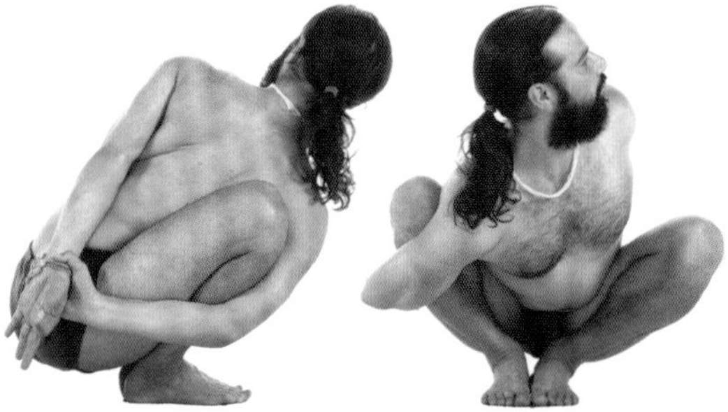

313
काग आसन (एक जानु बद्ध)
Kāga āsana (eka jānu baddha)
Crow pose (one knee bound)

कागासन (एकजानुबद्ध)
Kāgāsana (ekajānubaddha)

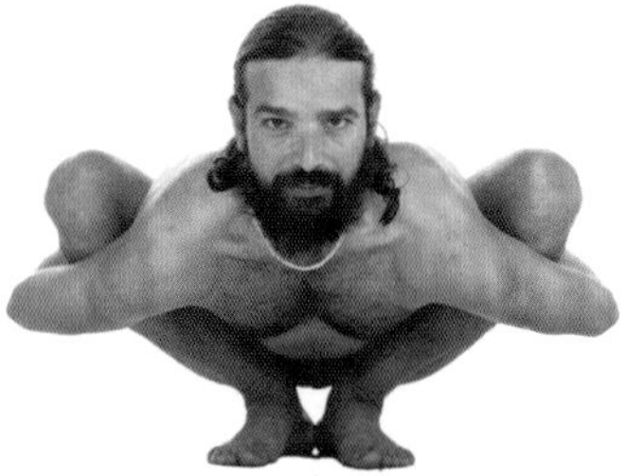

314
कूर्म काग आसन (जानु बद्ध)
Kūrma kāga āsana (jānu baddha)
Tortoise crow pose (bound knees)

कूर्मकागासन (जानुबद्ध)
Kūrmakāgāsana (jānubaddha)

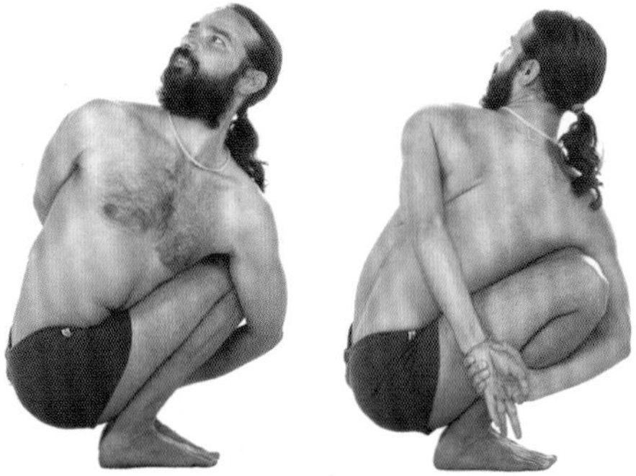

315
परिवृत्त काग आसन (जानु बद्ध)
Parivṙtta kāga āsana (jānu baddha)
Twisted crow pose (bound knee)

परिवृत्तकागासन (जानुबद्ध)
Parivṙttakāgāsana (jānubaddha)

Seated

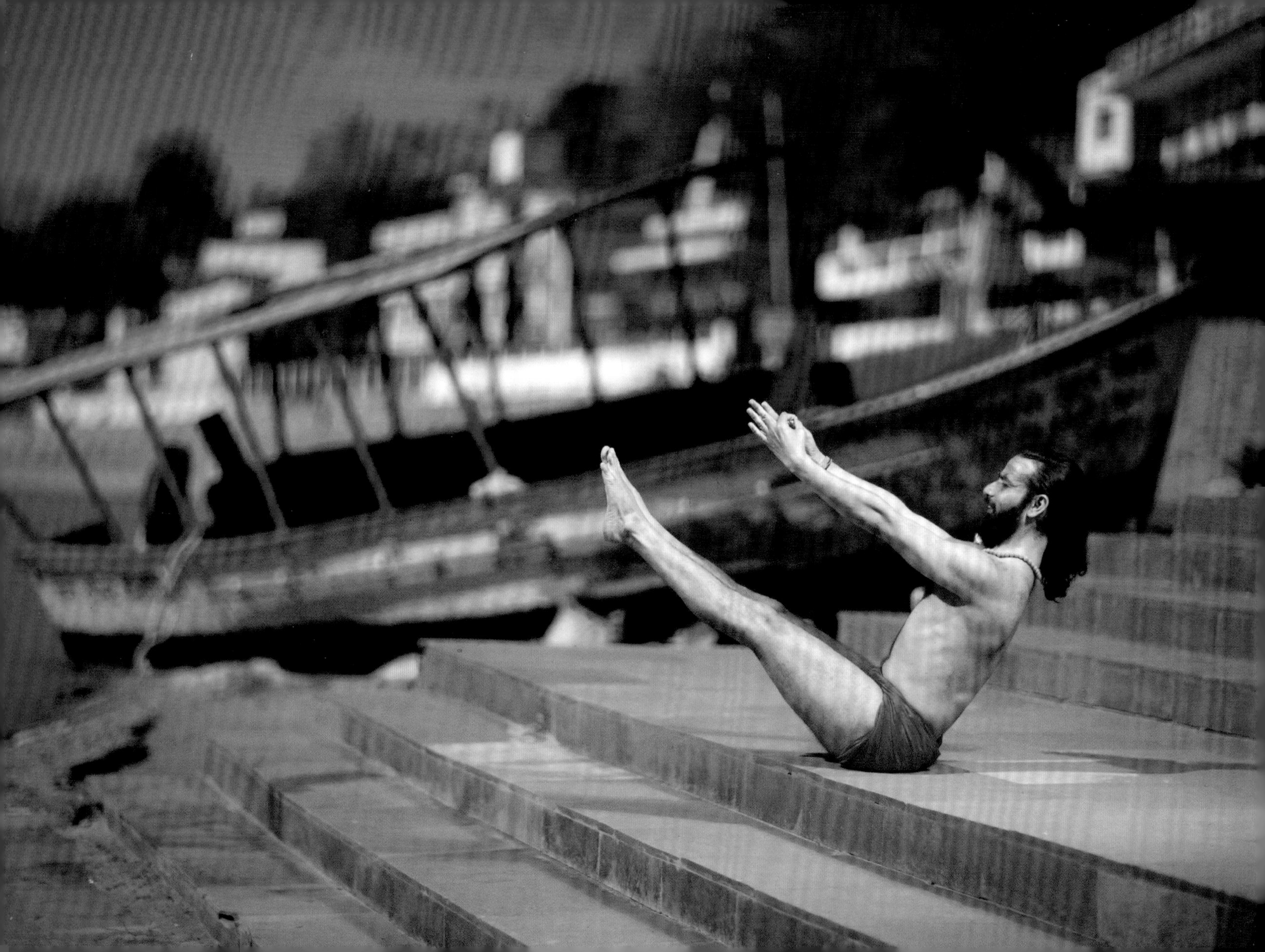

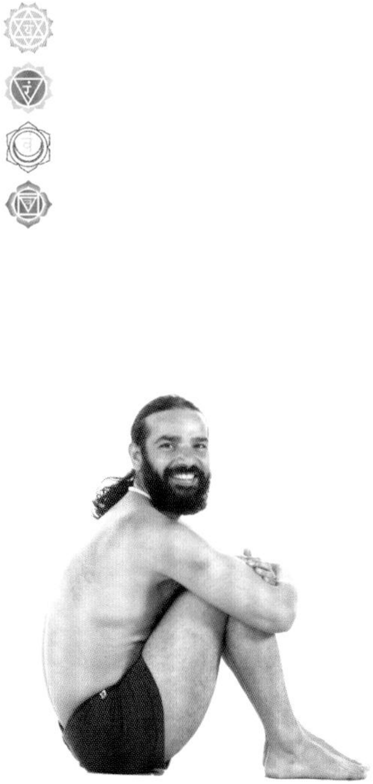

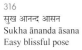

316
सुख आनन्द आसन
Sukha ānanda āsana
Easy blissful pose

सुखानन्दासन
Sukhānandāsana

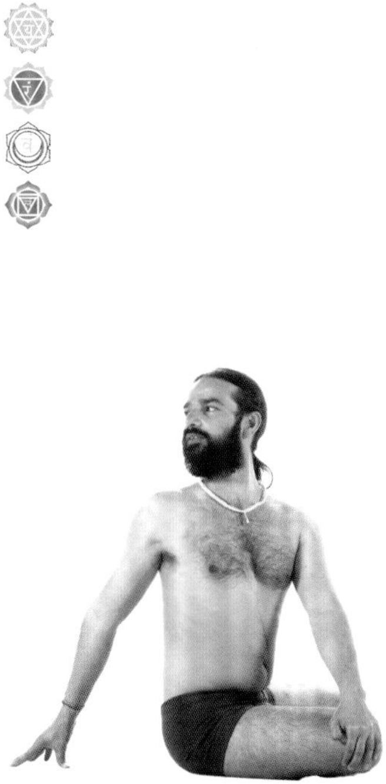

317
परिवृत्त सुख आसन
Parivṛtta sukha āsana
Twisted easy pose

परिवृत्तसुखासन
Parivṛttasukhāsana

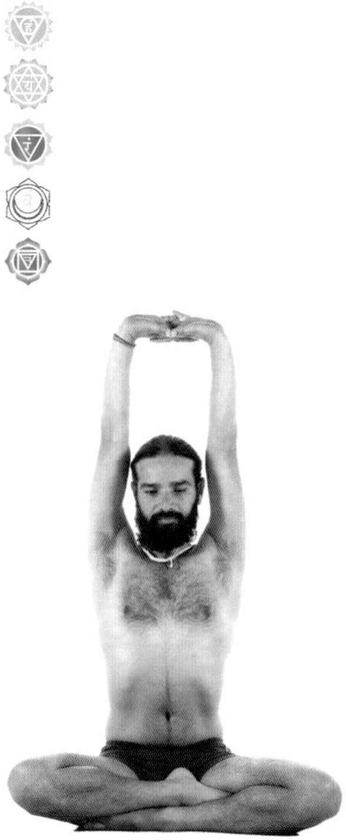

318
सुख आसन (ऊर्ध्व करतल)
Sukha āsana (ūrdhva karatala)
Easy pose (palms extended overhead)

सुखासन (ऊर्ध्वकरतल)
Sukhāsana (ūrdhvakaratala)

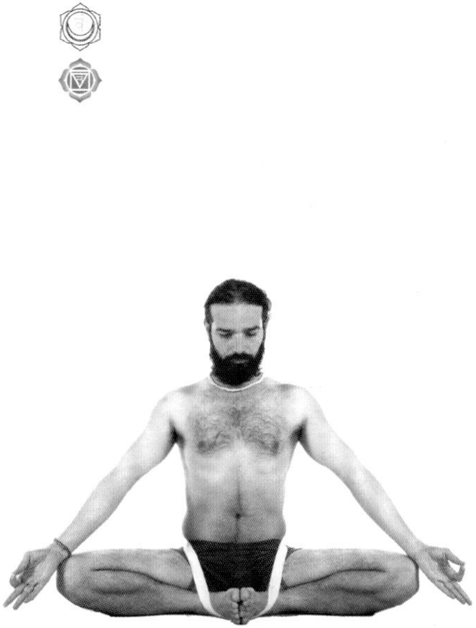

319
पार्वती आसन (सरज्जु)
Pārvatī āsana (sarajju)
Divine feminine pose (supported with straps)

पार्वत्यासन (सरज्जु)
Pārvatiyāsana (sarajju)

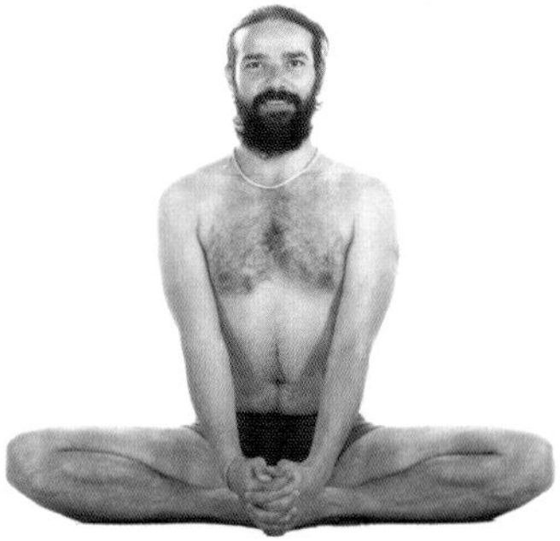

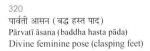

320
पार्वती आसन (बद्ध हस्त पाद)
Pārvatī āsana (baddha hasta pāda)
Divine feminine pose (clasping feet)

पार्वत्यासन (बद्धहस्तपाद)
Pārvatyāsana (baddhahastapāda)

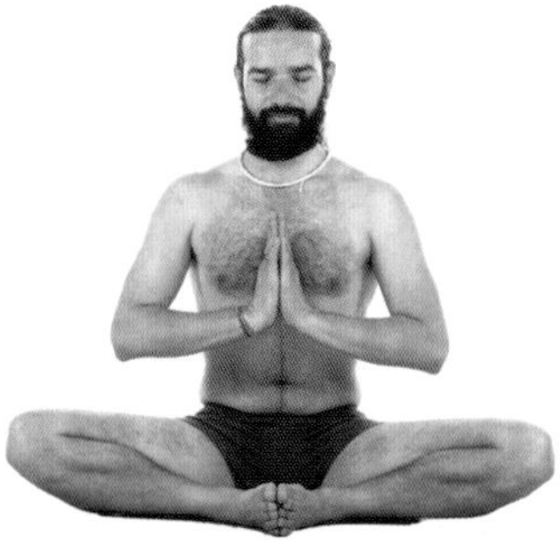

321
नमस्कार पार्वती आसन
Namaskāra pārvatī āsana
Praying divine feminine pose

नमस्कारपार्वत्यासन
Namaskārapārvatyāsana

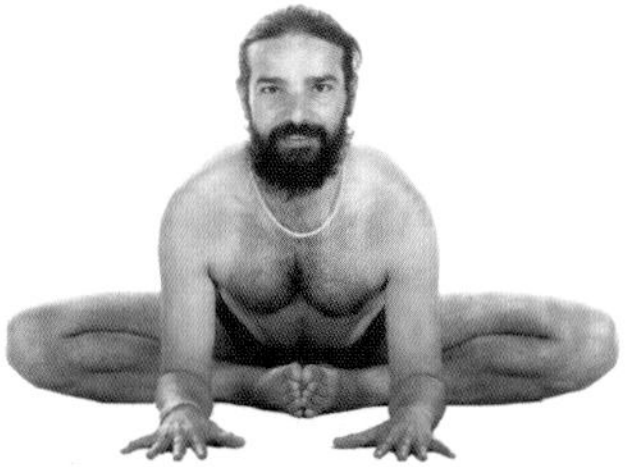

322
पार्वती आसन (कफोणि भू)
Pārvatī āsana (kaphoṇi bhū)
Divine feminine pose (elbows on the earth)

पार्वत्यासन (कफोणिभू)
Pārvatyāsana (kaphoṇibhū)

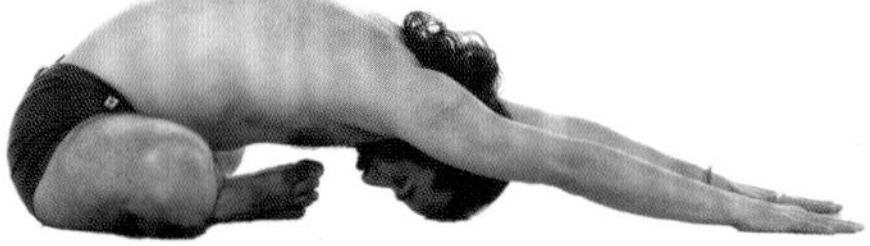

323
पार्वती आसन (ललाट भू)
Pārvatī āsana (lalāṭa bhū)
Divine feminine pose (forehead on the earth)

पार्वत्यासन (ललाटभू)
Pārvatyāsana (lalāṭabhū)

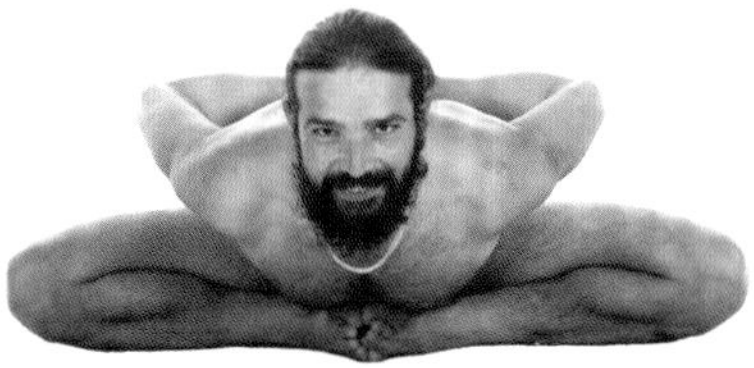

324
पार्वती आसन (हृदय पाद ,पृष्ठ नमस्कार)
Pārvatī āsana (hṛdayaḥ pāda, pṛṣṭha namaskāra)
Divine feminine pose (heart to feet, hands in prayer behind)

पार्वत्यासन (हृदयपाद ,पृष्ठनमस्कार)
Pārvatyāsana (hṛdayapāda, pṛṣṭhanamaskāra)

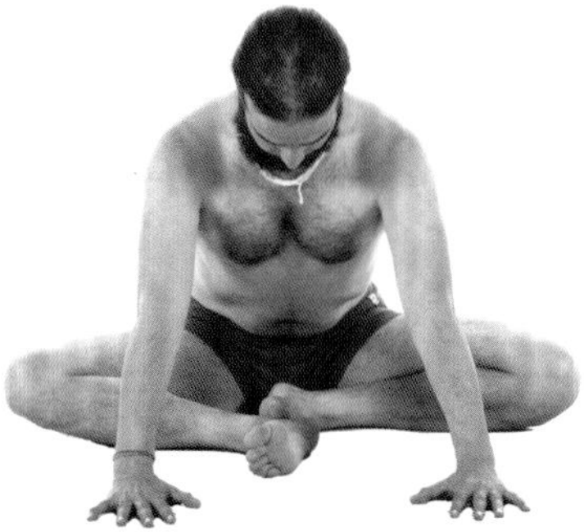

325
पार्वती आसन (पाद पृष्ठ, कर तल भू)
Pārvatī āsana (pāda pṛṣṭha, karatala bhū)
Divine feminine pose (one foot behind the other, palms on the earth)

पार्वत्यासन (पादपृष्ठ, करतलभू)
Pārvatyāsana (pādapṛṣṭha, karatalabhū)

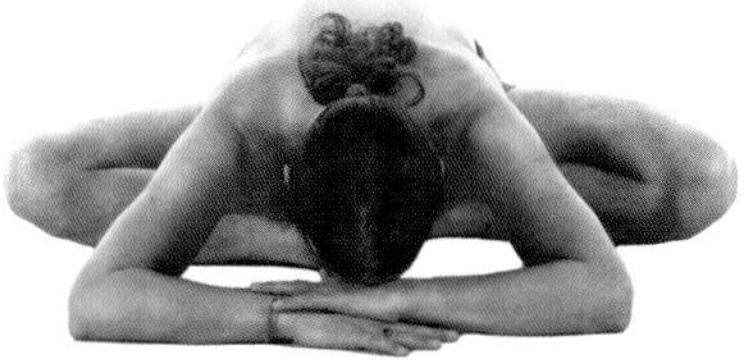

326
पार्वती आसन (पाद पृष्ठ, ललाट हस्त भू)
Pārvatī āsana (pāda pṛṣṭha, lalāṭa hasta bhū)
Divine feminine pose (one foot behind the other, forehead on the earth)

पार्वत्यासन (पादपृष्ठ, ललाटहस्तभू)
Pārvatyāsana (pādapṛṣṭha, lalāṭahastabhū)

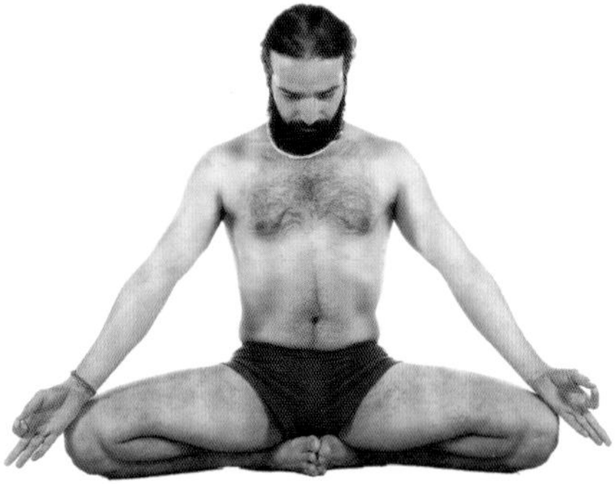

327
गोरक्ष नाथ आसन
Gorakṣa Nātha āsana
Sage Goraksa Nātha pose

गोरक्षनाथासन
Gorakṣanāthāsana

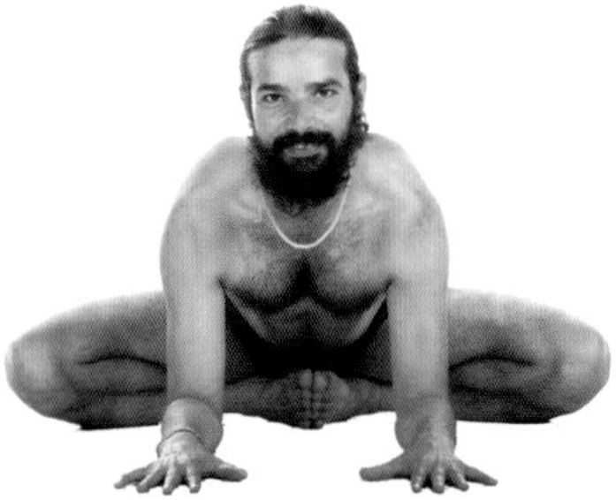

328
गोरक्ष नाथ आसन (कफोणि भू)
Gorakṣa Nātha āsana (kaphoṇi bhū)
Sage Goraksa Nātha pose (elbows on the earth)

गोरक्षनाथासन (कफोणिभू)
Gorakṣanāthāsana (kaphoṇibhū)

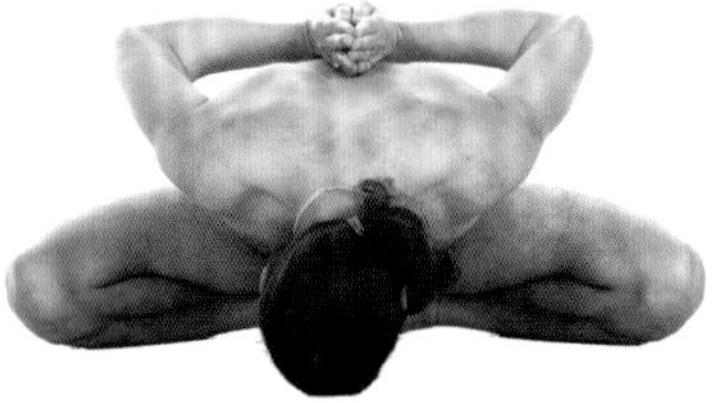

329
गोरक्ष नाथ आसन (ललाट भू पृष्ठ नमस्कार)
Gorakṣa Nātha āsana (lalāṭa bhū, pṛṣṭha namaskāra)
Sage Goraksa Nātha pose (forehead on the earth, hands behind in prayer)

गोरक्षनाथासन (ललाटभू ,पृष्ठनमस्कार)
Gorakṣanāthāsana (lalāṭabhū, pṛṣṭhanamaskāra)

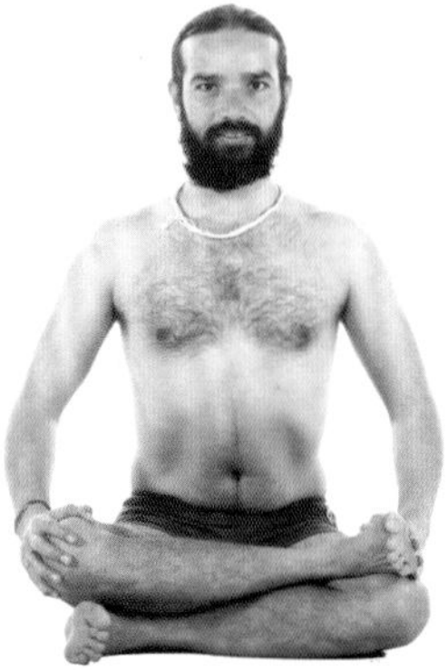

330
समिधा स्थापन आसन (जानु हस्त)
Samidhā sthāpana āsana (jānu hasta)
Sacred fire log pose (hands on knees)

समिधास्थापनासन (जानुहस्त)
Samidhāsthāpanāsana (jānuhasta)

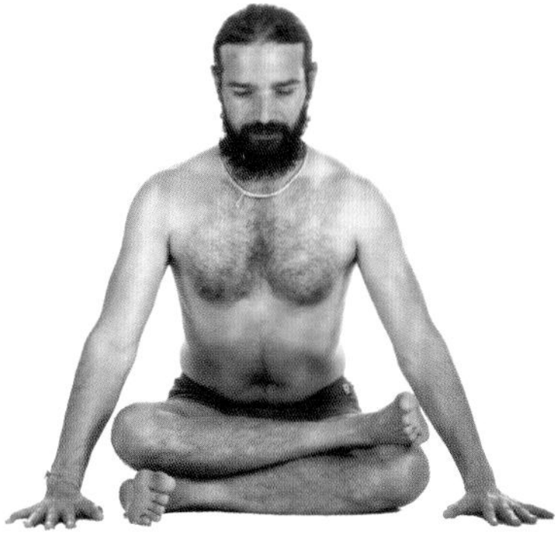

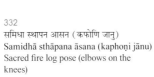

331
समिधा स्थापन (हस्त भू)
Samidhā sthāpana āsana (hasta bhū)
Sacred fire log pose (hands on the earth)

समिधास्थापन (हस्तभू)
Samidhāsthāpanāsana (hastabhū)

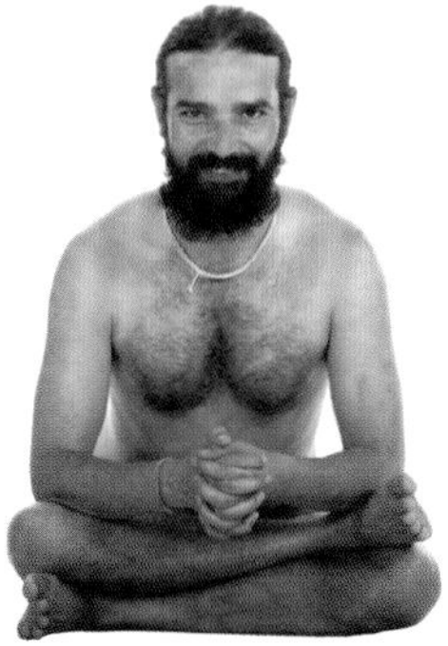

332
समिधा स्थापन आसन (कफोणि जानु)
Samidhā sthāpana āsana (kaphoṇi jānu)
Sacred fire log pose (elbows on the knees)

समिधास्थापनासन (कफोणिजानु)
Samidhāsthāpanāsana (kaphoṇijānu)

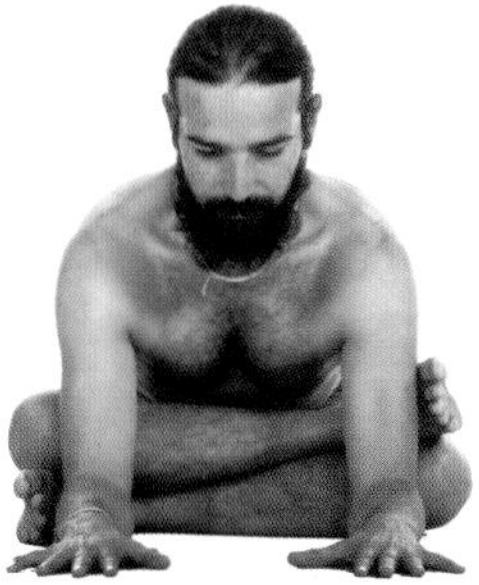

333
समिधा स्थापन आसन (कफोणि भू)
Samidhā sthāpana āsana (kaphoṇi bhū)
Sacred fire log pose (elbows on the earth)

समिधास्थापनासन (कफोणिभू)
Samidhāsthāpanāsana (kaphoṇibhū)

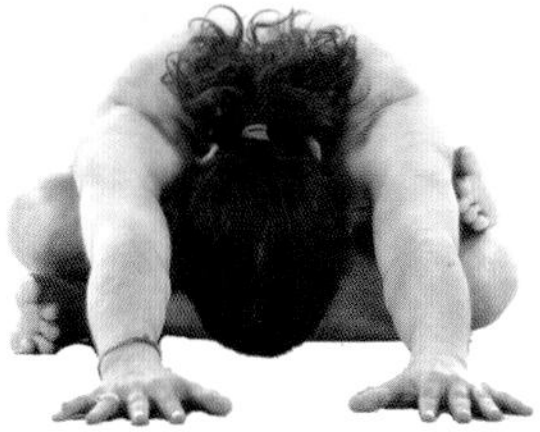

334
समिधा स्थापन आसन (हस्त ललाट भू)
Samidhā sthāpana āsana (hasta lalāṭa bhū)
Sacred fire log pose (hands and forehead on the earth)

समिधास्थापनासन (हस्तललाटभू)
Samidhāsthāpanāsana (hastalalāṭabhū)

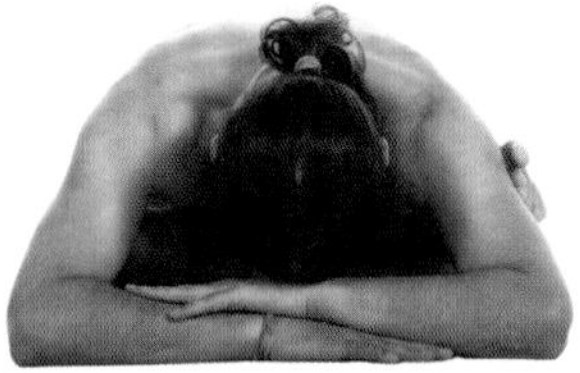

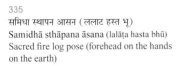

335
समिधा स्थापन आसन (ललाट हस्त भू)
Samidhā sthāpana āsana (lalāṭa hasta bhū)
Sacred fire log pose (forehead on the hands on the earth)

समिधास्थापनासन (ललाटहस्तभू)
Samidhāsthāpanāsana (lalāṭahastabhū)

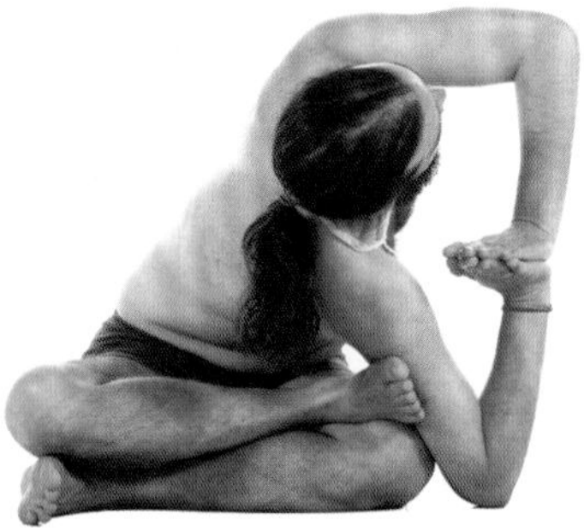

336
परिवृत्त समिधा स्थापन आसन (नमस्कार)
Parivṛtta samidhā sthāpana āsana (namaskāra)
Twisted sacred fire log pose (hands in prayer)

परिवृत्तसमिधास्थापनासन (नमस्कार)
Parivṛttasamidhāsthāpanāsana (namaskāra)

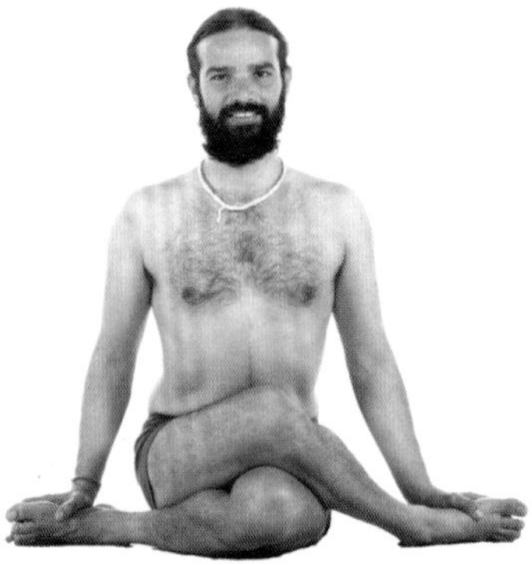

337
गो मुख आसन (हस्त पाद)
Go mukha āsana (hasta pāda)
Cow face pose (hands on the feet)

गोमुखासन (हस्तपाद)
Gomukhāsana (hastapāda)

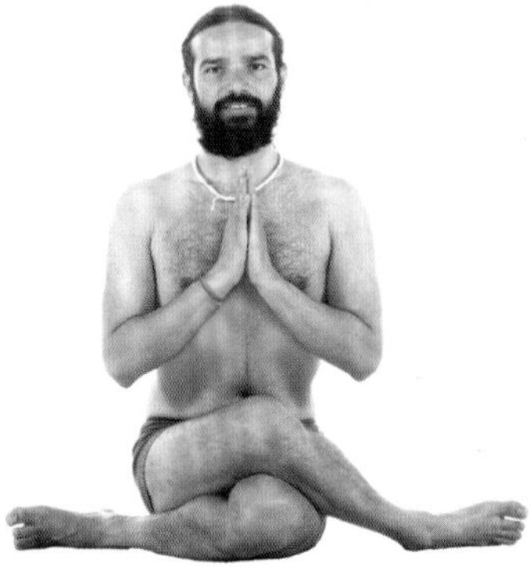

338
नमस्कार गो मुख आसन
Namaskāra go mukha āsana
Praying cow face pose

नमस्कारगोमुखासन
Namaskāragomukhāsana

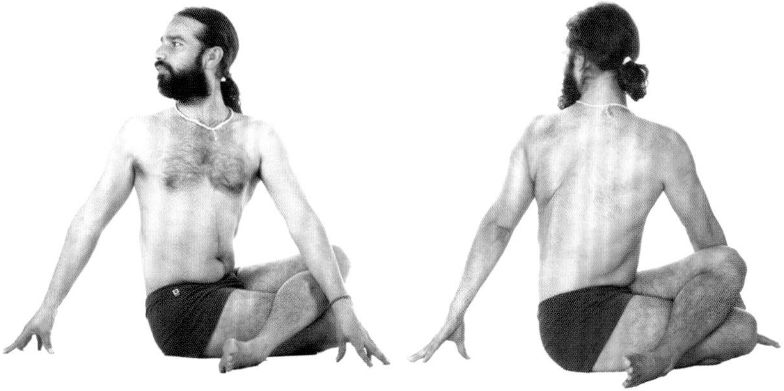

339
परिवृत्त गो मुख आसन (हस्त अङ्गुल भू)
Parivṛtta go mukha āsana (hasta aṅgula bhū)
Twisted cow face pose (fingers on the earth)

परिवृत्तगोमुखासन (हस्ताङ्गुलभू)
Parivṛttagomukhāsana (hastāṅgulabhū)

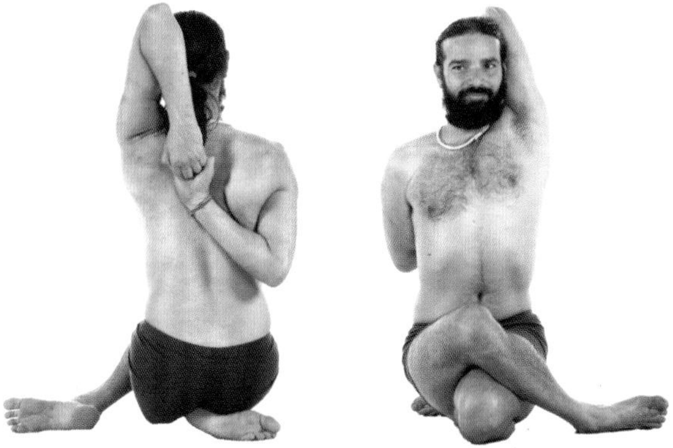

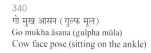

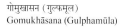

340
गो मुख आसन (गुल्फ मूल)
Go mukha āsana (gulpha mūla)
Cow face pose (sitting on the ankle)

गोमुखासन (गुल्फमूल)
Gomukhāsana (Gulphamūla)

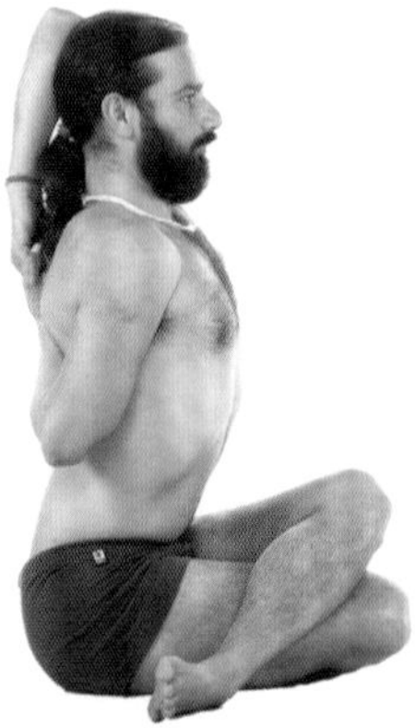

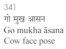

341
गो मुख आसन
Go mukha āsana
Cow face pose

गोमुखासन
Gomukhāsana

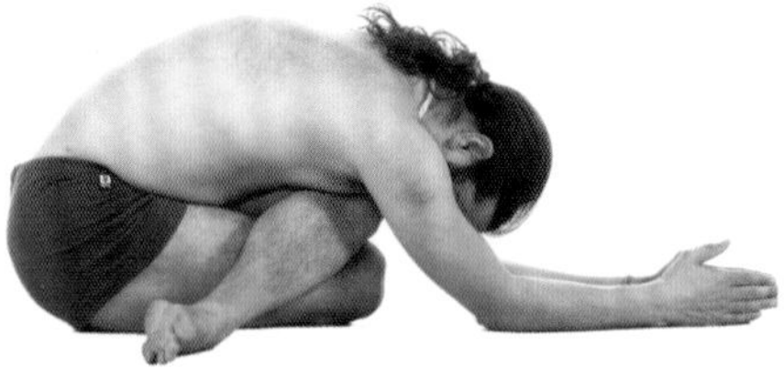

342
गो मुख आसन (भू नमन)
Go mukha āsana (bhū namana)
Cow face pose (honoring the earth)

गोमुखासन (भूनमन)
Gomukhāsana (bhūnamana)

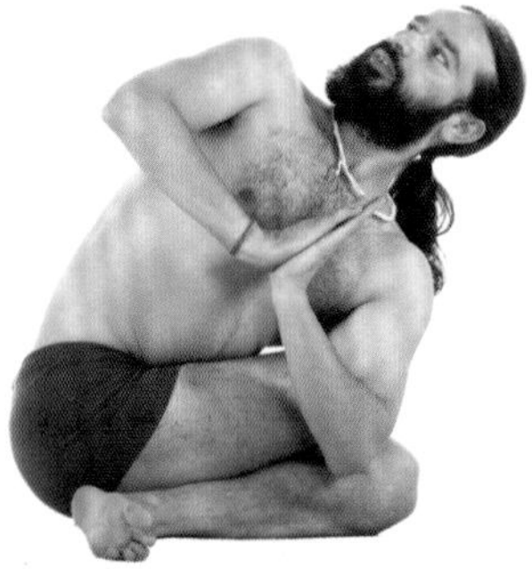

343
परिवृत्त गो मुख आसन (नमस्कार)
Parivṛtta go mukha āsana (namaskāra)
Twisted cow face pose (hands in prayer)

परिवृत्तगोमुखासन (नमस्कार)
Parivṛttagomukhāsana (namaskāra)

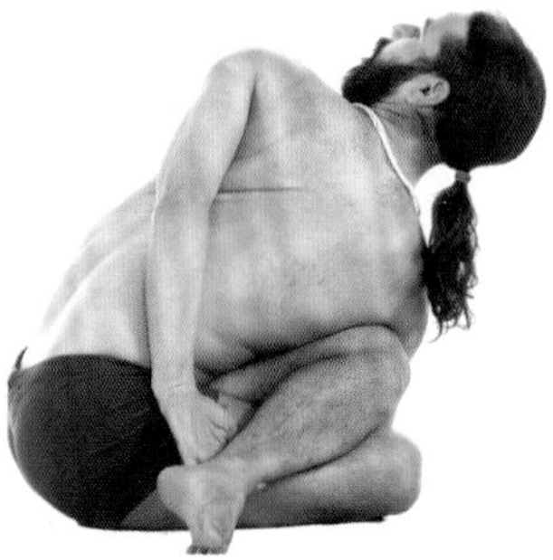

344
परिवृत्त गो मुख आसन (विपरीत बद्ध गुल्फ)
Parivṛitta go mukha āsana
(viparīta baddha gulpha)
Twisted cow face pose (holding opposite ankle)

परिवृत्तगोमुखासन (विपरीतबद्धगुल्फ)
Parivṛittagomukhāsana (viparītabaddhagulpha)

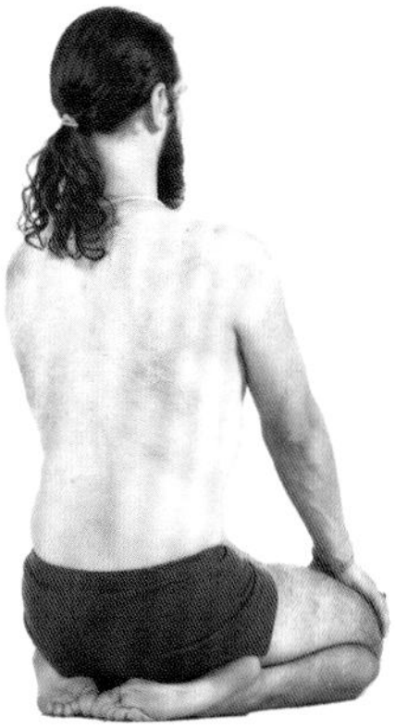

345
वज्र आसन (पाद अङ्गुष्ठ स्पर्श)
Vajra āsana (pāda aṅguṣṭha sparśa)
Thunderbolt pose (toes touching)

वज्रासन (पादाङ्गुष्ठस्पर्श)
Vajrāsana (pādāṅguṣṭhasparśa)

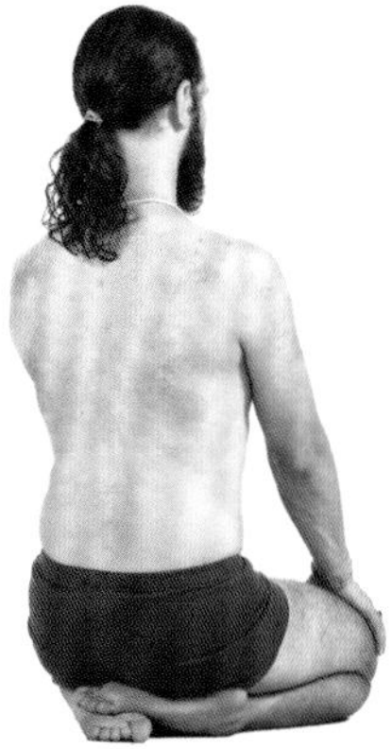

346
वज्र आसन (पाद उपरि पाद)
Vajra āsana (pāda upari pāda)
Thunderbolt pose (feet stacked)

वज्रासन (पादोपरिपाद)
Vajrāsana (pādoparipāda)

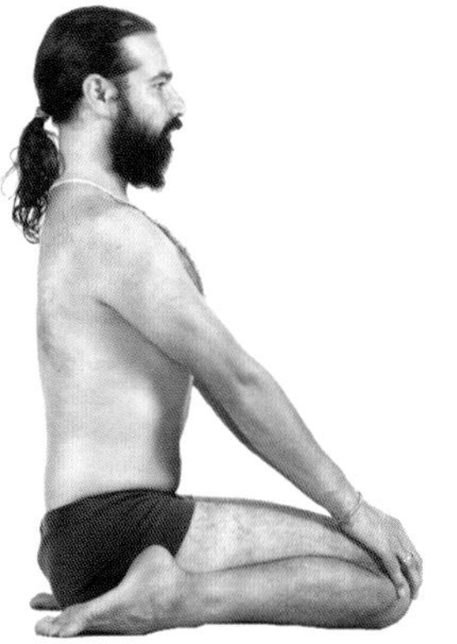

347
वज्र आसन(नितम्ब भू)
Vajra āsana (nitamba bhū)
Thunderbolt pose (hips on the earth)

वज्रासन (नितम्बभू)
Vajrāsana (nitambabhū)

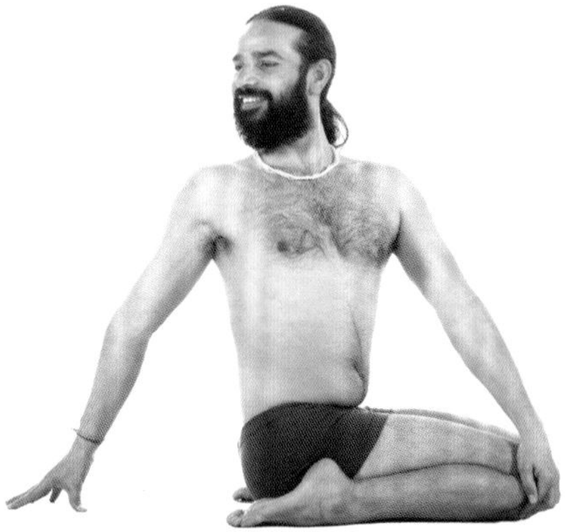

348
परिवृत्त वज्र आसन (नितम्ब भू)
Parivṛtta vajra āsana (nitamba bhū)
Twisted thunderbolt pose (hips on the earth)

परिवृत्तवज्रासन (नितम्बभू)
Parivṛttavajrāsana (nitambabhū)

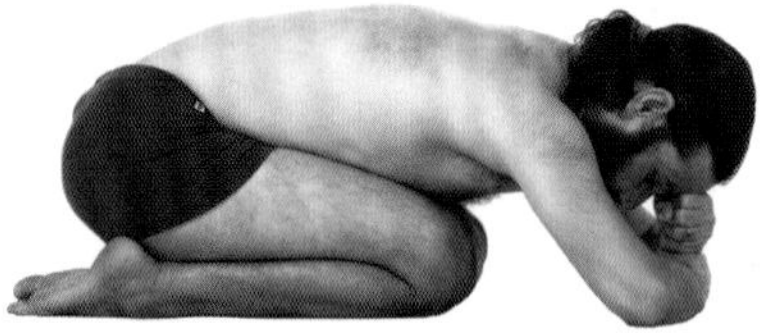

349
वज्र योग मुद्रा आसन (मुष्टिका ललाट धर)
Vajra yoga mudrā āsana (muṣṭikā lalāṭa dhara)
Thunderbolt yoga mudrā pose
(forehead on stacked fists)

वज्रयोगमुद्रासन (मुष्टिकाललाटधर)
Vajrayogamudrāsana (muṣṭikālalāṭadhara)

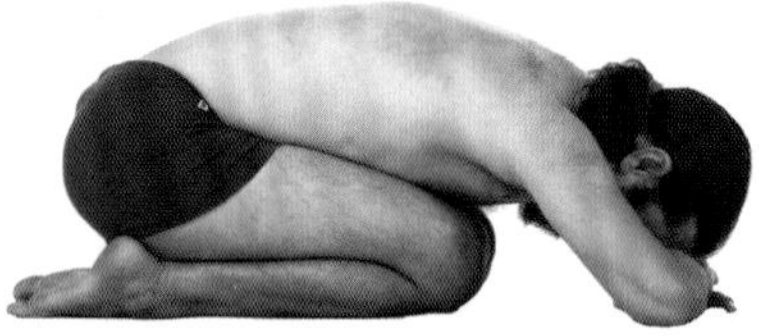

350
वज्र योग मुद्रा आसन (हस्त ललाट धर)
Vajra yoga mudrā āsana (hasta lalāṭa dhara)
Thunderbolt yoga mudrā pose
(forehead on stacked hands)

वज्रयोगमुद्रासन (हस्तललाटधर)
Vajrayogamudrāsana (hastalalāṭadhara)

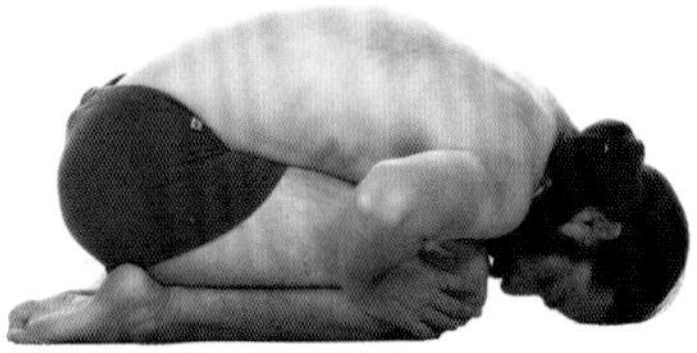

351
वज्र योग मुद्रा आसन (हस्त जानु)
Vajra yoga mudrā āsana (hasta jānu)
Thunderbolt yoga mudrā pose
(hands on knees)

वज्रयोगमुद्रासन (हस्तजानु)
Vajrayogamudrāsana (hastajānu)

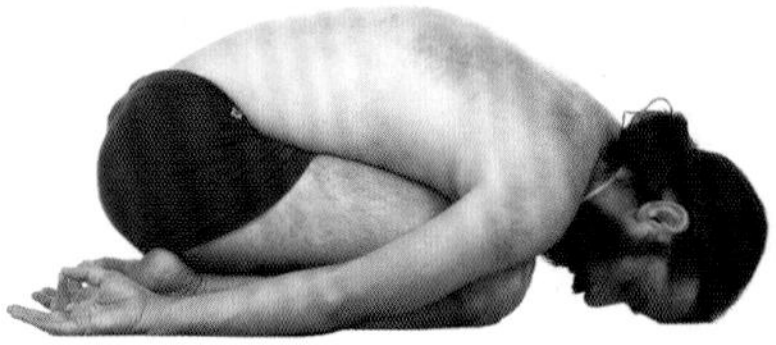

352
वज्र योग मुद्र आसन (पृष्ठ हस्त,)
Vajra yoga mudrā āsana (pṛṣṭha hasta)
Thunderbolt yoga mudrā pose
(hands behind)

वज्रयोगमुद्रासन (पृष्ठहस्त)
Vajrayogamudrāsana (pṛṣṭhahasta)

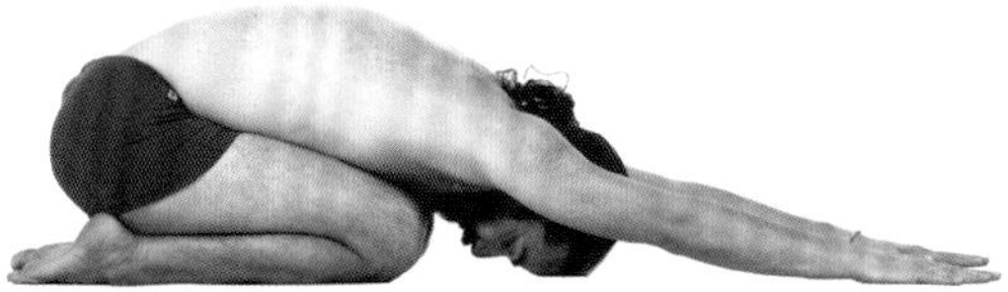

353
वज्र योग मुद्रा आसन
Vajra yoga mudrā āsana
Thunderbolt yoga mudrā pose

वज्रयोगमुद्रासन
Vajrayogamudrāsana

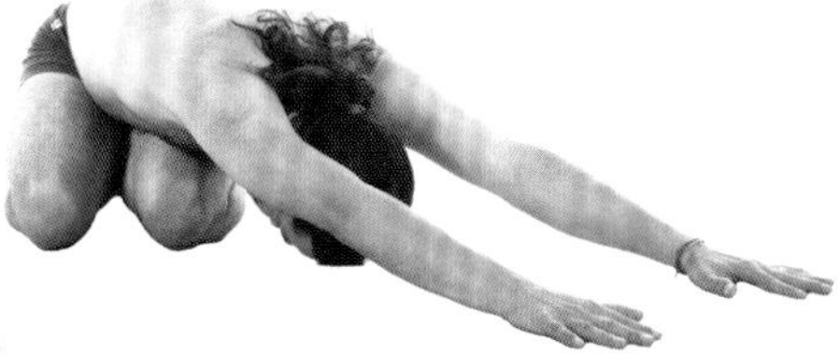

354
पार्श्ववज्र योग मुद्रा आसन
Pārśva vajra yoga mudrā āsana
Side thunderbolt yoga mudrā pose

पार्श्ववज्रयोगमुद्रासन
Pārśvavajrayogamudrāsana

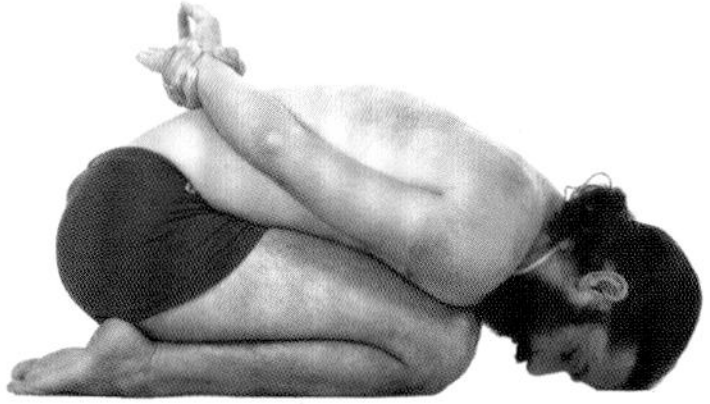

355
वज्र योग मुद्रा आसन (पृष्ठ हस्त बद्ध)
Vajra yoga mudrā āsana (pṛṣṭha hasta baddha)
Thunderbolt yoga mudrā pose (hands bound behind)

वज्रयोगमुद्रासन (पृष्ठहस्तबद्ध)
Vajrayogamudrāsana (pṛṣṭhahastabaddha)

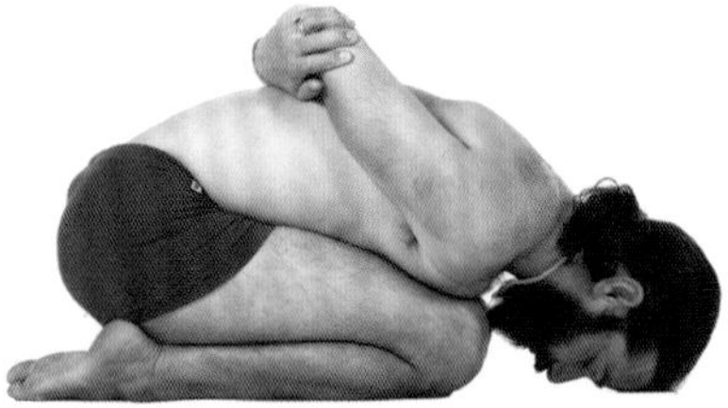

356
वज्र योग मुद्रा (पृष्ठ कफोणि बद्ध)
Vajra yoga mudrā (pṛṣṭha kaphoṇi baddha)
Thunderbolt yoga mudrā pose
(bound elbows behind the back)

वज्रयोगमुद्रा (पृष्ठकफोणिबद्ध)
Vajrayogamudrā (pṛṣṭhakaphoṇibaddha)

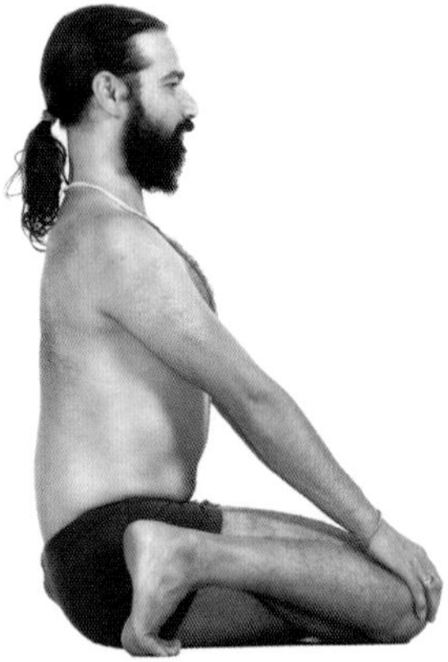

357
विकट वज्र आसन (नितम्ब भू)
Vikaṭa vajra āsana (nitamba bhū)
Challenging thunderbolt pose (hips on the earth)

विकटवज्रासन (नितम्बभू)
Vikaṭavajrāsana (nitambabhū)

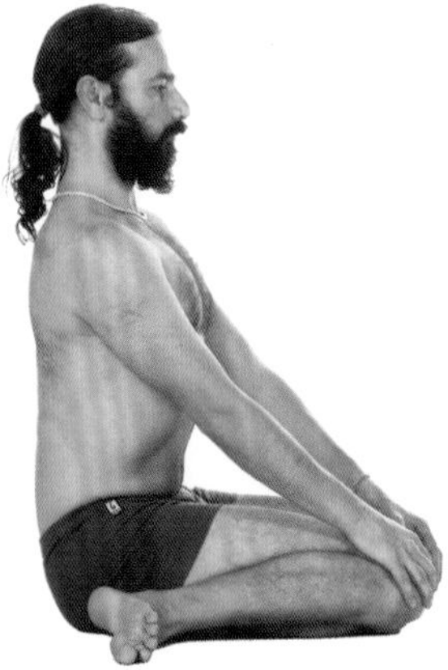

358
ब्रह्मचर्य आसन
Brahmacarya āsana
Containment of vital energy pose

ब्रह्मचर्यासन
Brahmacaryāsana

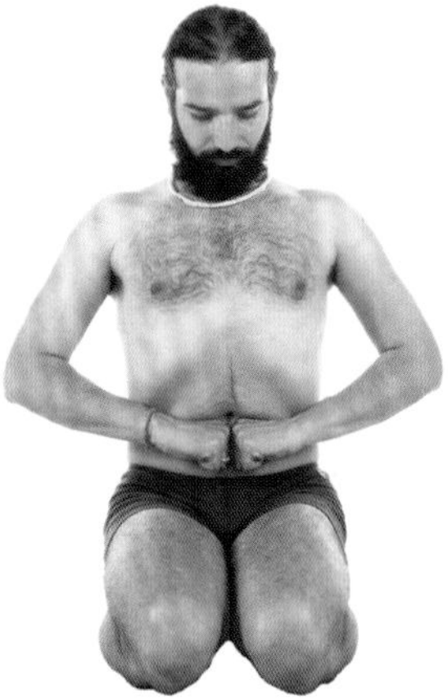

359
मण्डूक आसन(मुष्टि नाभ, आरम्भ अवस्था)
Maṇḍūka āsana (muṣṭi nābha, ārambha avasthā)
Frog pose (fists at the navel, starting position)

मण्डूकासन (मुष्टिनाभ, आरम्भावस्था)
Maṇḍūkāsana (muṣṭinābha, ārambhavasthā)

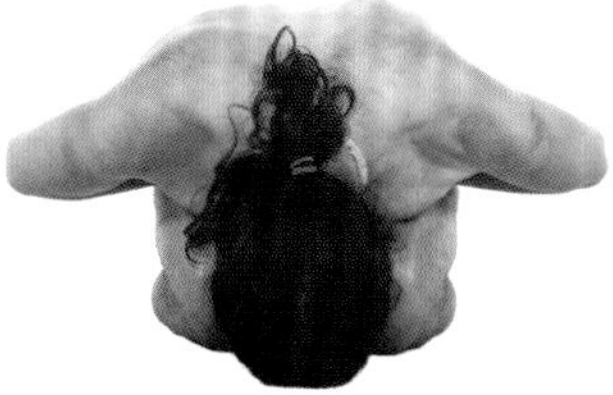

360
मण्डूक आसन (मुष्टि नाभ ललाट भू)
Maṇḍūka āsana (muṣṭi nābha, lalāṭa bhū)
Frog pose (fists at the navel, forehead on the earth)

मण्डूकासन (एकमुष्टिनाभ, ललाटभू)
Maṇḍūkāsana (muṣṭinābha, lalāṭabhū)

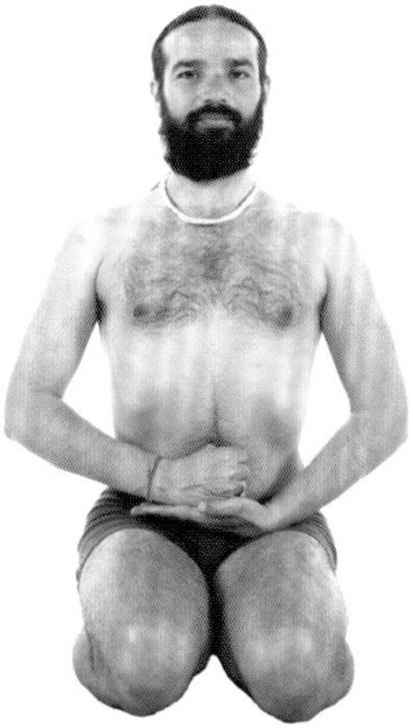

361
मण्डूक आसन (एक मुष्टि नाभ, आरम्भ अवस्था)
Maṇḍūka āsana (eka muṣṭi nābha, ārambha avasthā)
Frog pose (one fist at the navel, starting position)

मण्डूकासन (एकमुष्टिनाभ, आरम्भावस्था)
Maṇḍūkāsana (ekamuṣṭinābha, ārambhavasthā)

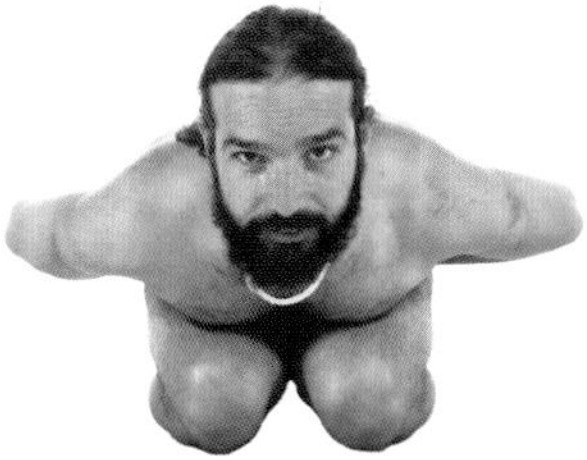

362
मण्डूक आसन (एक मुष्टि नाभ)
Maṇḍūka āsana (eka muṣṭi nābha)
Frog pose (one fist at the navel)

मण्डूकासन (एकमुष्टिनाभ)
Maṇḍūkāsana (ekamuṣṭinābha)

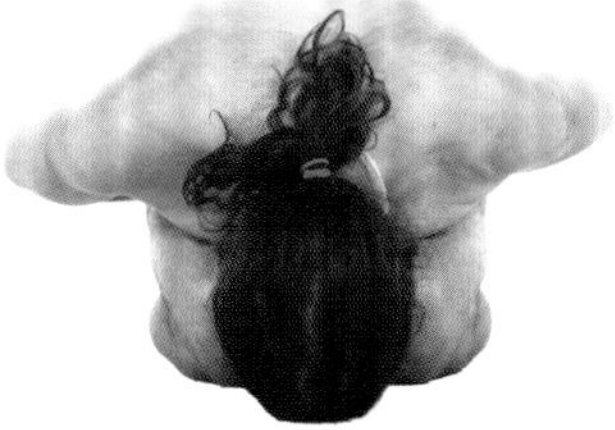

363
मण्डूक आसन (एक मुष्टि नाभ ललाट भू)
Maṇḍūka āsana (eka muṣṭi nābha, lalāṭa bhū)
Frog pose (one fist at the navel, forehead on the earth)

मण्डूकासन (एकमुष्टिनाभ, ललाटभू)
Maṇḍūkāsana (ekamuṣṭinābha, lalāṭabhū)

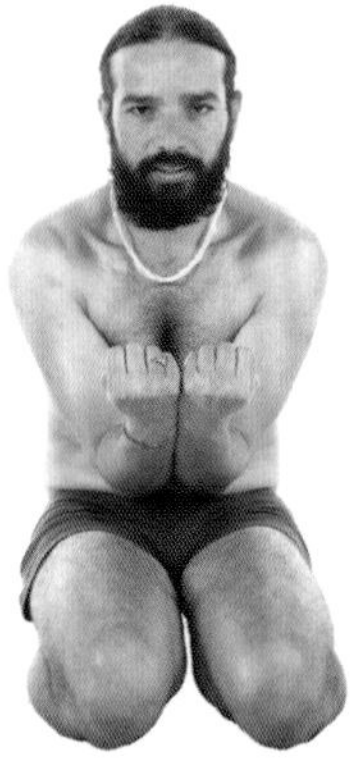

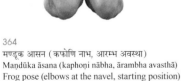

364
मण्डूक आसन (कफोणि नाभ, आरम्भ अवस्था)
Maṇḍūka āsana (kaphoṇi nābha, ārambha avasthā)
Frog pose (elbows at the navel, starting position)

मण्डूकासन (कफोणिनाभ, आरम्भावस्था)
Maṇḍūkāsana (kaphoṇinābha, ārambhāvasthā)

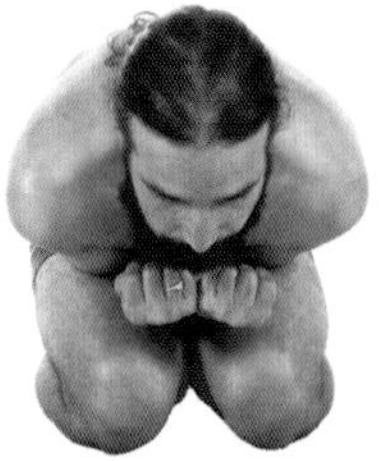

365
मण्डूक आसन (कफोणि नाभ)
Maṇḍūka āsana (kaphoṇi nābha)
Frog pose (elbows at the navel)

मण्डूकासन (कफोणिनाभ)
Maṇḍūkāsana (kaphoṇinābha)

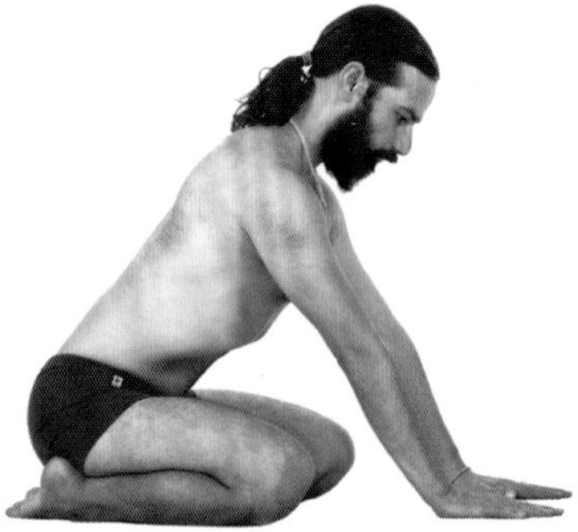

366
बालक आसन (आरम्भ अवस्था)
Bālaka āsana (ārambha avasthā)
Baby pose (starting position)

बालकासन (आरम्भावस्था)
Bālakāsana (ārambhāvasthā)

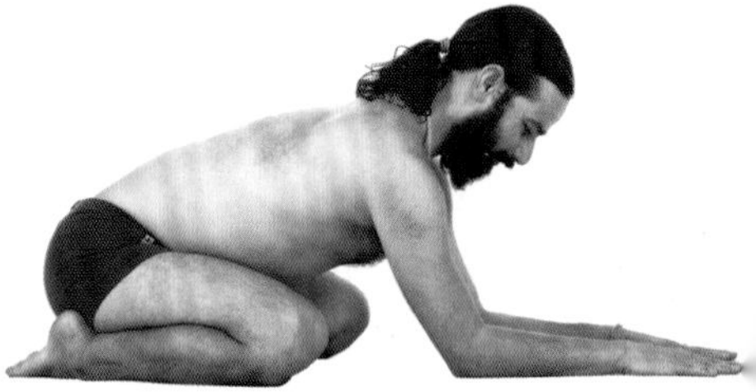

367
बालक आसन (कफोणि भू)
Bālaka āsana (kaphoṇi bhū)
Baby pose (elbows on the earth)

बालकासन (कफोणिभू)
Bālakāsana (kaphoṇibhū)

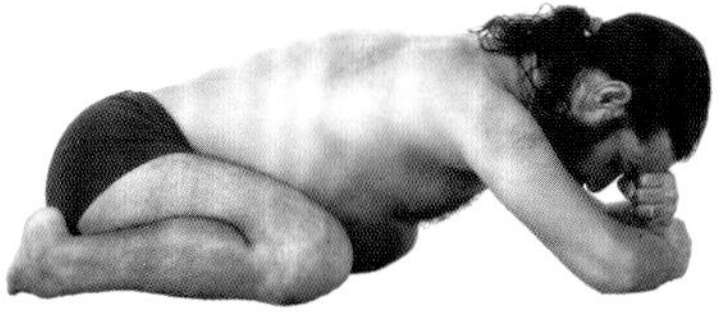

368
बालक आसन (मुष्टिका ललाट धर)
Bālaka āsana (muṣṭika lalāṭa dhara)
Baby pose (forehead on stacked fists)

बालकासन (मुष्टिकाललाटधर)
Bālakāsana (muṣṭikalalāṭadhara)

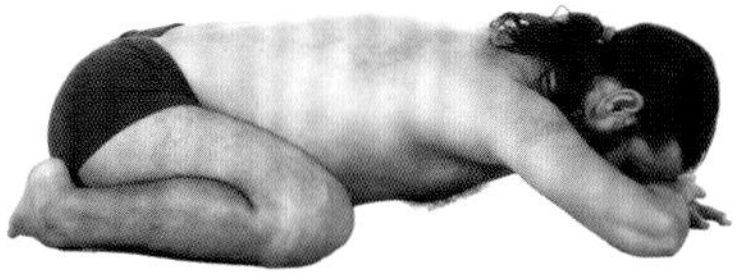

369
बालक आसन (हस्त ललाट धर)
Bālaka āsana (hasta lalāṭa dhara)
Baby pose (forehead on stacked hands)

बालकासन (हस्तललाटधर)
Bālakāsana (hastalalāṭadhara)

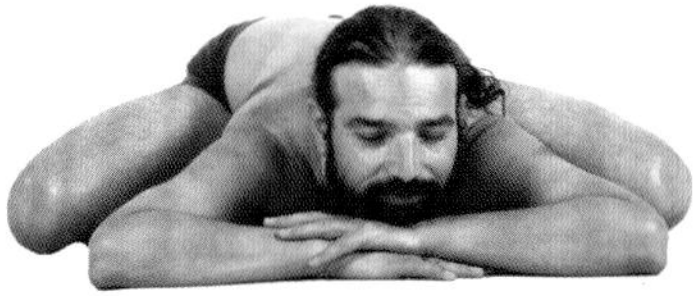

370
बालक आसन (कर पृष्ठ हनु धर)
Bālaka āsana (kara pṛṣṭha hanu dhara)
Baby pose (chin on the hands)

बालकासन (करपृष्ठहनुधर)
Bālakāsana (karapṛṣṭhahanudhara)

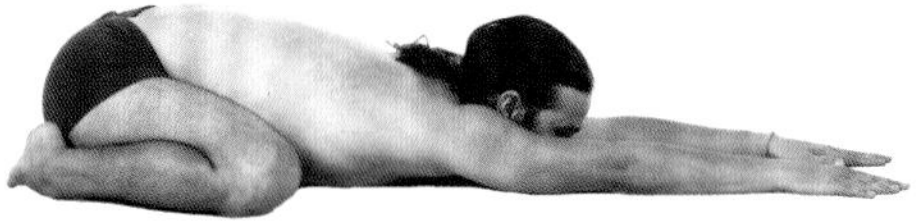

371
बालक आसन (हनु भू)
Bālaka āsana (hanu bhū)
Baby pose (chin on the earth)

बालकासन (हनुभू)
Bālakāsana (hanubhū)

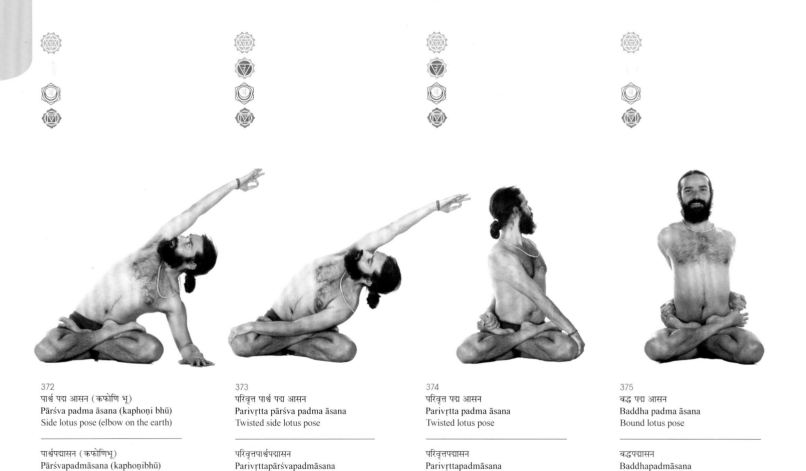

372
पार्श्व पद्म आसन (कफोणि भू)
Pārśva padma āsana (kaphoṇi bhū)
Side lotus pose (elbow on the earth)

पार्श्वपद्मासन (कफोणिभू)
Pārśvapadmāsana (kaphoṇibhū)

373
परिवृत्त पार्श्व पद्म आसन
Parivṛtta pārśva padma āsana
Twisted side lotus pose

परिवृत्तपार्श्वपद्मासन
Parivṛttapārśvapadmāsana

374
परिवृत्त पद्म आसन
Parivṛtta padma āsana
Twisted lotus pose

परिवृत्तपद्मासन
Parivṛttapadmāsana

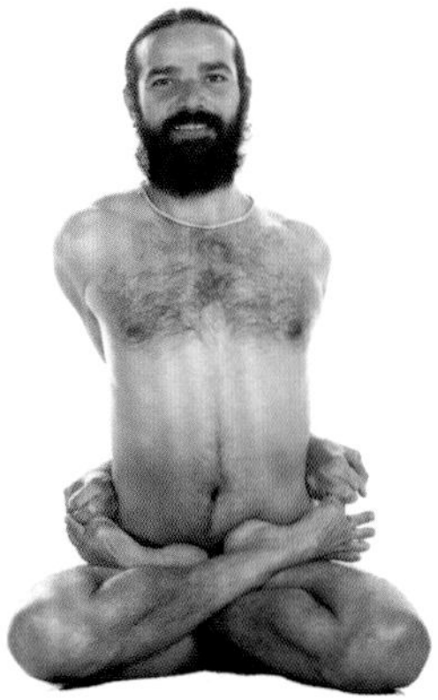

375
बद्ध पद्म आसन
Baddha padma āsana
Bound lotus pose

बद्धपद्मासन
Baddhapadmāsana

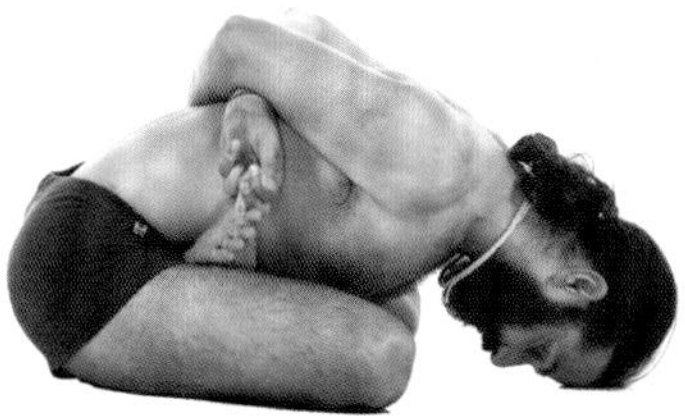

376
योग मुद्रा आसन
Yoga mudrā āsana
Seal of yoga pose

योगमुद्रासन
Yogamudrāsana

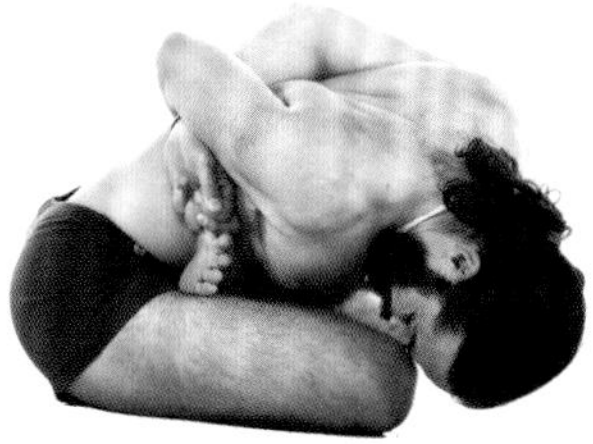

377
सुश्रुत योग मुद्रा आसन (जानु ललाट)
Suśruta yoga mudrā āsana (jānu lalāṭa)
Seal of Sage Suśruta pose (forehead to knee)

सुश्रुतयोगमुद्रासन (जानुललाट)
Suśrutayogamudrāsana (jānulalāṭa)

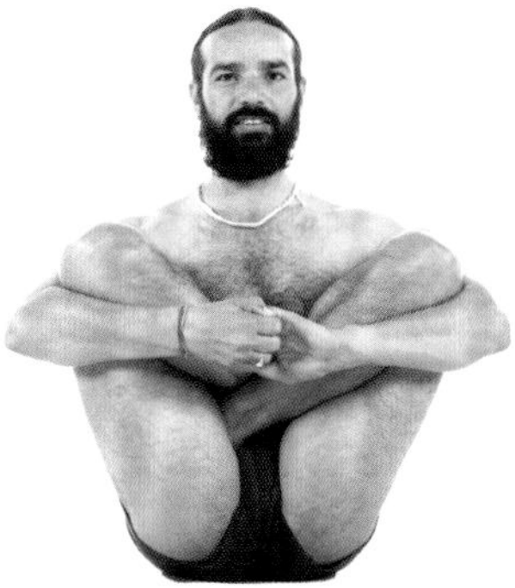

378
उत्तोलन पद्म नाभि आसन (रज्जु हस्त)
Uttolana padma nābhi āsana (rajju hasta)
Balancing lotus navel pose (bound hands)

उत्तोलनपद्मनाभ्यासन (रज्जुहस्त)
Uttolanapadmanābhyāsana (rajjuhasta)

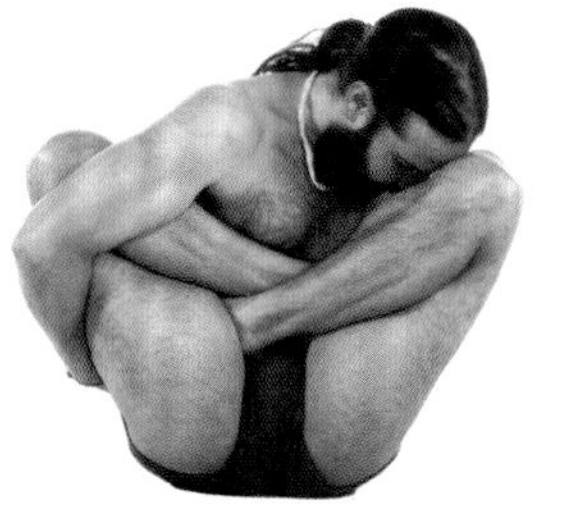

379
उत्तोलन पद्म नाभि आसन (एक जानु ललाट रज्जु हस्त)
Uttolana padma nābhi āsana (eka jānu lalāṭa rajju hasta)
Balancing lotus navel pose (bound, one knee to forehead)

उत्तोलनपद्मनाभ्यासन (एकजानुललाटरज्जुहस्त)
Uttolanapadmānābhyāsana (ekajānulalāṭarajjuhasta)

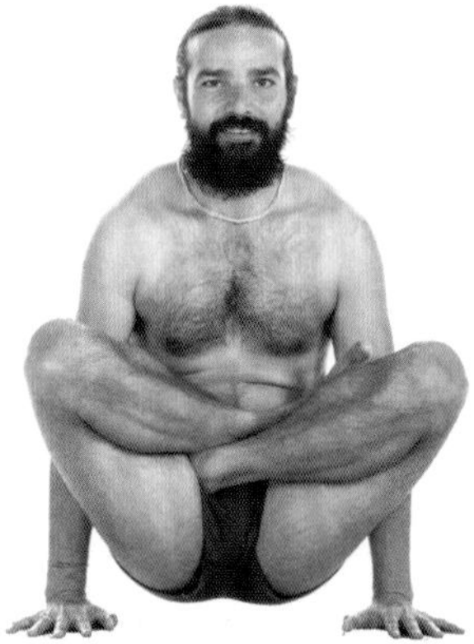

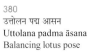

380
उत्तोलन पद्म आसन
Uttolana padma āsana
Balancing lotus pose

उत्तोलनपद्मासन
Uttolanapadmāsana

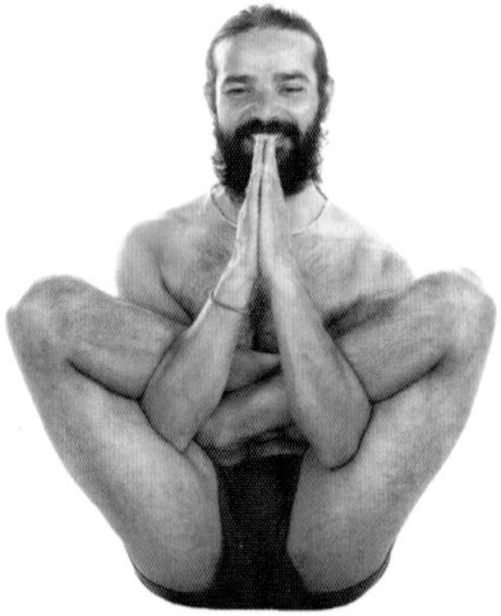

381
उपविष्ट गर्भ पिण्ड आसन (नमस्कार)
Upaviṣṭa garbha piṇḍa āsana (namaskāra)
Sitting womb pose (hands in prayer)

उपविष्टगर्भपिण्डासन (नमस्कार)
Upaviṣṭagarbhapiṇḍāsana (namaskāra)

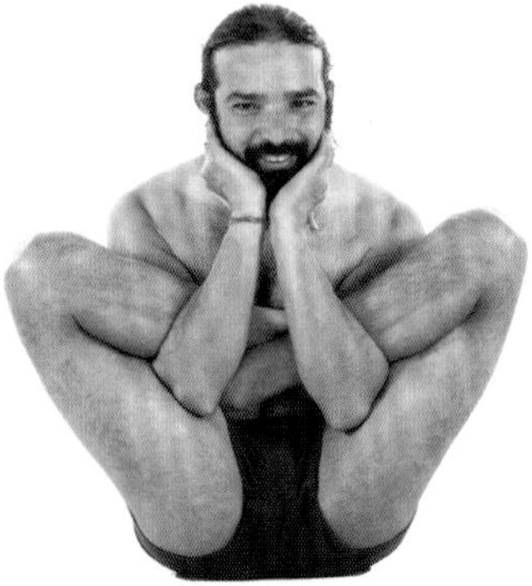

382
उपविष्ट गर्भ पिण्ड आसन
Upaviṣṭa garbha piṇḍa āsana
Sitting womb pose

उपविष्टगर्भपिण्डासन
Upaviṣṭagarbhapiṇḍāsana

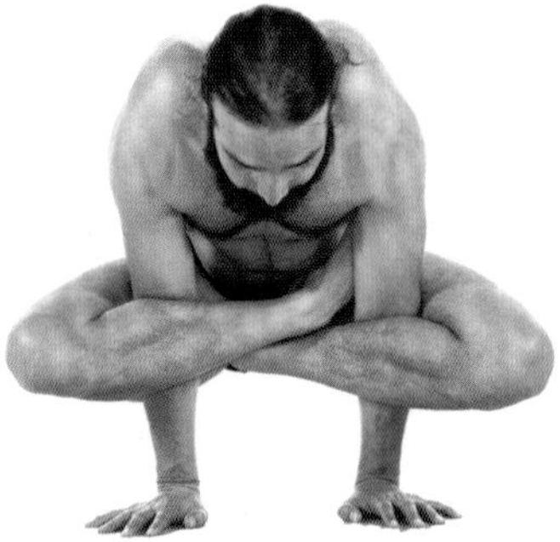

383
कुक्कुट आसन
Kukkuṭa āsana
Rooster pose

कुक्कुटासन
Kukkuṭāsana

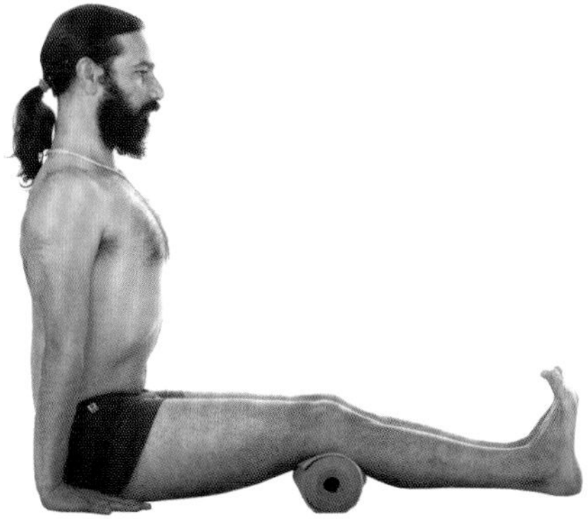

384
दण्ड आसन (सालम्ब)
Daṇḍa āsana (sālamba)
Staff pose (supported)

दण्डासन (सालम्ब)
Daṇḍāsana (sālamba)

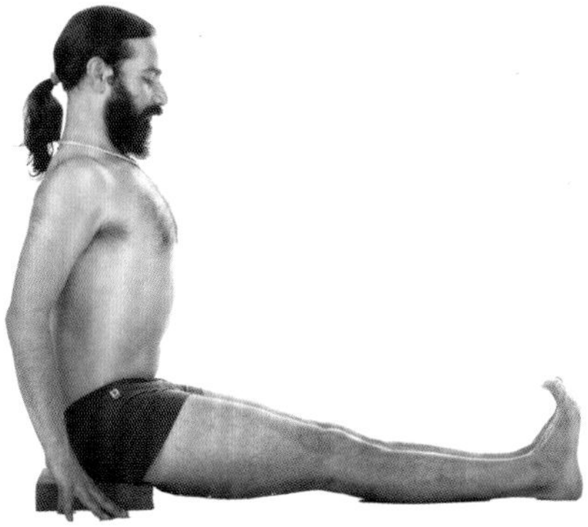

385
दण्ड आसन (सालम्ब मूल)
Daṇḍa āsana (sālamba mūla)
Staff pose (supported root)

दण्डासन (सालम्बमूल)
Daṇḍāsana (sālambamūla)

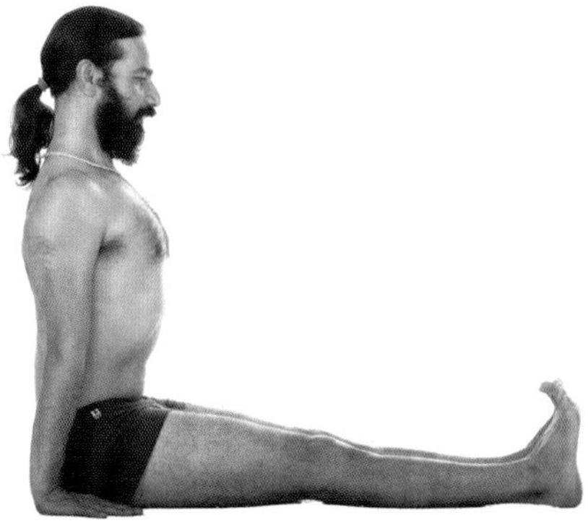

386
दण्ड आसन
Daṇḍa āsana
Staff pose

दण्डासन
Daṇḍāsana

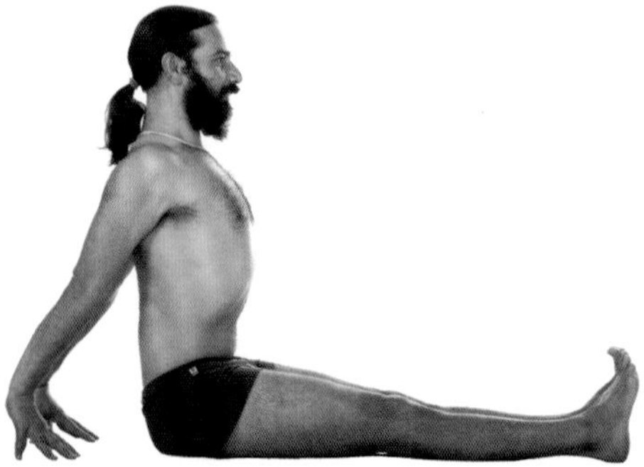

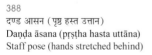

387
दण्ड आसन (पृष्ठ अङ्गुल भू)
Daṇḍa āsana (pṛṣṭha aṅgula bhū)
Staff pose (fingers on the earth behind)

दण्डासन (पृष्ठाङ्गुलभू)
Daṇḍāsana (pṛṣṭhāṅgulabhū)

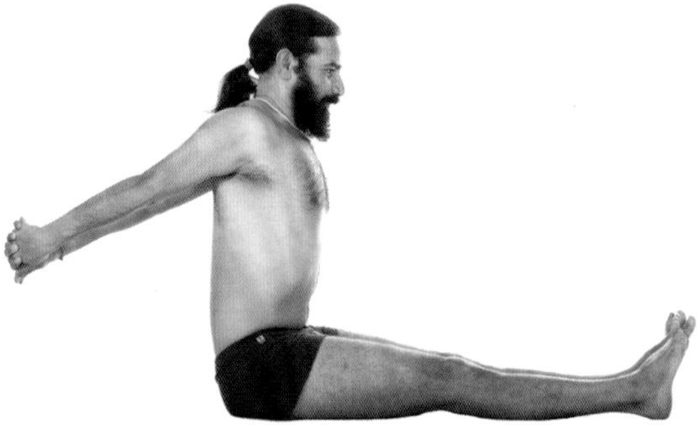

388
दण्ड आसन (पृष्ठ हस्त उत्तान)
Daṇḍa āsana (pṛṣṭha hasta uttāna)
Staff pose (hands stretched behind)

दण्डासन (पृष्ठहस्तोत्तान)
Daṇḍāsana (pṛṣṭhahastottāna)

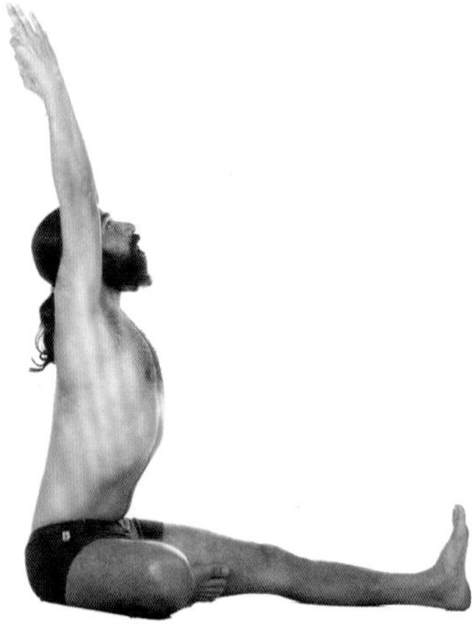

389
जानु शीर्ष आसन (आरम्भ अवस्था)
Jānu śīrṣa āsana (ārambha āvasthā)
Head to knee pose (starting position)

जानुशीर्षासन (आरम्भावस्था)
Jānuśīrṣāsana (ārambhāvasthā)

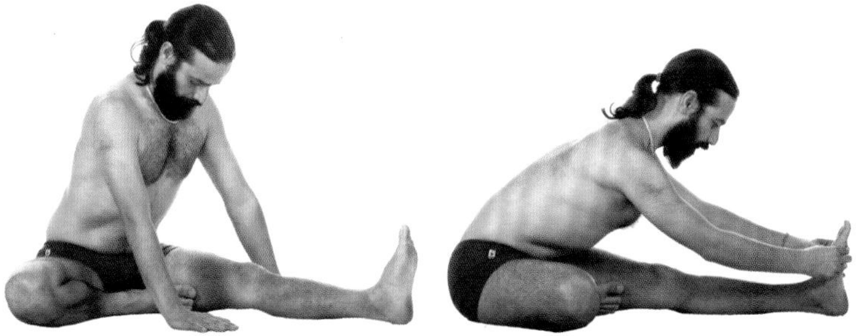

390
अर्ध जानु शीर्ष आसन
Ardha jānu śīrṣa āsana
Halfway head to knee pose

अर्धजानुशीर्षासन
Ardhajānuśīrṣāsana

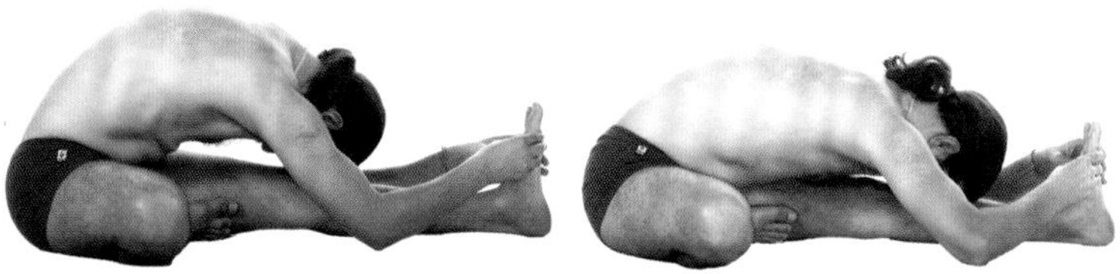

391
जानु शीर्ष आसन (कफोणि भू)
Jānu śīrṣa āsana (kaphoṇi bhū)
Head to knee pose (elbows on the earth)

जानुशीर्षासन (कफोणिभू)
Jānuśīrśāsana (kaphoṇibhū)

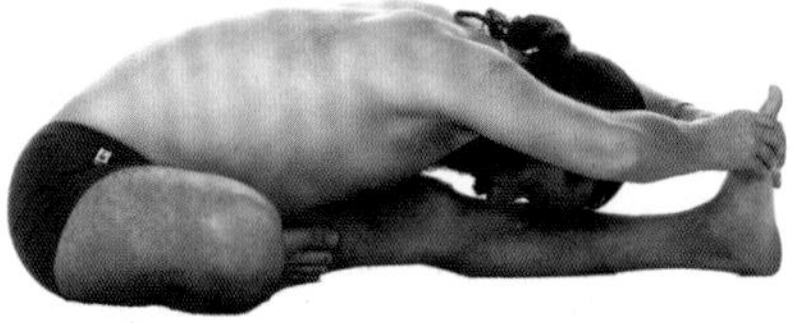

392
जानु शीर्ष आसन (उत्कफोणि)
Jānu śīrṣa āsana (utkaphoṇi)
Head to knee pose (elbows up)

जानुशीर्षासन (उत्कफोणि)
Jānuśīrṣāsana (utkaphoṇi)

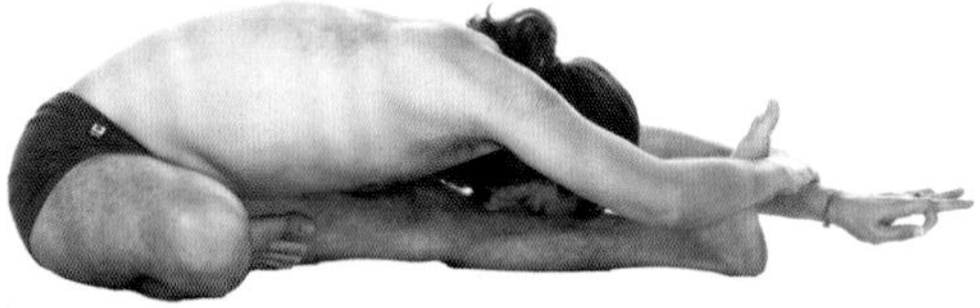

393
जानु शीर्ष आसन (बद्ध हस्त)
Jānu śīrṣa āsana (baddha hasta)
Head to knee pose (bound hands)

जानुशीर्षासन (बद्धहस्त)
Jānuśīrṣāsana (baddhahasta)

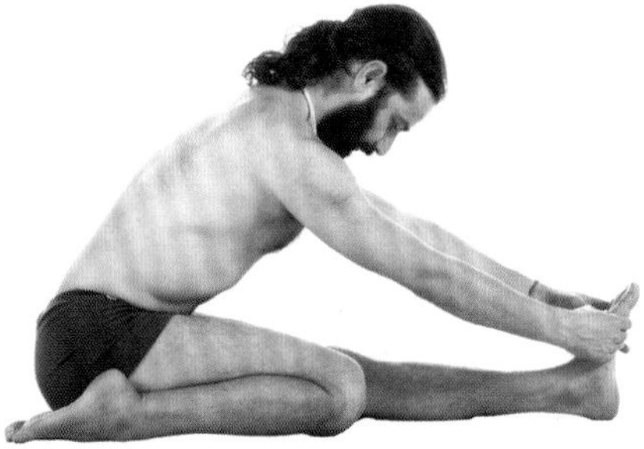

394
अर्ध वज्र जानु शीर्ष आसन
Ardha vajra jānu śīrṣa āsana
Halfway thunderbolt head to knee pose

अर्धवज्रजानुशीर्षासन
Ardhavajrajānuśīrṣāsana

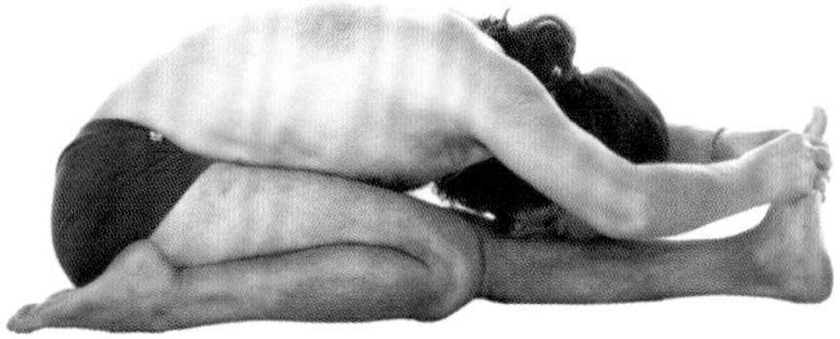

395
वज्र जानु शीर्ष आसन (उत्कफोणि)
Vajra jānu śīrṣa āsana (utkaphoṇi)
Thunderbolt head to knee pose (elbows up)

वज्रजानुशीर्षासन (उत्कफोणि)
Vajrajānuśīrṣāsana (utkaphoṇi)

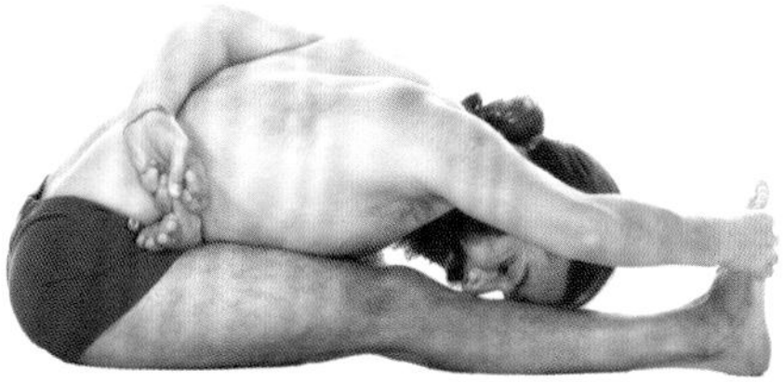

396
अर्ध बद्ध पद्म जानु शीर्ष आसन (उत्कफोणि)
Ardha baddha padma jānu śīrṣa āsana (utkaphoṇi)
Half bound lotus head to knee pose (elbows up)

अर्धबद्धपद्मजानुशीर्षासन (उत्कफोणि)
Ardhabaddhapadmajānuśīrṣāsana (utkaphoṇi)

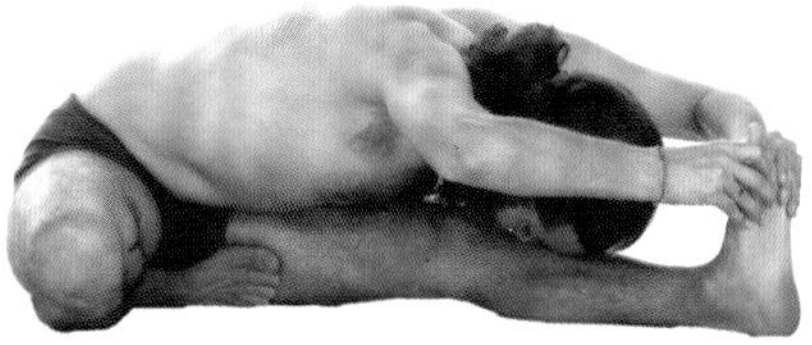

397
जानु शीर्ष आसन (एक पाद उपरि मूल, उत्कफोणि)
Jānu śīrṣa āsana (eka pāda upari mūla, utkaphoṇi)
Head to knee pose (sitting on one foot, elbows up)

जानुशीर्षासन (एकपादोपरिमूल, उत्कफोणि)
Jānuśīrṣāsana (ekapādoparimūla, utkaphoṇi)

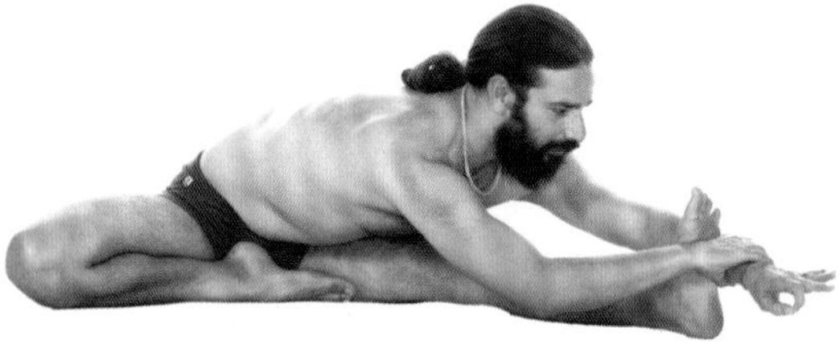

398
पार्श्व जानु शीर्ष आसन (बद्ध हस्त,आरम्भ अवस्था)
Pārśva jānu śīrṣa āsana (baddha hasta, ārambha āvasthā)
Side head to knee pose (bound hands, starting position)

पार्श्वजानुशीर्षासन (बद्धहस्तारम्भावस्था)
Pārśvajānuśīrṣāsana (baddhahasta, ārambhāvasthā)

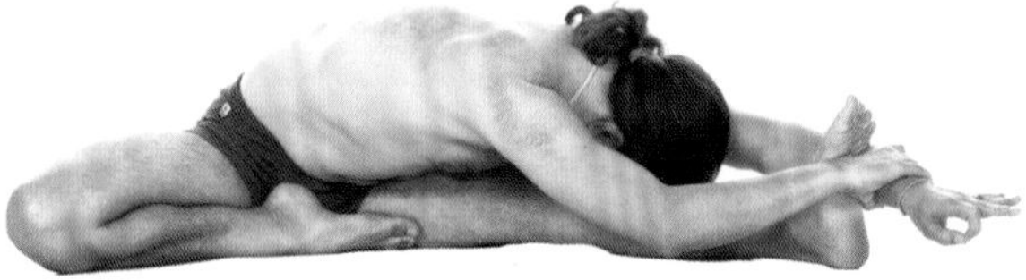

399
पार्श्व जानु शीर्ष आसन (बद्ध हस्त)
Pārśva jānu śīrṣa āsana (baddha hasta)
Side head to knee pose (bound hands)

पार्श्वजानुशीर्षासन (बद्धहस्त)
Pārśvajānuśīrṣāsana (baddhahasta)

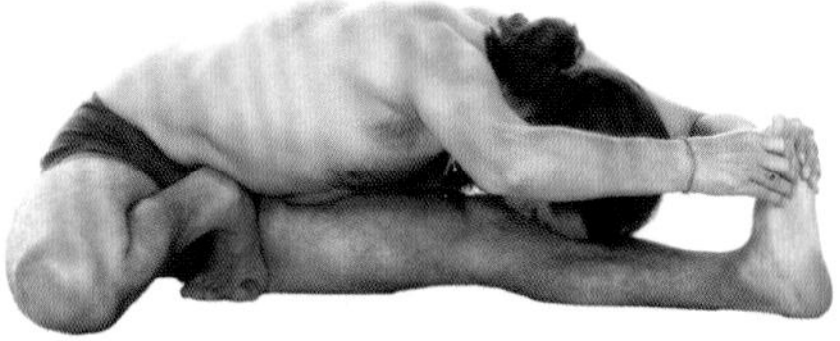

400
पाद अङ्गुल भू जानु शीर्ष आसन
Pāda aṅgula bhū jānu śīrṣa āsana
Toes on the earth head to knee pose

पादाङ्गुलभूजानुशीर्षासन
Pādāṅgulabhūjānuśīrṣāsana

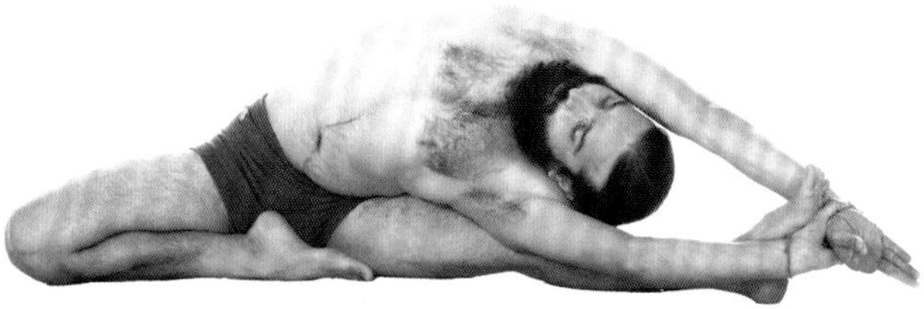

401
परिवृत्त पार्श्व जानु शीर्ष आसन (बद्ध हस्त)
Parivṛtta pārśva jānu śīrṣa āsana (baddha hasta)
Twisted side head to knee pose (bound hands)

परिवृत्तपार्श्वजानुशीर्षासन (बद्धहस्त)
Parivṛttapārśvajānuśīrṣāsana (baddhahasta)

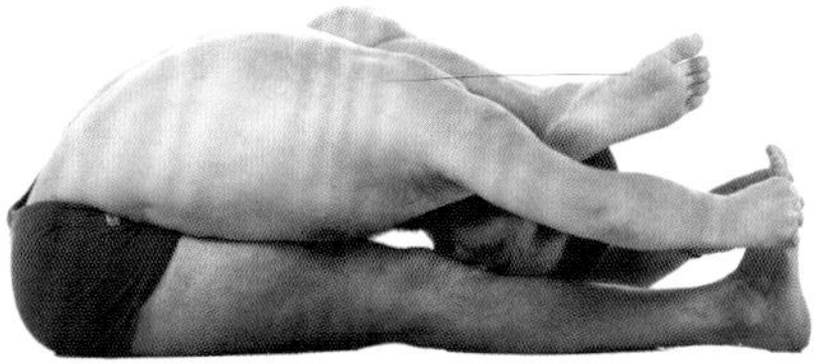

402
जानु शिर भैरव आसन (उत्कफोणि)
Jānu śira bhairava āsana (utkaphoṇi)
Head to knee fearless pose (elbows up)

जानुशिरभैरवासन (उत्कफोणि)
Jānuśirabhairavāsana (utkaphoṇi)

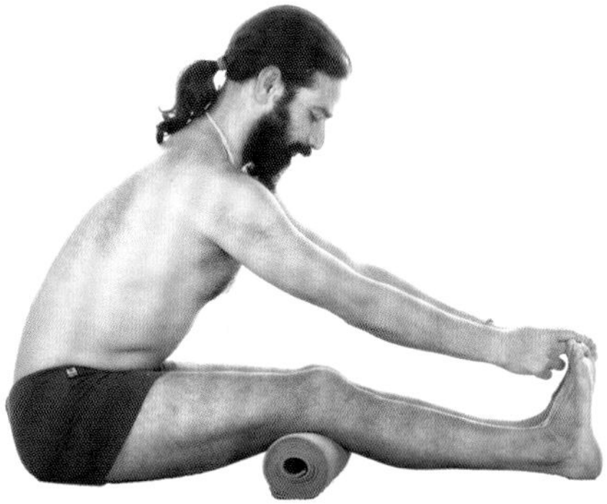

403
अर्ध पश्चिम उत्तान आसन (सालम्ब)
Ardha paścima uttāna āsana (sālamba)
Half back stretch pose (supported)

अर्धपश्चिमोत्तानासन (सालम्ब)
Ardhapaścimottānāsana (sālamba)

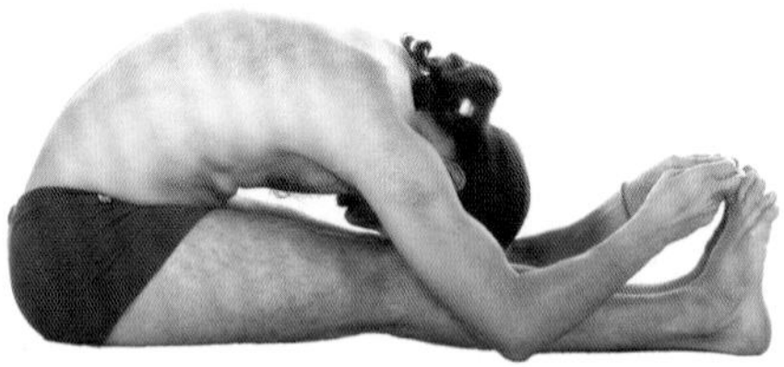

404
पश्चिम उत्तान आसन (कफोणि भू जानु शीर्ष)
Paścima uttāna āsana (kaphoṇi bhū jānu śīrṣa)
Back stretch pose (elbows on the earth, head to knee, chin to throat, round back)

पश्चिमोत्तानासन (कफोणिभूजानुशीर्ष)
Paścimottānāsana (kaphoṇibhūjānuśīrṣa)

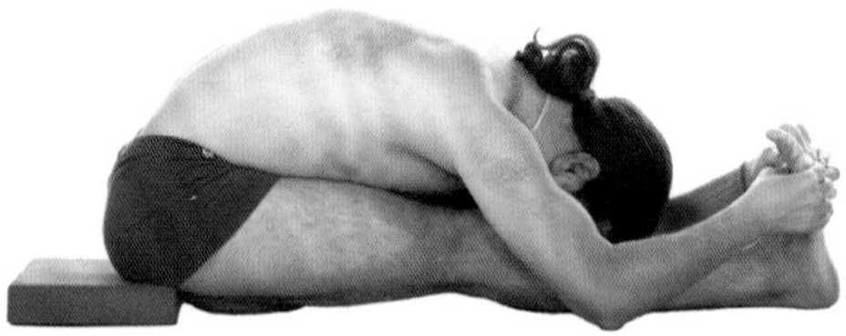

405
पश्चिम उत्तान आसन (कफोणि भू, सालम्बमूल)
Paścima uttāna āsana (kaphoṇi bhū, sālamba mūla)
Back stretch pose (elbows on the earth, supported root)

पश्चिमोत्तानासन (कफोणिभू, सालम्बमूल)
Paścimottānāsana (kaphoṇibhū, sālambamūla)

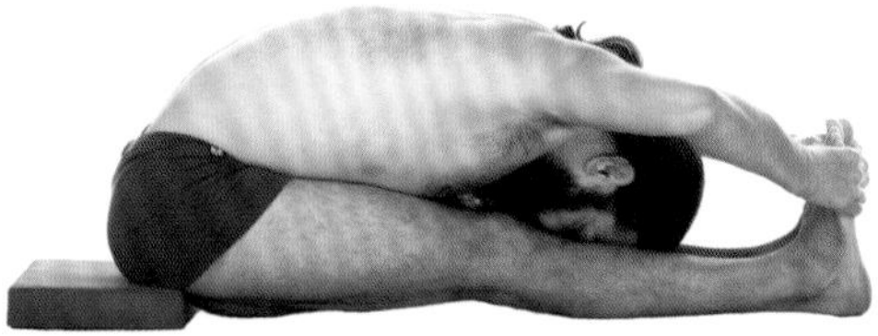

406
पश्चिम उत्तान आसन (उत्कफोणि, सालम्ब मूल)
Paścima uttāna āsana (utkaphoṇi bhū, sālamba mūla)
Back stretch pose (elbows up, supported root)

पश्चिमोत्तानासन (उत्कफोणि, सालम्बमूल)
Paścimottānāsana (utkaphoṇibhū, sālambamūla)

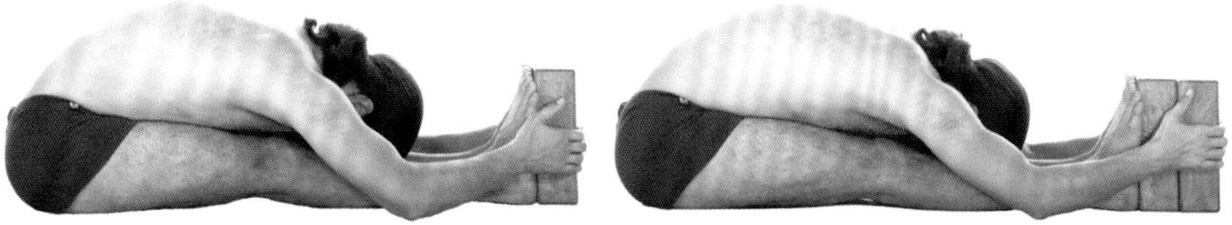

407
पश्चिम उत्तान आसन (कफोणि भू सालम्ब पाद)
Paścima uttāna āsana (kaphoṇi bhū, sālamba pāda)
Back stretch pose (elbows on the earth, supported feet)

पश्चिमोत्तानासन (कफोणिभूसालम्बपाद)
Paścimottānāsana (kaphoṇibhūsālambapāda)

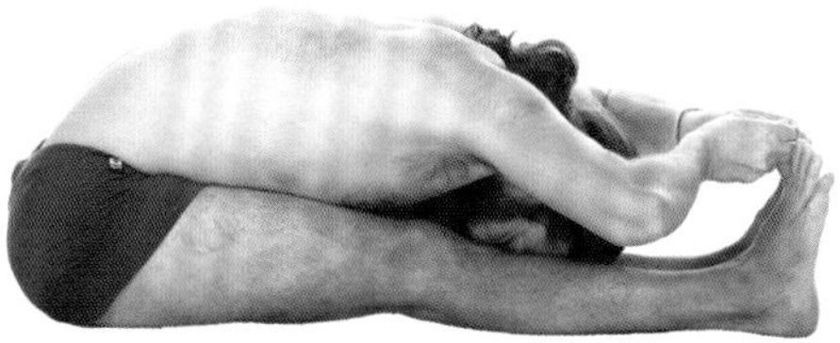

408
पश्चिम उत्तान आसन (उत्कफोणि, बद्ध पाद अङ्गुष्ठ)
Paścima uttāna āsana (utkaphoṇi, baddha pāda aṅguṣṭha)
Back stretch pose (elbows up, bound toes)

पश्चिमोत्तानासन (उत्कफोणि, बद्धपादाङ्गुष्ठ)
Paścimottānāsana (utkaphoṇi baddhapādāṅguṣṭha)

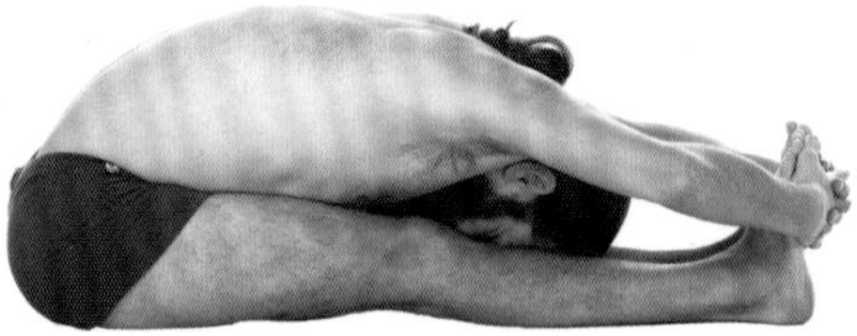

409
पश्चिम उत्तान आसन (उत्कफोणि, हस्त पाद बद्ध)
Paścima uttāna āsana (utkaphoṇi, hasta pāda baddha)
Back stretch pose (elbows up, bound feet)

पश्चिमोत्तानासन (उत्कफोणि, हस्तपादबद्ध)
Paścimottānāsana (utkaphoṇi, hastapādabaddha)

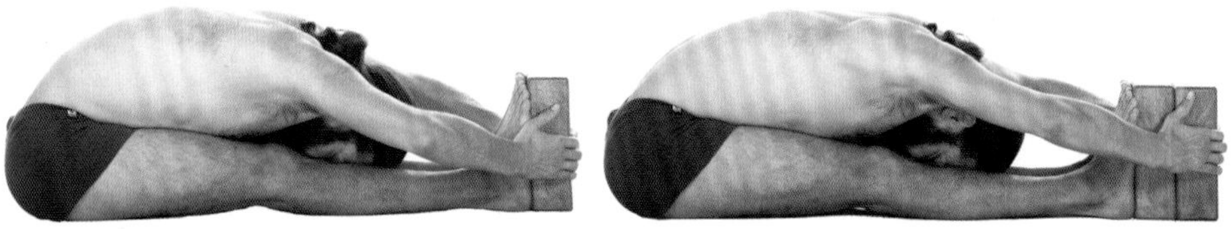

410
पश्चिम उत्तान आसन (उत्कफोणि, सालम्ब पाद)
Paścima uttāna āsana (utkaphoṇi, sālamba pāda)
Back stretch pose (elbows up, supported feet)

पश्चिमोत्तानासन (उत्कफोणि, सालम्बपाद)
Paścimottānāsana (utkaphoṇi, sālambapāda)

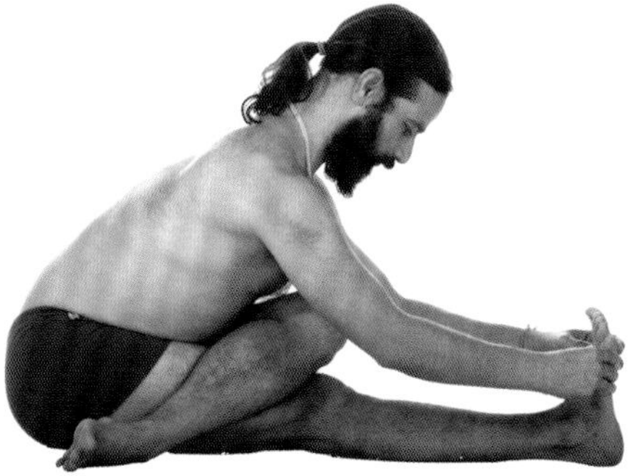

411
गो मुख पश्चिम उत्तान आसन
Go mukha paścima uttāna āsana
Cow face back stretch pose

गोमुखपश्चिमोत्तानासन
Gomukhapaścimottānāsana

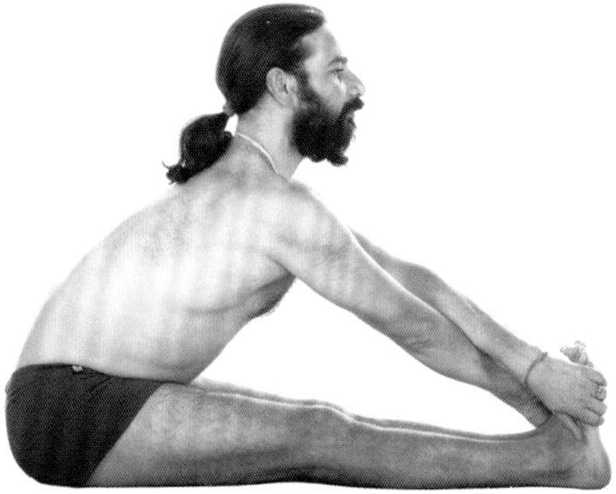

412
अर्ध पश्चिम उत्तान (विपरीत हस्त पाद बद्ध)
Ardha paścima uttāna (viparīta hasta pāda baddha)
Half back stretch pose (hands bound to opposite feet)

अर्धपश्चिमोत्तान (विपरीतहस्तपादबद्ध)
Ardhapaścimottāna (viparītahastapādabaddha)

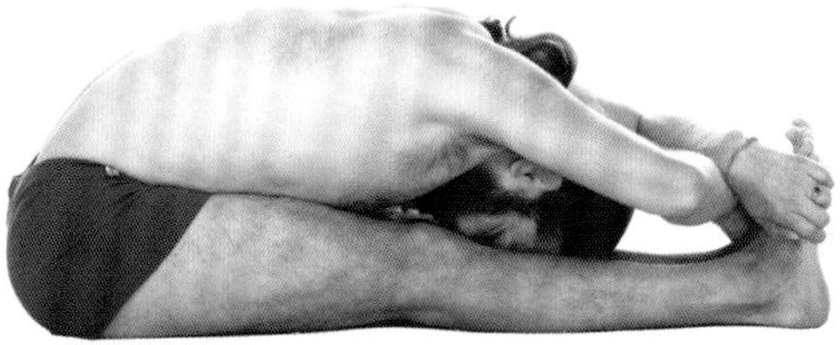

413
पश्चिम उत्तान (विपरीत हस्त पाद बद्ध)
Paścima uttāna (viparīta hasta pāda baddha)
Back stretch pose (hands bound to opposite feet)

पश्चिमोत्तान (विपरीतहस्तपादबद्ध)
Paścimottāna (viparītahastapādabaddha)

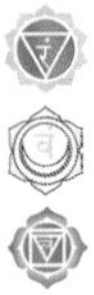

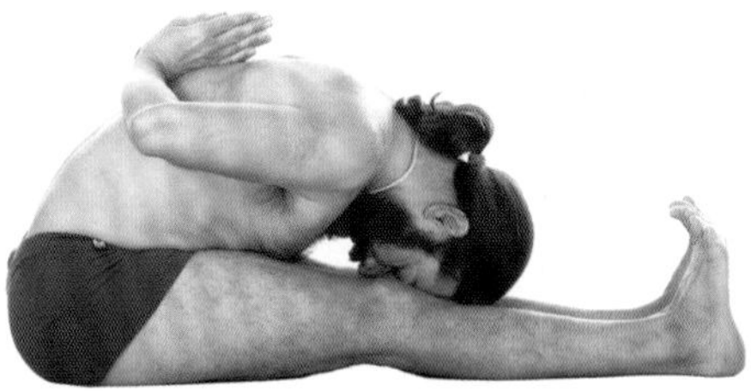

414
पश्चिम उत्तान आसन (पृष्ठ नमस्कार)
Paścima uttāna āsana (pṛṣṭha namaskāra)
Back stretch pose (hands behind in prayer)

पश्चिमोत्तानासन (पृष्ठनमस्कार)
Paścimottānāsana (pṛṣṭhanamaskāra)

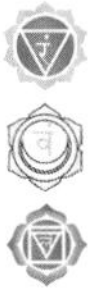

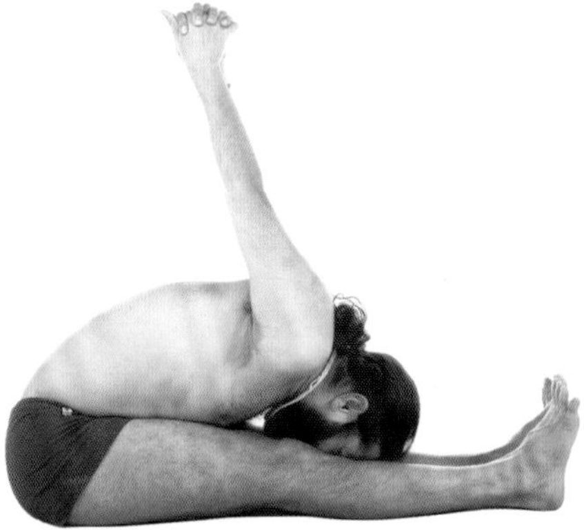

415
पश्चिम उत्तान आसन (पृष्ठ हस्त उत्तान)
Paścima uttāna āsana (pṛṣṭha hasta uttāna)
Back stretch pose (hands stretched behind)

पश्चिमोत्तानासन (पृष्ठहस्तोत्तान)
Paścimottānāsana (pṛṣṭhahastottāna)

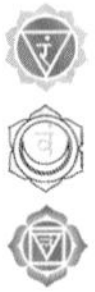

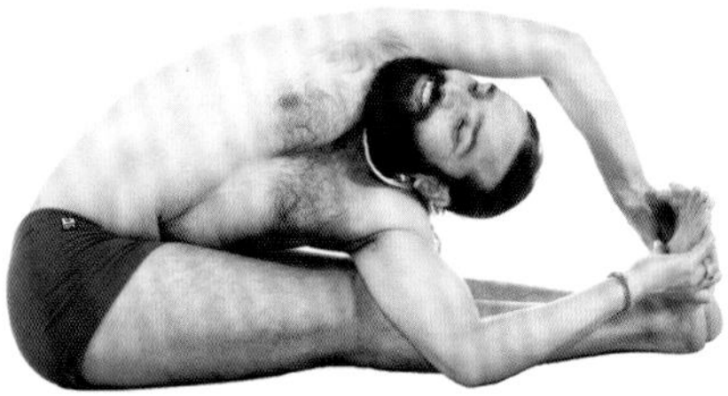

416
परिवृत्त पश्चिम उत्तान आसन
Parivṛtta paścima uttāna āsana
Twisted back stretch pose

परिवृत्तपश्चिमोत्तानासन
Parivṛttapaścimottānāsana

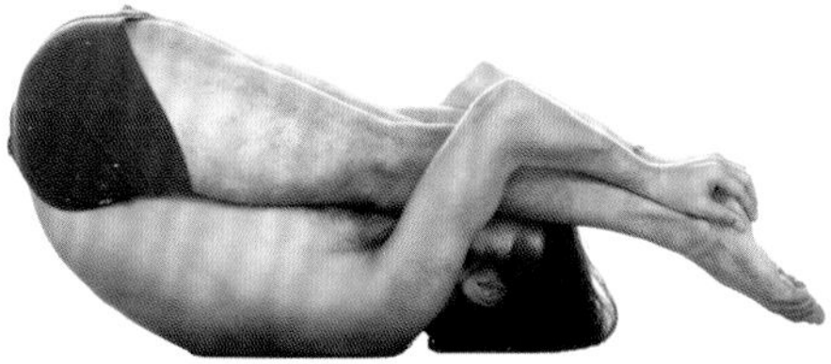

417
पश्चिम उत्तान आसन (मेरु भू)
Paścima uttāna āsana (meru bhū)
Back stretch pose (spine on the earth)

पश्चिमोत्तानासन (मेरुभू)
Paścimottānāsana (merubhū)

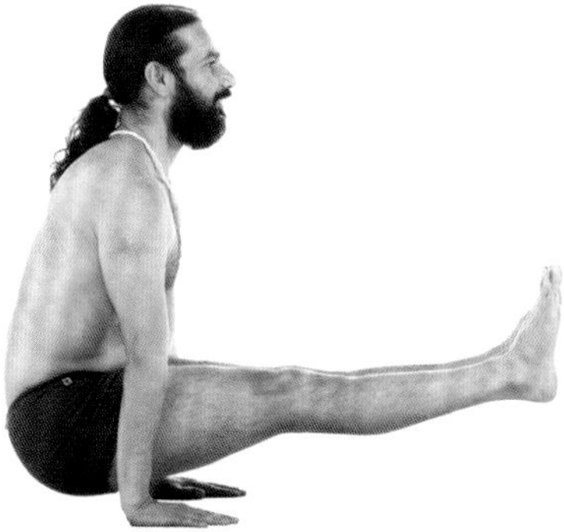

418
दण्ड तुला आसन (कर तल भू)
Daṇḍa tulā āsana (karatala bhū)
Balancing staff pose (palms on the earth)

दण्डतुलासन (करतलभू)
Daṇḍatulāsana (karatalabhū)

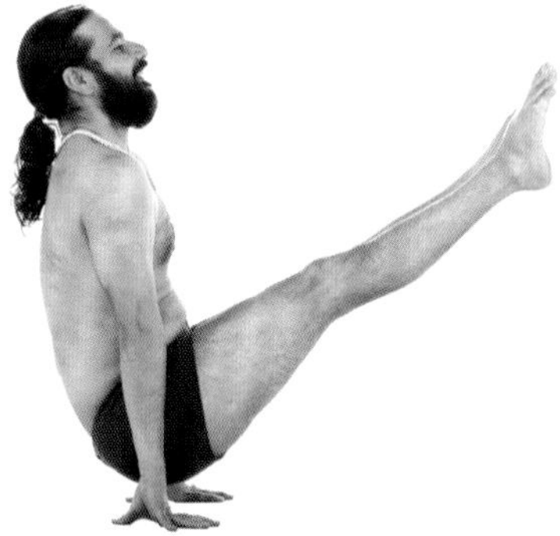

419
दण्ड तुला आसन (उत्तान पाद, हस्त अङ्गुल भू)
Daṇḍa tulā āsana (uttāna pāda, hasta aṅgula bhū)
Balancing staff pose (legs lifted, fingers on the earth)

दण्डतुलासन (उत्तानपाद, हस्ताङ्गुलभू)
Daṇḍatulāsana (uttānapāda, hastāṅgulabhū)

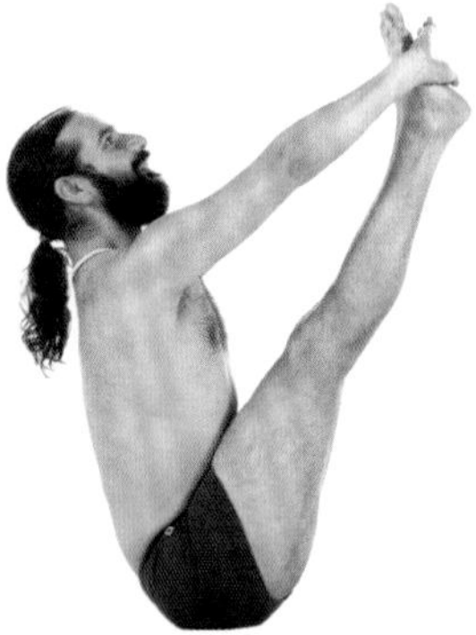

420
उत्तोलन पश्चिम उत्तान आसन (आरम्भ अवस्था)
Uttolana paścima uttāna āsana (ārambha avasthā)
Balancing back stretch pose (starting position)

उत्तोलनपश्चिमोत्तानासन (आरम्भावस्था)
Uttolanapaścimottānāsana (ārambhāvasthā)

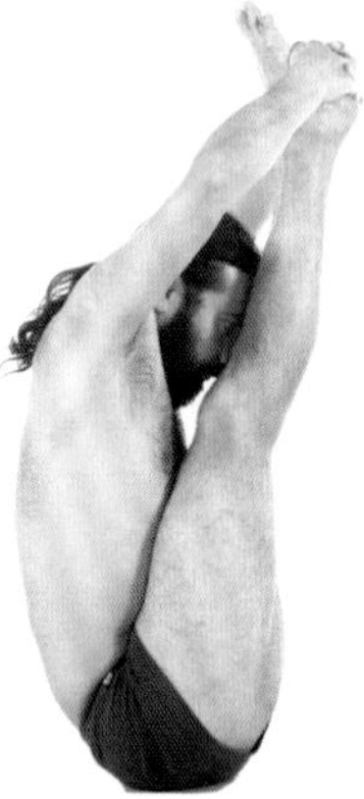

421
उत्तोलन पश्चिम उत्तान आसन
Uttolana paścima uttāna āsana
Balancing back stretch pose

उत्तोलनपश्चिमोत्तानासन
Uttolanapaścimottānāsana

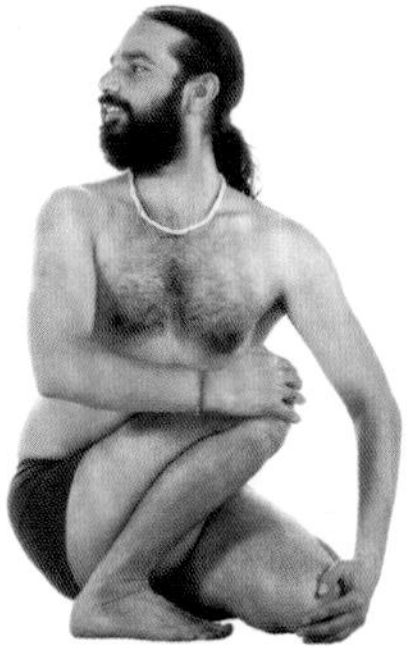

422
उदर आकुञ्चन आसन
Udara ākuñcana āsana
Abdominal cleansing pose

उदराकुञ्चनासन
Udarākuñcanāsana

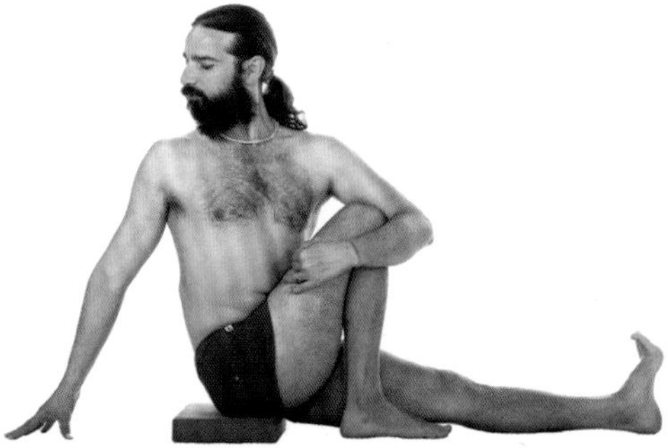

423
परिवृत्त वक्र आसन (अन्तर्पार्श्व पाद, सालम्ब मूल)
Parivṛtta vakra āsana (antarpārśva pāda, sālamba mūla)
Seated twist pose (foot inside, supported root)

परिवृत्तवक्रासन (अन्तर्पार्श्वपाद, सालम्बमूल)
Parivṛttavakrāsana (antarpārśvapāda, sālambamūla)

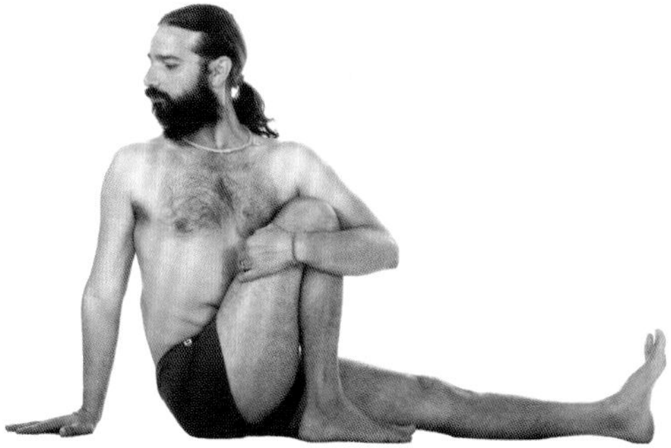

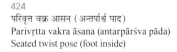

424
परिवृत्त वक्र आसन (अन्तर्पार्श्व पाद)
Parivṛtta vakra āsana (antarpārśva pāda)
Seated twist pose (foot inside)

परिवृत्तवक्रासन (अन्तर्पार्श्वपाद)
Parivṛttavakrāsana (antarpārśvapāda)

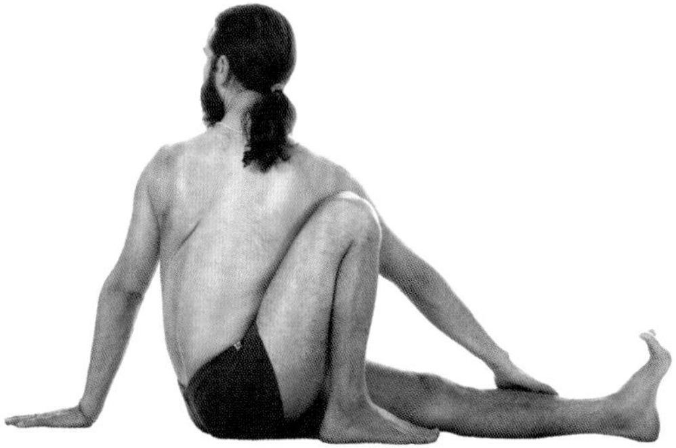

425
विपरीत परिवृत्त वक्र आसन (अन्तर्पार्श्व पाद)
Viparīta parivṛtta vakra āsana (antarpārśva pāda)
Reverse seated twist pose (foot inside)

विपरीतपरिवृत्तवक्रासन (अन्तर्पार्श्वपाद)
Viparītaparivṛttavakrāsana (antarpārśvapāda)

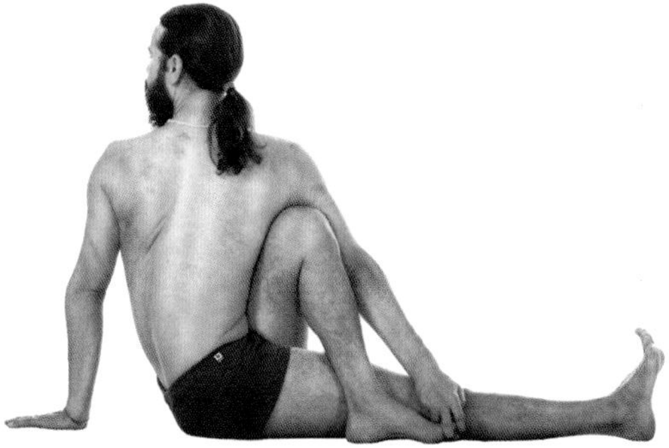

426
परिवृत्त वक्र आसन (बद्ध पाद अङ्गुष्ठ)
Parivṛtta vakra āsana (baddha pāda aṅguṣṭha)
Seated twist pose (holding big toe)

परिवृत्तवक्रासन (बद्धपादाङ्गुष्ठ)
Parivṛttavakrāsana (badhapādāṅguṣṭha)

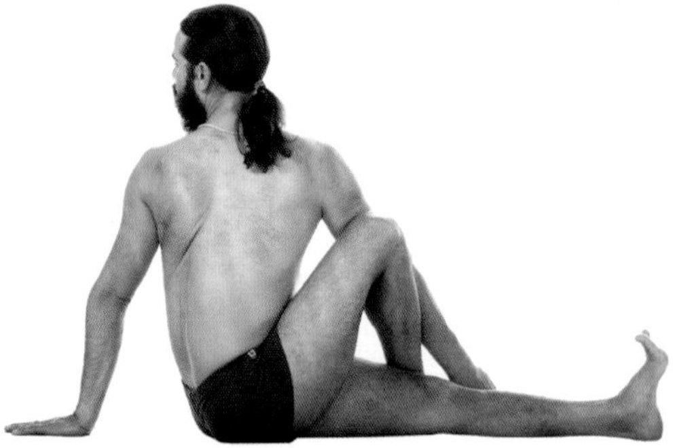

427
विपरीत परिवृत्त वक्र आसन
Viparīta parivṛtta vakra āsana
Reverse seated twist pose

विपरीतपरिवृत्तवक्रासन
Viparītaparivṛttavakrāsana

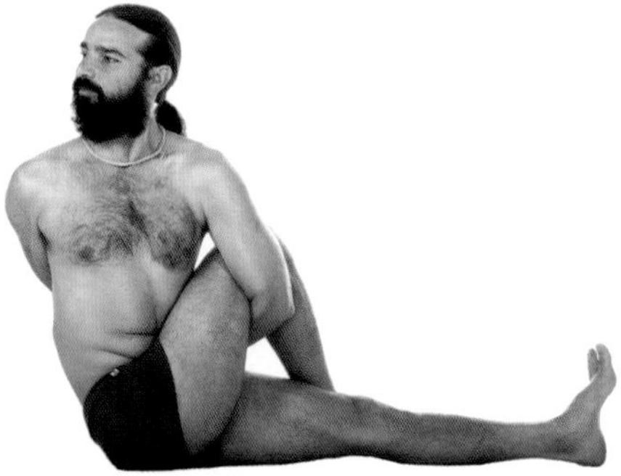

428
परिवृत्त वक्र आसन (रज्जु हस्त)
Parivṛtta vakra āsana (rajju hasta)
Bound seated twist pose (clasped hands)

परिवृत्तवक्रासन (रज्जुहस्त)
Parivṛttavakrāsana (rajjuhasta)

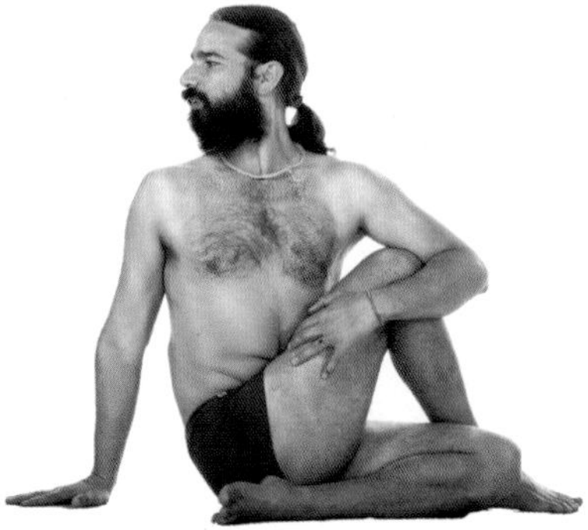

429
अर्ध मत्स्येन्द्र आसन (बद्ध जानु)
Ardha Matsyendra āsana (baddha jānu)
Half pose of the sage Matsyendra (bound knee)

अर्धमत्स्येन्द्रासन (बद्धजानु)
Ardhamatsyendrāsana (baddhajānu)

Start from where you are. It is never too late.

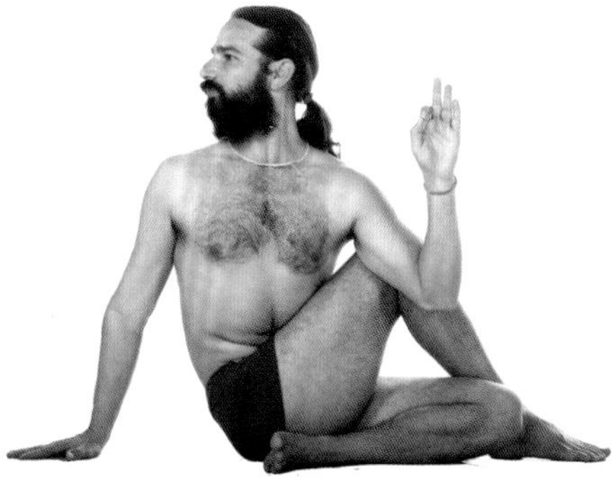

430
अर्ध मत्स्येन्द्र आसन (ज्ञान मुद्रा, पृष्ठ)
Ardha Matsyendra āsana (jñāna mudrā)
Half pose of the sage Matsyendra (jñāna mudrā)

अर्धमत्स्येन्द्रासन (ज्ञानमुद्रा)
Ardhamatsyendrāsana (jñānamudrā)

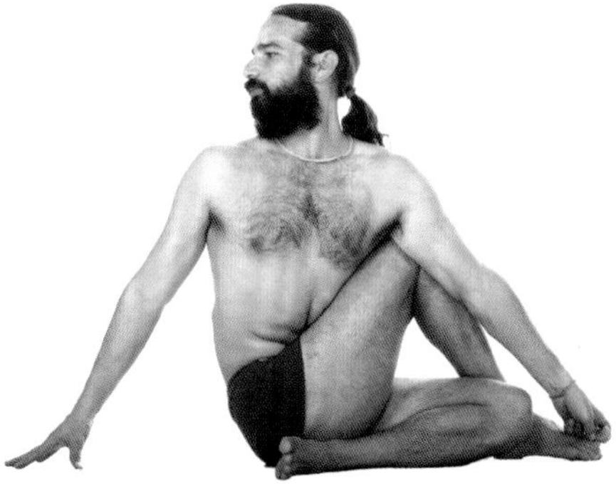

431
अर्ध मत्स्येन्द्र आसन
Ardha Matsyendra āsana
Half pose of the sage Matsyendra

अर्धमत्स्येन्द्रासन
Ardhamatsyendrāsana

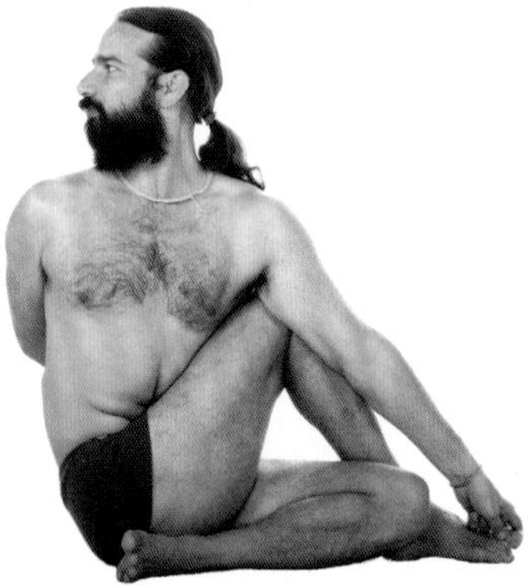

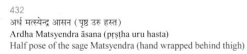

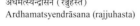

432
अर्ध मत्स्येन्द्र आसन (पृष्ठ उरु हस्त)
Ardha Matsyendra āsana (pṛṣṭha uru hasta)
Half pose of the sage Matsyendra (hand wrapped behind thigh)

अर्धमत्स्येन्द्रासन (पृष्ठोरुहस्त)
Ardhamatsyendrāsana (pṛṣṭhoruhasta)

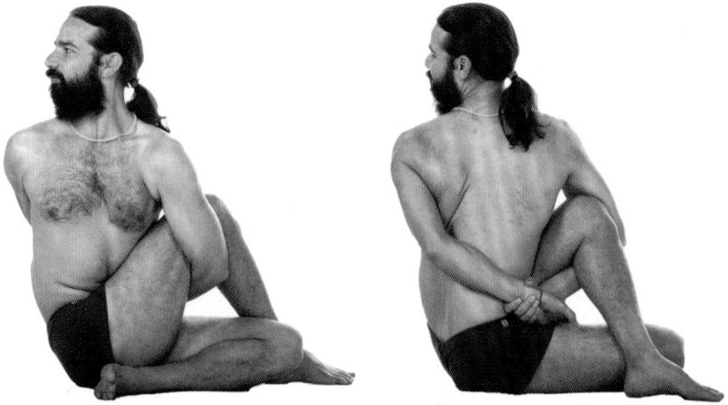

433
अर्ध मत्स्येन्द्र आसन (रज्जु हस्त)
Ardha Matsyendra āsana (rajju hasta)
Half pose of the sage Matsyendra (bound hands)

अर्धमत्स्येन्द्रासन (रज्जुहस्त)
Ardhamatsyendrāsana (rajjuhasta)

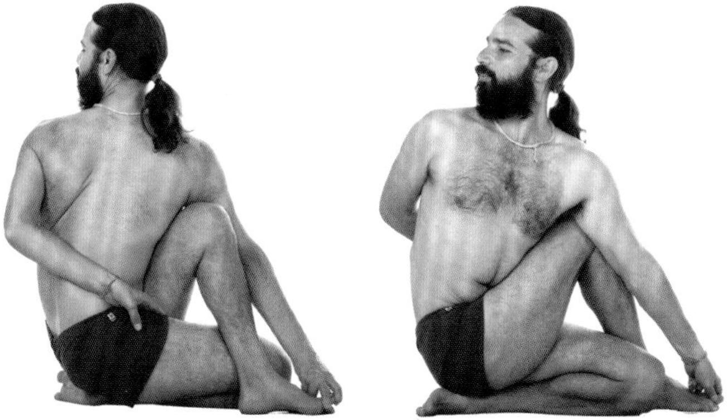

434
वज्र अर्ध मत्स्येन्द्र आसन (पृष्ठ उरु हस्त)
Vajra ardha Matsyendra āsana (pṛṣṭha uru hasta)
Half thunderbolt pose of the sage Matsyendra (hand wrapped behind thigh)

वज्रार्धमत्स्येन्द्रासन (पृष्ठोरुहस्त)
Vajrārdhamatsyendraāsana (pṛṣṭhoruhasta)

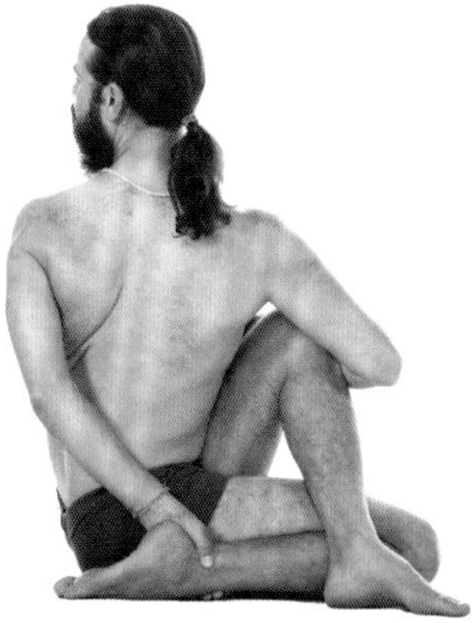

435
अर्ध वज्र मत्स्येन्द्र आसन (बद्ध जानु, बद्ध हस्त गुल्फ)
Ardha vajra Matsyendra āsana (baddha jānu, baddha hasta gulpha)
Half thunderbolt pose of the sage Matsyendra (holding knee and ankle)

अर्धवज्रमत्स्येन्द्रासन (बद्धजानु,बद्धहस्तगुल्फ)
Ardhavajrāmatsyendrāsana (baddhajānu, baddhahastagulpha)

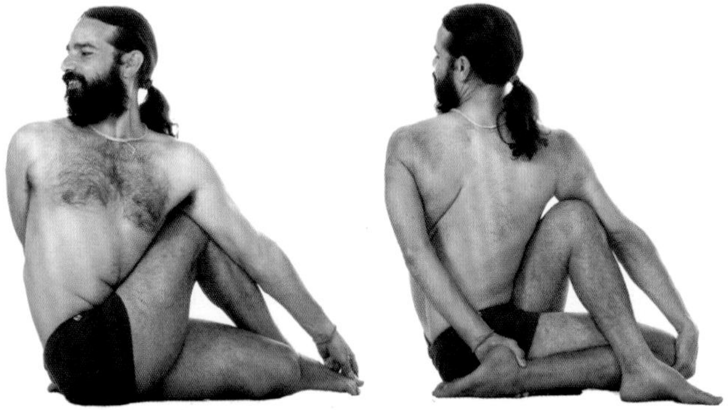

436
अर्ध वज्र मत्स्येन्द्र आसन (बद्ध पाद, बद्ध हस्तगुल्फ)
Ardha vajrā Matsyendra āsana (baddha pāda, baddha hasta gulpha)
Half thunderbolt pose of the sage Matsyendra (holding knee and ankle)

अर्धवज्रमत्स्येन्द्रासन (बद्धपाद, बद्धहस्तगुल्फ)
Ardhavajrāmatsyendrāsana (baddhapāda, baddhastagulpha)

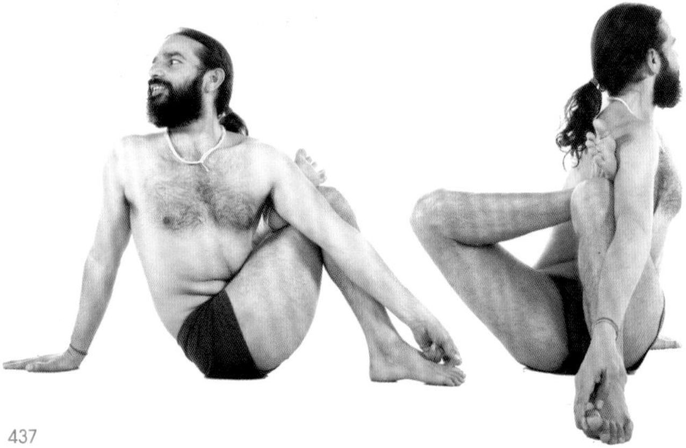

437
योग दण्ड मत्स्यइन्द्र आसन
Yoga daṇḍa Matsyendra āsana
Sage Matsyendra yoga staff pose

योगदण्डमत्स्येन्द्रासन
Yogadaṇḍamatsyendrāsana

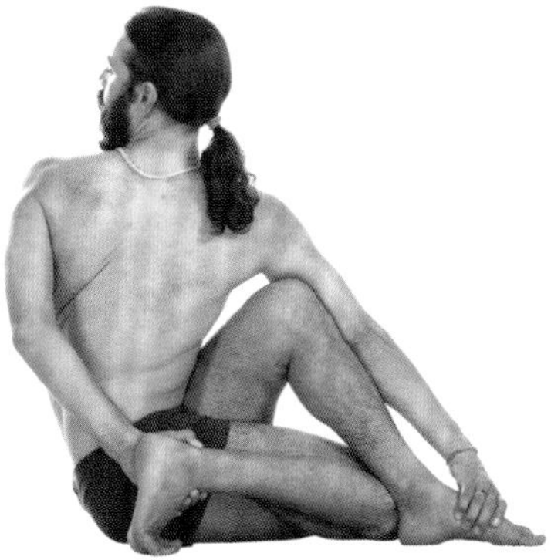

438
विकट मत्स्येन्द्र आसन
Vikaṭa Matsyendra āsana
Challenging pose of the sage Matsyendra

विकटमत्स्येन्द्रासन
Vikaṭamatsyendrāsana

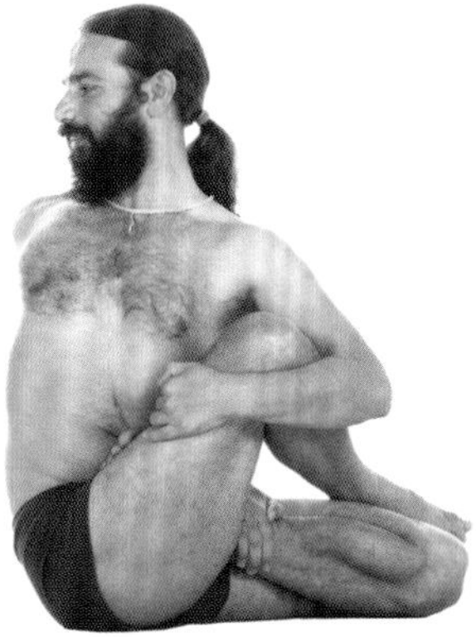

439
पूर्णमत्स्येन्द्रआसन (बद्ध जानु)
Pūrṇa Matsyendra āsana (baddha jānu)
Full pose of the sage Matsyendra (holding knee)

पूर्णमत्स्येन्द्रासन (बद्धजानु)
Pūrṇamatsyendrāsana (baddhajānu)

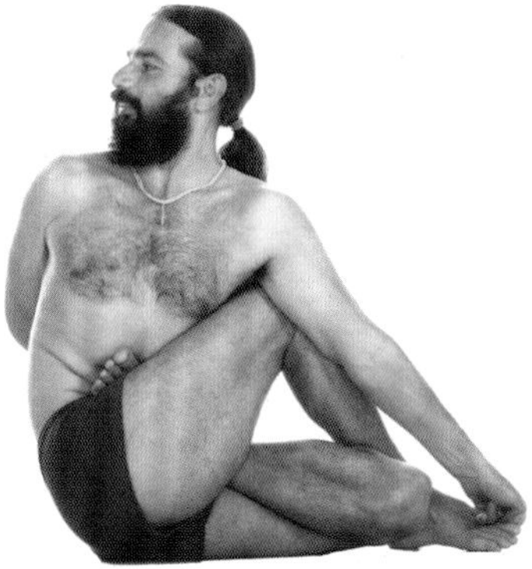

440
पूर्णमत्स्येन्द्र आसन
Pūrṇa Matsyendra āsana āsana
Full pose of the sage Matsyendra

पूर्णमत्स्येन्द्रासन
Pūrṇamatsyendraāsanāsana

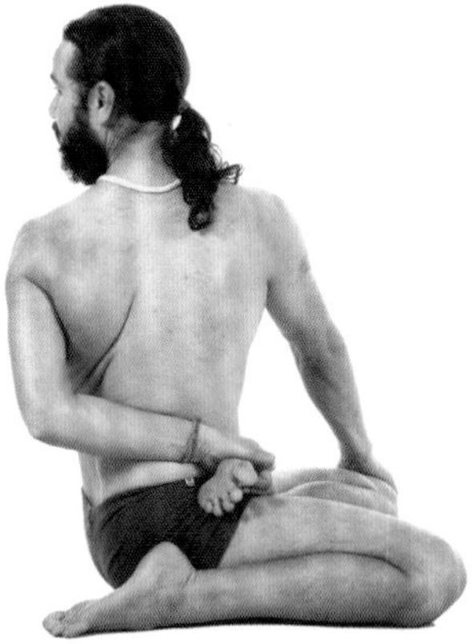

441
परिवृत्त भारद्वाज आसन
Parivṛtta Bhārdvāja āsana
Twisted sage Bhārdvāja pose

परिवृत्तभारद्वाजासन
Parivṛttabhārdvājāsana

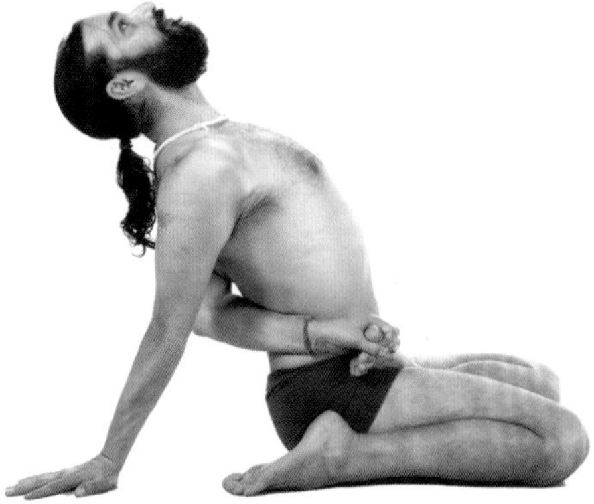

442
ऊर्ध्व मुख भारद्वाज आसन
Ūrdhva mukha Bhārdvāja āsana
Upward facing sage Bhārdvāja pose

ऊर्ध्वमुखभारद्वाजासन
Ūrdhvamukhabhāradvājāsana

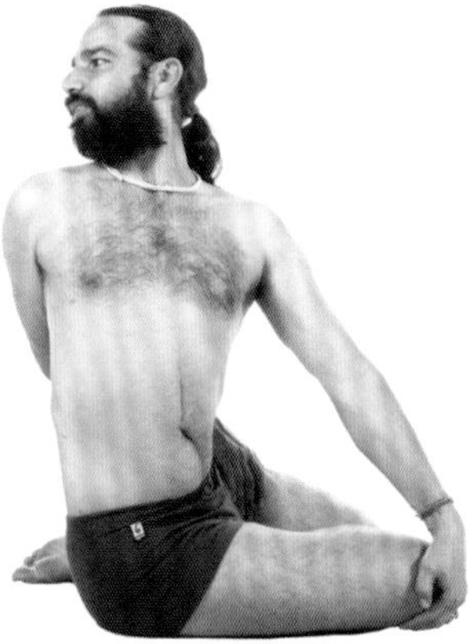

443
परिवृत्त भारद्वाज आसन (जानु हस्त, उरु हस्त)
Parivṛtta Bhārdvāja āsana (jānu hasta, uru hasta)
Twisted sage Bhārdvāja pose (hand on knee and thigh)

परिवृत्तभारद्वाजासन (जानुहस्त,उरुहस्त)
Parivṛttabhārdvājāsana (jānuhasta, uruhasta)

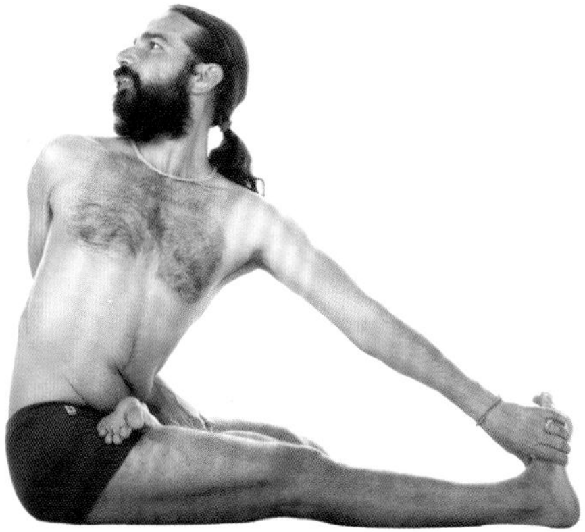

444
परिवृत्त भारद्वाज आसन (एक पाद दण्ड)
Parivṛtta Bhāradvāja āsana (eka pāda daṇḍa)
Twisted sage Bhārdvāja pose (one leg straight in staff position)

परिवृत्तभारद्वाजासन (एकपाददण्ड)
Parivṛttabhāradvājāsana (ekapādadaṇḍa)

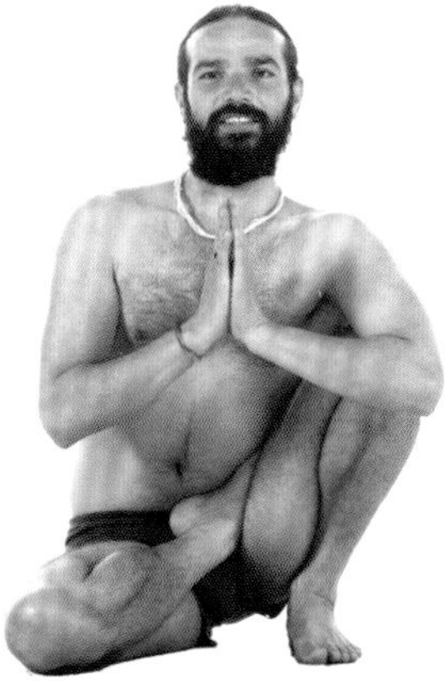

445
नमन मरीचि आसन
Namana Marīci āsana
Humble pose of the sage Marīci

नमनमरीच्यासन
Namanamarīcyāsana

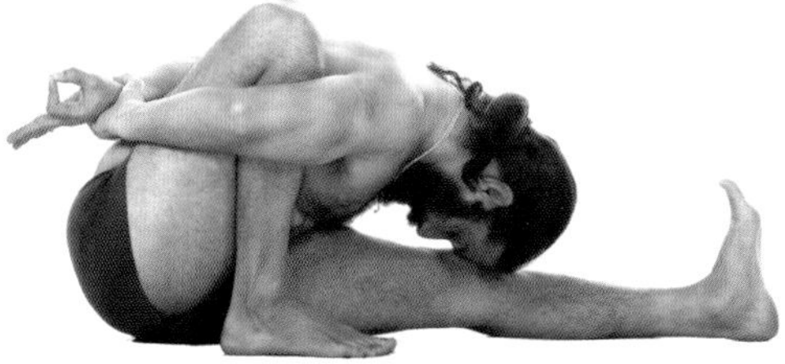

446
मरीचि आसन (जानु शीर्ष)
Marīci āsana (jānu śīrṣa)
Pose of the sage Marīci (head to knee)

मरीच्यासन (जानुशीर्ष)
Marīcyāsana (jānuśīrṣa)

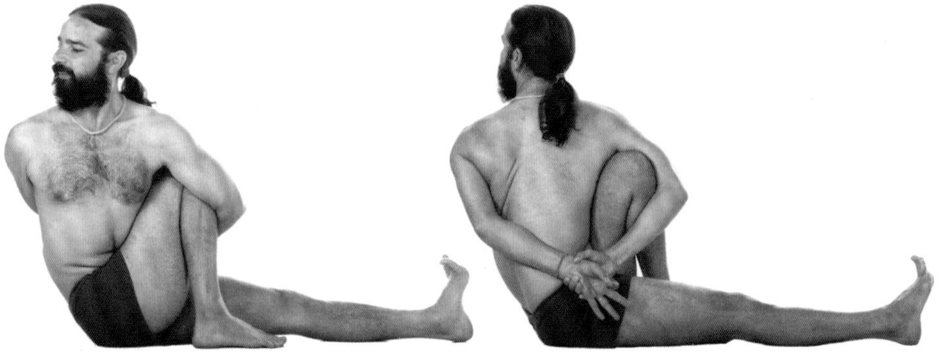

447
परिवृत्त मरीचि आसन
Parivṛtta Marīci āsana
Twisted pose of the sage Marīci

परिवृत्तमरीच्यासन
Parivṛttamarīcyāsana

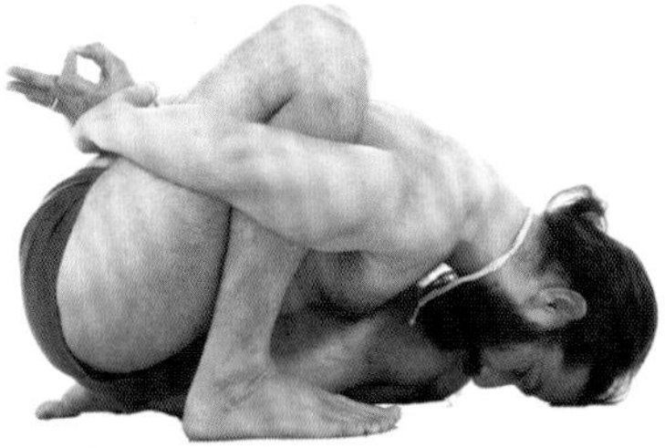

448
मरीचि आसन (एक पाद वज्र ,ललाट भू)
Marīci āsana (eka pāda vajra, lalāṭa bhū)
Pose of the sage Marīci (one leg thunderbolt, forehead on the earth)

मरीच्यासन (एकपादवज्र, ललाटभू)
Marīcyāsana (ekapādavajra, lalāṭabhū)

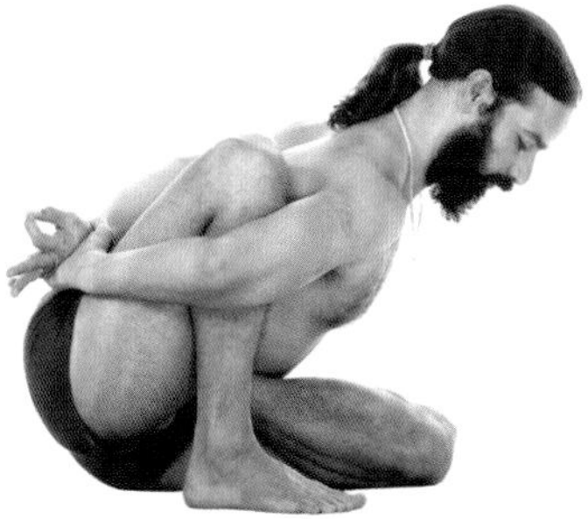

449
अर्धपद्म मरीचि आसन
Ardha padma Marīci āsana
Half lotus pose of the sage Marīci

अर्धपद्ममरीच्यासन
Ardhapadmamarīcyāsana

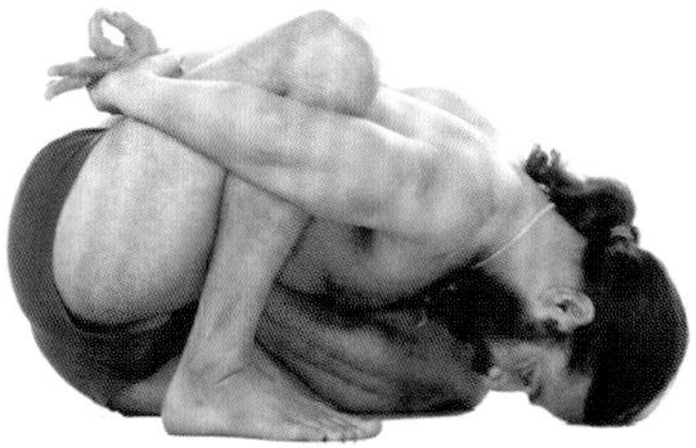

450
अर्धपद्म मरीचि आसन (ललाट भू)
Ardha padma Marīci āsana (lalāṭa bhū)
Half lotus pose of the sage Marīci (forehead on the earth)

अर्धपद्ममरीच्यासन (ललाटभू)
Ardhapadmamarīcyāsana (lalāṭabhū)

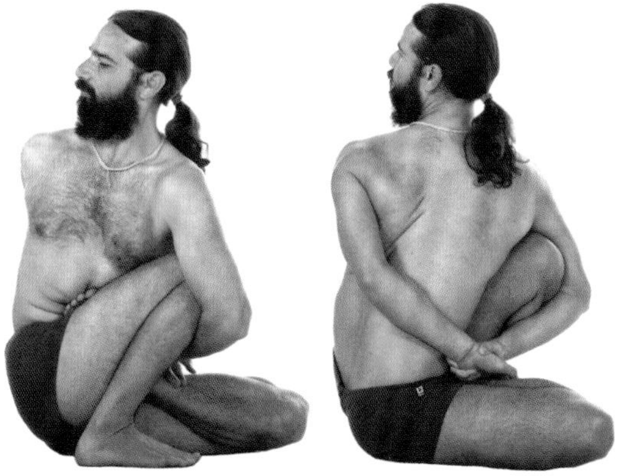

451
अर्ध पद्म परिवृत्त मरीचि आसन
Ardha padma parivṛtta Marīci āsana
Half lotus twisted pose of the sage Marīci

अर्धपद्मापरिवृत्तमरीच्यासन
Ardhapadmaparivṛttamarīcyāsana

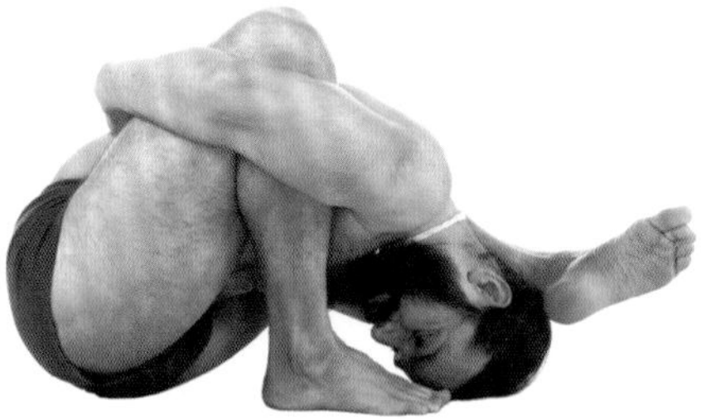

452
भैरव मरीचि आसन
Bhairava Marīci āsana
Fearless Sage Marīci pose

भैरवमरीच्यासन
Bhairavamarīcyāsana

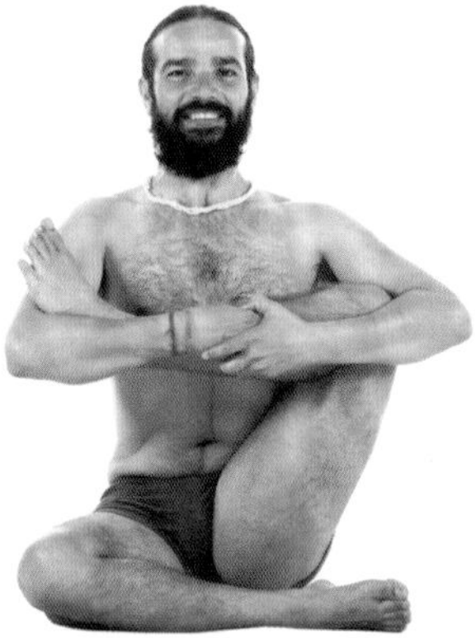

453
उपविष्ट शिशु वात्सल्य आसन
Upaviṣṭa śiśu vātsalya āsana
Seated cradle baby pose

उपविष्टशिशुवात्सल्यासन
Upaviṣṭaśiśuvātsalyāsana

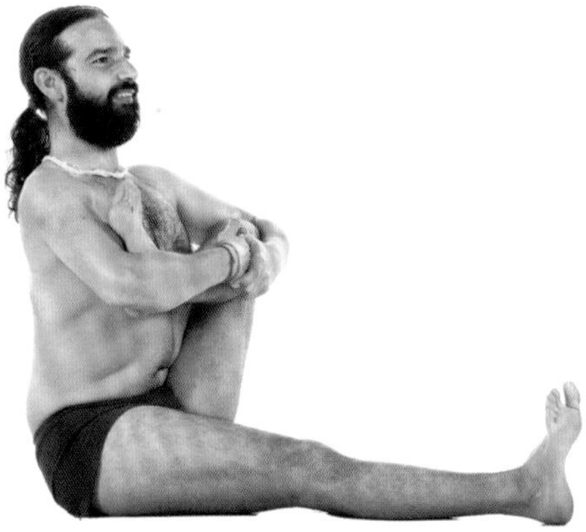

454
उपविष्ट शिशु वात्सल्य आसन (एक पाद दण्ड)
Upaviṣṭa śiśu vātsalya āsana (eka pāda daṇḍa)
Seated cradle baby pose (one leg in staff position)

उपविष्टशिशुवात्सल्यासन (एकपाददण्ड)
Upaviṣṭaśiśuvātsalyāsana (ekapādadaṇḍa)

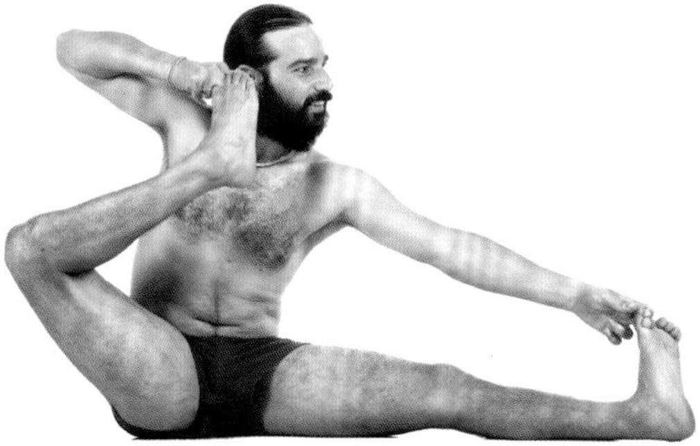

455
आकर्ण धनुः आसन
Ākarṇa dhanuḥ āsana
Drawn bow pose

आकर्णधनुरासन
Ākarṇadhanurāsana

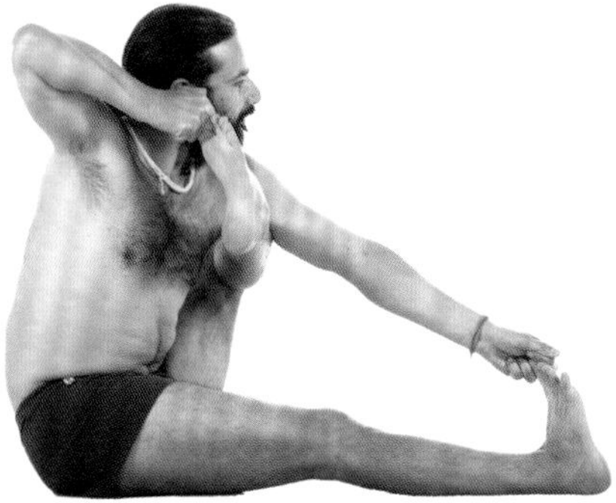

456
आकर्ण धनुः आसन (विपरीत एक पाद हस्त)
Ākarṇa dhanuḥ āsana (viparīta eka pāda hasta)
Drawn bow pose (opposite foot to hand)

आकर्णधनुरासन (विपरीतैकपादहस्त)
Akarṇadhanurāsana (viparītāaikapādahasta)

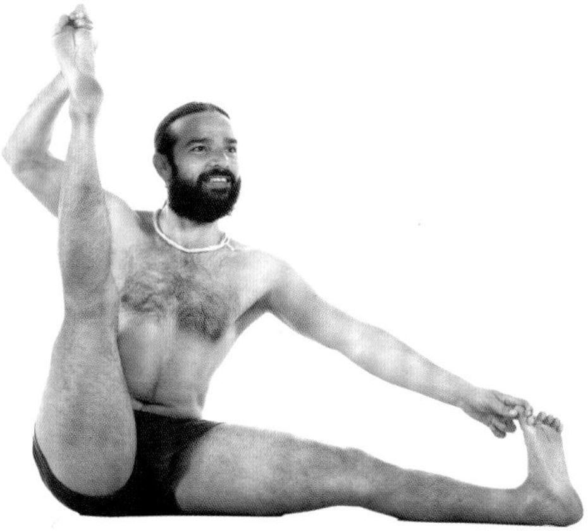

457
आकर्ण धनुः आसन (उत्तान एक पाद)
Ākarṇa dhanuḥ āsana (uttāna eka pāda)
Drawn bow pose (stretching one leg up)

आकर्णधनुरासन (उत्तानैकपाद)
Ākarṇadhanurāsana (uttānaikapāda)

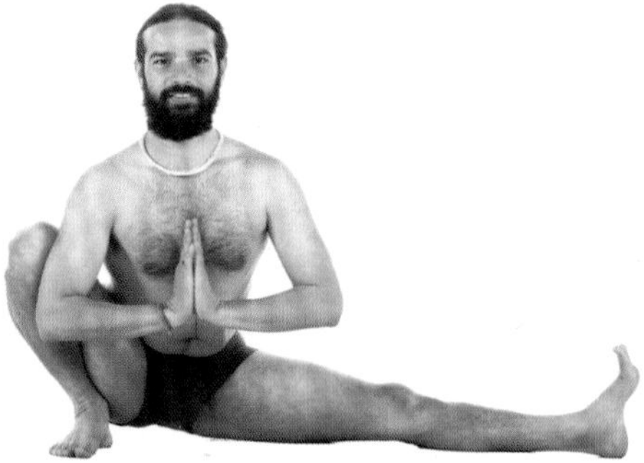

458
नमस्कार माला आसन (एक पाद दण्ड)
Namaskāra mālā āsana (eka pāda daṇḍa)
Praying garland pose (one leg in staff position)

नमस्कारमालासन (एकपाददण्ड)
Namaskāramālāsana (ekapādadaṇḍā)

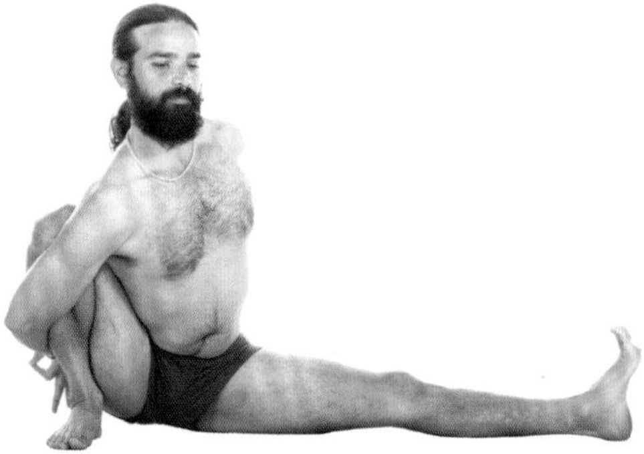

459
जानु बद्ध माला आसन (एक पाद दण्ड)
Jānu baddha mālā āsana (eka pāda daṇḍa)
Bound knee garland pose (one leg in staff position)

जानुबद्धमालासन (एकपाददण्ड)
Jānubaddhamālāsana (ekapādadaṇḍa)

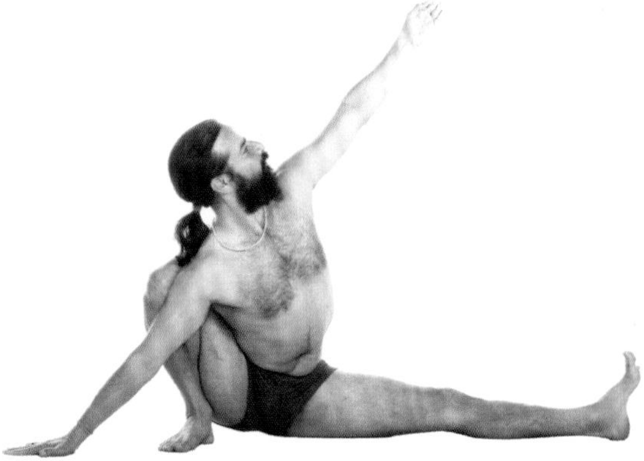

460
अर्जुन बाण आसन (एक पाद दण्ड)
Arjuna bāṇa āsana (eka pāda daṇḍa)
Focused arrow pose (one leg in staff position)

अर्जुनबाणासन (एकपाददण्ड)
Arjunabāṇāsana (ekapādadaṇḍa)

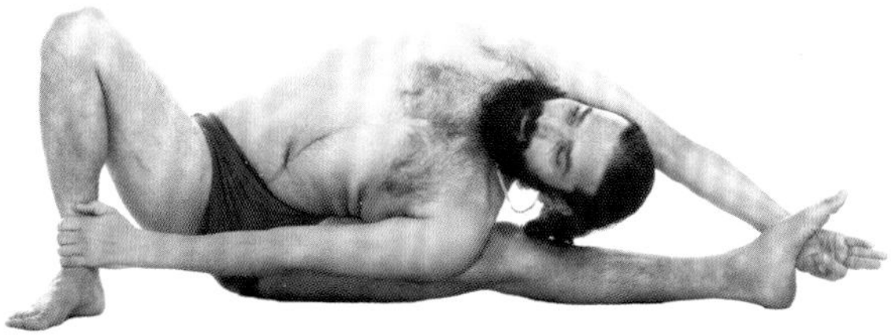

461
पार्श्व चौरङ्गी नाथ आसन (ज्ञान मुद्रा)
Pārśva Cauraṅgī Nātha āsana (jñāna mudrā)
Side sage Caurangī Nātha pose (hand in jñāna mudrā)

पार्श्वचौरङ्गीनाथासन (ज्ञानमुद्रा)
Pārśvacauraṅgīnāthāsana (jñānamudrā)

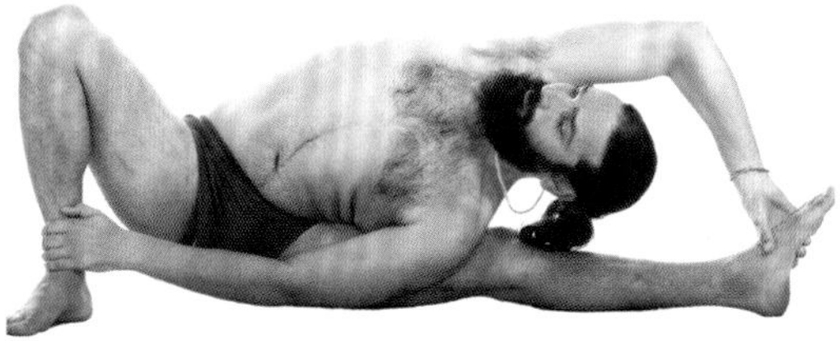

462
पार्श्व चौरङ्गी नाथ आसन (ज्ञान मुद्रा)
Pārśva Cauraṅgī Nātha āsana (baddha pāda)
Side sage Caurangī Nātha pose (holding foot)

पार्श्वचौरङ्गीनाथासन (ज्ञानमुद्रा)
Pārśvacauraṅgīnāthāsana (baddhapāda)

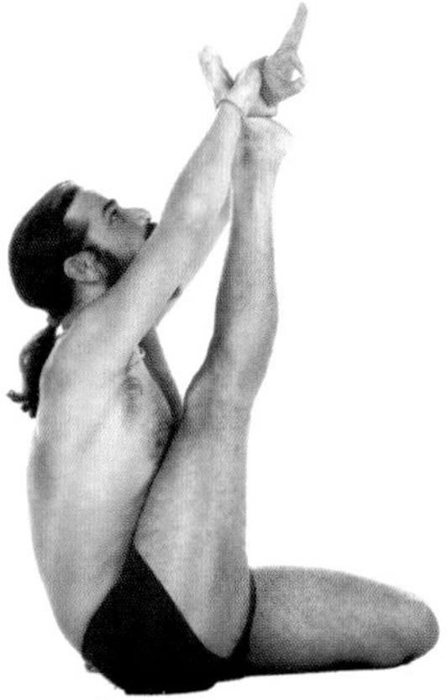

463
ऊर्ध्व मुख क्रौञ्च आसन
Ūrdhva mukha krauñca āsana
Upward facing curlew pose

ऊर्ध्वमुखक्रौञ्चासन
Ūrdhvamukhakrauñcāsana

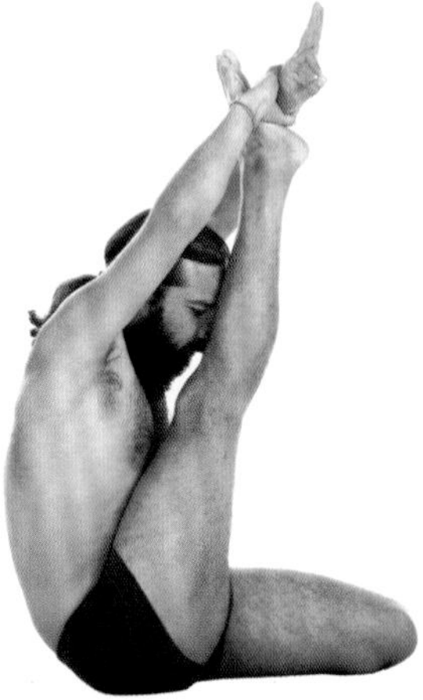

464
जानु शिर क्रौञ्च आसन
Jānu śira krauñca āsana
Head to knee curlew pose

जानुशिरक्रौञ्चासन
Jānuśirakrauñcāsana

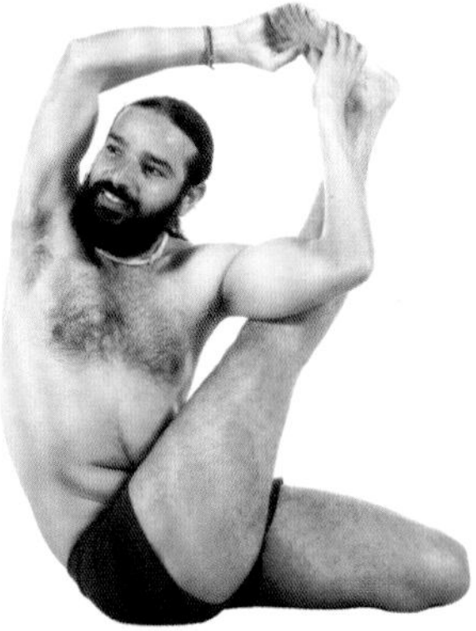

465
परिवृत्त क्रौञ्च आसन
Parivṛtta krauñca āsana
Twisted curlew pose

परिवृत्तक्रौञ्चासन
Parivṛttakrauñcāsana

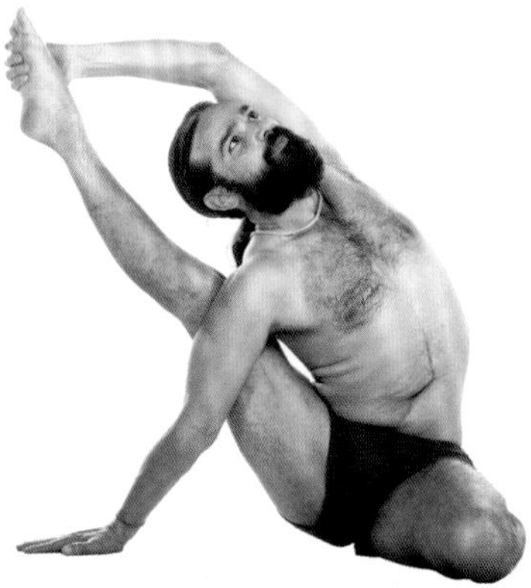

466
पार्श्व क्रौञ्च आसन (एक हस्त भू)
Pārśva krauñca āsana (eka hasta bhū)
Side curlew pose (one hand on the earth)

पार्श्वक्रौञ्चासन (एकहस्तभू)
Pārśvakrauñcāsana (ekahastabhū)

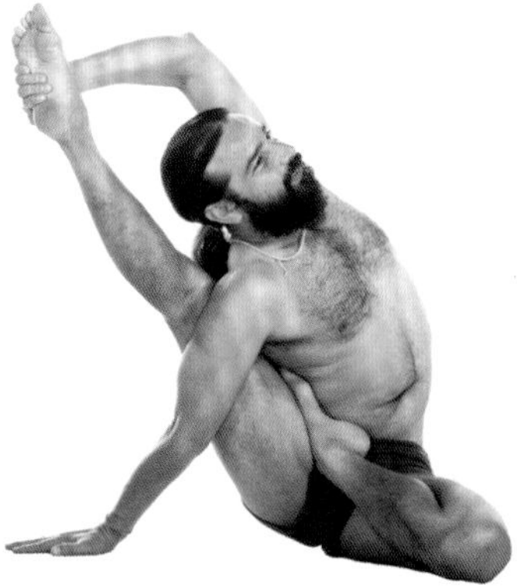

467
पार्श्व पद्म क्रौञ्च आसन (एक हस्त भू)
Pārśva padma krauñca āsana (eka hasta bhū)
Lotus side curlew pose (one hand on the earth)

पार्श्वपद्मक्रौञ्चासन (एकहस्तभू)
Pārśvapadmakrauñcāsana (ekahastabhū)

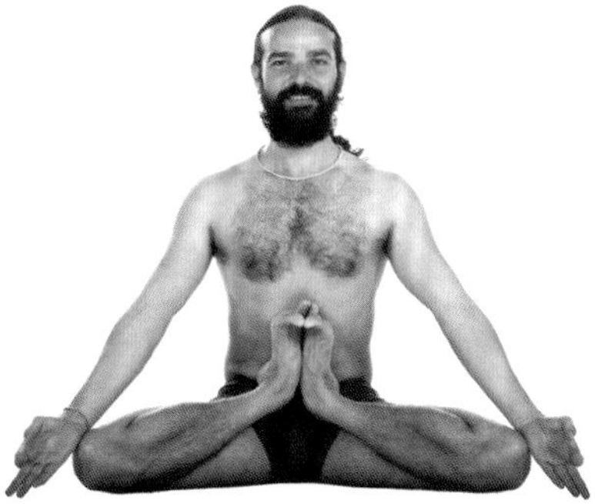

468
कन्द पीड आसन (ज्ञान मुद्रा)
Kanda pīḍa āsana (jñāna mudrā)
Energy releasing pose (hands in jñāna mudrā)

कन्दपीडासन (ज्ञानमुद्रा)
Kandapīḍaāsana (jñānamudrā)

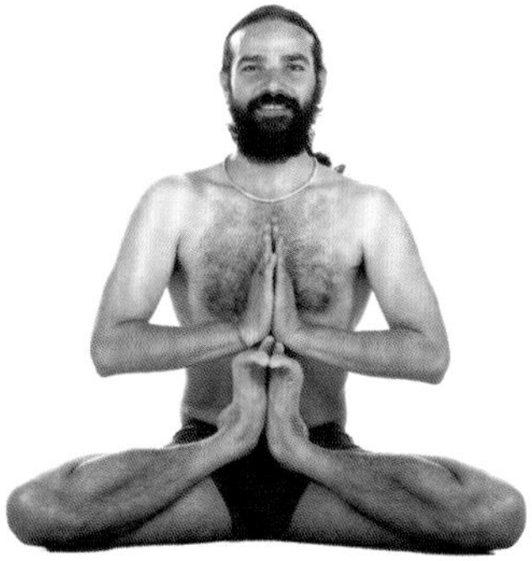

469
नमस्कार कन्द पीड आसन
Namaskāra kanda pīḍa āsana
Praying energy releasing pose

नमस्कारकन्दपीडासन
Namaskārakandapīḍāsana

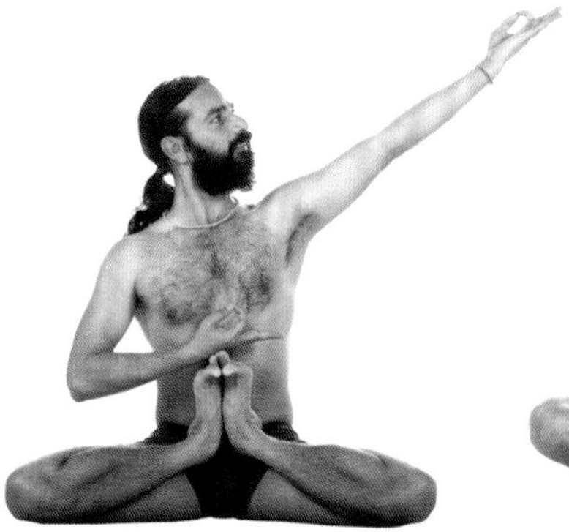

470
भद्र कन्द पीड आसन
Bhadra kanda pīḍa āsana
Beautiful energy releasing pose

भद्रकन्दपीडासन
Bhadrakandapīḍāsana

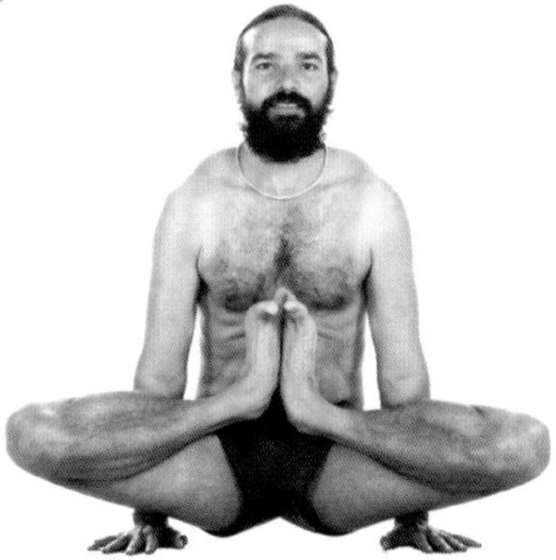

471
उत्तोलन कन्द पीड आसन
Uttolana kanda pīḍa āsana
Balancing energy releasing pose

उत्तोलनकन्दपीडासन
Uttolanakandapīḍāsana

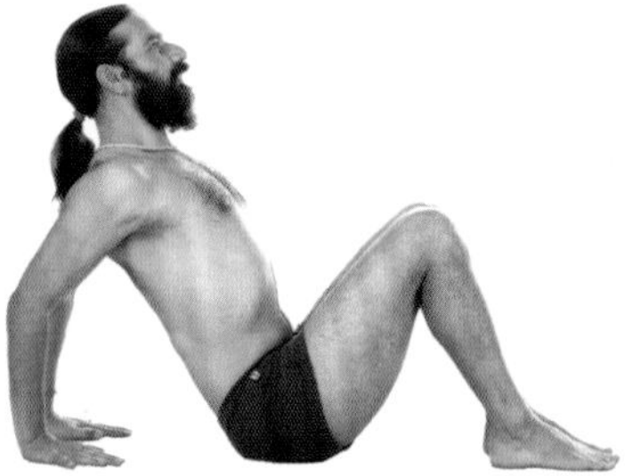

472
अर्ध नौका आसन (आरम्भ अवस्था)
Ardha naukā āsana (ārambha avasthā)
Half boat pose (starting position)

अर्धनौकासन (आरम्भावस्था)
Ardhanaukāsana (ārambhāvasthā)

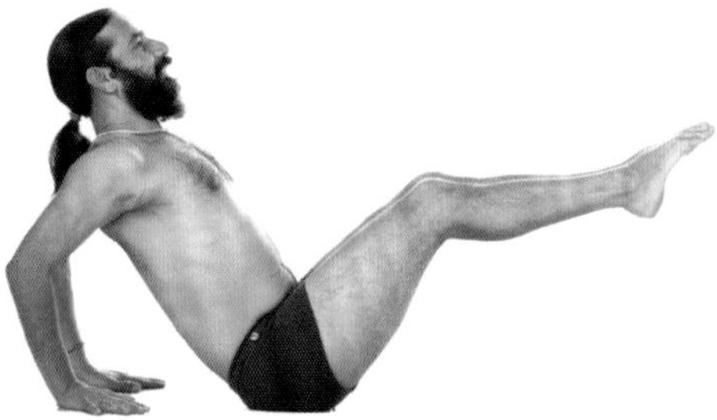

473
अर्ध नौका आसन (पृष्ठ हस्त भू)
Ardha naukā āsana (pṛṣṭha hasta bhū)
Half boat pose (hands on the earth behind)

अर्धनौकासन (पृष्ठहस्तभू)
Ardhanaukāsana (pṛṣṭhahastabhū)

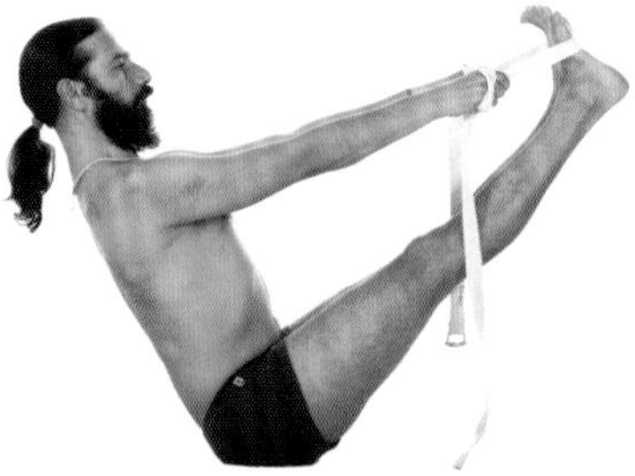

474
नौका आसन (सालम्ब रज्जु)
Naukā āsana (sālamba rajju)
Boat pose (supported with strap)

नौकासन (सालम्बरज्जु)
Naukāsana (sālambarajju)

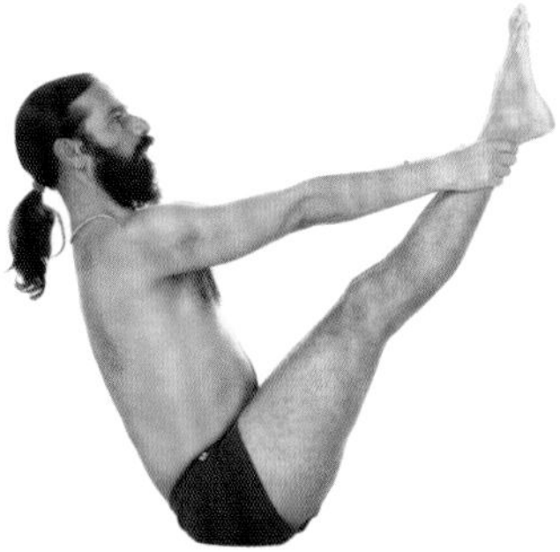

475
नौका आसन (हस्त गुल्फ बद्ध)
Naukā āsana (hasta gulpha baddha)
Boat pose (holding ankles)

नौकासन (हस्तगुल्फबद्ध)
Naukāsana (hastagulphabaddha)

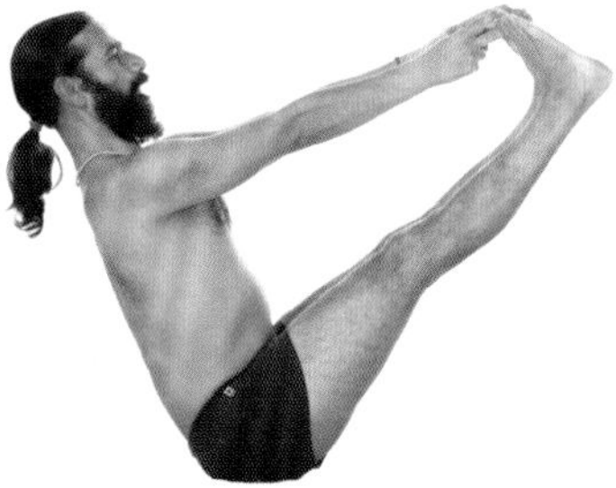

476
नौका आसन (हस्त पाद अङ्गुष्ठ)
Naukā āsana (hasta pāda aṅguṣṭha)
Boat pose (holding big toes)

नौकासन (हस्तपादाङ्गुष्ठ)
Naukāsana (hastapādāṅguṣṭha)

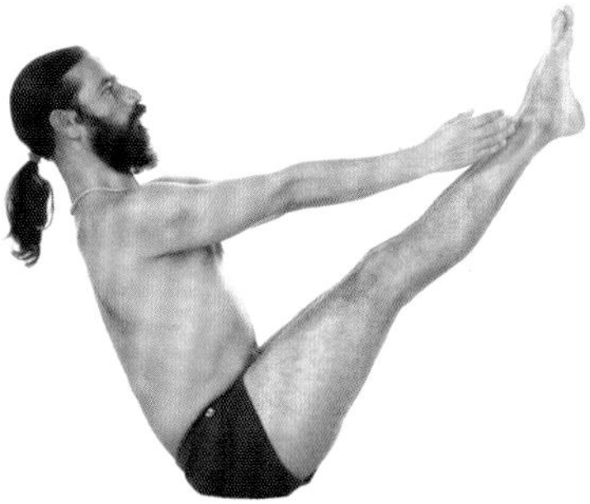

477
नौका आसन
Naukā āsana
Boat pose

नौकासन
Naukāsana

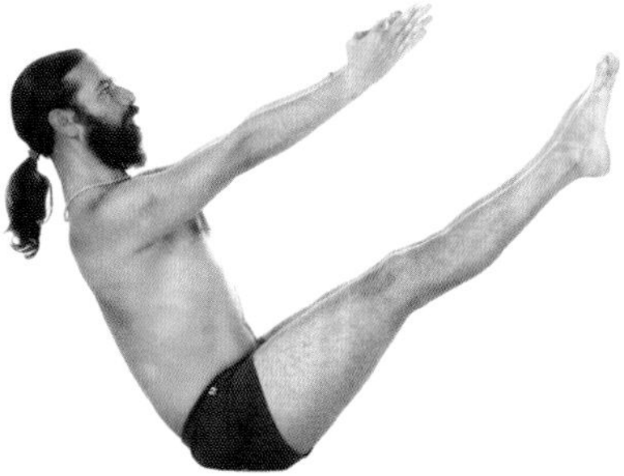

478
नौका आसन (क्षितिज हस्त)
Naukā āsana (kṣitija hasta)
Boat pose (hands reaching for horizon)

नौकासन (क्षितिजहस्त)
Naukāsana (kṣitijahasta)

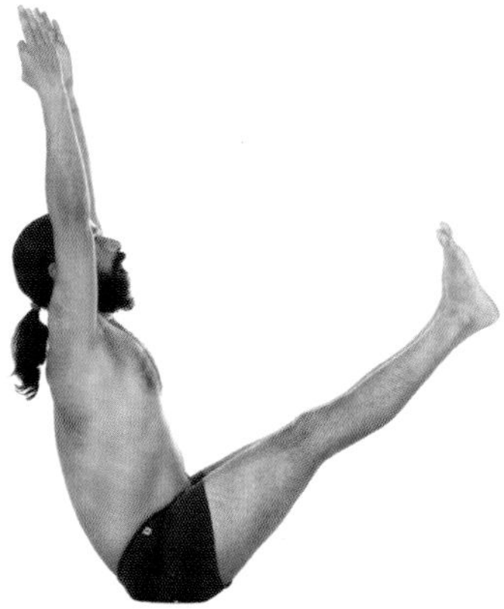

479
नौका आसन (ऊर्ध्व हस्त)
Naukā āsana (urdhva hasta)
Boat pose (arms overhead)

नौकासन (ऊर्ध्वहस्त)
Naukāsana (urdhvahasta)

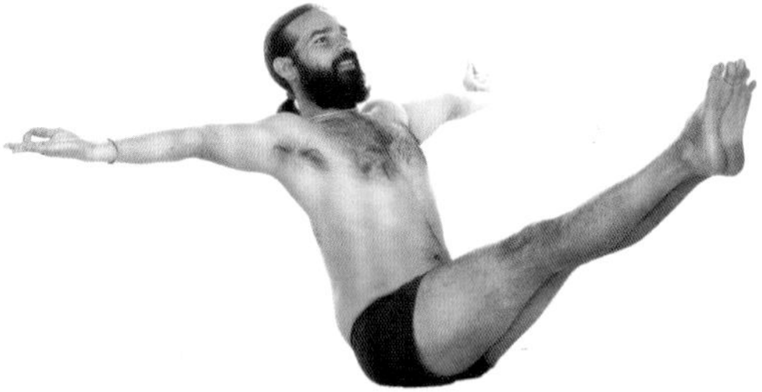

480
नौका आसन (विराट हस्त)
Naukā āsana (virāṭa hasta)
Boat pose (arms extended wide)

नौकासन (विराटहस्त)
Naukāsana (virāṭahasta)

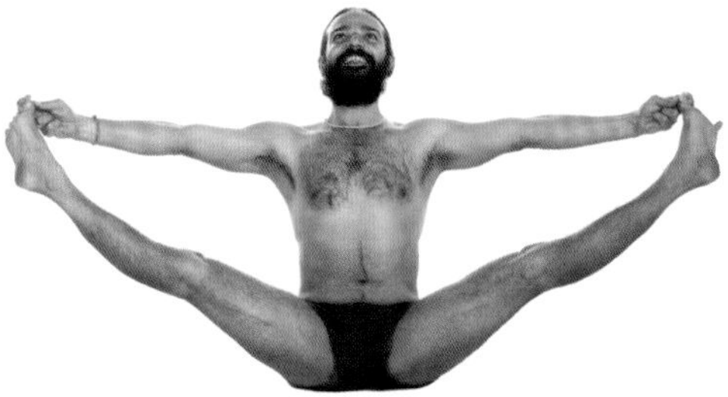

481
प्रसरित पाद नौका आसन (हस्त पाद अङ्गुष्ठ)
Prasarita pāda naukā āsana (hasta pāda aṅguṣṭha)
Wide leg boat pose (holding big toes)

प्रसरितपादनौकासन (हस्तपादाङ्गुष्ठ)
Prasaritapādanaukāsana (hastapādāṅguṣṭha)

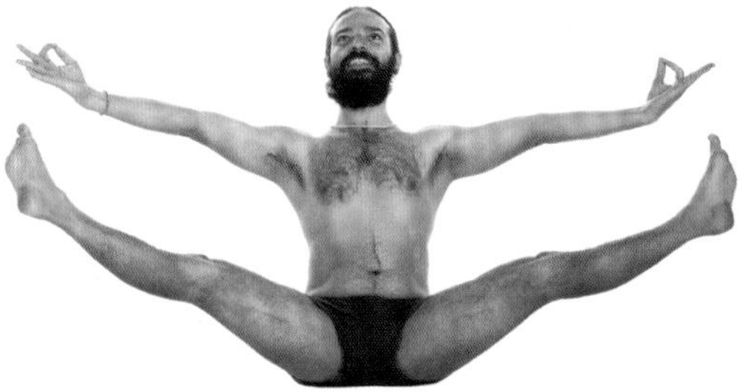

482
प्रसरित पाद कोण नौका आसन (विराट हस्त)
Prasarita pāda naukā āsana (virāṭa hasta)
Wide leg boat pose (arms extended wide)

प्रसरितपादकोणनौकासन (विराटहस्त)
Prasaritapādanaukāsana (virāṭahasta)

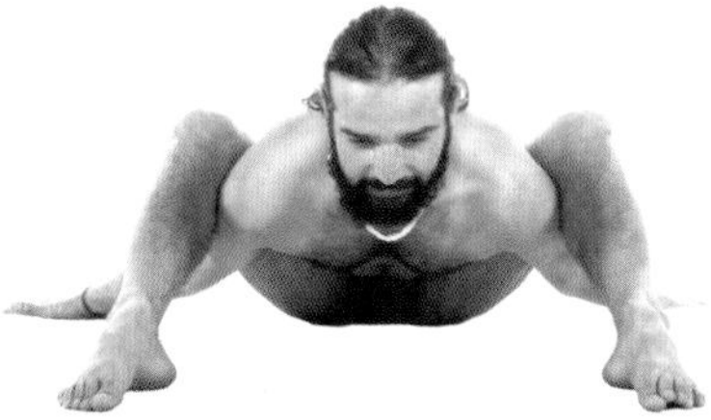

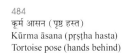

483
अर्ध कूर्म आसन
Ardha kūrma āsana
Half tortoise pose

अर्धकूर्मासन
Ardhakūrmāsana

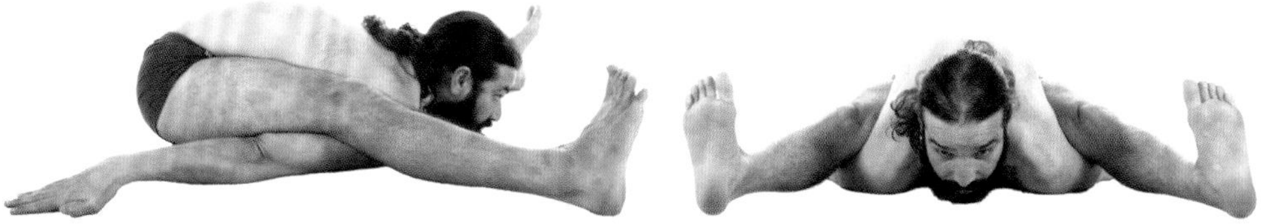

484
कूर्म आसन (पृष्ठ हस्त)
Kūrma āsana (pṛṣṭha hasta)
Tortoise pose (hands behind)

कूर्मासन (पृष्ठहस्त)
Kūrmāsana (pṛṣṭhahasta)

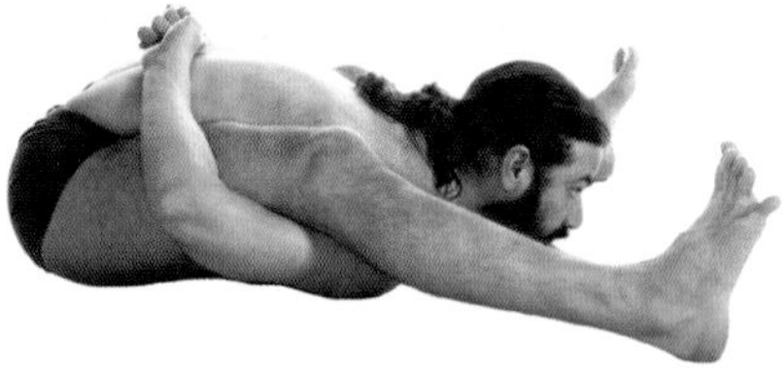

485
कूर्म आसन (रज्जु हस्त)
Kūrma āsana (rajju hasta)
Tortoise pose (bound hands)

कूर्मासन (रज्जुहस्त)
Kūrmāsana (rajjuhasta)

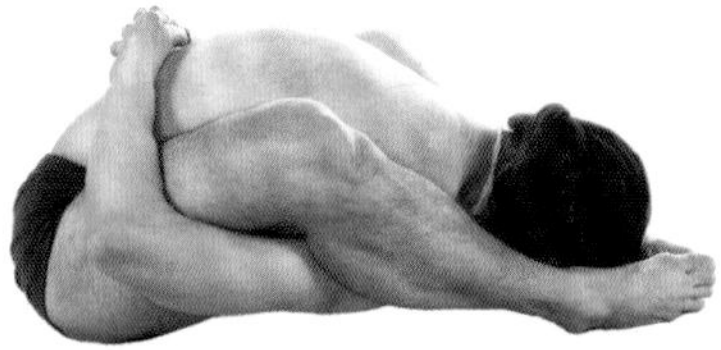

486
कूर्म आसन (शिर भू)
Kūrma āsana (śira bhū)
Tortoise pose (head on the earth)

कूर्मासन (शिरभू)
Kūrmāsana (śirabhū)

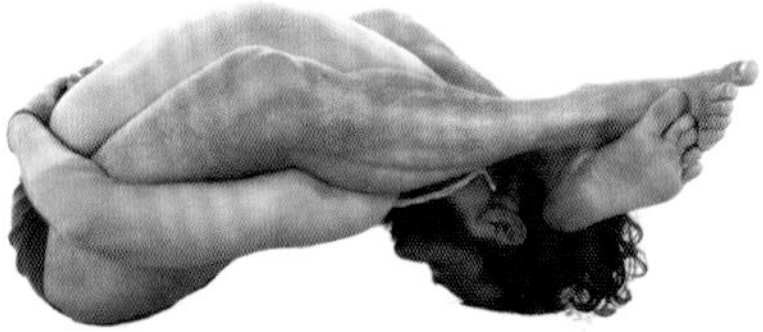

487
पूर्ण गुप्त कूर्म आसन
Pūrṇa gupta kūrma āsana
Fully concealed tortoise pose

पूर्णगुप्तकूर्मासन
Pūrṇaguptakūrmāsana

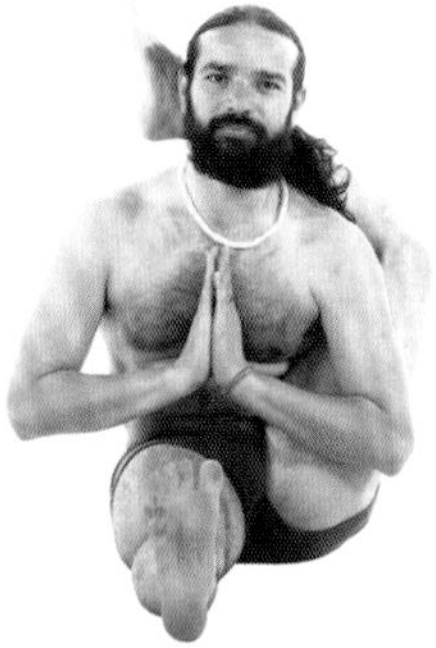

488
एक पाद स्कन्ध आसन
Eka pāda skandha āsana
One leg behind shoulders pose

एकपादस्कन्धासन
Ekapādaskandhāsana

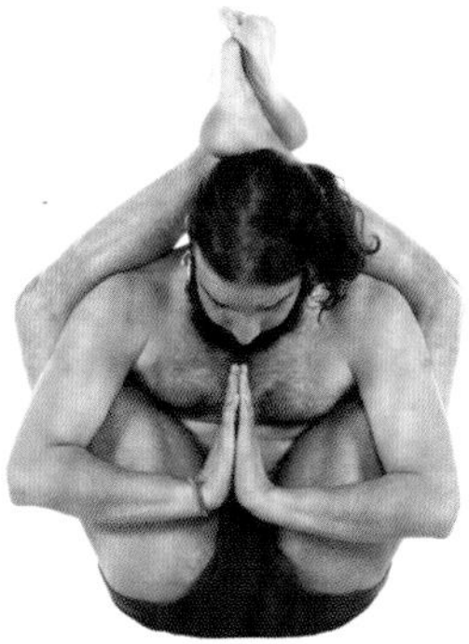

489
द्वि पाद स्कन्ध आसन
Dvi pāda skandha āsana
Two legs behind shoulders pose

द्विपादस्कन्धासन
Dvipādaskandhāsana

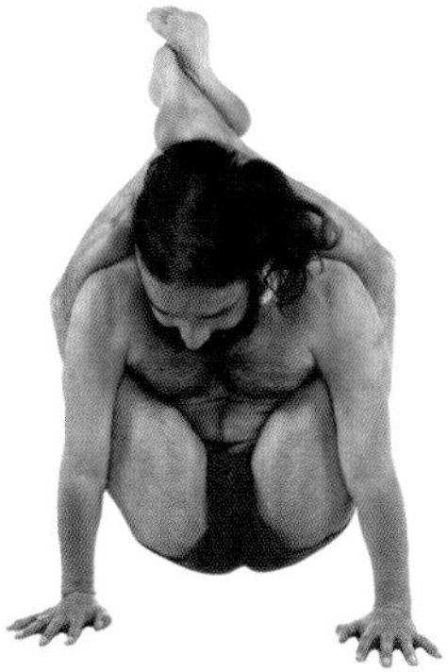

490
उत्थित द्वि पाद स्कन्ध आसन
Utthita dvi pāda skandha āsana
Lifted two legs behind shoulders pose

उत्थितद्विपादस्कन्धासन
Utthitadvipādaskandhāsana

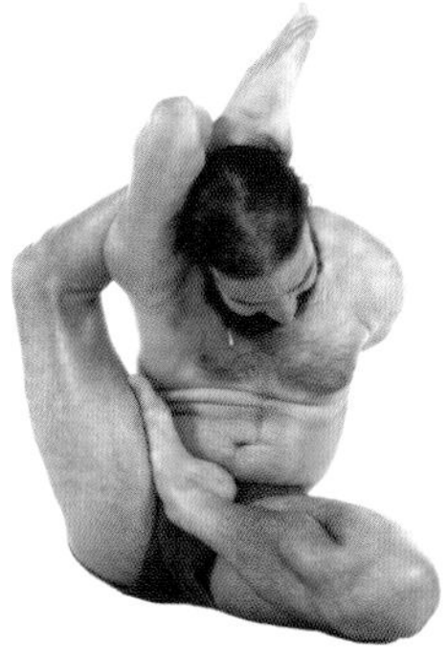

491
विरञ्चि आसन
Virañci āsana
Lord Brahma pose

विरञ्चिासन
Virañciāsana

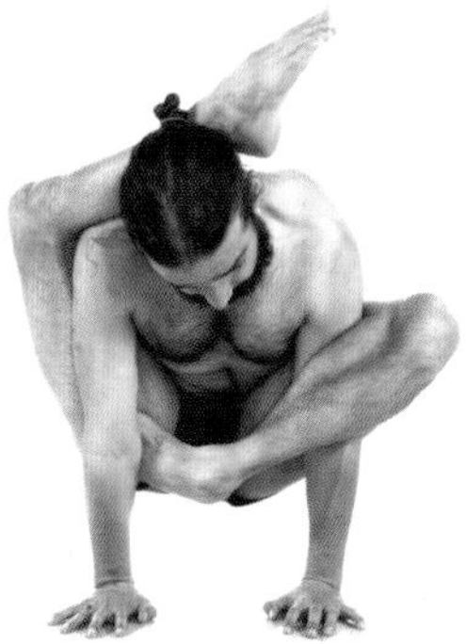

492
ओमकार आसन
Oṇkāra āsana
Shape of Om pose

ओङ्कारासन
Oṇkārāsana

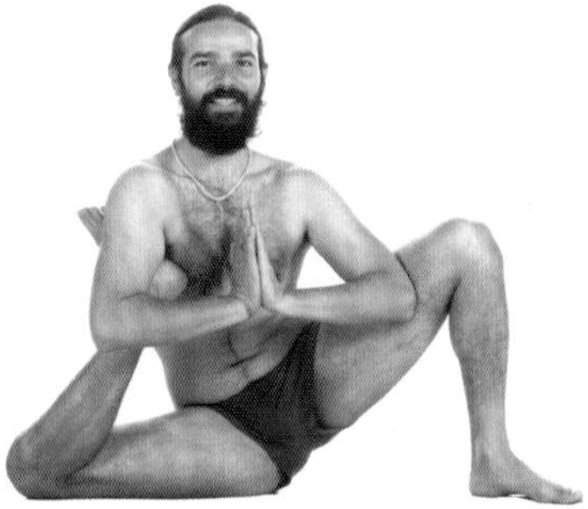

493
नमस्कार योग दण्ड आसन
Namaskāra yoga daṇḍa āsana
Praying yoga staff pose

नमस्कारयोगदण्डासन
Namaskārayogadaṇḍāsana

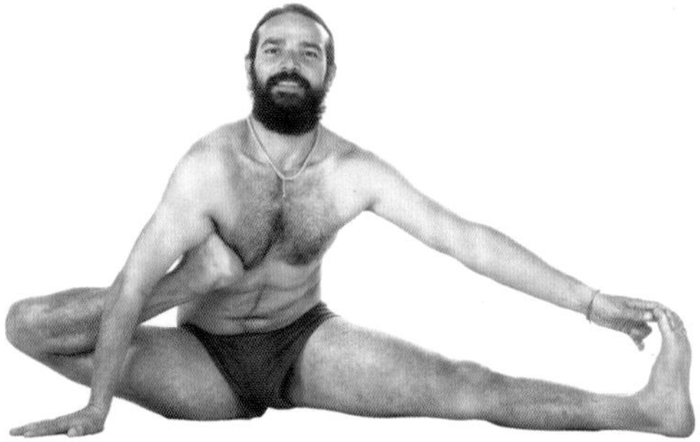

494
बद्ध पाद अङ्गुष्ठ योग दण्ड आसन
Baddha pāda aṅguṣṭha yoga daṇḍa āsana
Bound big toe yoga staff pose

बद्धपादाङ्गुष्ठयोगदण्डासन
Baddhapādāṅguṣṭhayogadaṇḍāsana

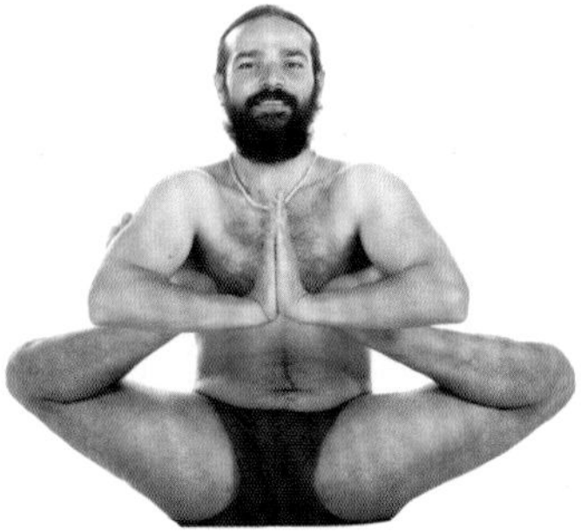

495
नमस्कार द्वि पाद योग दण्ड आसन
Namaskāra dvi pāda yoga daṇḍa āsana
Praying two leg yoga staff pose

नमस्कारद्विपादयोगदण्डासन
Namaskāradvipādayogadaṇḍāsana

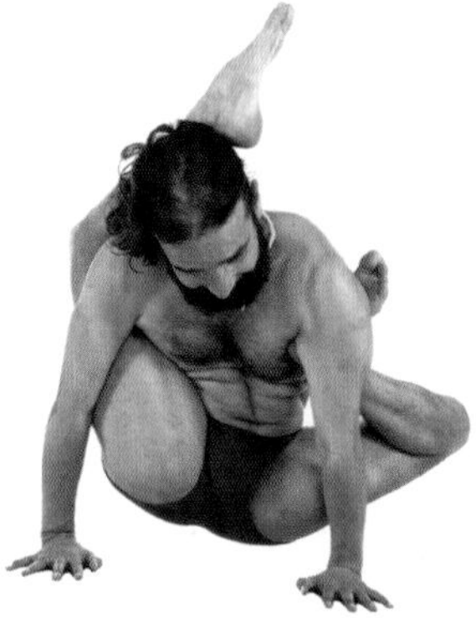

496
उत्थित योग दण्ड भैरव आसन
Utthita yoga daṇḍa bhairava āsana
Lifted fearless yoga staff pose

उत्थितयोगदण्डभैरवासन
Utthitayogadaṇḍabhairavāsana

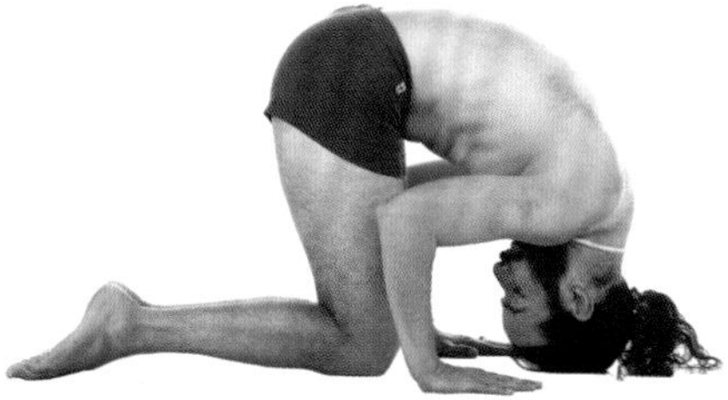

497
अर्ध शशाङ्क आसन (आरम्भ अवस्था)
Ardha śaśāṅka āsana (ārambha avasthā)
Half rabbit pose (starting position)

अर्धशशाङ्कासन (आरम्भावस्था)
Ardhaśaśāṅkāsana (ārambhāvasthā)

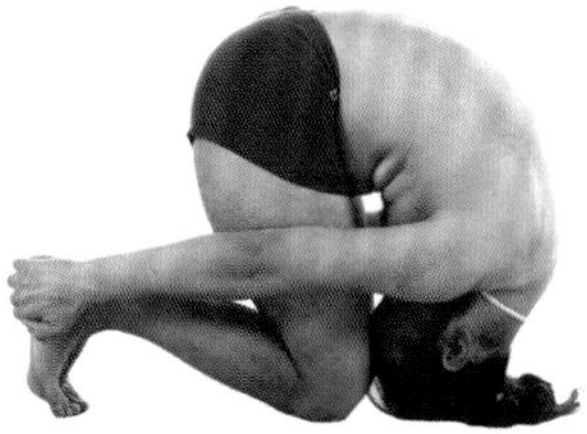

498
शशाङ्क आसन (प्रपदिक)
Śaśāṅka āsana (prapadika)
Rabbit pose (ball of toes on the earth)

शशाङ्कासन (प्रपदिक)
Śaśāṅkāsana (prapadika)

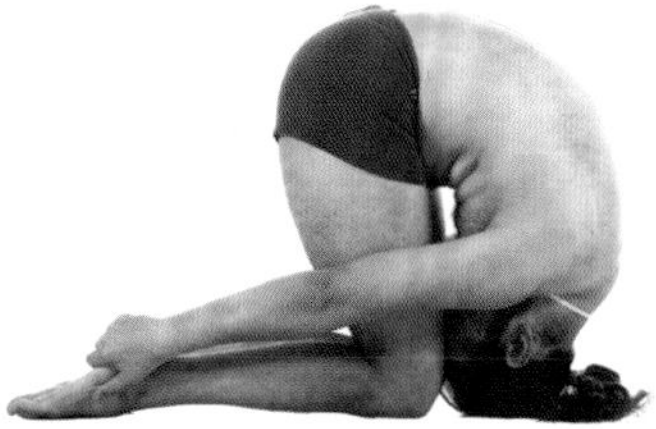

499
शशाङ्क आसन
Śaśāṅka āsana
Rabbit pose

शशाङ्कासन
Śaśāṅkāsana

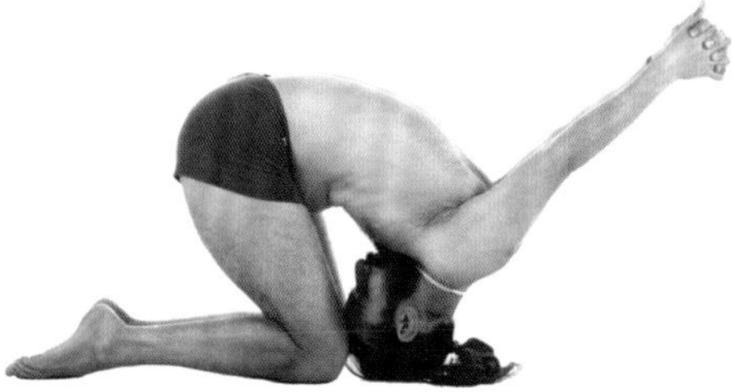

500
शशाङ्क आसन (पृष्ठ हस्त उत्तान)
Śaśāṅka āsana (pṛṣṭha hasta uttāna)
Rabbit pose (hands extended behind)

शशाङ्कासन (पृष्ठहस्तोत्तान)
Śaśāṅkāsana (pṛṣṭhahastauttāna)

Breathe deeply,
smile proudly.

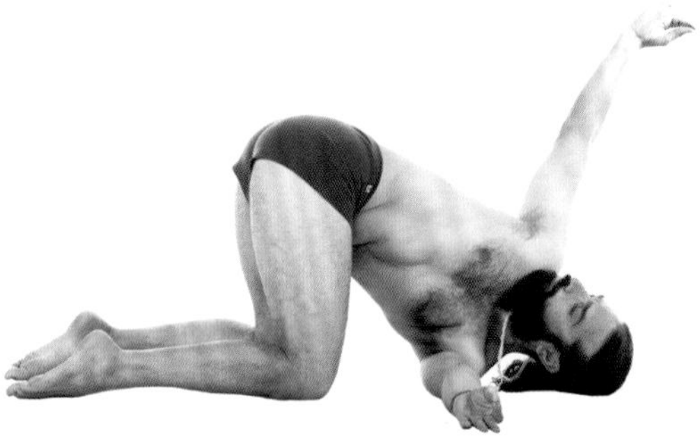

501
बाल वक्र नाथ आसन (विराट हस्त)
Bāla vakra nātha āsana (virāṭa hasta)
Baby yogi pose (arms extended wide)

बालवक्रनाथासन (विराटहस्त)
Bālavakranāthāsana (virāṭahasta)

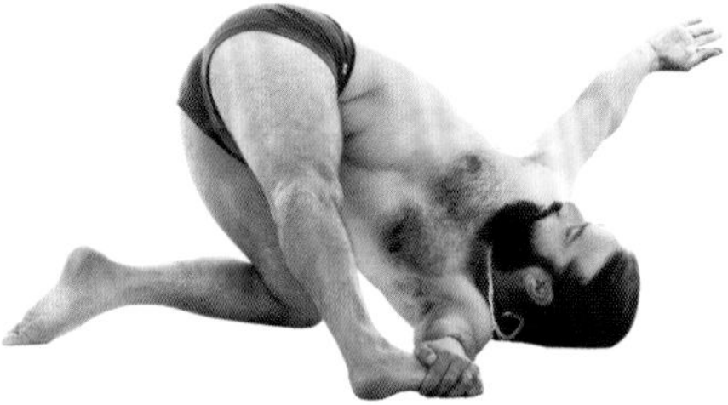

502
बाल वक्र नाथ आसन (बद्ध पाद अङ्गुष्ठ)
Bāla vakra nātha āsana (baddha pāda aṅguṣṭha)
Baby yogi pose (holding the big toe)

बालवक्रनाथासन (बद्धपादाङ्गुष्ठ)
Bālavakranāthāsana (baddhapādāṅguṣṭha)

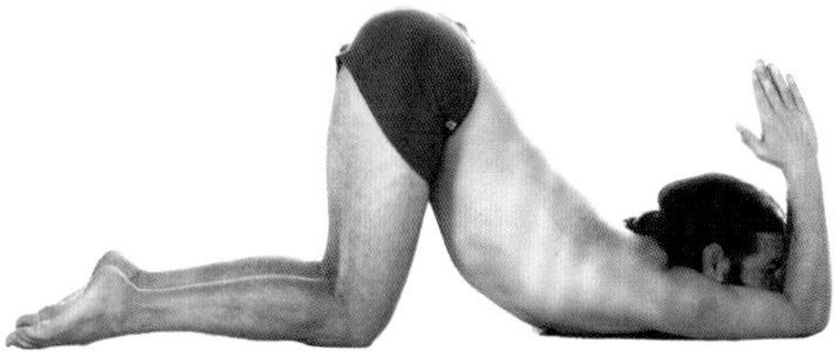

503
पल्लव कृमि आसन (ऊर्ध्व हस्त नमस्कार)
Pallava kṛmi āsana (ūrdhva hasta namaskāra)
Worm pose (arms overhead in prayer)

पल्लवकृमि आसन (ऊर्ध्वहस्तनमस्कार)
Pallavakṛmiāsana (ūrdhvahastanamaskāra)

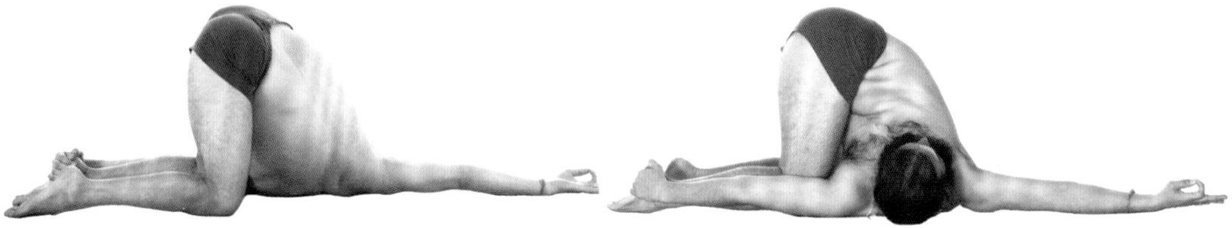

504
चरक आसन (विपरीत हस्त पाद बद्ध)
Caraka āsana (viparīta hasta pāda baddha)
Sage Caraka pose (hand bound to opposite foot)

चरकासन (विपरीतहस्तपादबद्ध)
Carakāsana (viparītahastapādabaddha)

Arm Balances

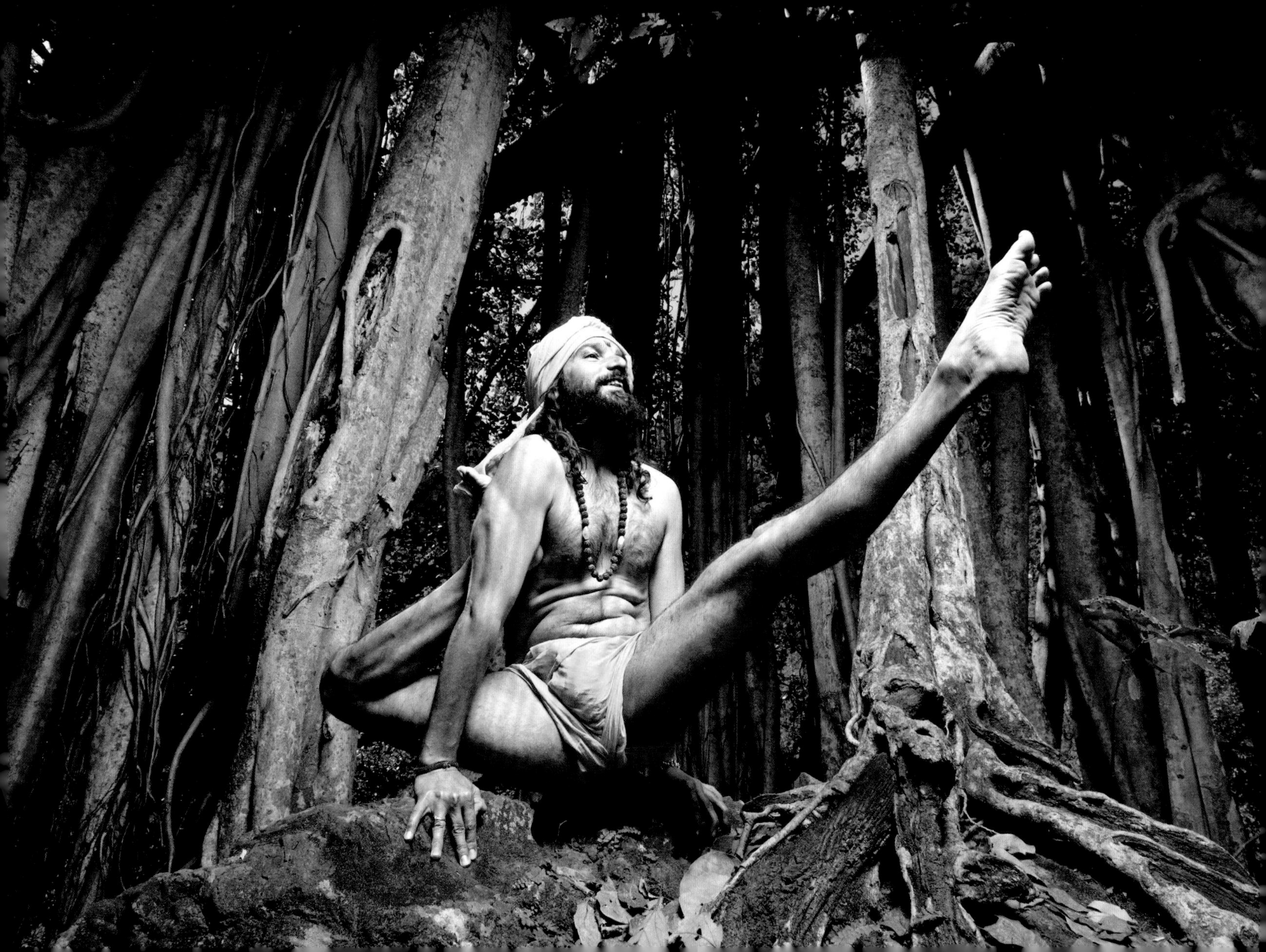

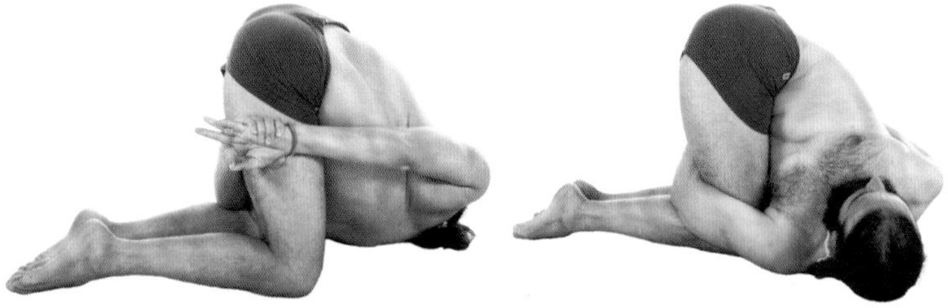

505
पूर्ण चरक आसन (रज्जु हस्त)
Pūrṇa Caraka āsana (rajju hasta)
Full sage Caraka pose (bound hands)

पूर्णचरकासन (रज्जुहस्त)
Pūrṇacarakāsana (rajjuhasta)

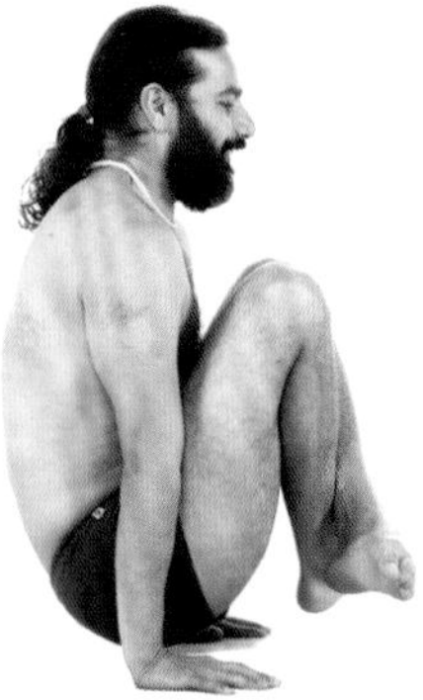

506
लोल आसन
Lola āsana
Swinging pose

लोलासन
Lolāsana

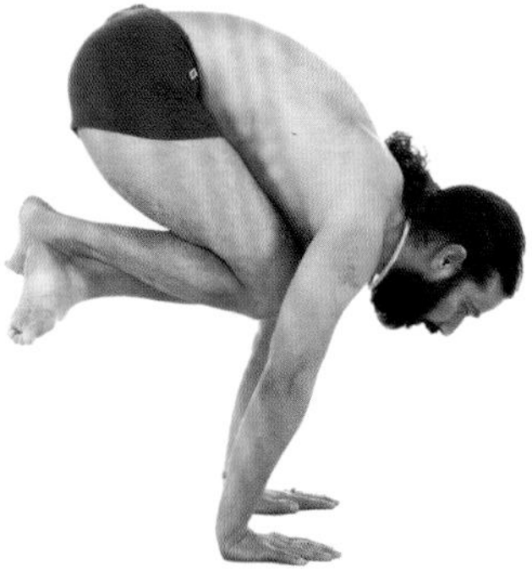

507
उड्डियान लोल आसन
Uḍḍiyāna lola āsana
Lifted swinging pose

उड्डियानलोलासन
Uḍḍiyānalolāsana

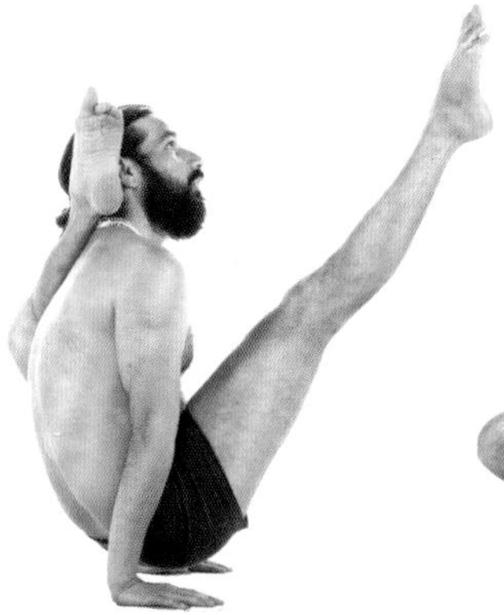

508
चातक आसन
Cātaka āsana
Skylark pose

चातकासन
Cātakāsana

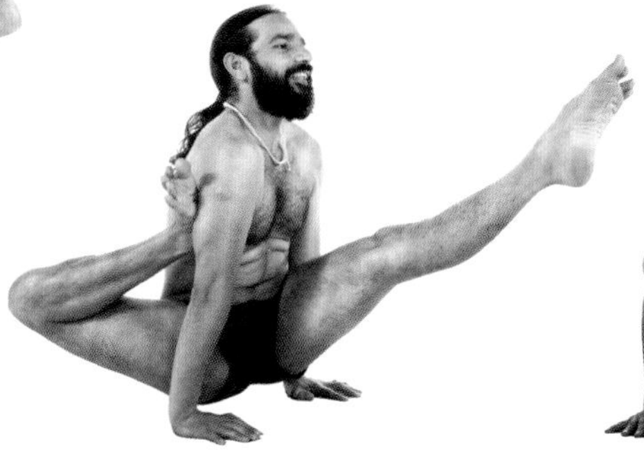

509
चर्पट नाथ आसन
Carpaṭa Nātha āsana
Sage Carpaṭa Nātha pose

चर्पटनाथासन
Carpaṭanāthāsana

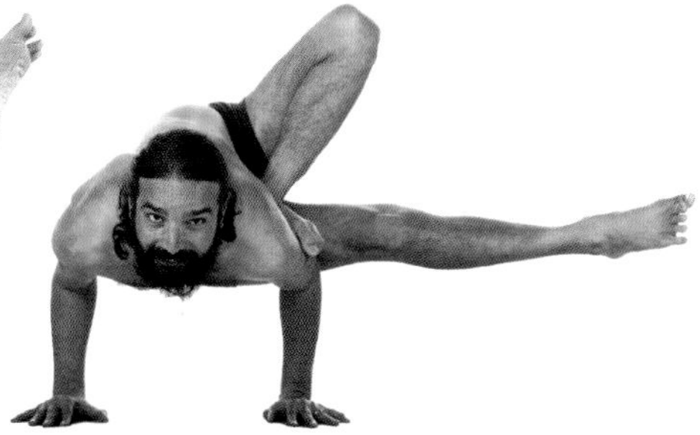

510
परिवृत्त चर्पट नाथ आसन
Parivṛtta Carpaṭa Nātha āsana
Twisted sage Carpata Nātha pose

परिवृत्तचर्पटनाथासन
Parivṛttacarpaṭanāthāsana

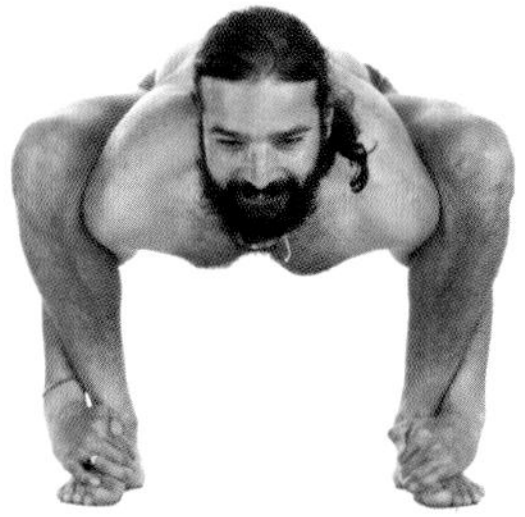

511
खञ्जन आसन
Khañjana āsana
Wagtail pose

खञ्जनासन
Khañjanāsana

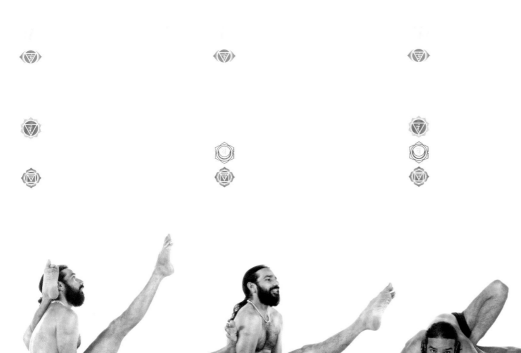

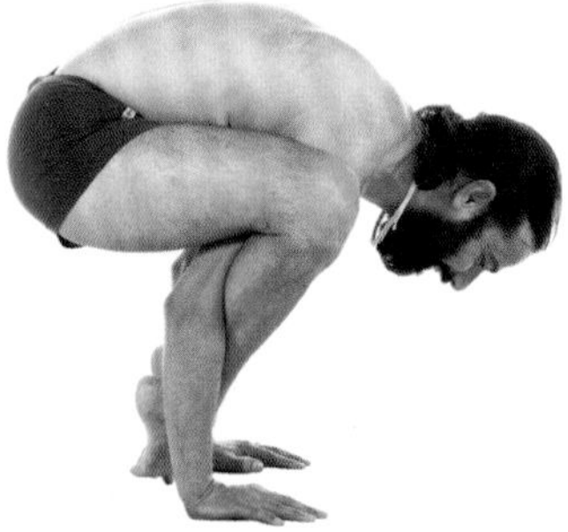

512
भुज पीड आसन (भू पाद)
Bhuja pīḍa āsana (bhū pāda)
Arm pressure pose (feet on the earth)

भुजपीडासन (भूपाद)
Bhujapīḍāsana (bhūpāda)

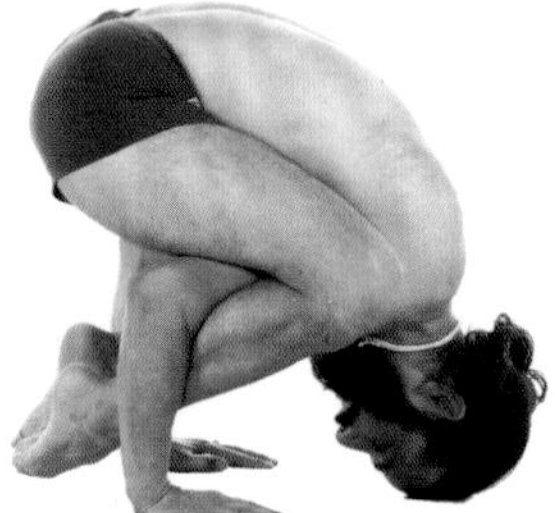

513
भुज पीड आसन (भू शिर)
Bhuja pīḍa āsana (bhū śira)
Arm pressure pose (head on the earth)

भुजपीडासन (भूशिर)
Bhujapīḍāsana (bhūśira)

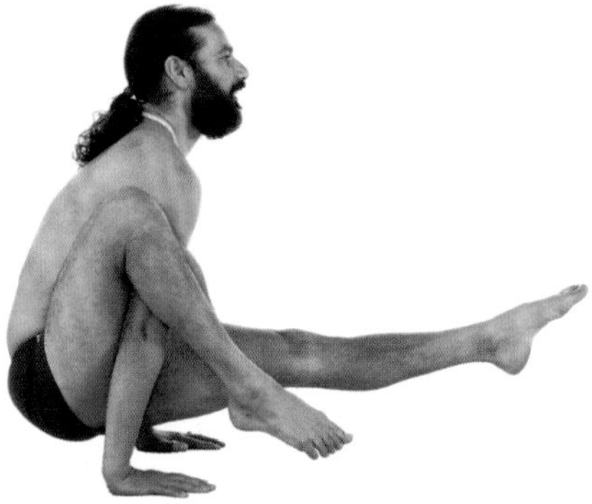

514
भुज पीड आसन (एक पाद दण्ड तुला)
Bhuja pīḍa āsana (eka pāda daṇḍa tulā)
Arm pressure pose (one leg balancing staff variation)

भुजपीडासन (एकपाददण्डतुला)
Bhujapīḍāsana (ekapādadaṇḍatulā)

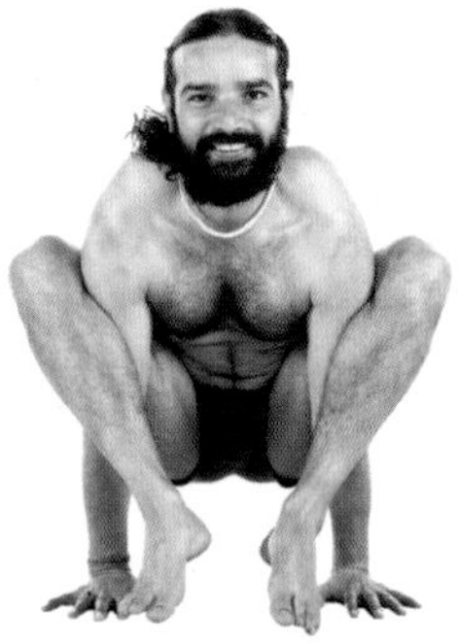

515
भुज पीड आसन
Bhuja pīḍa āsana
Arm pressure pose

भुजपीडासन
Bhujapīḍāsana

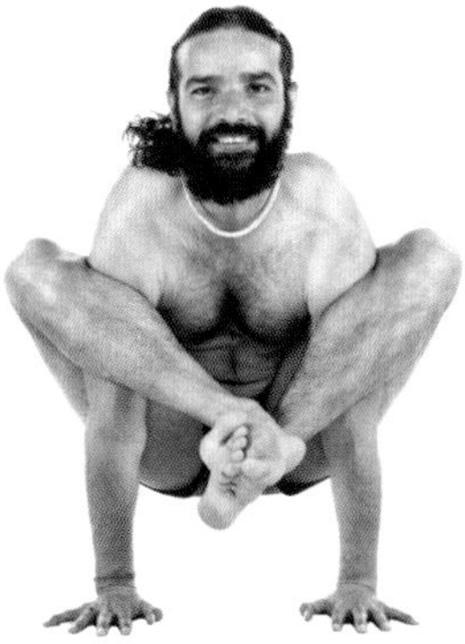

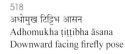

516
भुज पीड आसन (विकट)
Bhuja pīḍa āsana (vikaṭa)
Arm pressure pose (challenging variation)

भुजपीडासन (विकट)
Bhujapīḍāsana (vikaṭa)

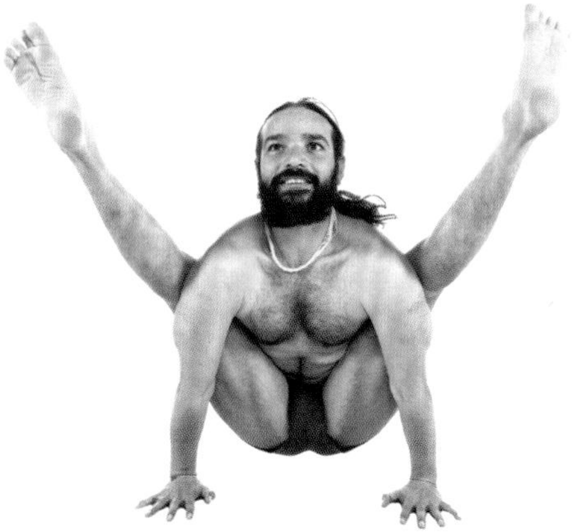

517
ऊर्ध्व मुख टिट्टिभ आसन
Ūrdhva mukha ṭiṭṭibha āsana
Upward facing firefly pose

ऊर्ध्वमुखटिट्टिभासन
Ūrdhvamukhaṭiṭṭibhāsana

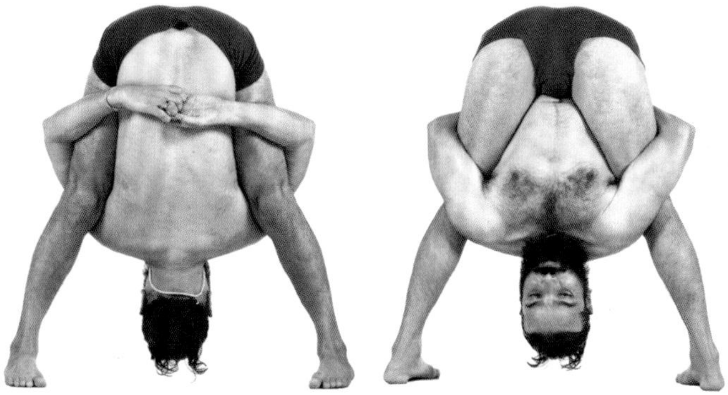

518
अधोमुख टिट्टिभ आसन
Adhomukha ṭiṭṭibha āsana
Downward facing firefly pose

अधोमुखटिट्टिभासन
Adhomukhaṭiṭṭibhāsana

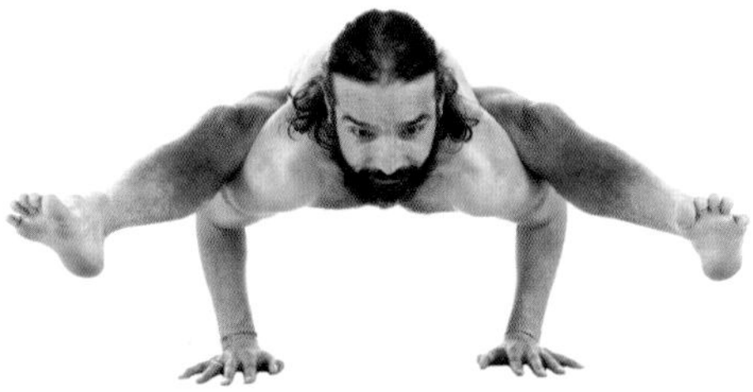

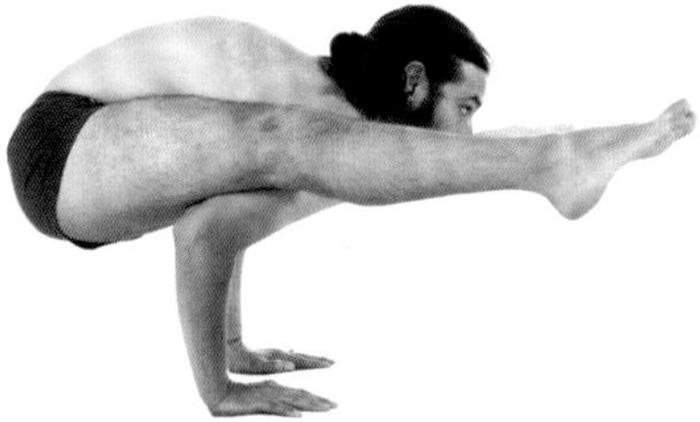

519
टिट्टिभ आसन (कफोणि उत्तोलन)
Ṭiṭṭibha āsana (kaphoṇi uttolana)
Firefly pose (balancing on the elbows)

टिट्टिभासन (कफोणिउत्तोलन)
Ṭiṭṭibhāsana (kaphoṇiuttolana)

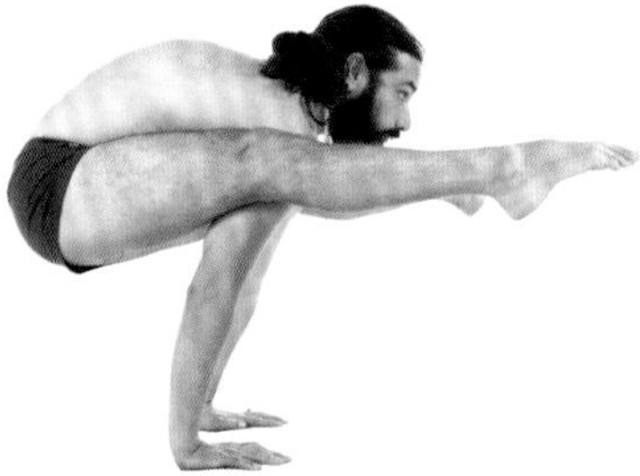

520
टिट्टिभ आसन
Ṭiṭṭibha āsana
Firefly pose

टिट्टिभासन
Ṭiṭṭibhāsana

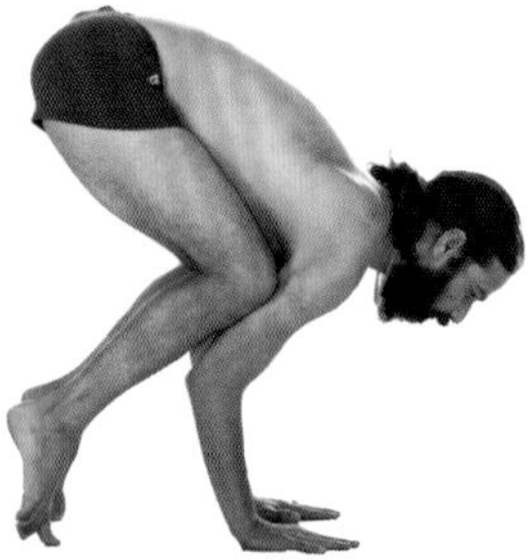

521
अर्ध बक आसन (पाद अङ्गुल भू)
Ardha baka āsana (pāda āṅgula bhū)
Half crane pose (toes on the earth)

अर्धबकासन (पादाङ्गुलभू)
Ardhabakāsana (pādāṅgulabhū)

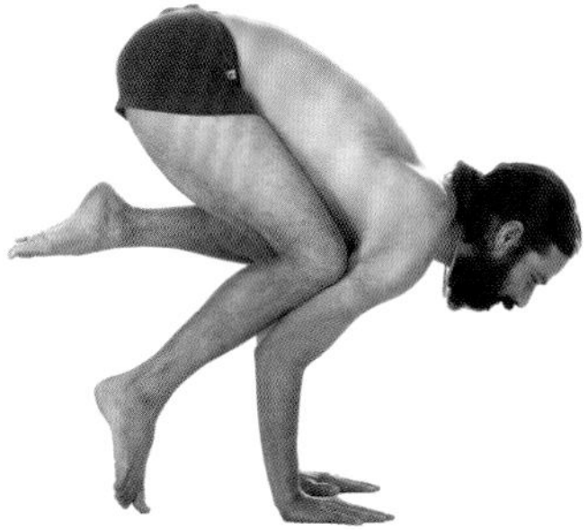

522
अर्ध बक आसन (एक पाद अङ्गुल भू)
Ardha baka āsana (eka pāda aṅgula bhū)
Half crane pose (toes of one foot on the earth)

अर्धबकासन (एकपादाङ्गुलभू)
Ardhabakāsana (ekapādāṅgulabhū)

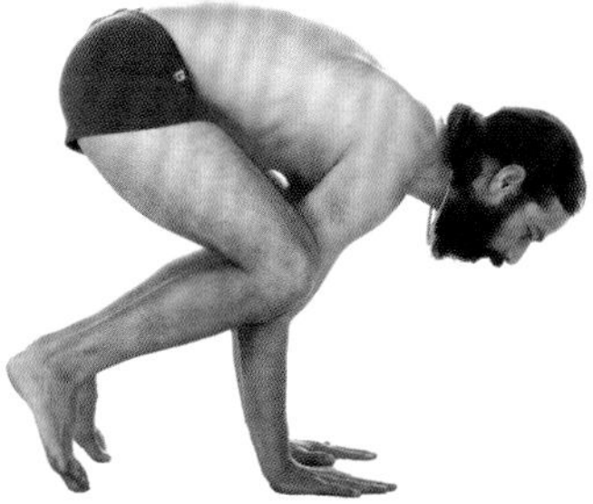

523
अर्ध बक आसन (पाद अङ्गुल भू, बहिर्जानु)
Ardha baka āsana (pāda aṅgula bhū, bahirjānu)
Half crane pose (toes on the earth, knees outside)

अर्धबकासन (पादाङ्गुलभू, बहिर्जानु)
Ardhabakāsana (pādāṅgulabhū, bahirjānu)

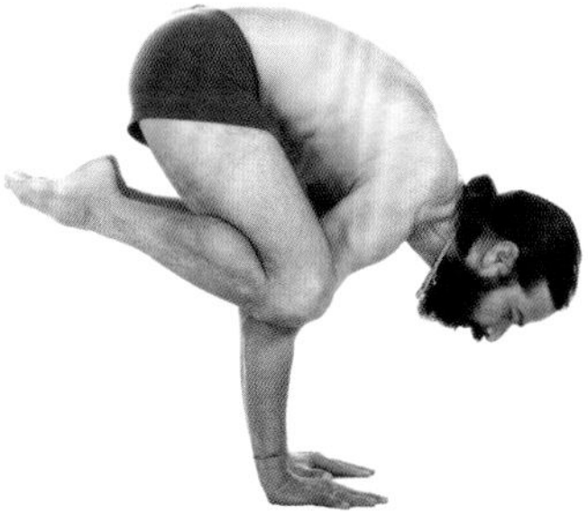

524
बक आसन (बहिर्जानु)
Baka āsana (bahirjānu)
Crane pose (knees outside)

बकासन (बहिर्जानु)
Bakāsana (bahirjānu)

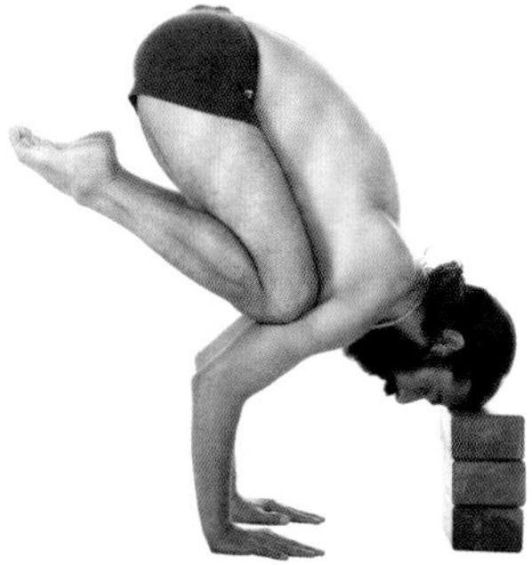

525
बक आसन (सालम्ब)
Baka āsana (sālamba)
Crane pose (supported)

बकासन (सालम्ब)
Bakāsana (sālamba)

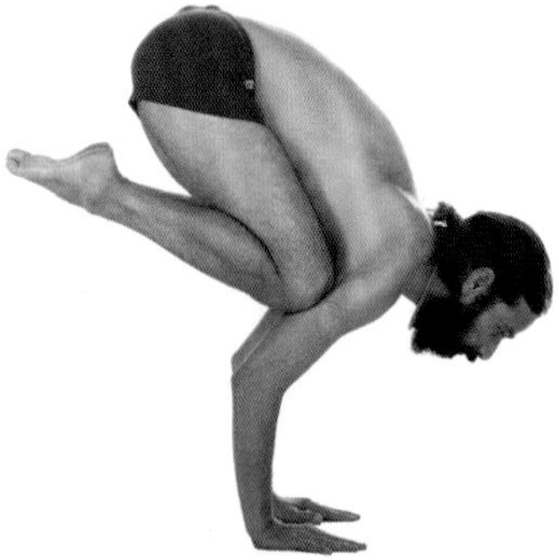

526
बक आसन
Baka āsana
Crane pose

बकासन
Bakāsana

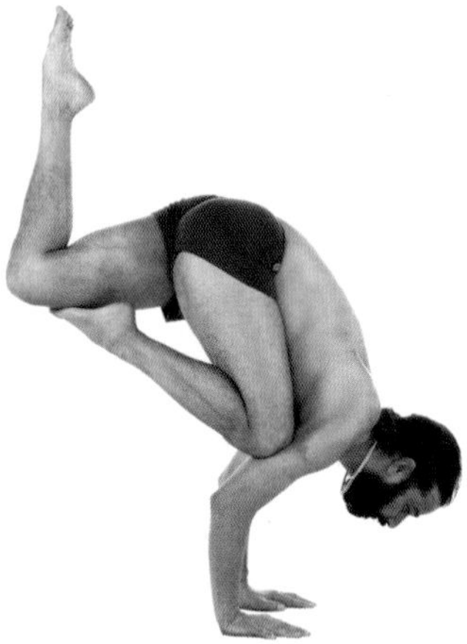

527
महा बक आसन
Mahā baka āsana
Great crane pose

महाबकासन
Mahābakāsana

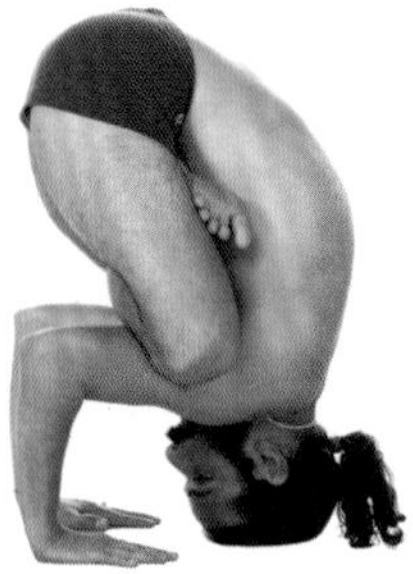

528
पद्म बक आसन (आरम्भ अवस्था)
Padma baka āsana (ārambha avasthā)
Lotus crane pose (starting position)

पद्मबकासन (आरम्भावस्था)
Padmabakāsana (ārambhavasthā)

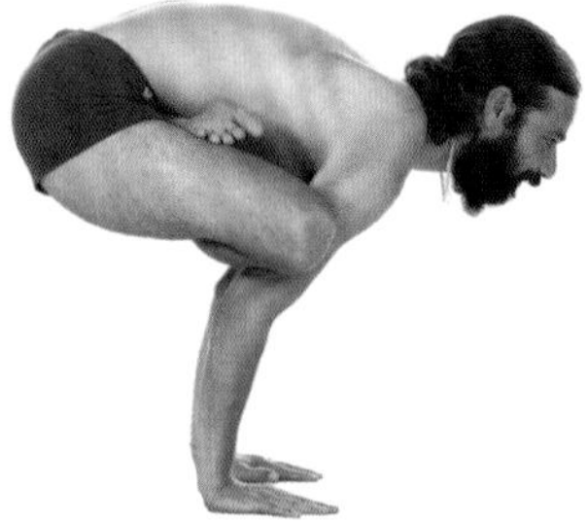

529
पद्म बक आसन
Padma baka āsana
Lotus crane pose

पद्मबकासन
Padmabakāsana

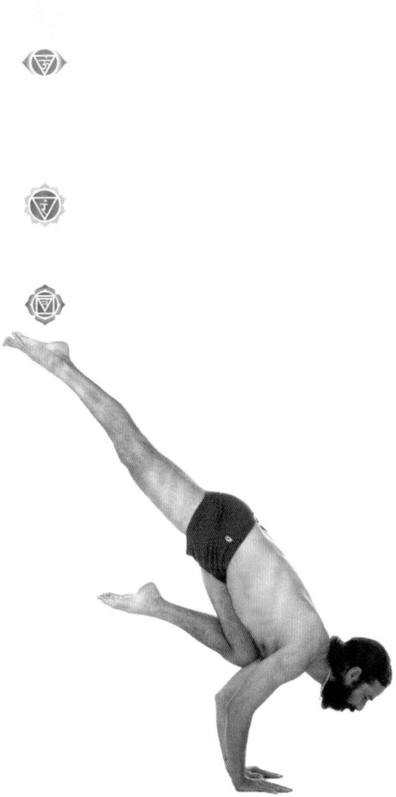

530
बक आसन (ऊर्ध्व एक पाद)
Baka āsana (ūrdhva eka pāda)
Crane pose (one leg lifted)

बकासन (ऊर्ध्वैकपाद)
Bakāsana (ūrdhvaikapāda)

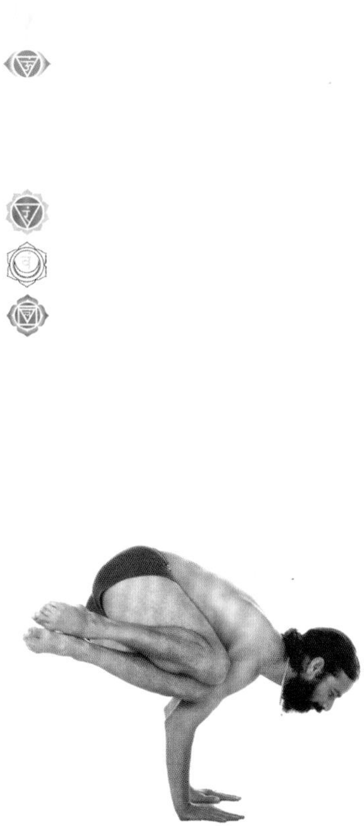

531
परिवृत्त बक आसन
Parivṛtta baka āsana
Twisted crane pose

परिवृत्तबकासन
Parivṛttabakāsana

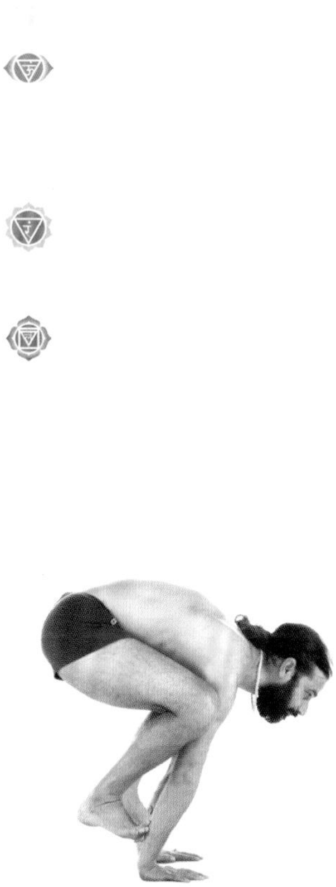

532
बक आसन (मणि बन्ध)
Baka āsana (maṇi bandha)
Crane pose (toes to wrists)

बकासन (मणिबन्ध)
Bakāsana (maṇibandha)

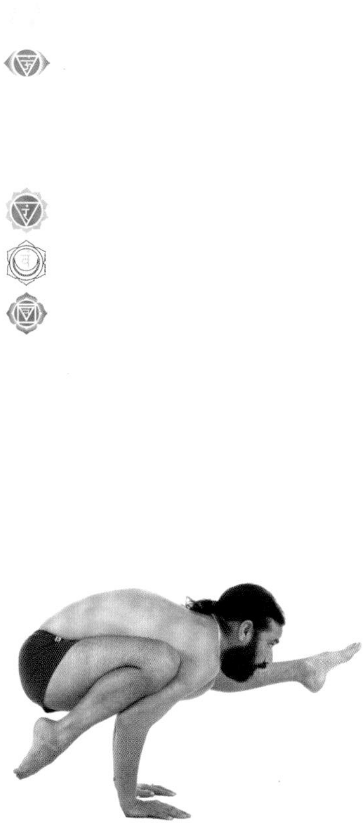

533
टिट्टिभ बक आसन
Ṭiṭṭibha baka āsana
Firefly crane pose

टिट्टिभबकासन
Ṭiṭṭibhabakāsana

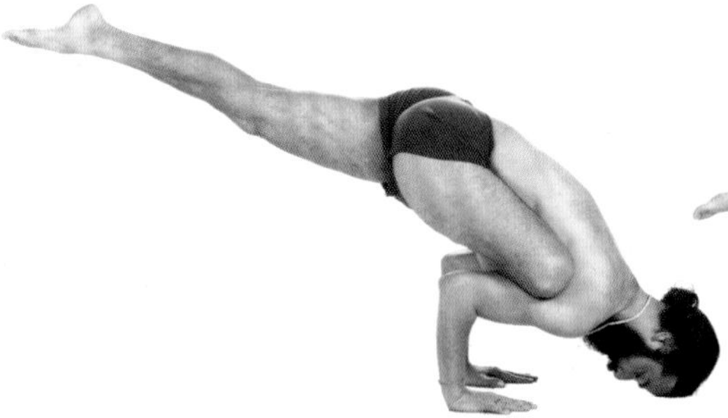

534
गालव आसन (ललाट भू)
Gālava āsana (lalāṭa bhū)
Sage Gālava pose (forehead on the earth)

गालवासन (ललाटभू)
Gālavāsana (lalāṭabhū)

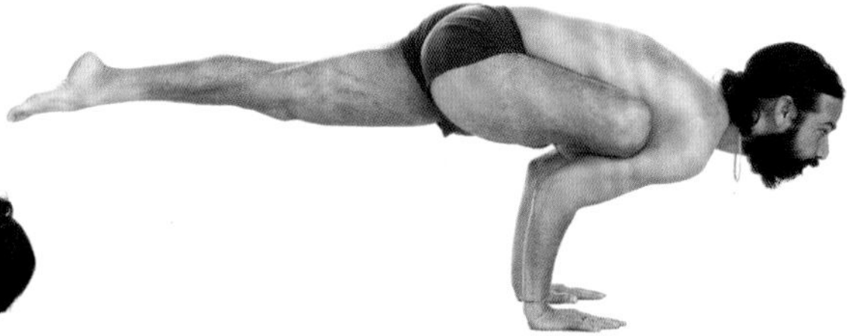

535
गालव आसन
Gālava āsana
Sage Gālava pose

गालवासन
Gālavāsana

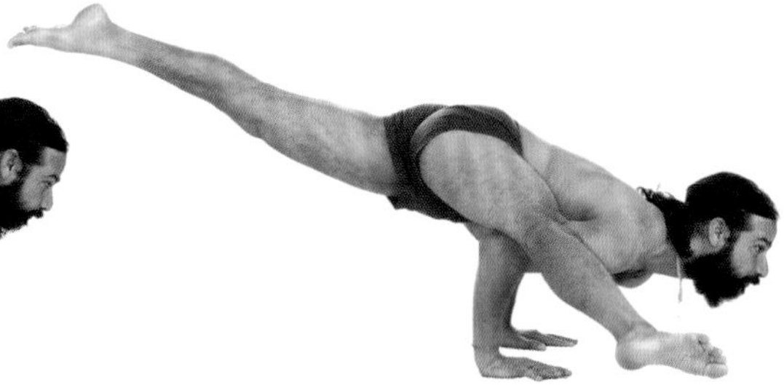

536
एक पाद कौण्डीन्य आसन
Eka pāda Kauṇḍīnya āsana
One leg Sage Kaundīnya pose

एकपादकौण्डीन्यासन
Ekapādakauṇḍīnyāsana

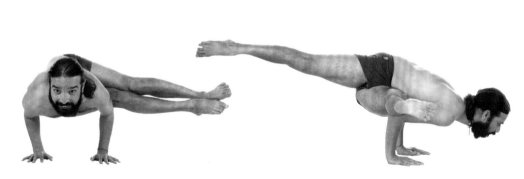

537
परिवृत्त कौण्डीन्य आसन
Parivṛtta Kauṇḍīnya āsana
Twisted sage Kaundīnya pose

परिवृत्तकौण्डीन्यासन
Parivṛttakauṇḍīnyāsana

538
परिवृत्त कौण्डीन्य आसन
Parivṛtta eka pāda Kauṇḍīnya āsana
Twisted one leg Sage Kaundīnya pose

परिवृत्तैकपादकौण्डीन्यासन
Parivṛttaikapādakauṇḍīnyāsana

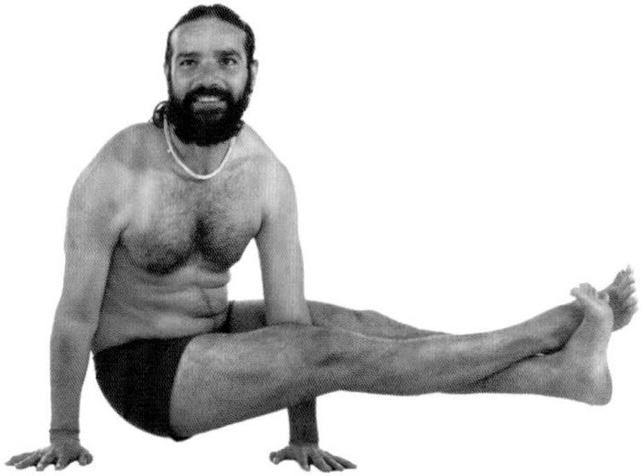

539
अष्टावक्र आसन
Aṣṭāvakra āsana
Sage Astāvakra pose

अष्टावक्रासन
Aṣṭāvakrāsana

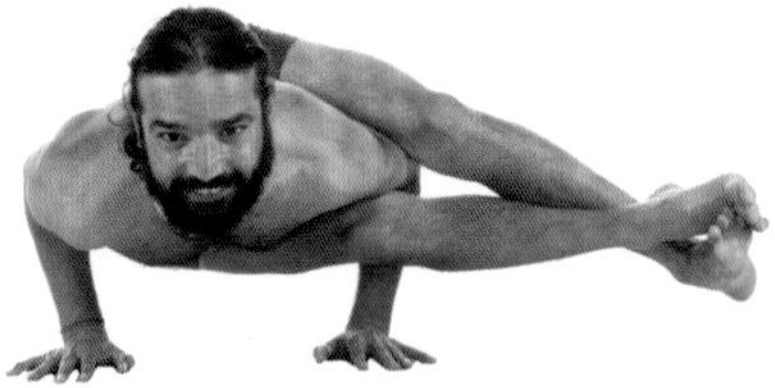

540
अष्टावक्र आसन (विकट)
Aṣṭāvakra āsana (vikaṭa)
Sage Astāvakra pose (challenging variation)

अष्टावक्रासन (विकटा)
Aṣṭāvakrāsana (vikaṭa)

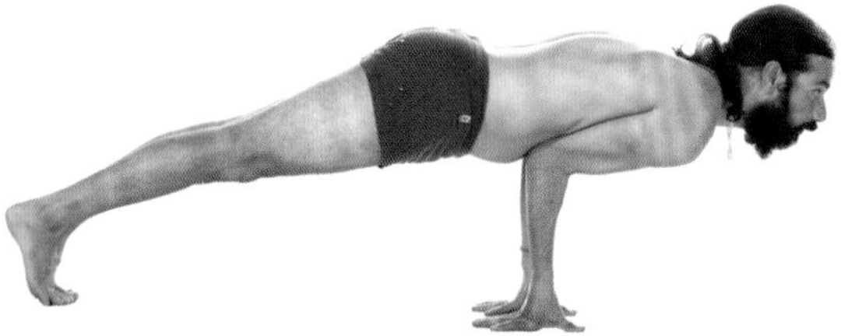

541
मयूर आसन (आरम्भ अवस्था)
Mayūra āsana (ārambha avasthā)
Peacock pose (starting position)

मयूरासन (आरम्भावस्था)
Mayūrāsana (ārambhāvasthā)

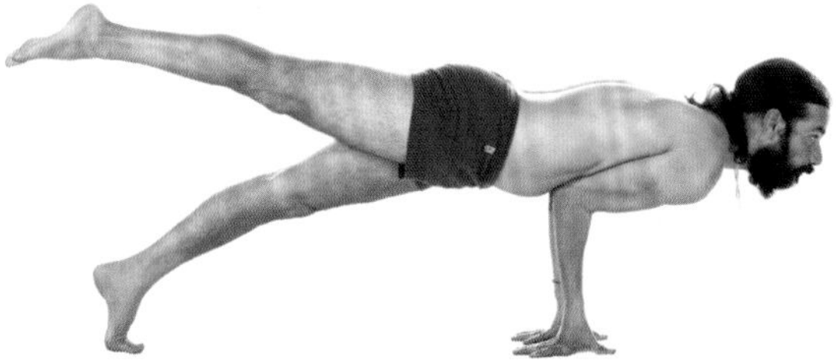

542
मयूर आसन (एक पाद ऊर्ध्व)
Mayūra āsana (eka pāda ūrdhva)
Peacock pose (one leg lifted)

मयूरासन (एकपादऊर्ध्व)
Mayūrāsana (ekapādordhva)

Yoga is about finding the right balance.

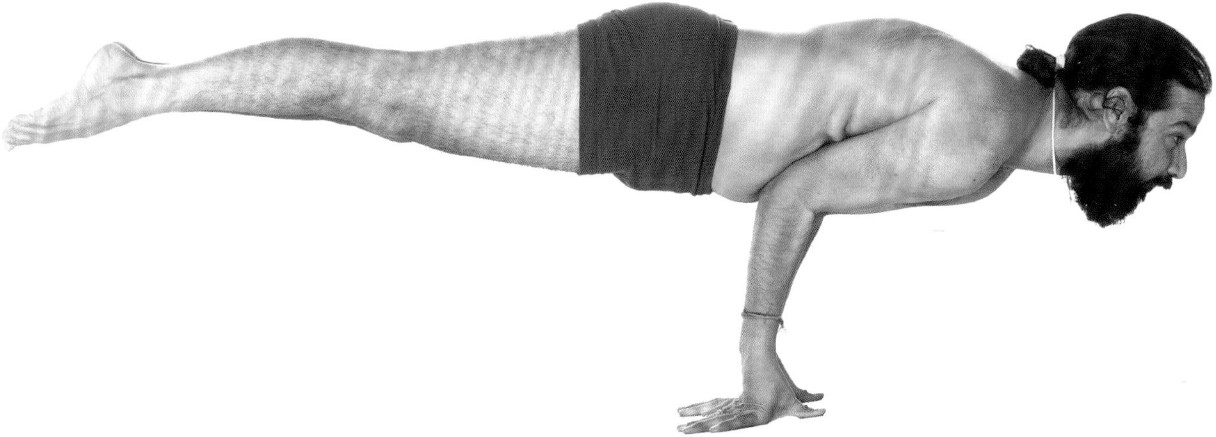

543
मयूर आसन (हस्त अङ्गुल भू)
Mayūra āsana (hasta aṅgula bhū)
Peacock pose (fingers on the earth)

मयूरासन (हस्ताङ्गुलभू)
Mayūrāsana (hastāṅgulabhū)

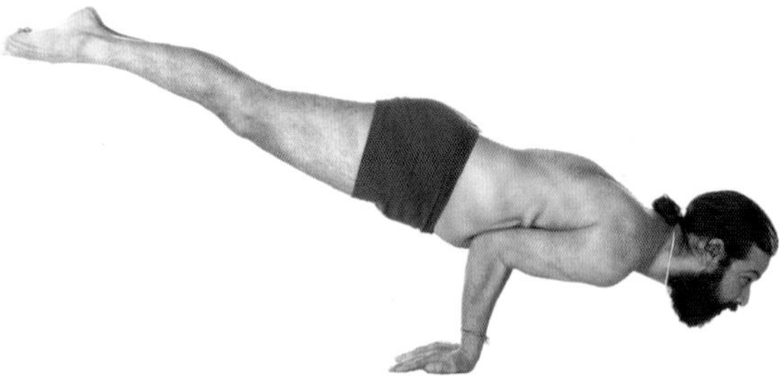

544
मयूर आसन (करतल भू)
Mayūra āsana (karatala bhū)
Peacock pose (palms on the earth)

मयूरआसन (करतलभू)
Mayūrāsana (karatalabhū)

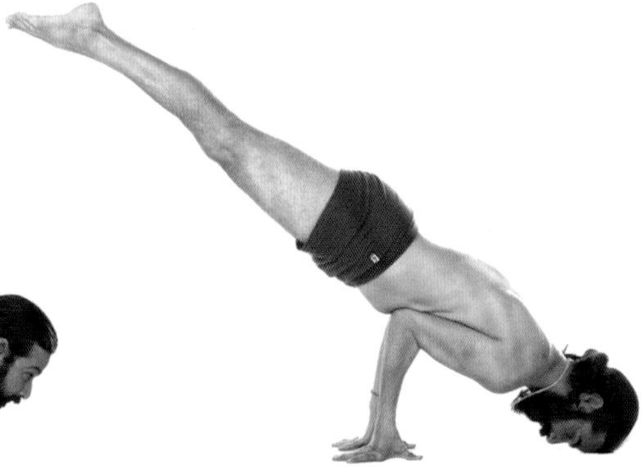

545
मयूर आसन (ललाट भू)
Mayūra āsana (lalāṭa bhū)
Peacock pose (forehead on the earth)

मयूरासन (ललाटभू)
Mayūrāsana (lalāṭabhū)

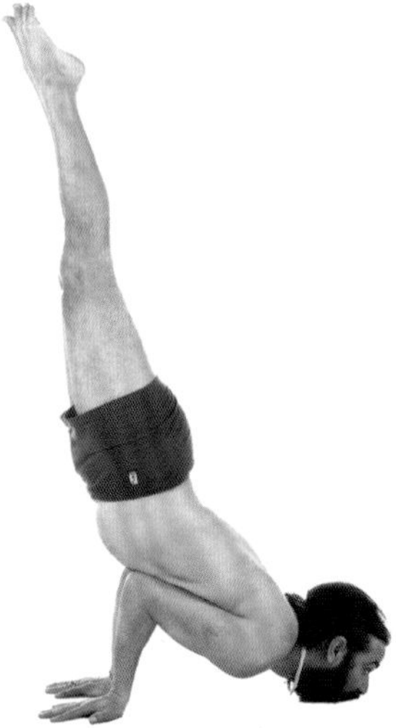

546
मयूर आसन (हनु भू)
Mayūra āsana (hanu bhū)
Peacock pose (chin on the earth)

मयूरासन (हनुभू)
Mayūrāsana (hanubhū)

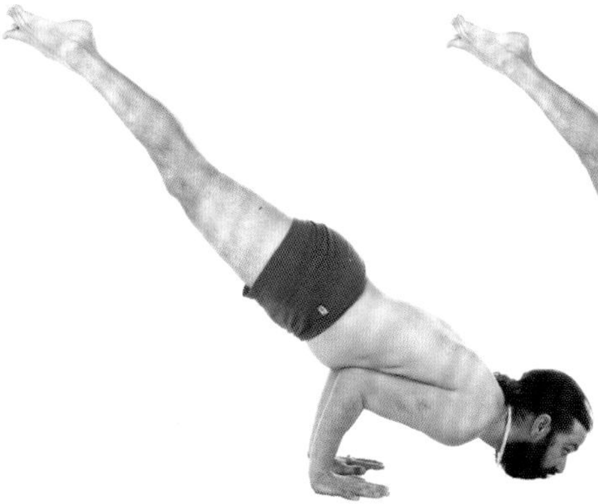

547
मयूर आसन (हनु भू अन्तर्हस्त)
Mayūra āsana (hanu bhū antarhasta)
Peacock pose (chin on the earth, fingers pointed in)

मयूरासन (हनुभ्वान्तर्हस्त)
Mayūrāsana (hanubhūantarhasta)

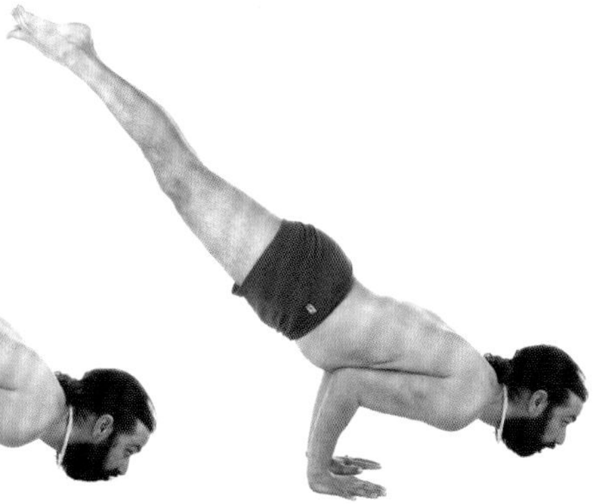

548
मयूर आसन (अन्तर्हस्त)
Mayūra āsana (antarhasta)
Peacock pose (fingers pointed in)

मयूरासन (अन्तर्हस्त)
Mayūrāsana (antarhasta)

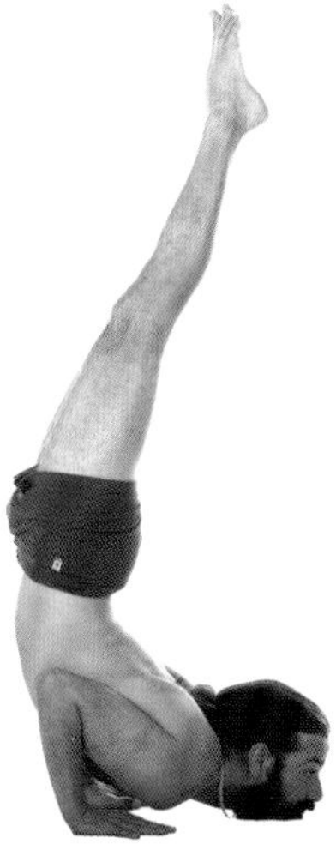

549
पुच्छ मयूर आसन (करतल भू)
Puccha mayūra āsana (karatala bhū)
Peacock feather pose (palms on the earth)

पुच्छमयूरासन (करतलभू)
Pucchamayūrāsana (karatalabhū)

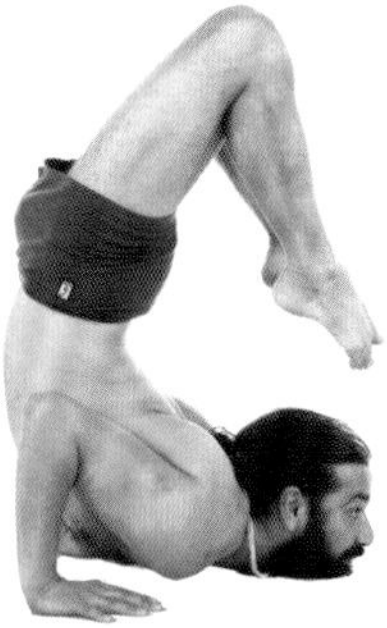

550
नृत्य मयूर आसन (करतल भू)
Nṛtya mayūra āsana (karatala bhū)
Dancing peacock feather pose (palms on the earth)

नृत्यमयूरासन (करतलभू)
Nṛtyamayūrāsana (karatalabhū)

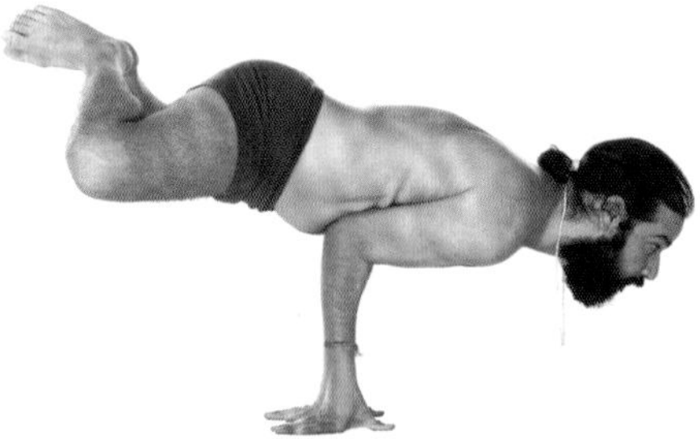

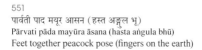

551
पार्वती पाद मयूर आसन (हस्त अङ्गुल भू)
Pārvati pāda mayūra āsana (hasta aṅgula bhū)
Feet together peacock pose (fingers on the earth)

पार्वतीपादमयूरासन (हस्ताङ्गुल भू)
Pārvatipādamayūrāsana (hastāṅgulabhū)

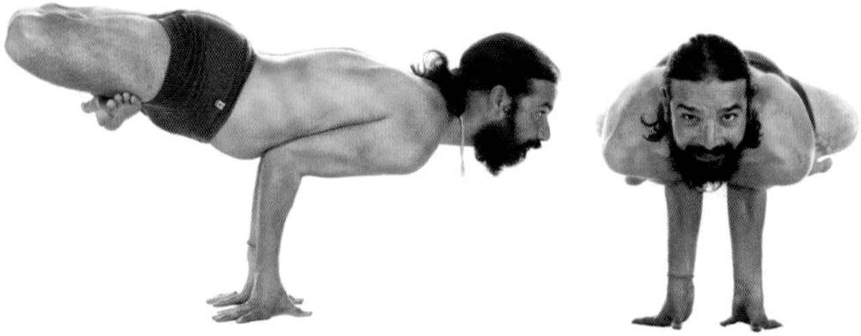

552
पद्म मयूर आसन
Padma mayūra āsana
Lotus peacock pose

पद्ममयूरासन
Padmamayūrāsana

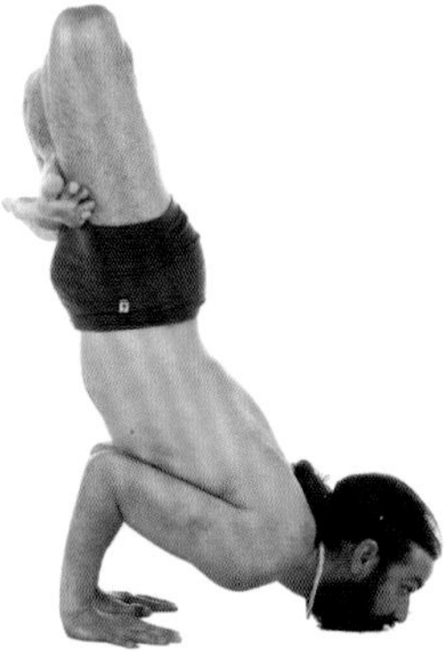

553
ऊर्ध्व पद्म मयूर आसन (हनु भू)
Ūrdhva padma mayūra āsana (hanu bhū)
Lifted lotus peacock pose (chin on the earth)

ऊर्ध्वपद्ममयूरासन (हनुभू)
Ūrdhvapadmamayūrāsana (hanubhū)

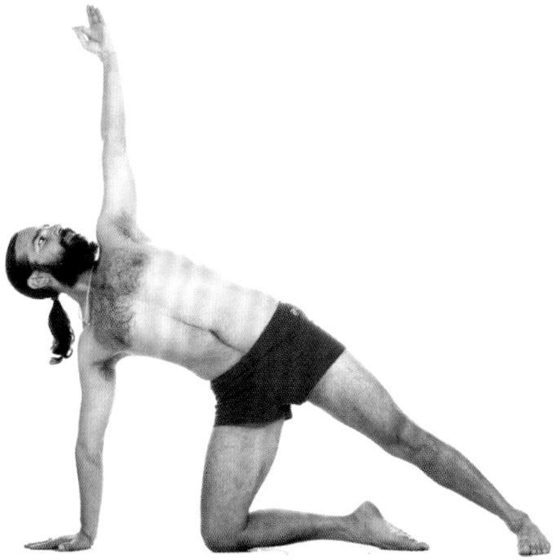

554
वशिष्ठ आसन (जानु भू)
Vaśiṣṭha āsana (jānu bhū)
Sage Vasistha pose (knee on the earth)

वशिष्ठासन (जानुभू)
Vaśiṣṭhāsana (jānubhū)

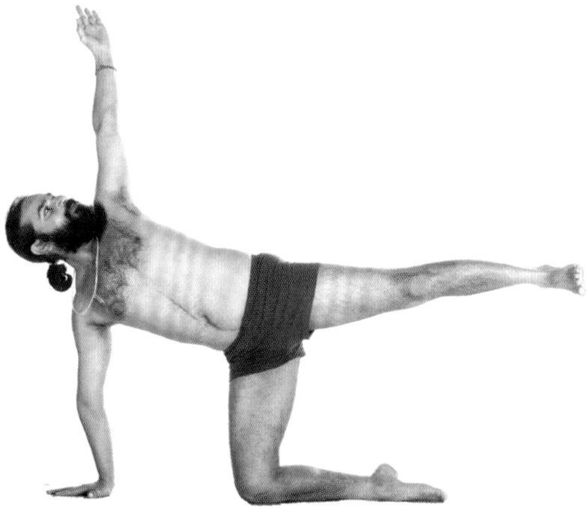

555
उत्तोलन एक पाद वशिष्ठ आसन (जानु भू)
Uttolana eka pāda Vaśiṣṭha āsana (jānu bhū)
Balancing one leg Sage Vasistha pose (knee on the earth)

उत्तोलनैकपादवशिष्ठासन (जानुभू)
Uttolanaikapādavaśiṣṭhāsana (jānubhū)

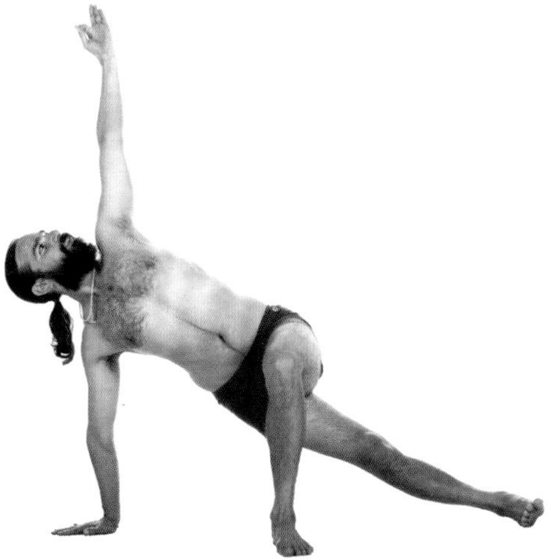

556
वशिष्ठ आसन (त्रि अङ्ग भू)
Vaśiṣṭha āsana (tri aṅga bhū)
Sage Vasistha pose (three limbs on the earth)

वशिष्ठासन (त्र्यङ्गभू)
Vaśiṣṭhāsana (Triaṅgabhū)

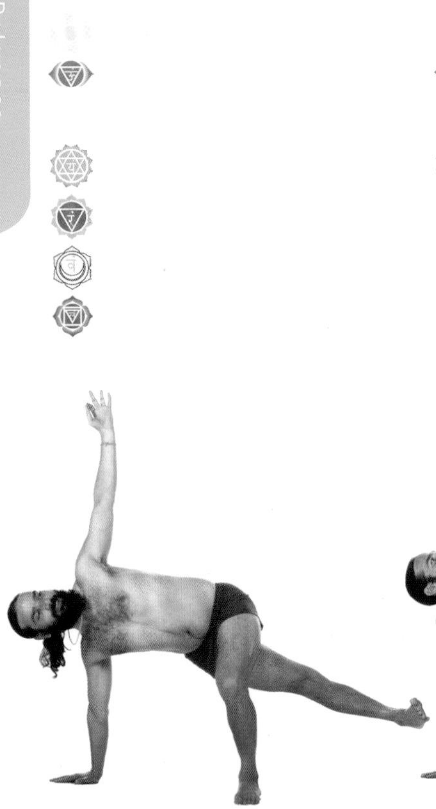

557
उत्तोलन वशिष्ठ आसन (विपरीत हस्त पाद)
Uttolana Vaśiṣṭha āsana (viparīta hasta pāda)
Balancing Sage Vasistha pose (opposite hand and leg)

उत्तोलनवशिष्ठासन (विपरीतहस्तपाद)
Uttolanavaśiṣṭhāsana (viparītahastapāda)

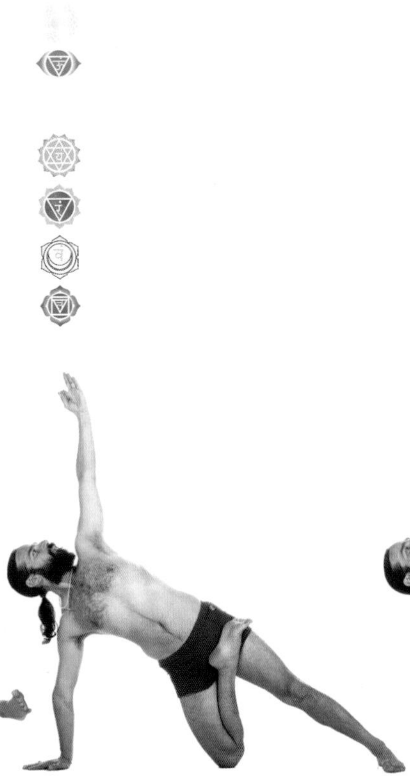

558
अर्ध पद्म वशिष्ठ आसन (जानु भू)
Ardha padma Vaśiṣṭha āsana (jānu bhū)
Half lotus Sage Vasistha pose (knee on the earth)

अर्धपद्मवशिष्ठासन (जानुभू)
Ardhapadmaśiṣṭhāsana (jānubhū)

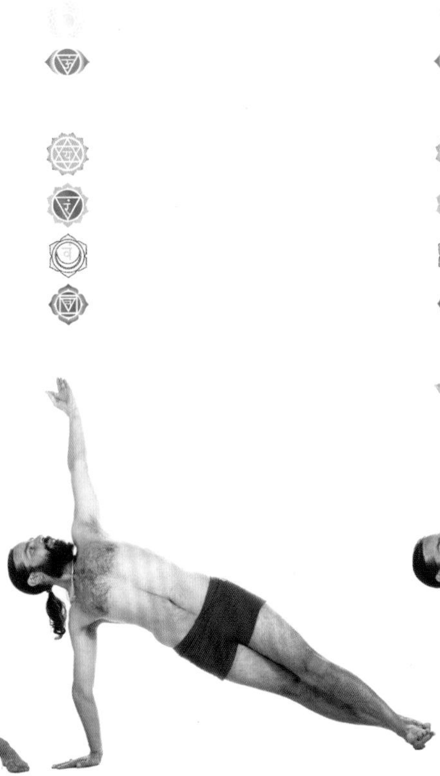

559
वशिष्ठ आसन (समक्षपाद)
Vaśiṣṭha āsana (samakṣapāda)
Sage Vasistha pose (one foot in front of the other)

वशिष्ठासन (समक्षपाद)
Vaśiṣṭhāsana (samakṣapāda)

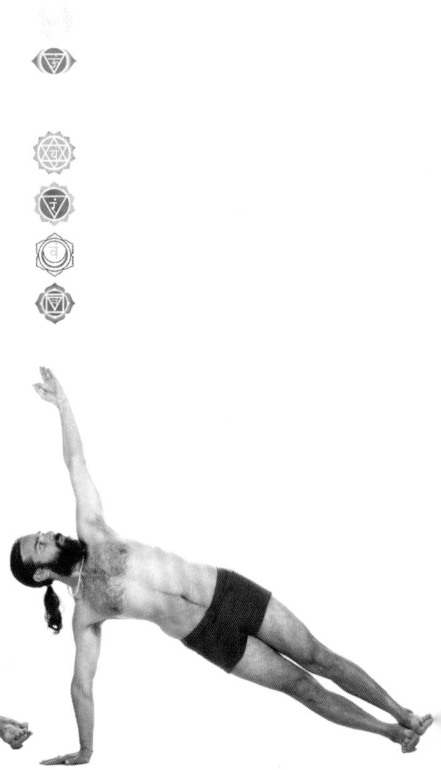

560
वशिष्ठ आसन
Vaśiṣṭha āsana
Sage Vasistha pose

वशिष्ठासन
Vaśiṣṭhāsana

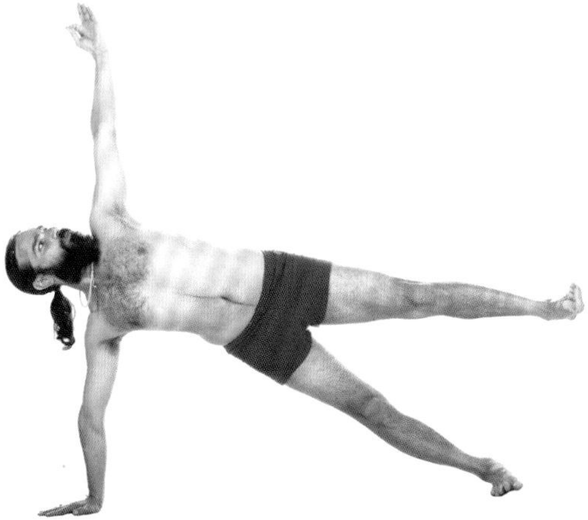

561
वशिष्ठ आसन (एक पाद उत्तान)
Vaśiṣṭha āsana (eka pāda uttāna)
Sage Vasistha pose (one leg lifted)

वशिष्ठासन (एकपादोत्तान)
Vaśiṣṭhāsana (ekapādottāna)

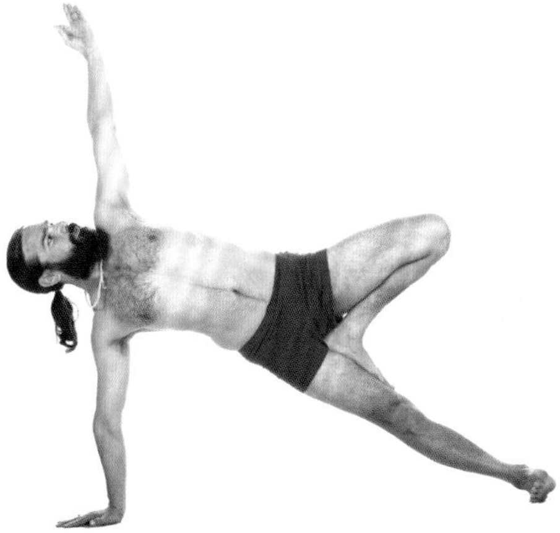

562
वशिष्ठ आसन (ध्रुव)
Vaśiṣṭha āsana (dhruva)
Sage Vasistha pose (fig tree variation)

वशिष्ठासन (ध्रुव)
Vaśiṣṭhāsana (dhruva)

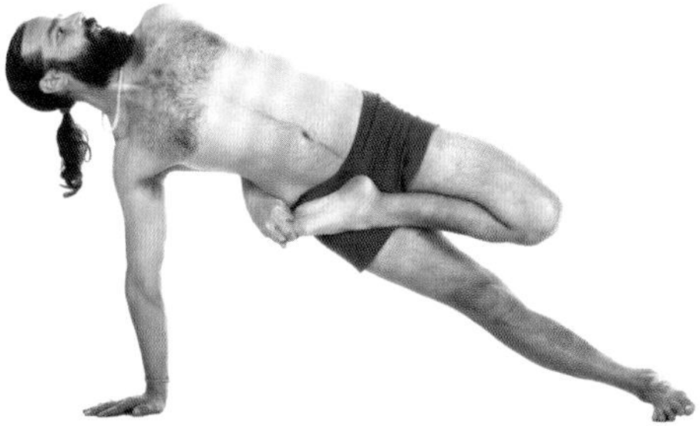

563
वशिष्ठ आसन (अर्धबद्ध पद्म)
Vaśiṣṭha āsana (ardha baddha padma)
Sage Vasistha pose (bound half lotus variation)

वशिष्ठासन (अर्धबद्धपद्म)
Vaśiṣṭhāsana (ardhabaddhapadma)

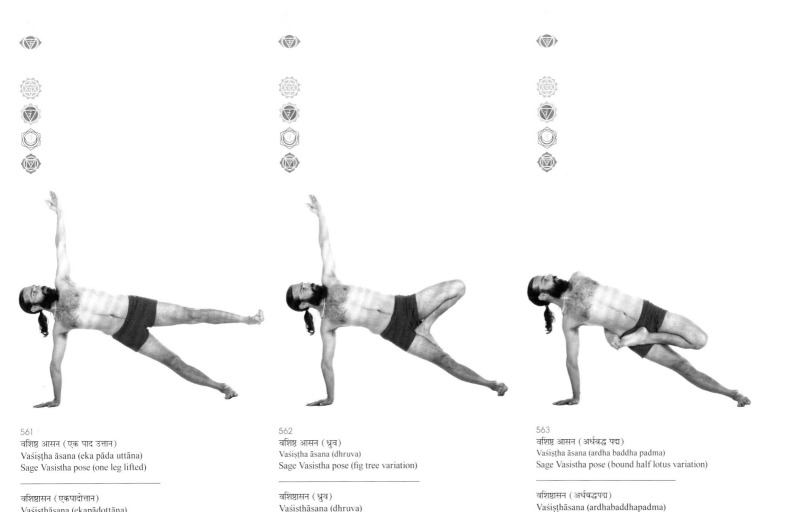

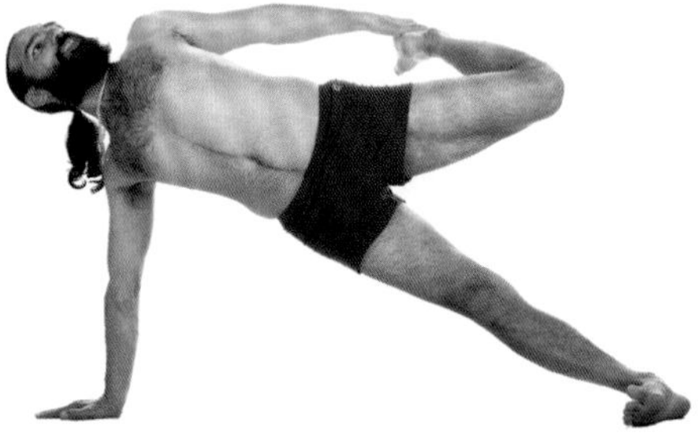

564
वशिष्ठ आसन (धनुः)
Vaśiṣṭha āsana (dhanuḥ)
Sage Vasistha pose (bow variation)

वशिष्ठासन (धनुः)
Vaśiṣṭhāsana (dhanuh)

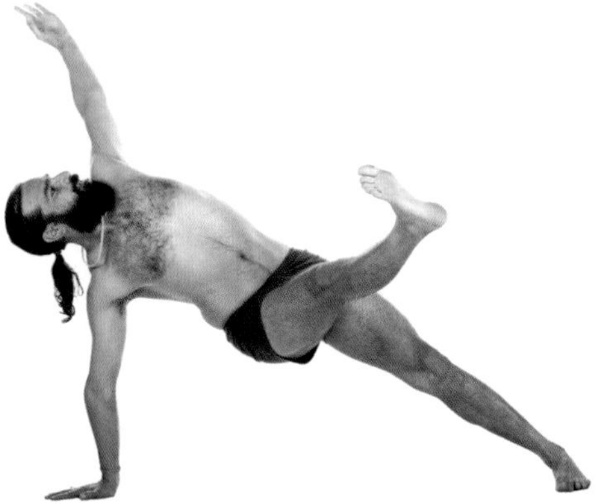

565
वशिष्ठ आसन (वायु यान)
Vaśiṣṭha āsana (vāyu yāna)
Sage Vasistha pose (airplane variation)

वशिष्ठासन(वायुयान)
Vaśiṣṭhāsana (vāyuyāna)

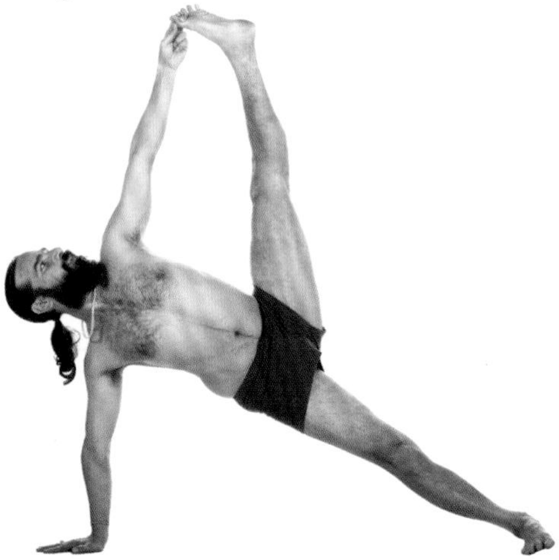

566
पूर्ण वशिष्ठ आसन (हस्त पाद अङ्गुष्ठ)
Pūrṇa Vaśiṣṭha āsana (hasta pāda āṅguṣṭha)
Full Sage Vasistha pose (holding big toe)

पूर्णवशिष्ठासन (हस्तपादाङ्गुष्ठ)
Pūrṇavaśiṣṭhāsana (hastapādāṅguṣṭha)

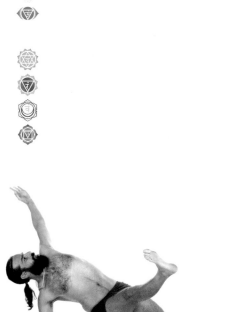

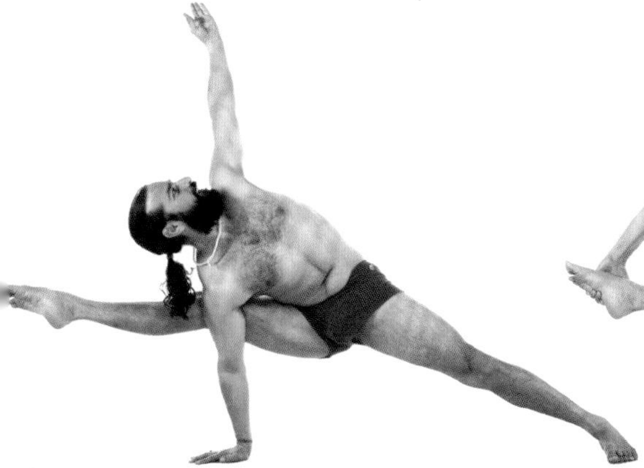

567
विश्वमित्र आसन
Viśvamitra āsana
Sage Viśvamitra pose

विश्वामित्रासन
Viśvāmitrāsana

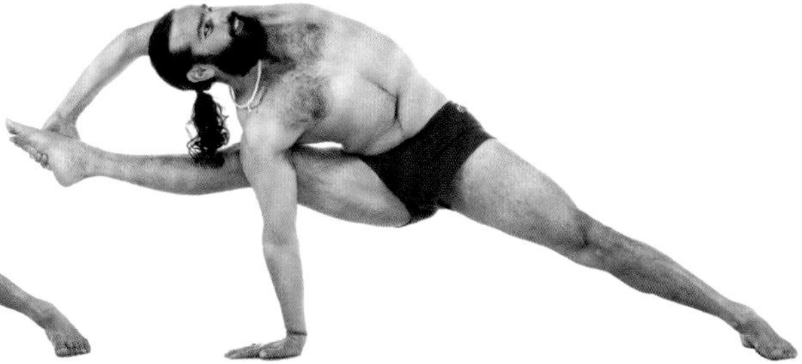

568
विश्वमित्र आसन (एक हस्त पाद बद्ध)
Viśvamitra āsana (eka hasta pāda baddha)
Sage Viśvamitra pose (one hand holding foot)

विश्वामित्रासन (एकहस्तपादबद्ध)
Viśvāmitrāsana (ekahastapādabaddha)

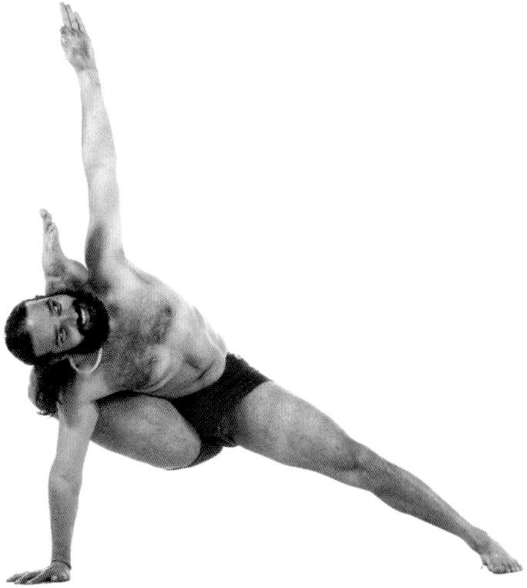

569
काल भैरव आसन
Kalā bhairava āsana
Timeless fearless pose

कालभैरवासन
Kalābhairavāsana

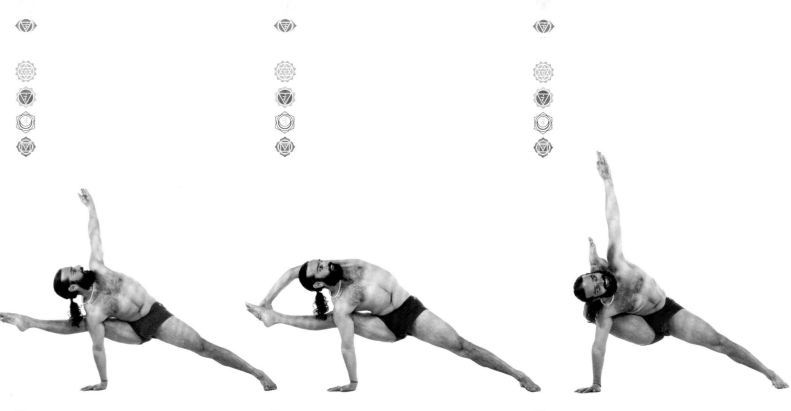

Backbends

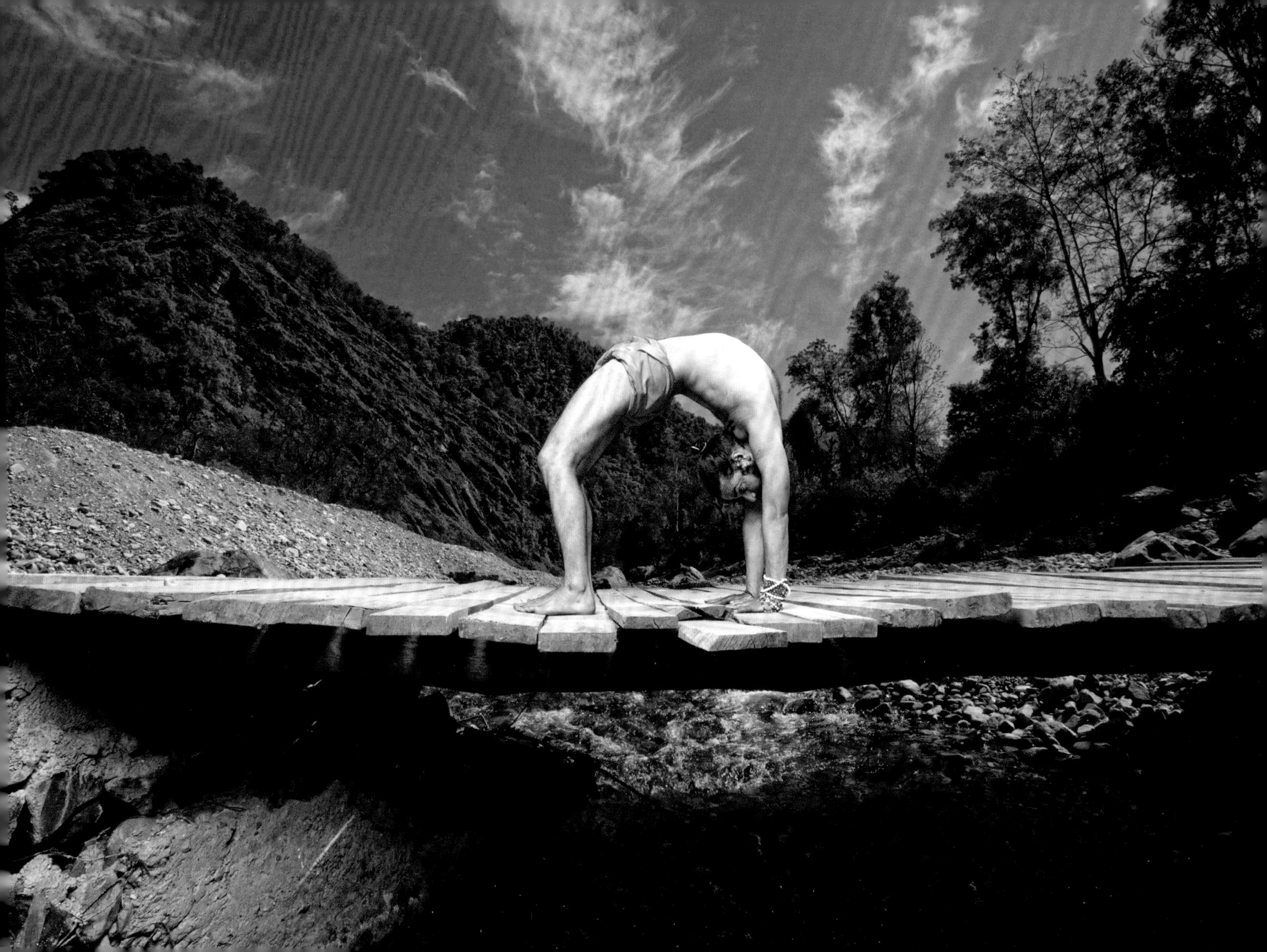

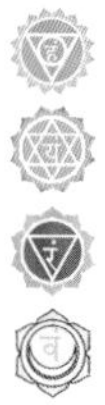

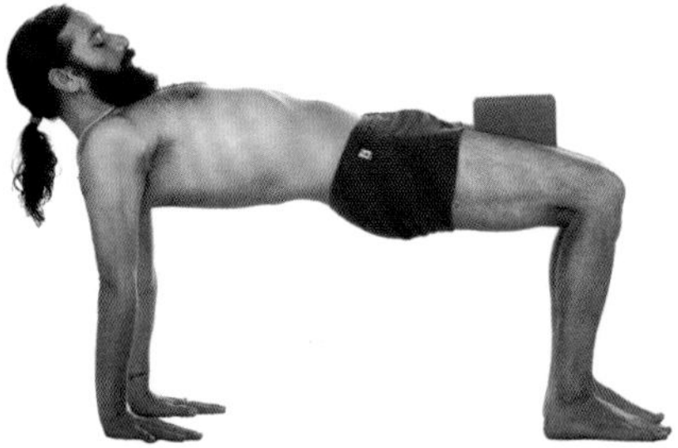

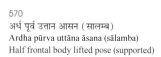

570
अर्ध पूर्व उत्तान आसन (सालम्ब)
Ardha pūrva uttāna āsana (sālamba)
Half frontal body lifted pose (supported)

अर्धपूर्वोत्तानासन (सालम्ब)
Ardhapūrvottānāsana (sālamba)

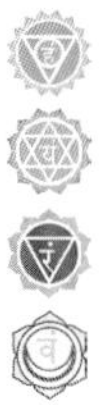

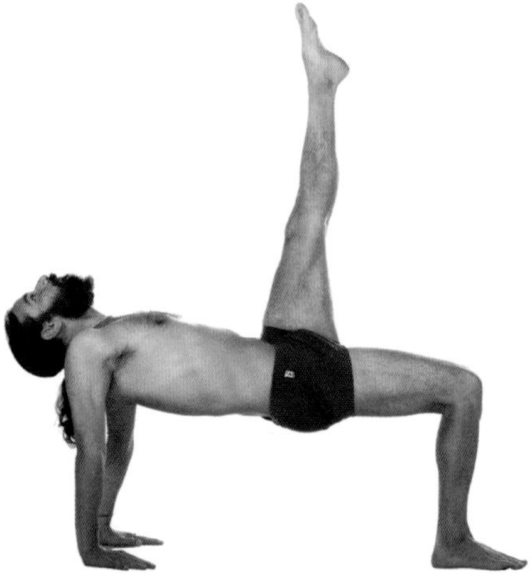

571
अर्ध पूर्व उत्तान आसन (ऊर्ध्व एक पाद)
Ardha pūrva uttāna āsana (ūrdhva eka pāda)
Half frontal body lifted pose (one leg lifted)

अर्धपूर्वोत्तानासन (ऊर्ध्वैकपाद)
Ardhapūrvottānāsana (ūrdhvaikapāda)

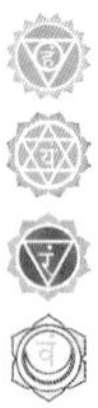

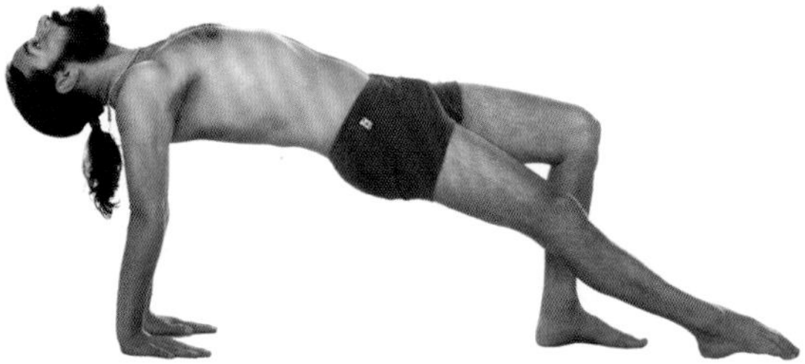

572
पूर्व उत्तान आसन (एक पाद)
Pūrva uttāna āsana (eka pāda)
Frontal body lifted pose (one leg)

पूर्वोत्तानासन (एकपाद)
Pūrvottānāsana (ekapāda)

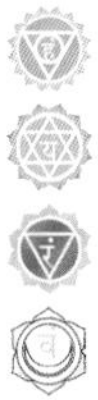

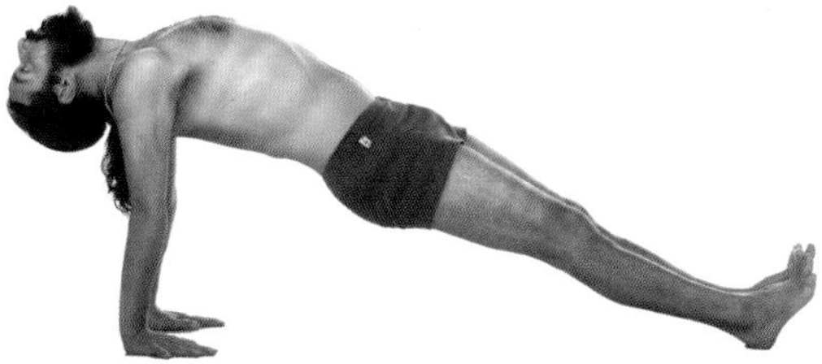

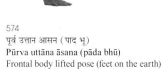

573
पूर्व उत्तान आसन (उत्तान पाद)
Pūrva uttāna āsana (uttāna pāda)
Frontal body lifted pose (lifted toes)

पूर्वोत्तानासन (उत्तानपाद)
Pūrvottānāsana (uttānapāda)

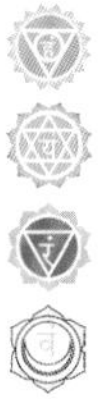

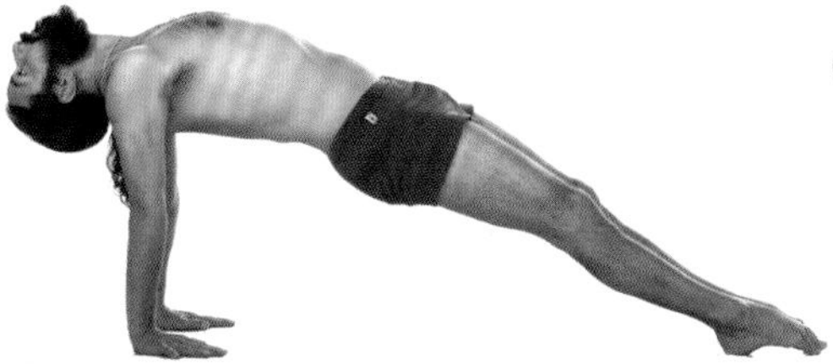

574
पूर्व उत्तान आसन (पाद भू)
Pūrva uttāna āsana (pāda bhū)
Frontal body lifted pose (feet on the earth)

पूर्वोत्तानासन (पादभू)
Pūrvottānāsana (pādabhū)

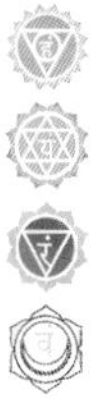

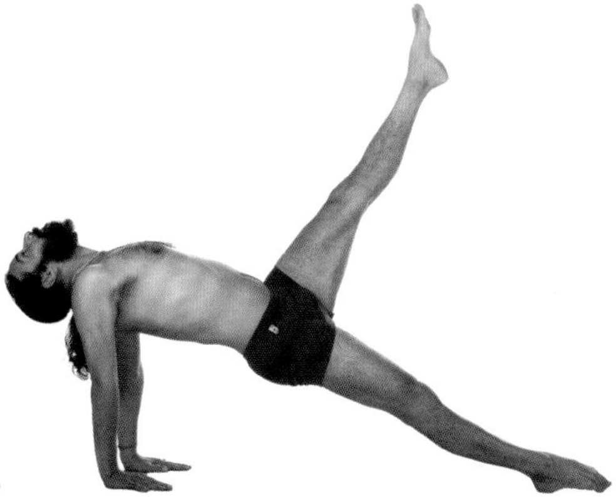

575
पूर्व उत्तान आसन (ऊर्ध्व एक पाद)
Pūrva uttāna āsana (ūrdhva eka pāda)
Frontal body lifted pose (one leg overhead)

पूर्वोत्तानासन (ऊर्ध्वैकपाद)
Pūrvottānāsana (ūrdhvaikapāda)

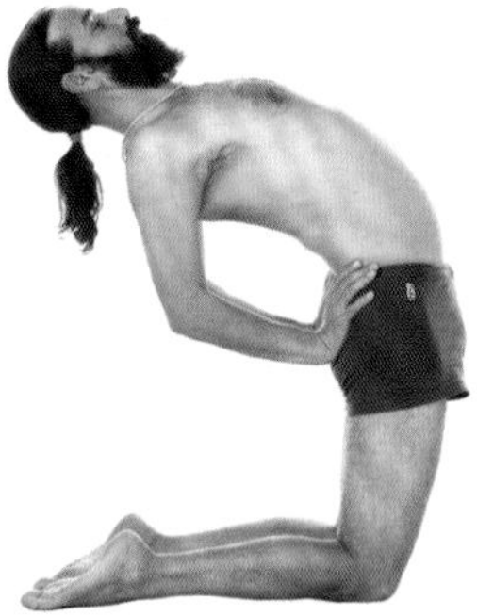

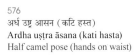

576
अर्ध उष्ट्र आसन (कटि हस्त)
Ardha uṣṭra āsana (kati hasta)
Half camel pose (hands on waist)

अर्द्धोष्ट्रासन (कटिहस्त)
Ardhaoṣṭrāsana (katihasta)

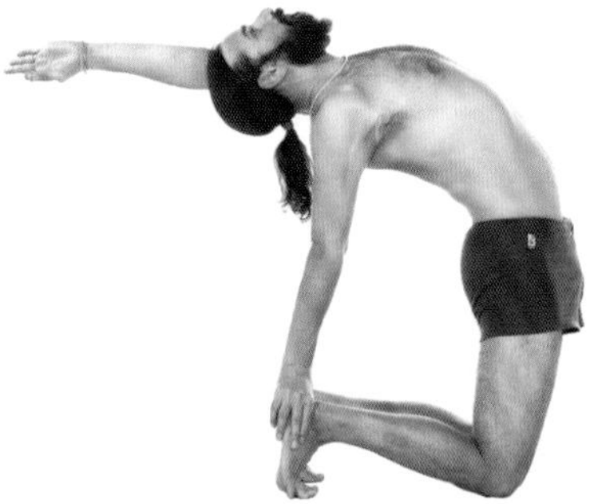

577
उष्ट्र आसन (प्रपदिक, विस्तृत एक हस्त)
Ūṣṭra āsana (prapadika, vistṛta eka hasta)
Camel pose (ball of toes on the earth, one hand extended)

उष्ट्रासन (प्रपदिक,विस्तृतैकहस्त)
Ūṣṭrāsana (prapadika, vistṛtaikahastapāda)

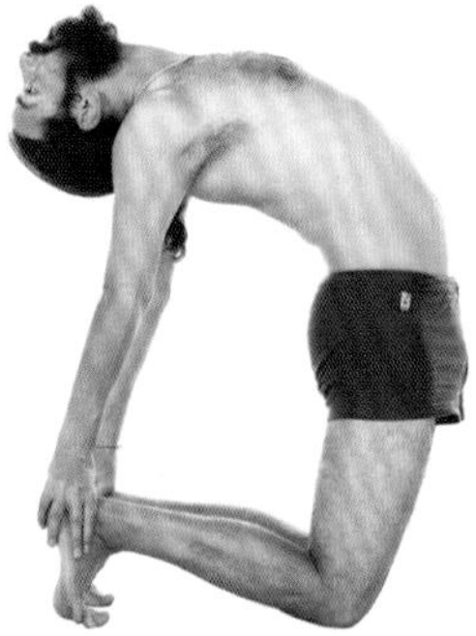

578
उष्ट्र आसन (प्रपदिक)
Ūṣṭra āsana (prapadika)
Camel pose (ball of toes on the earth)

उष्ट्रासन (प्रपदिक)
Ūṣṭrāsana (prapadika)

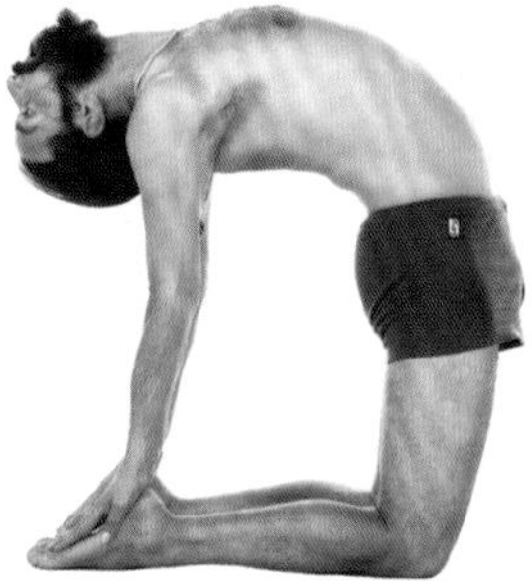

579
उष्ट्र आसन
Uṣṭra āsana
Camel pose

उष्ट्रासन
Uṣṭrāsana

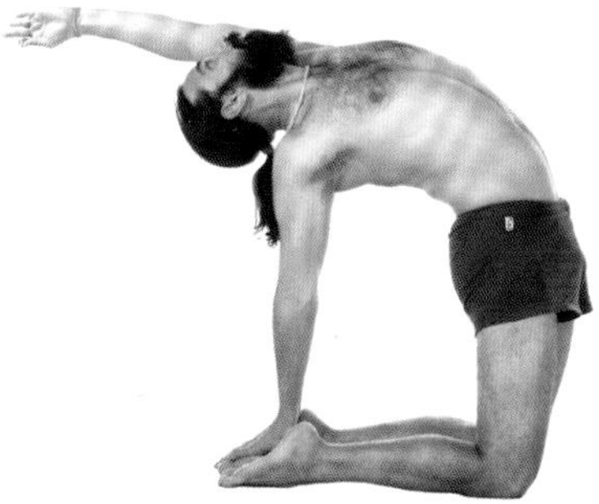

580
उष्ट्र आसन (विपरीत एक हस्त पाद)
Uṣṭra āsana (vistṛta eka hasta)
Camel pose (one hand extended)

उष्ट्रासन (विपरीतैकहस्त)
Uṣṭrāsana (vistṛtaikahastapāda)

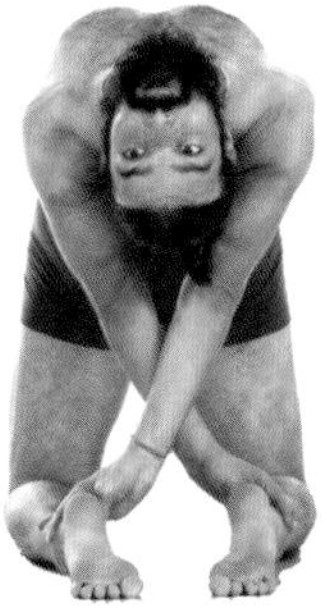

581
उष्ट्र आसन (कर्तरी हस्त)
Uṣṭra āsana (kartarī hasta)
Camel pose (scissor hands)

उष्ट्रासन (कर्तरीहस्त)
Ūṣṭrāsana (kartarīhasta)

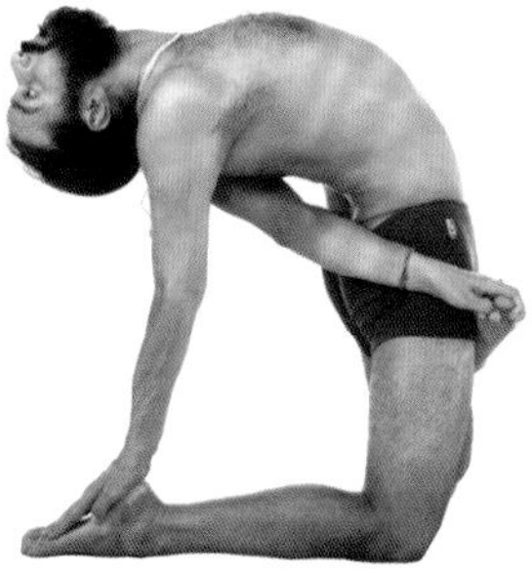

582
अर्ध बद्ध पद्म उष्ट्र आसन
Ardha baddha padma uṣṭra āsana
Bound half lotus camel pose

अर्धबद्धपद्मोष्ट्रासन
Ardhabaddhapadmoṣṭrāsana

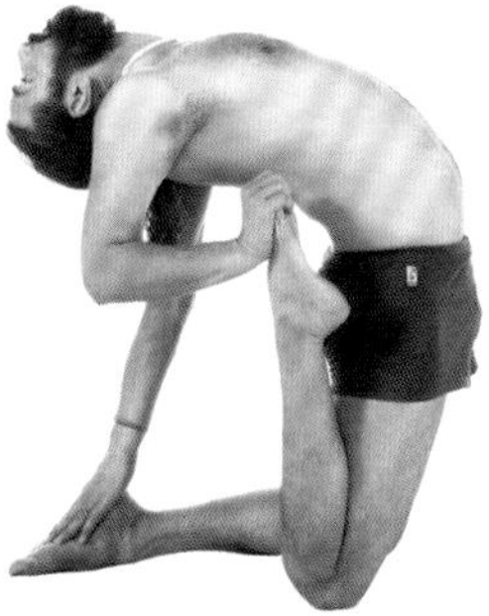

583
भेका उष्ट्र आसन (एक हस्त पाद)
Bhekā uṣṭra āsana (eka hasta pāda)
Frog camel pose (one hand on foot)

भेकोष्ट्रासन (एकहस्तपाद)
Bhekoṣṭrāsana (ekahastapāda)

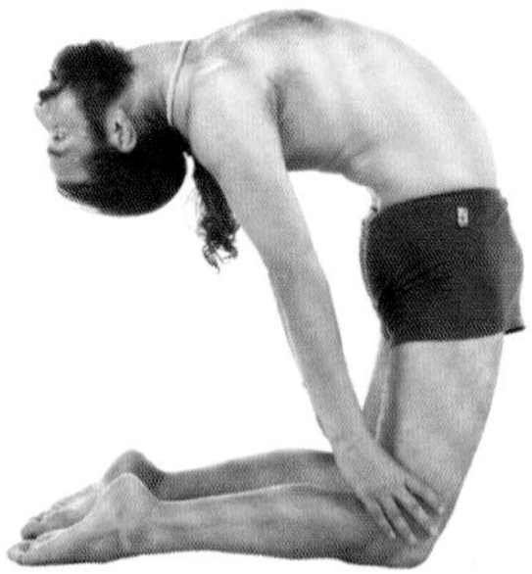

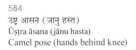

584
उष्ट्र आसन (जानु हस्त)
Ūṣṭra āsana (jānu hasta)
Camel pose (hands behind knee)

उष्ट्रासन (जानुहस्त)
Ūṣṭrāsana (jānuhasta)

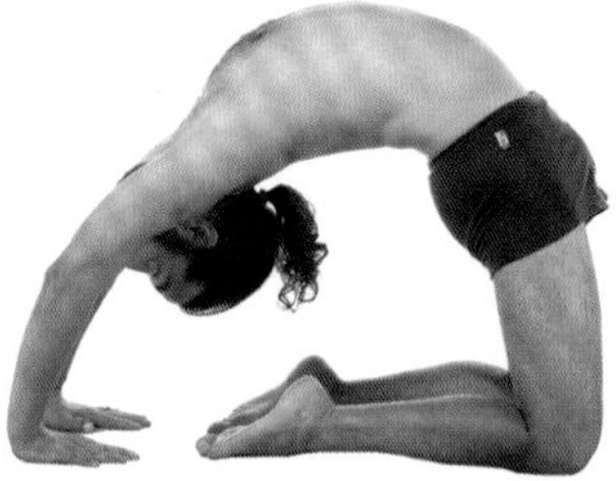

585
उष्ट्र कपोत आसन (हस्त भू)
Uṣṭra kapota āsana (hasta bhū)
Camel pigeon pose (hands on the earth)

उष्ट्रकपोतासन (हस्तभू)
Uṣṭrakapotāsana (hastabhū)

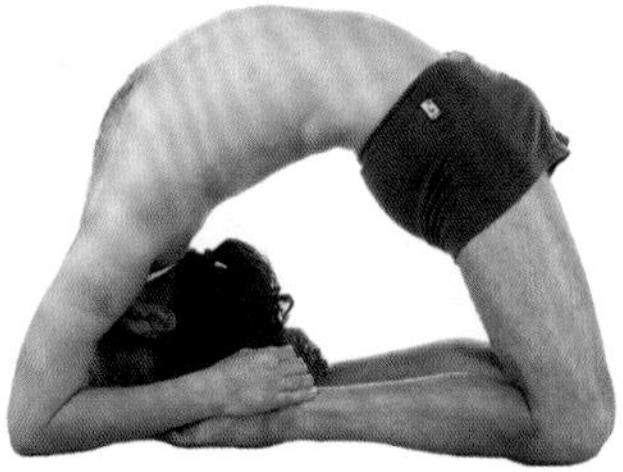

586
उष्ट्र कपोत राज आसन
Uṣṭra kapota rāja āsana
Camel king pigeon pose

उष्ट्रकपोतराजासन
Uṣṭrakapotarājāsana

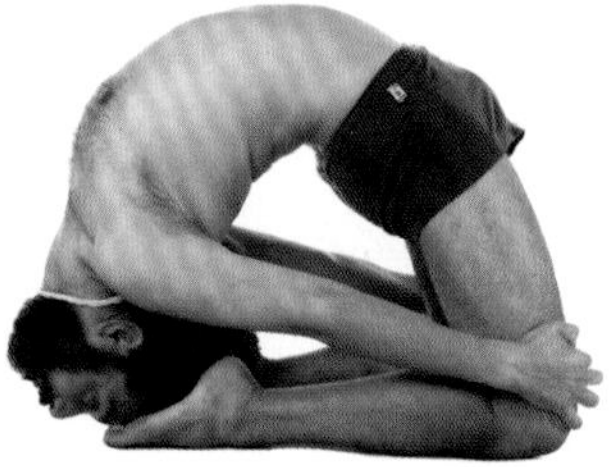

587
महा उष्ट्र कपोत राज आसन
Mahā uṣṭra kapota rāja āsana
Great camel king pigeon pose

महोष्ट्रकपोतराजासन
Mahoṣṭrakapotarājāsana

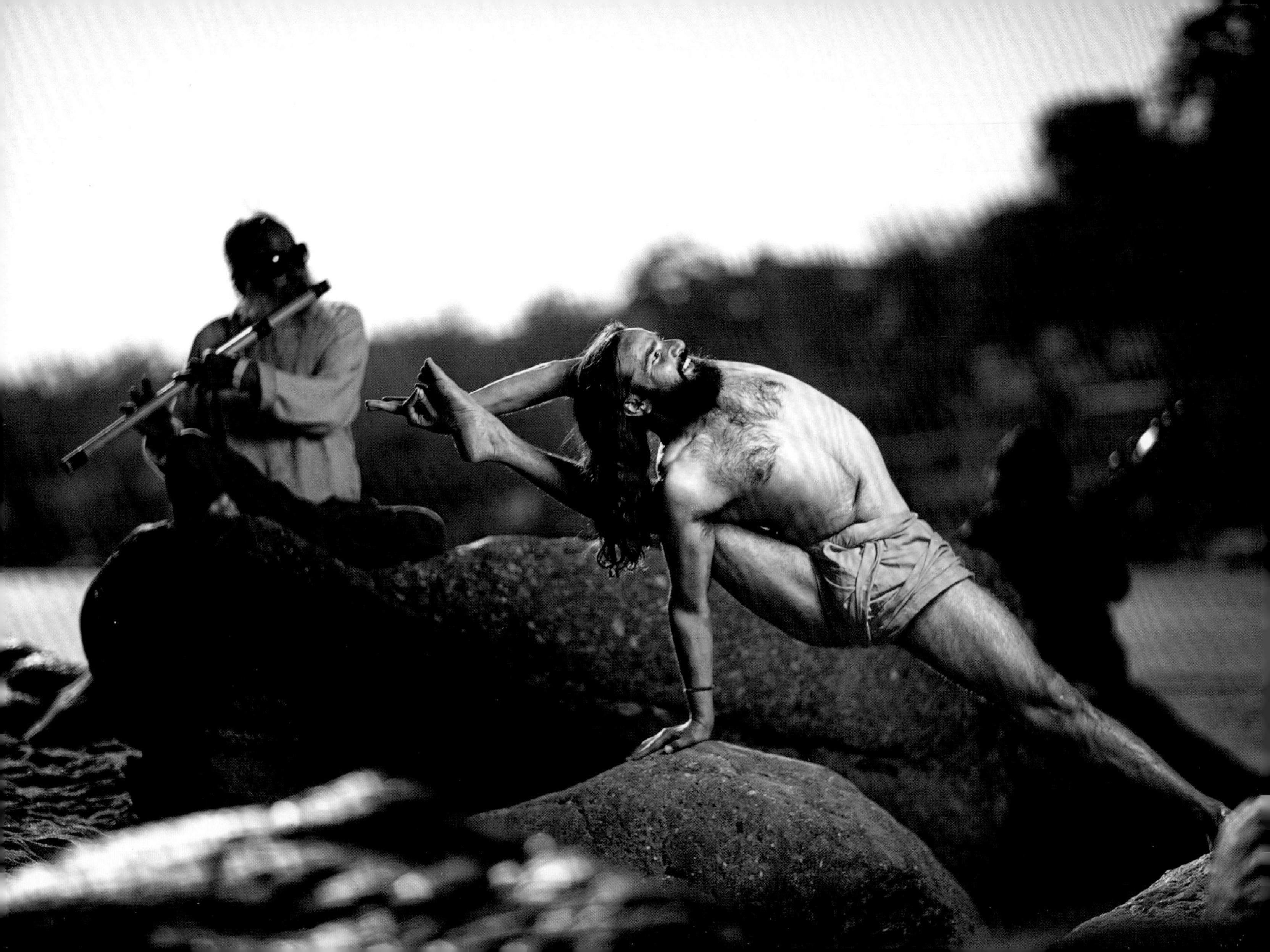

Life does not have a destination. Experience the fullness of every moment.

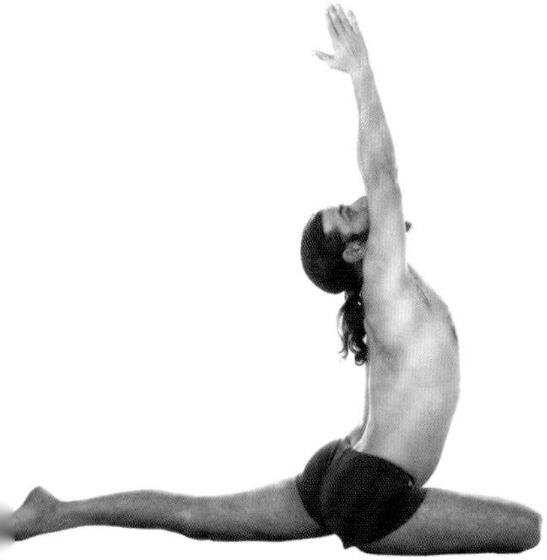

588
कपोत आसन (ऊर्ध्व हस्त नमस्कार)
Kapota āsana (ūrdhva hasta namaskāra)
Pigeon pose (hands ovehead in prayer)

कपोतासन (ऊर्ध्वहस्तनमस्कार)
Kapotāsana (ūrdhvahastanamaskāra)

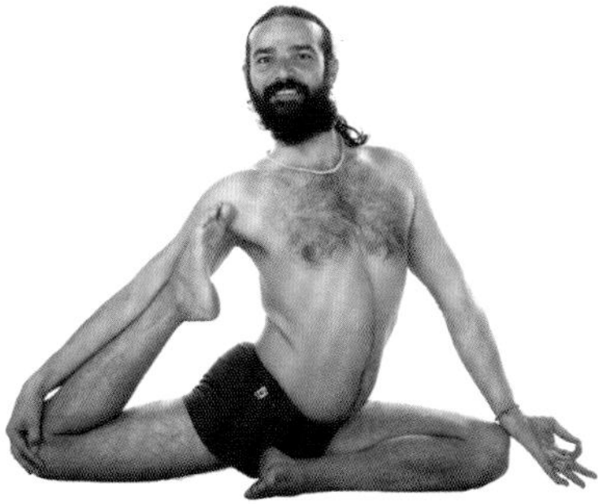

589
कपोत आसन (कुक्षि पाद जानु हस्त)
Kapota āsana (kukṣi pāda jānu hasta)
Pigeon pose (foot in armpit, holding knee)

कपोतासन (कुक्षिपादजानुहस्त)
Kapotāsana (kukṣipādajānuhasta)

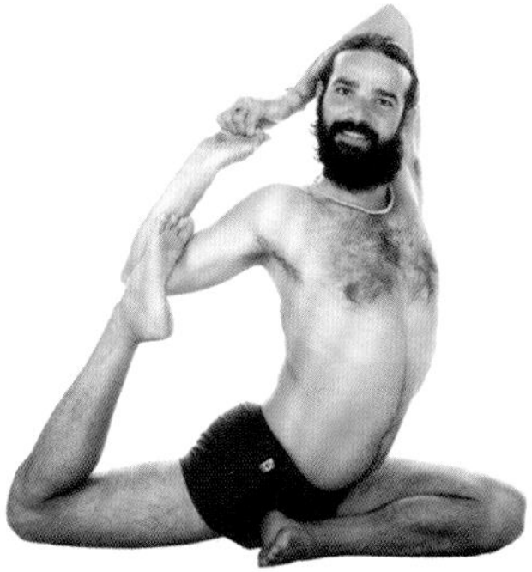

590
निर्भय कपोत आसन
Nirbhaya kapota āsana
Tranquil pigeon pose

निर्भयकपोतासन
Nirbhayakapotāsana

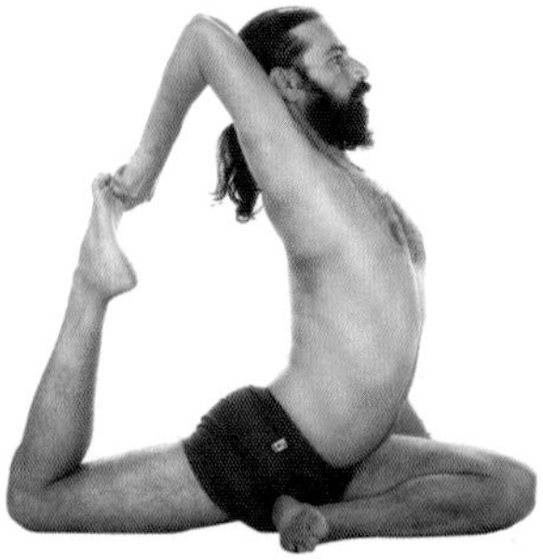

591
कपोत आसन (बद्ध एक हस्त पाद अङ्गुष्ठ)
Kapota āsana (baddha eka hasta pāda aṅguṣṭha)
Pigeon pose (one hand holding big toe)

कपोतासन (बद्धैकहस्तपादाङ्गुष्ठ)
Kapotāsana (baddhaikahastapādāṅguṣṭha)

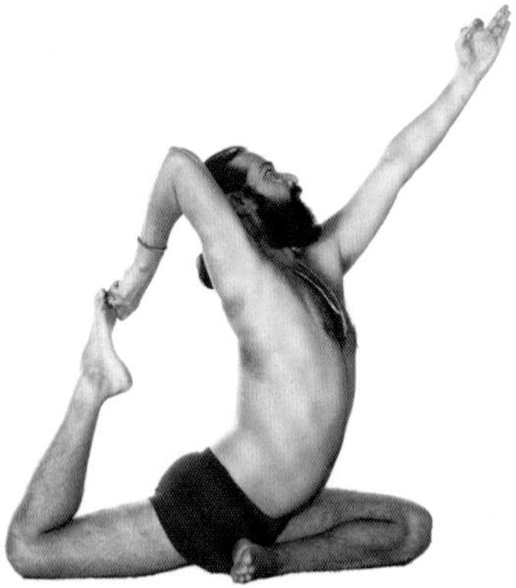

592
कपोत आसन (क्षितिज हस्त)
Kapota āsana (kṣitija hasta)
Pigeon pose (hand to the horizon)

कपोतासन(क्षितिजहस्त)
Kapotāsana (kṣitijahasta)

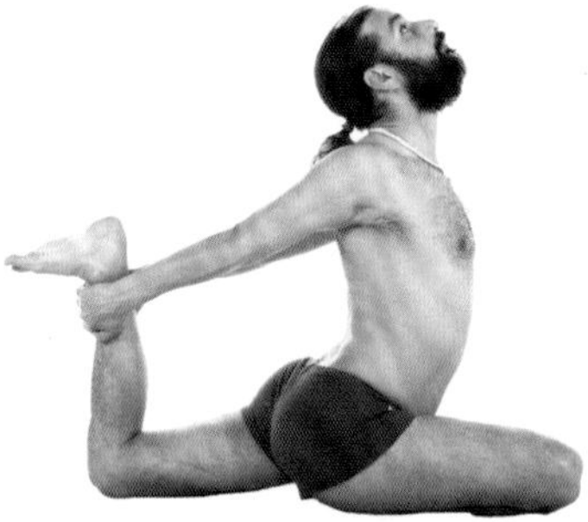

593
कपोत आसन (द्वि हस्त पाद बद्ध)
Kapota āsana (dvi hasta pāda baddha)
Pigeon pose (two hands holding foot)

कपोतासन (द्विहस्तपादबद्ध)
Kapotāsana (dvihastapādabaddha)

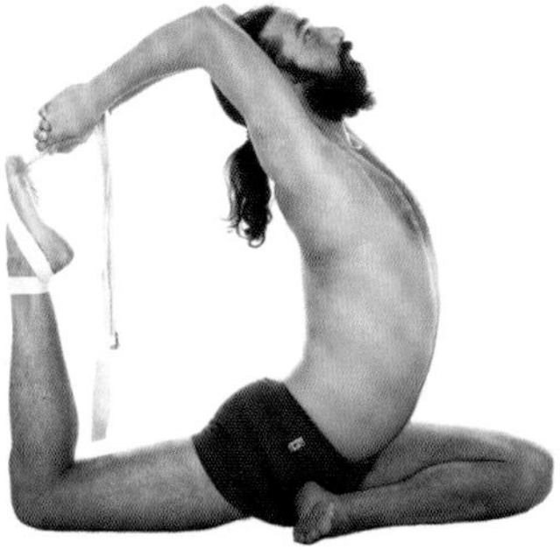

594
अर्ध राज कपोत आसन (सरज्जु)
Ardha rāja kapota āsana (sarajju)
Half king pigeon pose (with strap)

अर्धराजकपोतासन (सरज्जु)
Ardharājakapotāsana (sarajju)

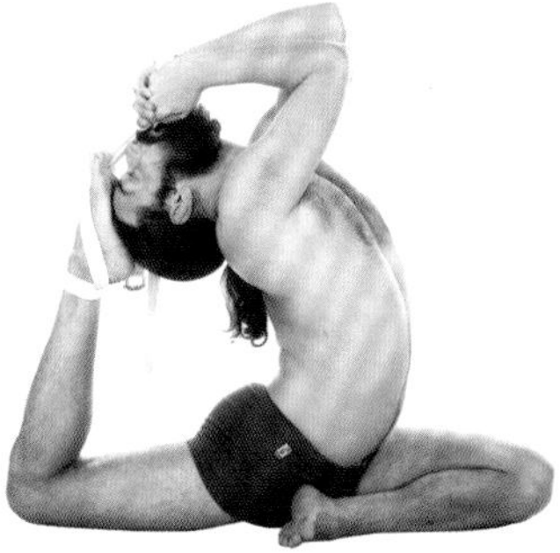

595
राज कपोत आसन (सरज्जु)
Rāja kapota āsana (sarajju)
King pigeon pose (with strap)

राजकपोतासन (सरज्जु)
Rājakapotāsana (sarajju)

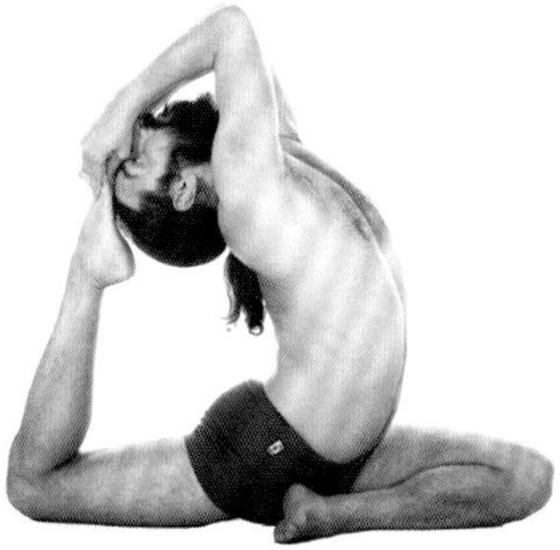

596
राज कपोत आसन
Rāja kapota āsana
King pigeon pose

राजकपोतासन
Rājakapotāsana

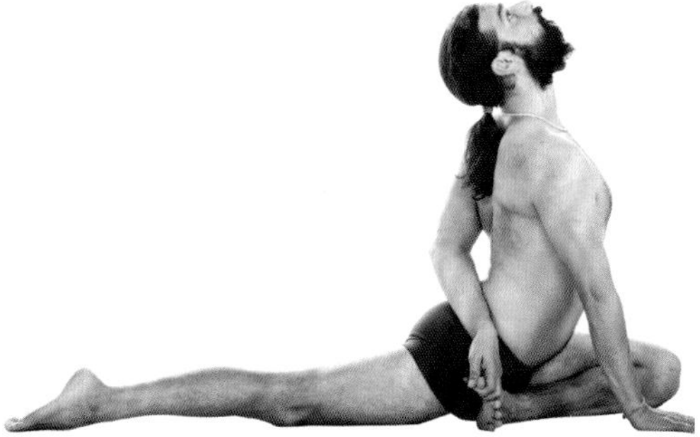

597
कपोत आसन (अर्ध बद्ध पद्म)
Kapota āsana (ardha baddha padma)
Pigeon pose (bound half lotus)

कपोतासन (अर्धबद्धपद्म)
Kapotāsana (ardhabaddhapadma)

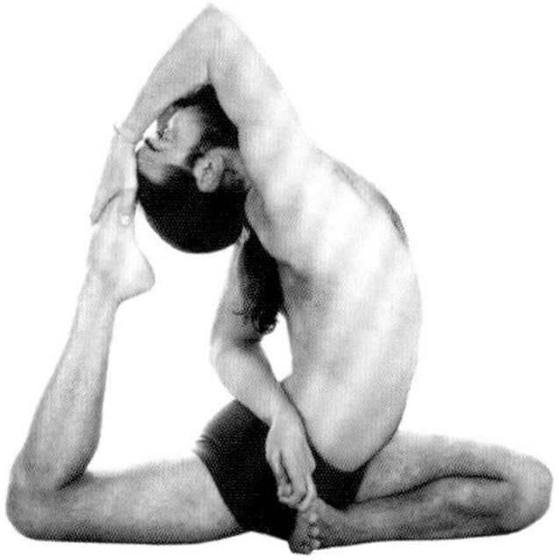

598
राज कपोत आसन (अर्ध बद्ध पद्म)
Rāja kapota āsana (ardha baddha padma)
King pigeon pose (bound half lotus)

राजकपोतासन (अर्धबद्धपद्म)
Rājakapotāsana (ardhabaddhapadma)

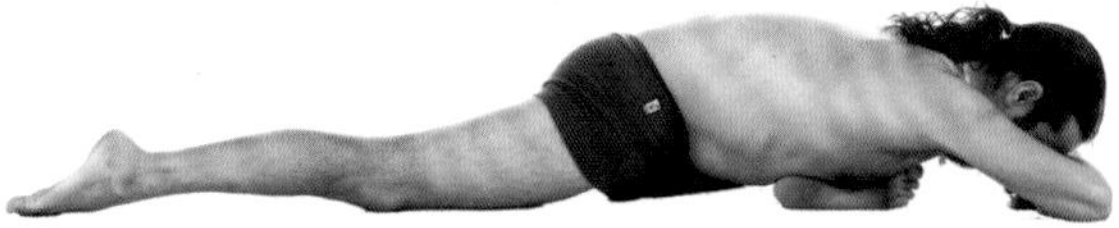

599
कपोत आसन (कर तल ललाट धर)
Kapota āsana (karatala lalāṭa dhara)
Pigeon pose (forehead on back of hands)

कपोतासन (करतलललाटधर)
Kapotāsana (karatalalalāṭadhara)

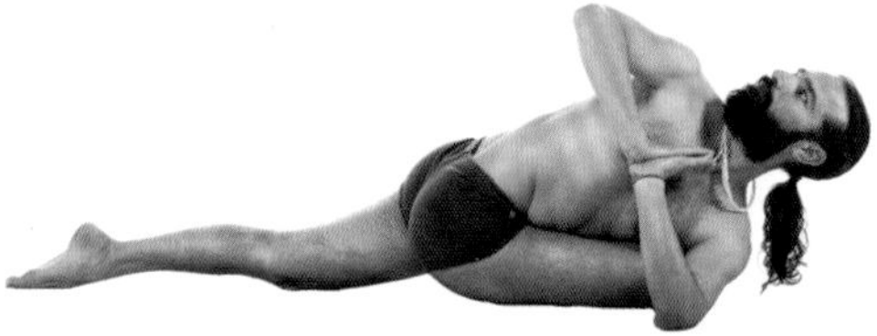

600
परिवृत्त नमस्कार कपोत आसन
Parivṛtta namaskāra kapota āsana
Twisted praying pigeon pose

परिवृत्तनमस्कारकपोतासन
Parivṛttanamaskārakapotāsana

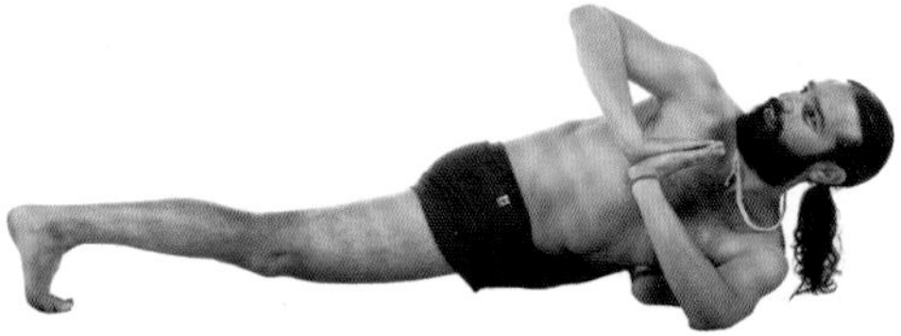

601
विपरीत परिवृत्त नमस्कार कपोत आसन
Viparīta parivṛtta namaskāra kapota āsana
Reverse twisted praying pigeon pose

विपरीतपरिवृत्तनमस्कारकपोतासन
Viparītaparivṛttanamaskārakapotāsana

602
बाल हनुमान आसन (हस्त भू)
Bāla Hanumāna āsana (hasta bhū)
Baby Hanumāna pose (hands on the earth)

बालहनुमानासन (हस्तभू)
Bālahanumānāsana (hastabhū)

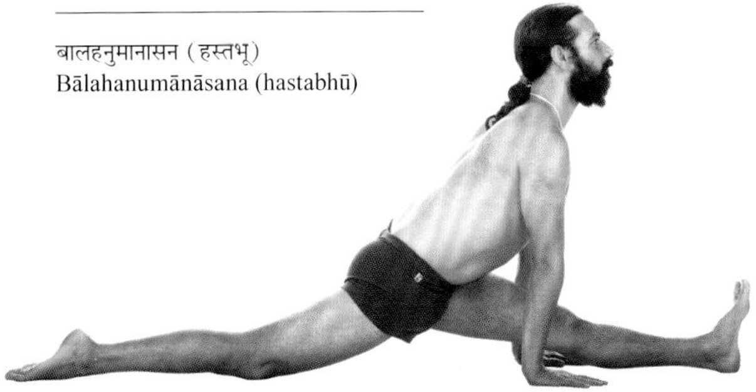

603
हनुमान आसन (हस्त अङ्गुल भू)
Hanumāna āsana (hasta aṅgula bhū)
Hanumāna pose (fingers on the earth)

हनुमानासन (हस्ताङ्गुलभू)
Hanumānāsana (hastāṅgulabhū)

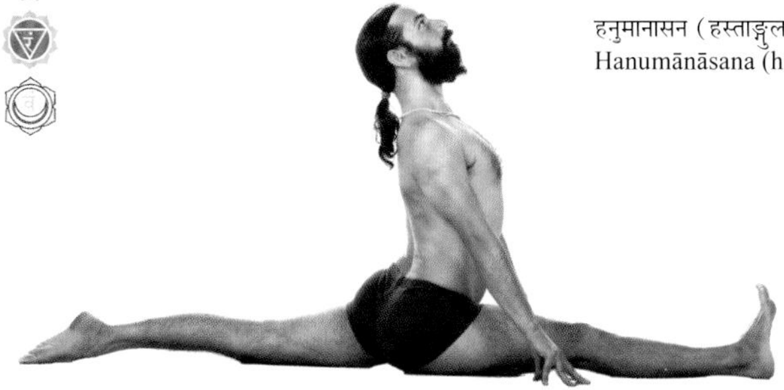

604
नमस्कार हनुमान आसन
Namaskāra Hanumāna āsana
Praying Hanumāna pose

नमस्कारहनुमानासन
Namaskārahanumānāsana

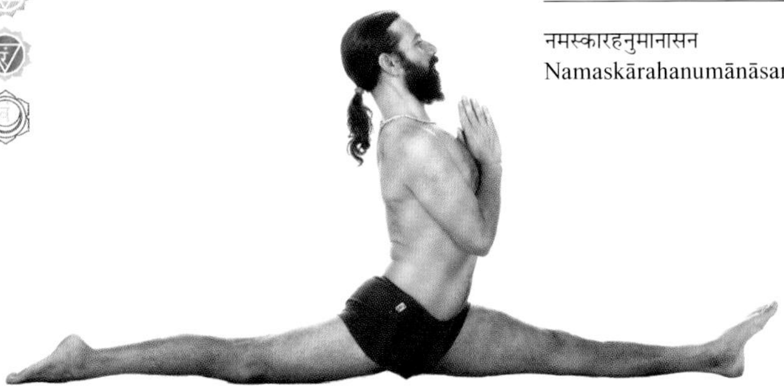

605
नमस्कार हनुमान आसन (ऊर्ध्व हस्त)
Namaskāra Hanumāna āsana (ūrdhva hasta)
Praying Hanumāna pose (arms overhead)

नमस्कारहनुमानासन (ऊर्ध्वहस्त)
Namaskārahanumānāsana (ūrdhvahasta)

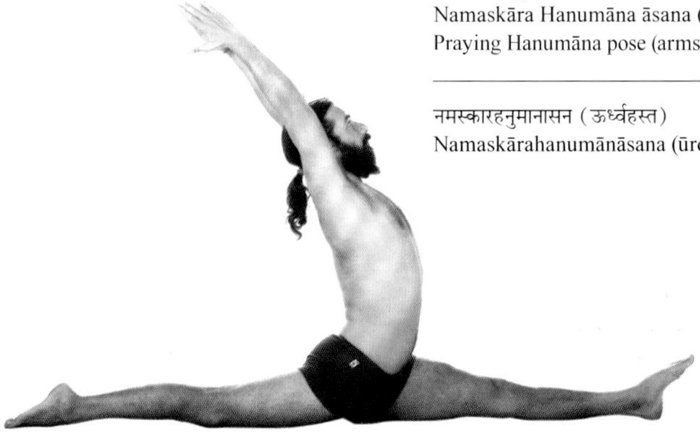

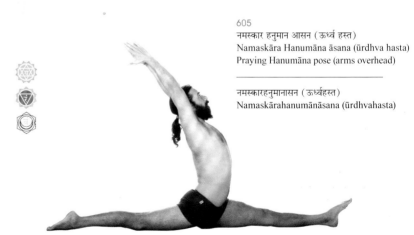

606
नमन हनुमान आसन (कफोणि भू)
Namana Hanumāna āsana (kaphoṇi bhū)
Humble Hanumāna pose (elbows on the earth)

नमनहनुमानासन (कफोणिभू)
Namanahanumānāsana (kaphoṇibhū)

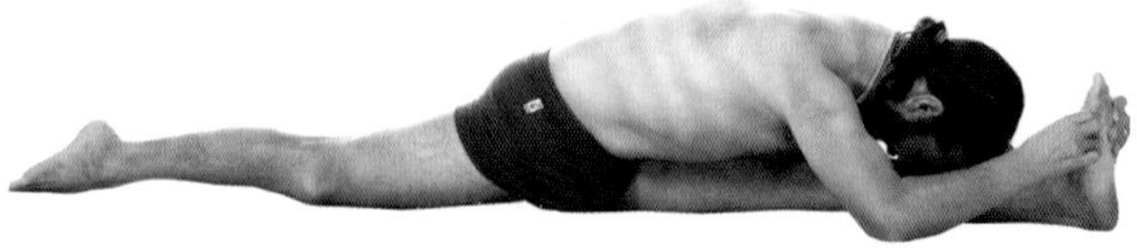

607
निर्भय कपोत हनुमान आसन
Nirbhaya kapota Hanumāna āsana
Tranquil pigeon Hanumāna pose

निर्भयकपोतहनुमानासन
Nirbhayakapotahanumānāsana

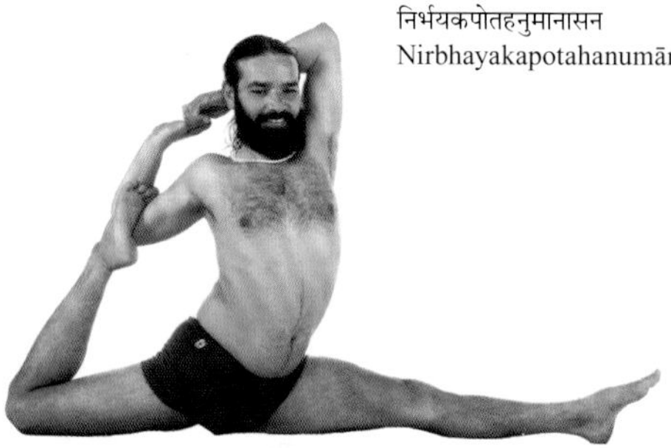

608
कपोत हनुमान आसन (द्वि हस्त पाद बद्ध)
Kapota Hanumāna āsana (dvi hasta pāda baddha)
Pigeon Hanumāna pose (two hands holding foot)

कपोतहनुमानासन (द्विहस्तपादबद्ध)
Kapotahanumānāsana (dvihastapādabaddha)

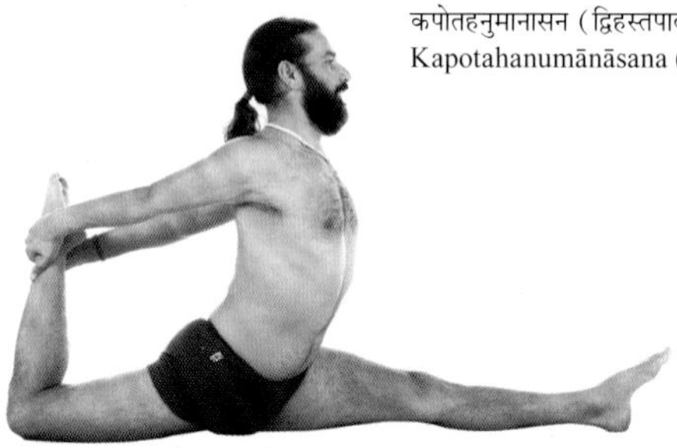

609
राज कपोत हनुमान आसन (एक हस्त भू)
Rāja kapota Hanumāna āsana (eka hasta bhū)
King pigeon Hanumāna pose (one hand on the earth)

राजकपोतहनुमानासन (एकहस्तभू)
Rājakapotahanumānāsana (ekahastabhū)

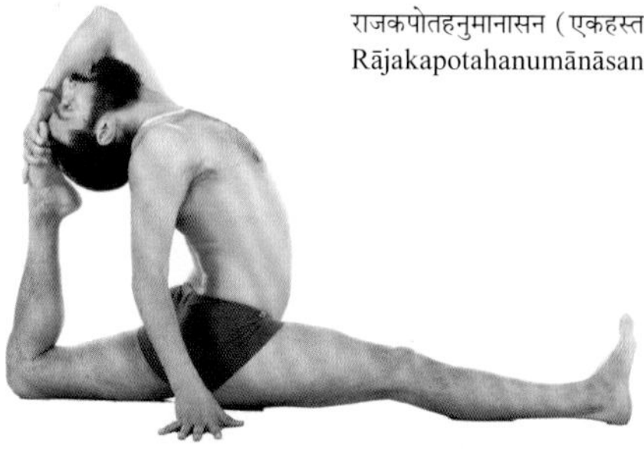

610
राज कपोत हनुमान आसन
Rāja kapota Hanumāna āsana
King pigeon Hanumāna pose

राजकपोतहनुमानासन
Rājakapotahanumānāsana

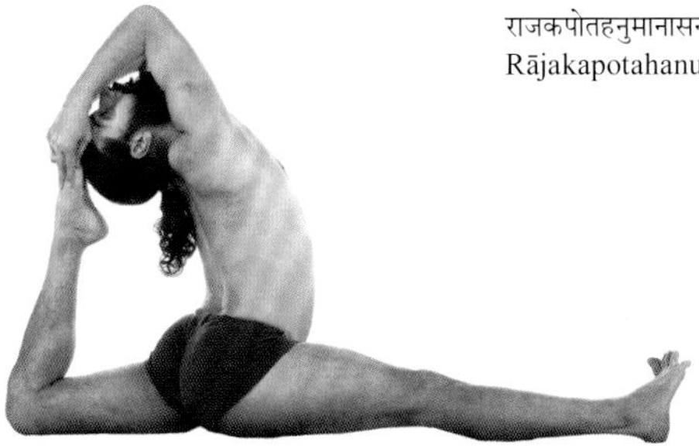

611
अर्ध समकोण पाद आसन (हस्त भू)
Ardha samakoṇa pāda āsana (hasta bhū)
Half side split pose (hands on the earth)

अर्धसमकोणपादासन (हस्तभू)
Ardhasamakoṇapādāsana (hastabhū)

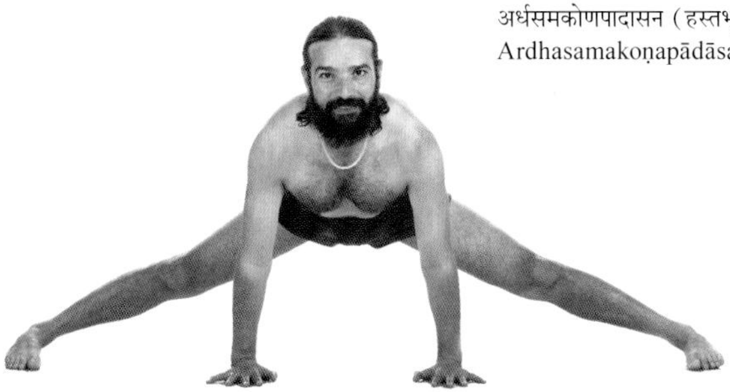

612
समकोण पाद आसन (हस्त भू)
Samakoṇa pāda āsana (hasta bhū)
Side split pose (hands on the earth)

समकोणपादासन (हस्तभू)
Samakoṇapādāsana (hastabhū)

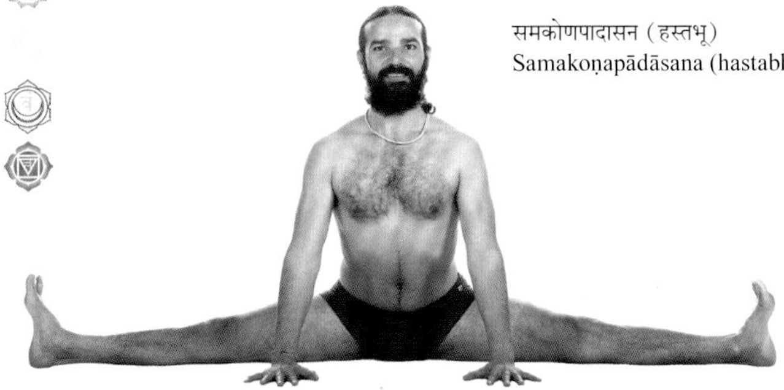

613
नमस्कार समकोण पाद आसन
Namaskāra samakoṇa pāda āsana
Praying side split pose

नमस्कारसमकोणपादासन
Namaskārasamakoṇapādāsana

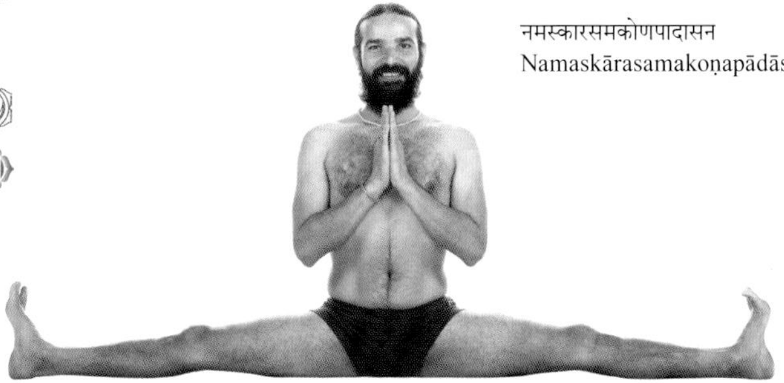

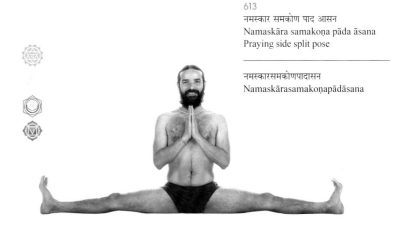

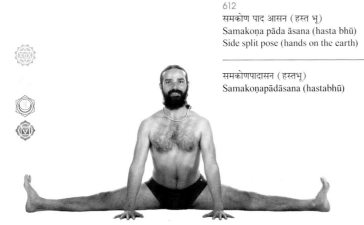

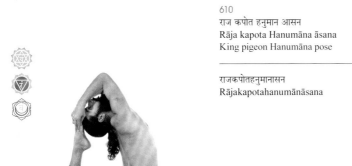

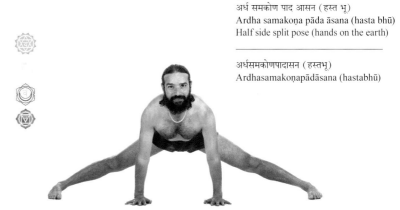

614
समकोण पाद आसन (विराट हस्त)
Samakoṇa pāda āsana (virāṭa hasta)
Side split pose (arms extended)

समकोणपादासन (विराटहस्त)
Samakoṇapādāsana (virāṭahasta)

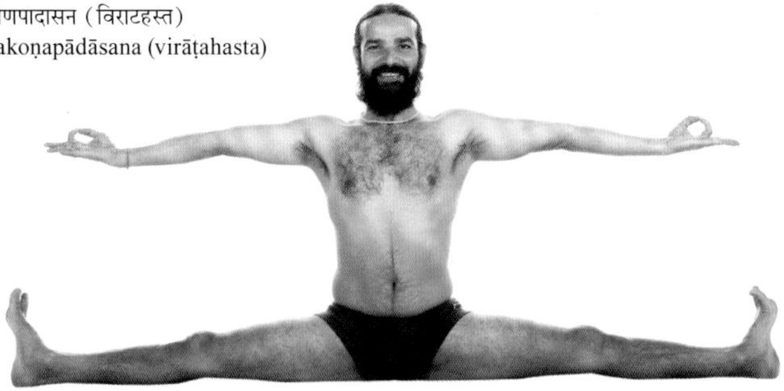

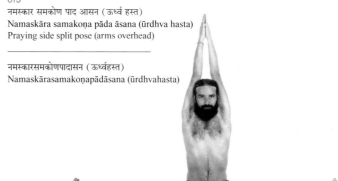

615
नमस्कार समकोण पाद आसन (ऊर्ध्व हस्त)
Namaskāra samakoṇa pāda āsana (ūrdhva hasta)
Praying side split pose (arms overhead)

नमस्कारसमकोणपादासन (ऊर्ध्वहस्त)
Namaskārasamakoṇapādāsana (ūrdhvahasta)

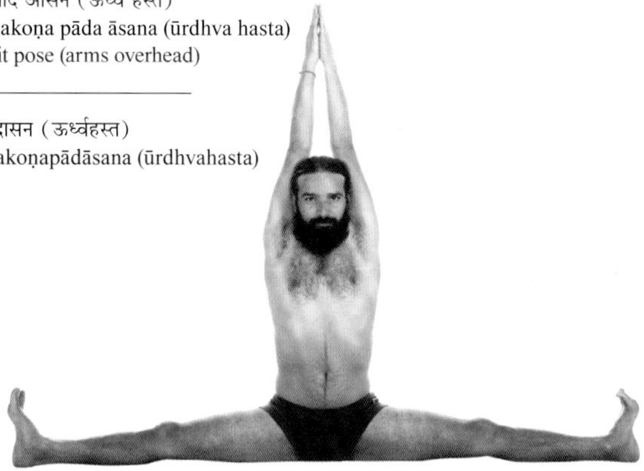

616
समकोण पाद आसन (हस्त हनु)
Samakoṇa pāda āsana (hasta hanu)
Side split pose (chin resting on hands)

समकोणपादासन (हस्तहनु)
Samakoṇapādāsana (hastahanu)

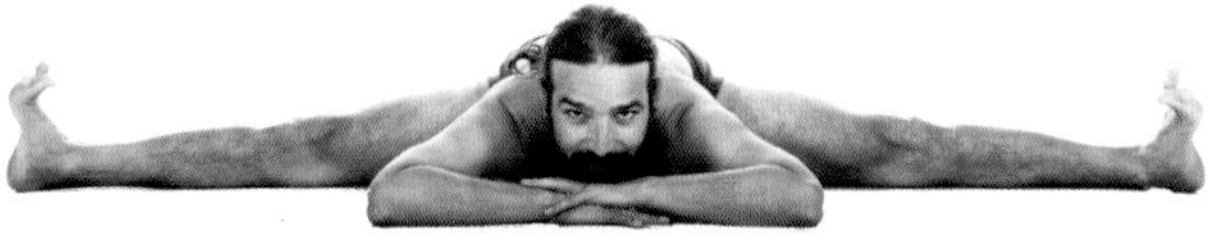

617
समकोण पाद आसन (बद्ध हस्त पाद अङ्गुष्ठ)
Samakoṇa pāda āsana (baddha hasta pāda aṅguṣṭha)
Side split pose (holding big toes)

समकोणपादासन (बद्धहस्तपादाङ्गुष्ठ)
Samakoṇapādāsana (baddhahastapādāṅguṣṭha)

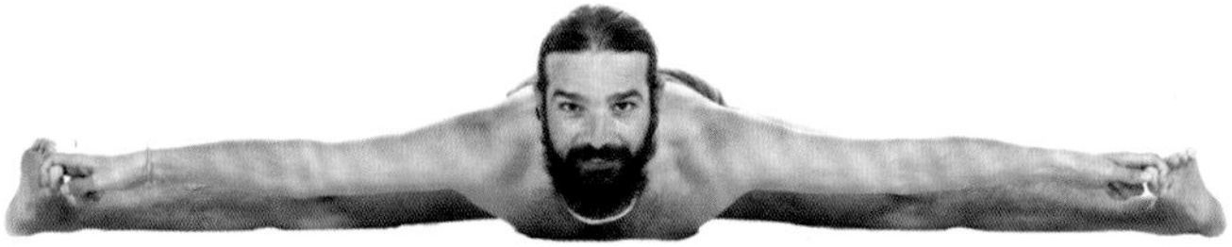

618
समकोण पाद आसन (पृष्ठ कफोणि बद्ध)
Samakoṇa pāda āsana (pṛṣṭha kaphoṇi baddha)
Side split pose (bound elbows behind back)

समकोणपादासन (पृष्ठकफोणिबद्ध)
Samakoṇapādāsana (pṛṣṭhakaphoṇibaddha)

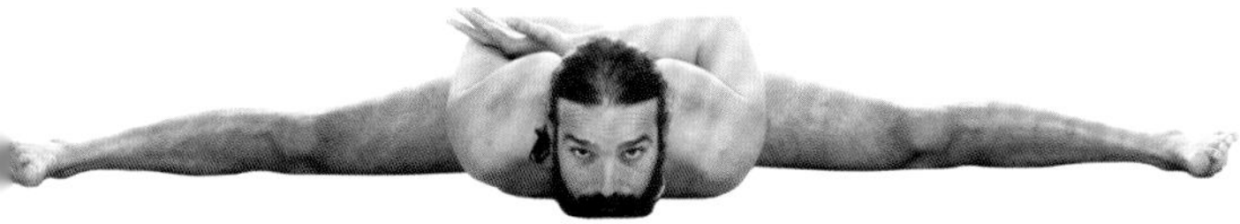

619
समकोण पाद आसन (ललाट भू, पृष्ठ नमस्कार)
Samakoṇa pāda āsana (lalāṭa bhū, pṛṣṭha namaskāra)
Side split pose (forehead on earth, hands in prayer behind back)

समकोणपादासन (ललाटभू, पृष्ठनमस्कार)
Samakoṇapādāsana (lalāṭabhū, pṛṣṭhanamaskāra)

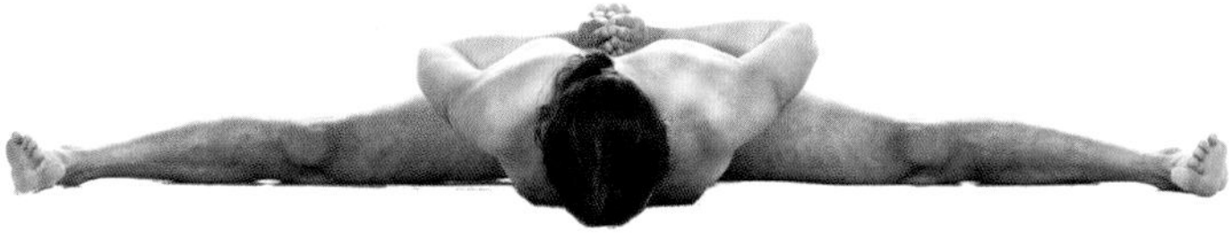

620
समकोण पाद आसन (उत् हनु ,पृष्ठ नमस्कार)
Samakoṇa pāda āsana (Ut hanu, pṛṣṭha namaskāra)
Side split pose (chin lifted, hands in prayer behind back)

समकोणपादासन (उत्हनु, पृष्ठनमस्कार)
Samakoṇapādāsana (uthanu, pṛṣṭhanamaskāra)

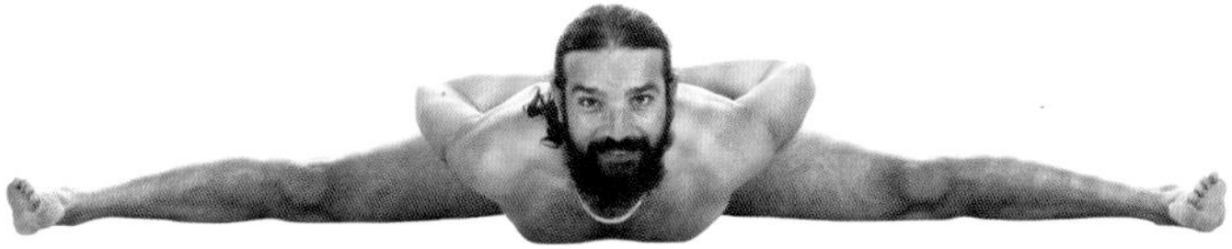

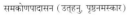

621
पार्श्व समकोण पाद आसन (बद्ध पाद मणि बन्ध)
Pārśva samakoṇa pāda āsana (baddha pāda maṇi bandha)
Side stretch split pose (clasping wrists around toes)

पार्श्वसमकोणपादासन (बद्धपादमणिबन्ध)
Pārśvasamakoṇapādāsana (baddhapādamaṇibandha)

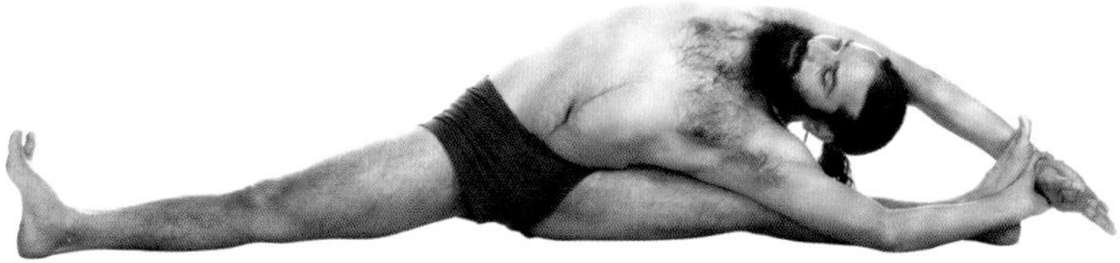

622
जानु शिर समकोण पाद आसन
Jānu śira samakoṇa pāda āsana
Head to knee side split pose

जानुशिरसमकोणपादासन
Jānuśirasamakoṇapādāsana

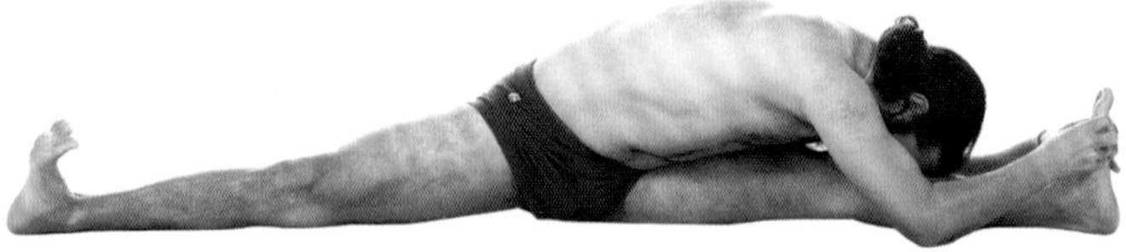

623
पार्श्व समकोण पाद आसन (बद्ध उरु हस्त)
Pārśva samakoṇa pāda āsana (baddha uru hasta)
Side stretch split pose (one arm bound around thigh)

पार्श्वसमकोणपादासन (बद्धोरुहस्त)
Pārśvasamakoṇapādāsana (baddhoruhasta)

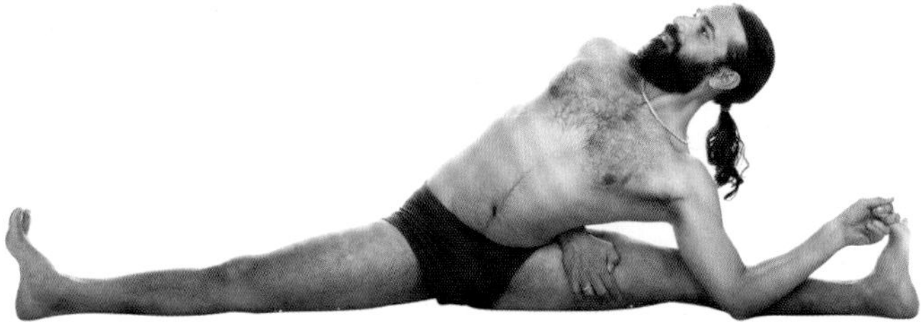

624
सुप्त पद्म नाभ आसन (रज्जु हस्त)
Supta padma nābha āsana (rajju hasta)
Reclined lotus at the navel pose (hands bound)

सुप्तपद्मनाभासन (रज्जुहस्त)
Suptapadmanābhāsana (rajjuhasta)

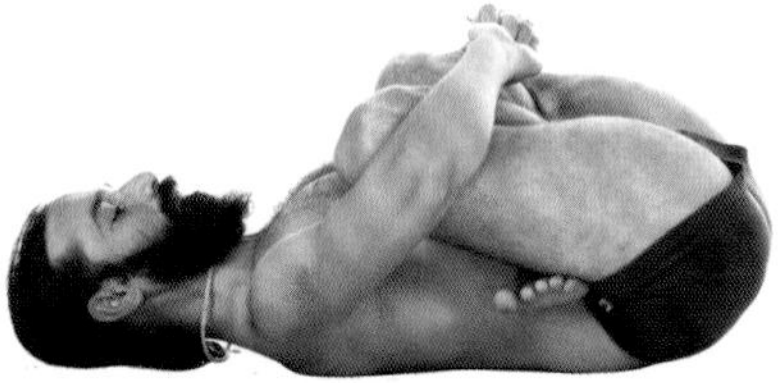

625
सुप्त पद्म आसन (शीर्ष कफोणि बद्ध)
Supta padma āsana (śīrṣa kaphoṇi baddha)
Reclined lotus pose (head and elbows bound)

सुप्तपद्मासन (शीर्षकफोणिबद्ध)
Suptapadmāsana (śīrṣakaphoṇibaddha)

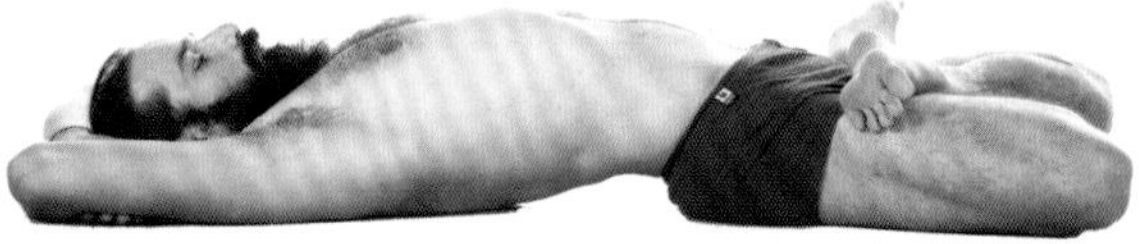

626
सुप्त पद्म आसन(पृष्ठ हस्त भू)
Supta padma āsana (pṛṣṭha hasta bhū)
Reclined lotus pose (hands on the earth above head)

सुप्तपद्मासन (पृष्ठहस्तभू)
Suptapadmāsana (pṛṣṭhahastabhū)

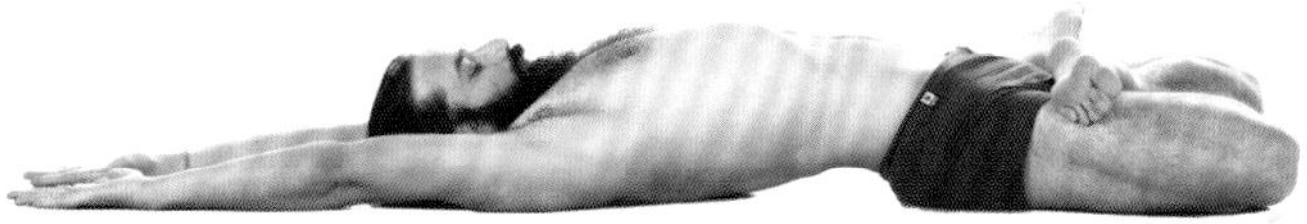

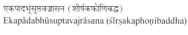

627
एक पाद भू सुप्त वज्र आसन (शीर्ष कफोणि बद्ध)
Eka pāda bhū supta vajra āsana (śīrṣa kaphoṇi baddha)
One foot on earth reclined thunderbolt pose (elbows bound behind the head)

एकपादभूसुप्तवज्रासन (शीर्षकफोणिबद्ध)
Ekapādabhūsuptavajrāsana (śīrṣakaphoṇibaddha)

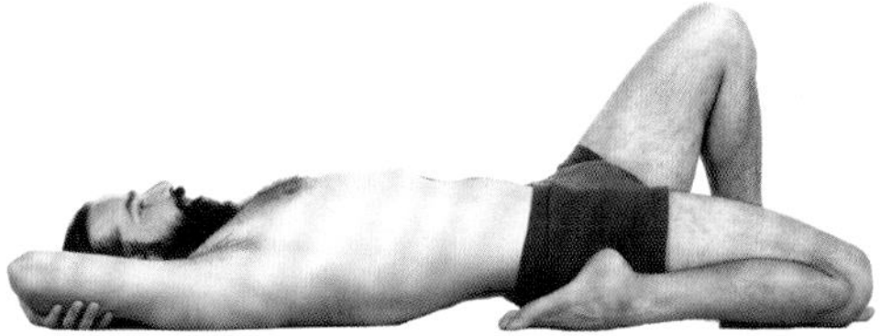

628
एक पाद सुप्त वज्र आसन (शीर्ष कफोणि बद्ध)
Eka pāda supta vajra āsana (śīrṣa kaphoṇi baddha)
One leg reclined thunderbolt pose (elbows bound behind the head)

एकपादसुप्तवज्रासन (शीर्षकफोणिबद्ध)
Ekapādasuptavajrāsana (śīrṣakaphoṇibaddha)

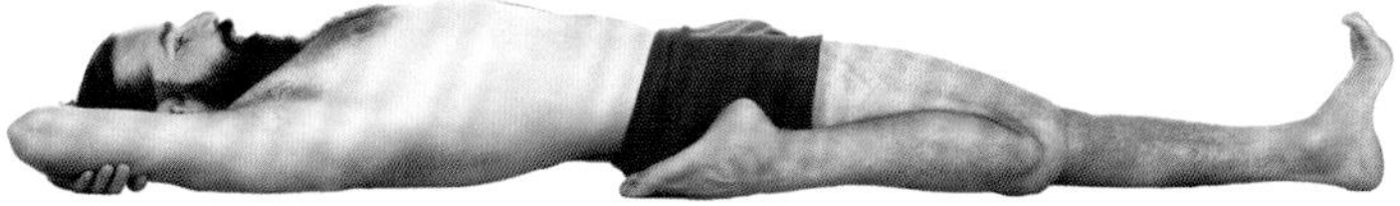

629
अर्ध सुप्त वज्र आसन (कफोणि भू)
Ardha supta vajra āsana (kaphoṇi bhū)
Half reclined thunderbolt pose (elbows on the earth)

अर्धसुप्तवज्रासन (कफोणिभू)
Ardhasuptavajrāsana (kaphoṇibhū)

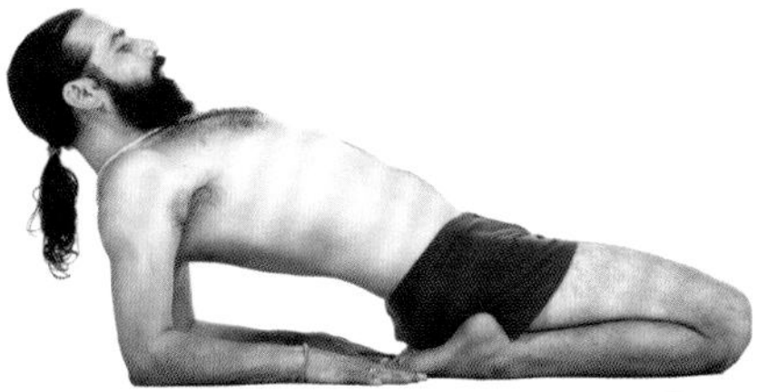

630
सुप्त वज्र आसन (कफोणि भू)
Supta vajra āsana (kaphoṇi bhū)
Reclined thunderbolt pose (elbows on the earth)

सुप्तवज्रासन (कफोणिभू)
Suptavajrāsana (kaphoṇibhū)

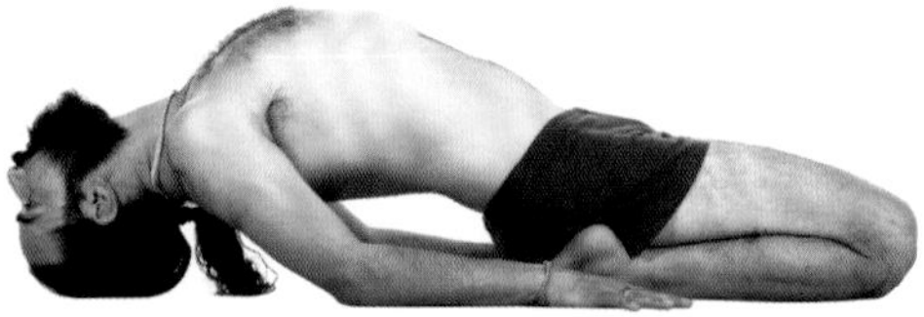

631
सुप्त वज्र आसन (हस्त भू)
Supta vajra āsana (hasta bhū)
Reclined thunderbolt pose (hands on the earth)

सुप्तवज्रासन (हस्तभू)
Suptavajrāsana (hastabhū)

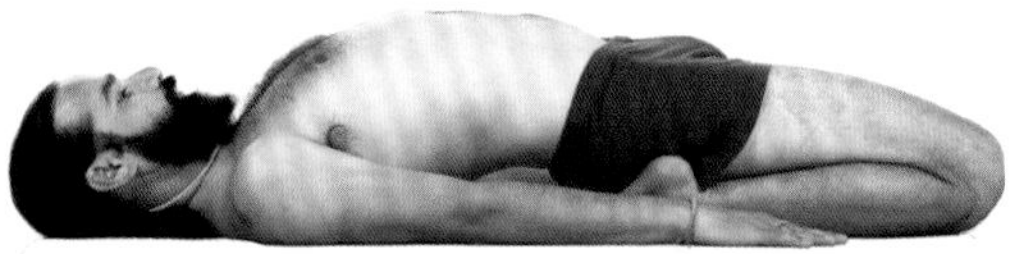

632
सुप्त वज्र आसन (उरु हस्त)
Supta vajra āsana (uru hasta)
Reclined thunderbolt pose (hands on thighs)

सुप्तवज्रासन (उरुहस्त)
Suptavajrāsana (uruhasta)

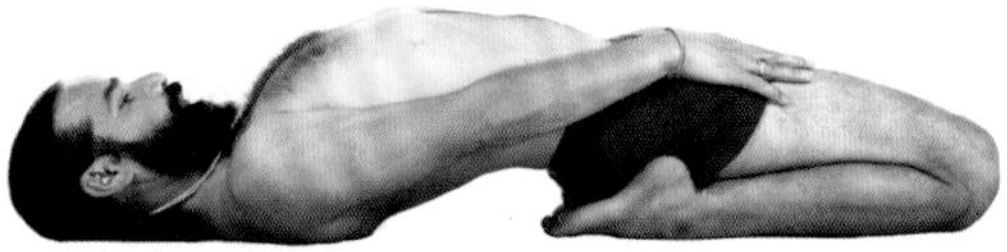

633
सुप्त वज्र आसन (शीर्ष कफोणि बद्ध)
Supta vajra āsana (śīrṣa kaphoṇi baddha)
Reclined thunderbolt pose (elbows bound behind head)

सुप्तवज्रासन (शीर्षकफोणिबद्ध)
Suptavajrāsana (śīrṣakaphoṇibaddha)

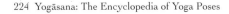

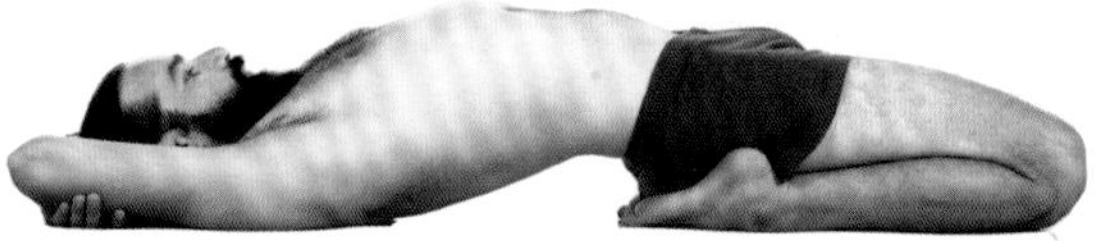

634
नमस्कार सुप्त वज्र आसन
Namaskāra supta vajra āsana
Praying reclined thunderbolt pose

नमस्कारसुप्तवज्रासन
Namaskārasuptavajrāsana

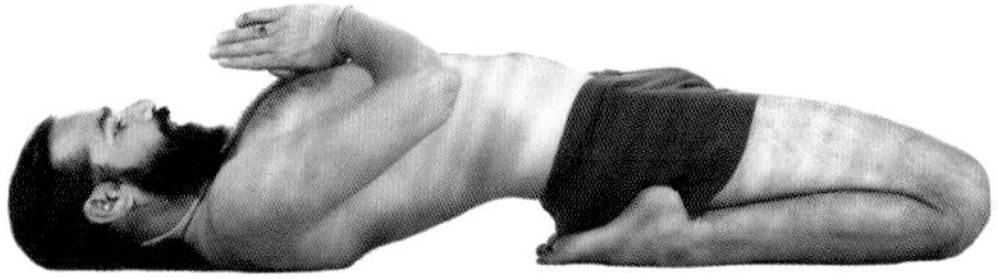

635
गरुड हस्त सुप्त वज्र आसन
Garuḍa hasta supta vajra āsana
Eagle hands reclined thunderbolt pose

गरुडहस्तसुप्तवज्रासन
Garuḍahastasuptavajrāsana

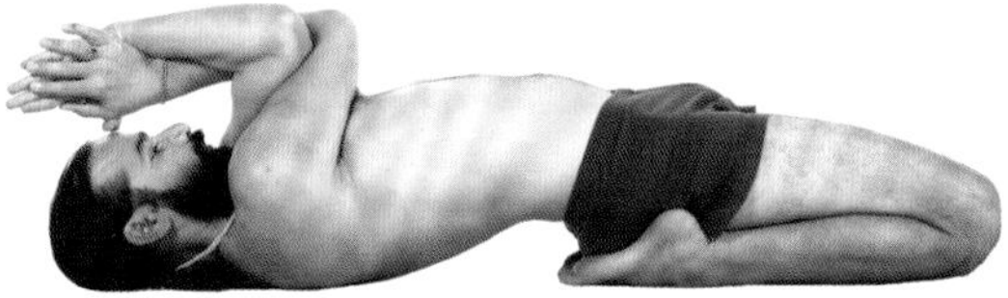

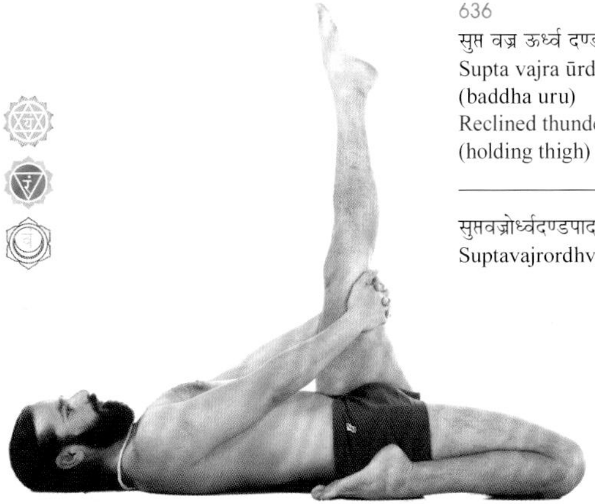

636
सुप्त वज्र ऊर्ध्व दण्ड पाद आसन (बद्ध उरु)
Supta vajra ūrdhva daṇḍa pāda āsana (baddha uru)
Reclined thunderbolt overhead staff pose (holding thigh)

सुप्तवज्रोर्ध्वदण्डपादासन (बद्धोरु)
Suptavajrordhvadaṇḍapādāsana (baddhoru)

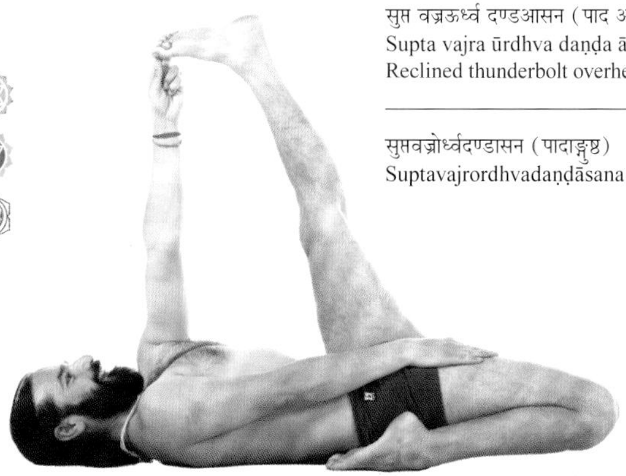

637
सुप्त वज्रऊर्ध्व दण्डआसन (पाद अङ्गुष्ठ)
Supta vajra ūrdhva daṇḍa āsana (pāda aṅguṣṭha)
Reclined thunderbolt overhead staff pose (holding big toe)

सुप्तवज्रोर्ध्वदण्डासन (पादाङ्गुष्ठ)
Suptavajrordhvadaṇḍāsana (pādāṅguṣṭha)

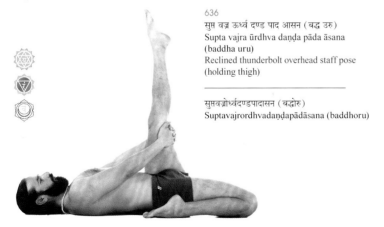

638
सुप्त वज्र पवन मुक्त आसन
Supta vajra pavana mukta āsana
Reclined thunderbolt wind relieving pose

सुप्तवज्रपवनमुक्तासन
Suptavajrapavanamuktāsana

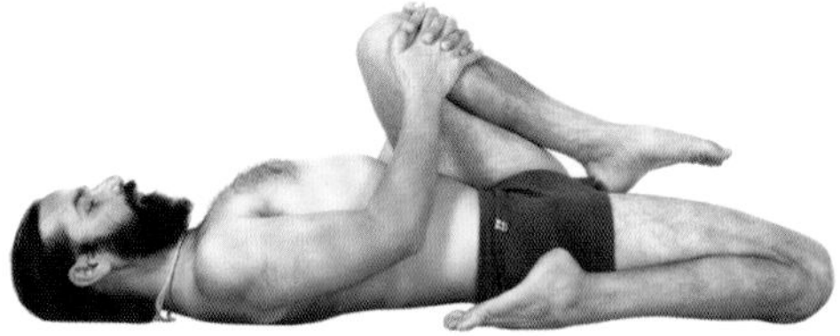

639
सुप्त वज्र पार्श्व दण्ड आसन (पाद अङ्गुष्ठ)
Supta vajra pārśva daṇḍa āsana (pāda aṅguṣṭha)
Reclined thunderbolt side staff pose (holding big toe)

सुप्तवज्रपार्श्वदण्डासन (पादाङ्गुष्ठ)
Suptavajrapārśvadaṇḍāsana (pādāṅguṣṭha)

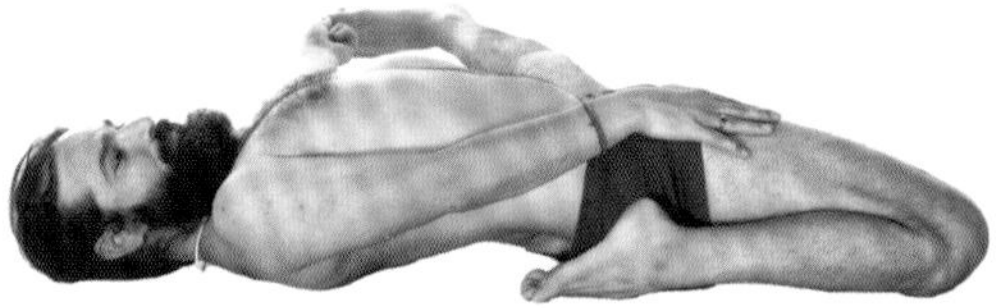

640
अर्ध पवन मुक्त आसन (एक पाद भू)
Ardha pavana mukta āsana (eka pāda bhū)
Half wind relieving pose (one foot on earth)

अर्धपवनमुक्तासन (एकपादभू)
Ardhapavanamuktāsana (ekapādabhū)

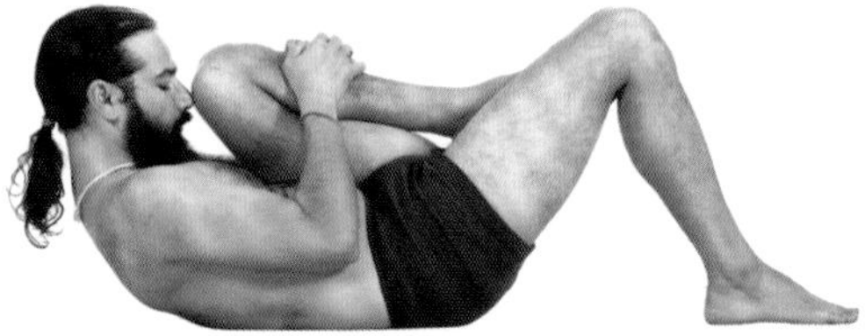

641
पवन मुक्त आसन (एक पाद)
Pavana mukta āsana (eka pāda)
Wind relieving pose (one leg)

पवनमुक्तासन (एकपाद)
Pavanamuktāsana (ekapāda)

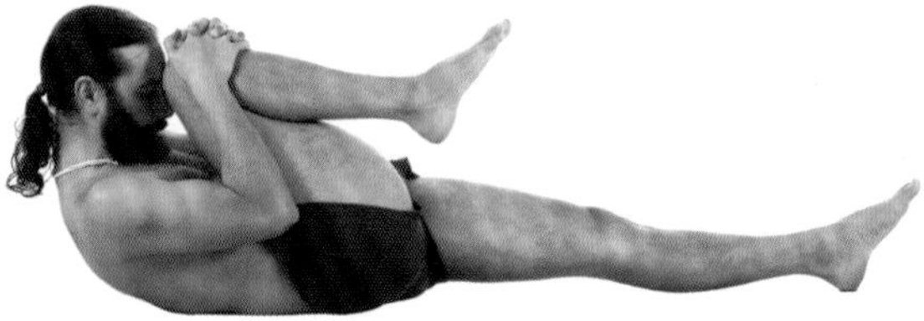

642
सुप्त पवन मुक्त आसन (एक पाद)
Supta pavana mukta āsana (eka pāda)
Reclined wind relieving pose (one leg)

सुप्तपवनमुक्तासन (एकपाद)
Suptapavanamuktāsana (ekapāda)

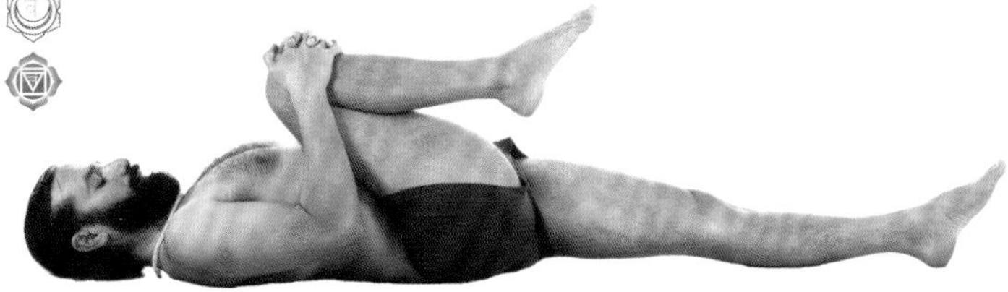

643
सुप्त पवन मुक्त आसन (एक पाद क्षितिज)
Supta pavana mukta āsana (eka pāda kṣitija)
Reclined wind relieving pose (one leg lifted toward the horizon)

सुप्तपवनमुक्तासन (एकपादक्षितिज)
Suptapavanamuktāsana (ekapādakṣitija)

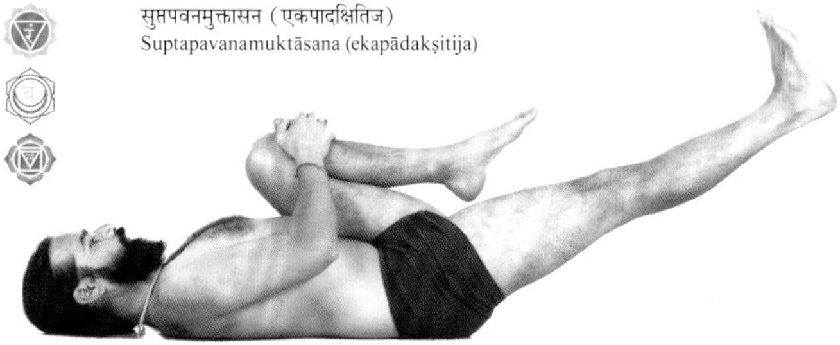

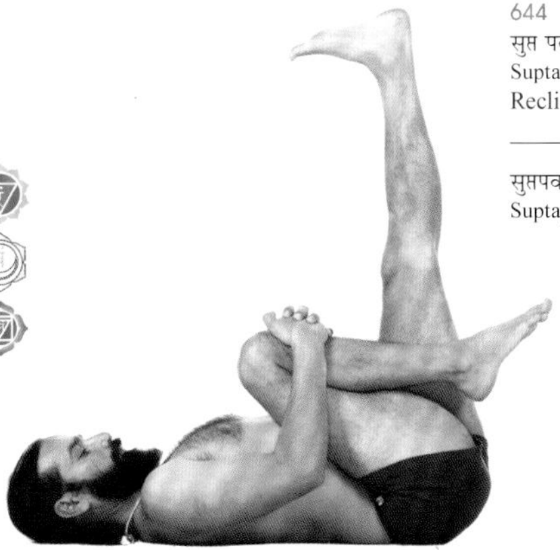

644
सुप्त पवन मुक्त आसन (एक ऊर्ध्व पाद)
Supta pavana mukta āsana (eka ūrdhva pāda)
Reclined wind relieving pose (one leg lifted)

सुप्तपवनमुक्तासन (एकोर्ध्वपाद)
Suptapavanamuktāsana (ekōrdhvapāda)

645
सुप्त पवन मुक्त आसन (पार्श्व जानु)
Supta pavana mukta āsana (pārśva jānu)
Reclined wind relieving pose (knee to the side)

सुप्तपवनमुक्तासन (पार्श्वजानु)
Suptapavanamuktāsana (pārśvajānu)

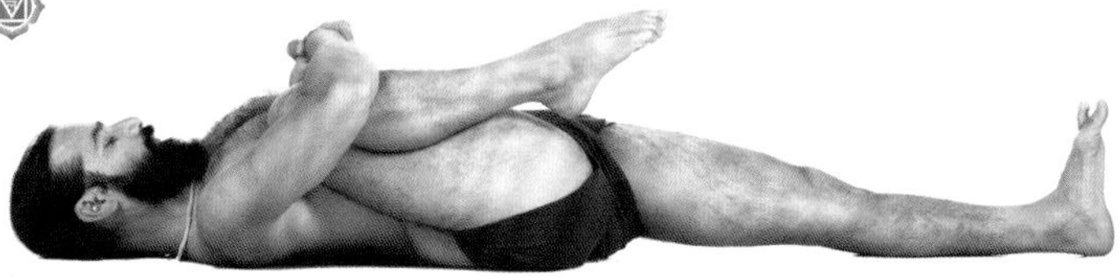

646
सुप्त पवन मुक्त आसन
Supta pavana mukta āsana
Reclined wind relieving pose

सुप्तपवनमुक्तासन
Suptapavanamuktāsana

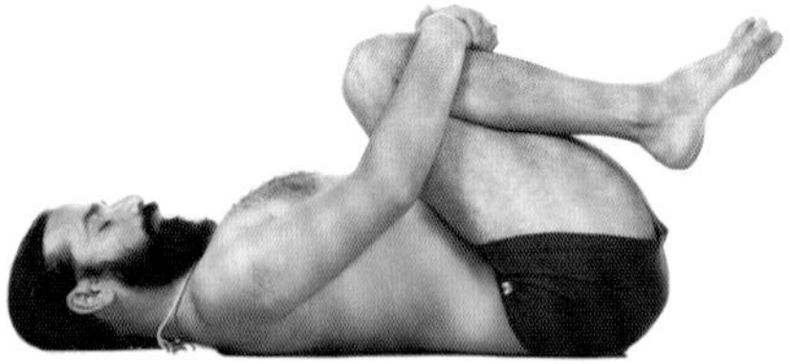

647
पूर्ण सुप्त पवन मुक्त आसन
Pūrṇa supta pavana mukta āsana
Full reclined wind relieving pose

पूर्णसुप्तपवनमुक्तासन
Pūrṇasuptapavanamuktāsana

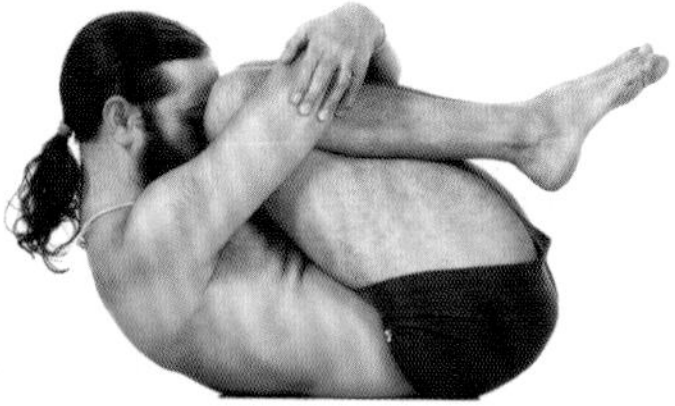

648
नाभि दर्शन आसन (एक पाद उत्तान)
Nābhi darśana āsana (eka pāda uttāna)
Navel gazing pose (one leg lifted)

नाभिदर्शनासन (एकपादोत्तान)
Nābhidarśanāsana (ekapādottāna)

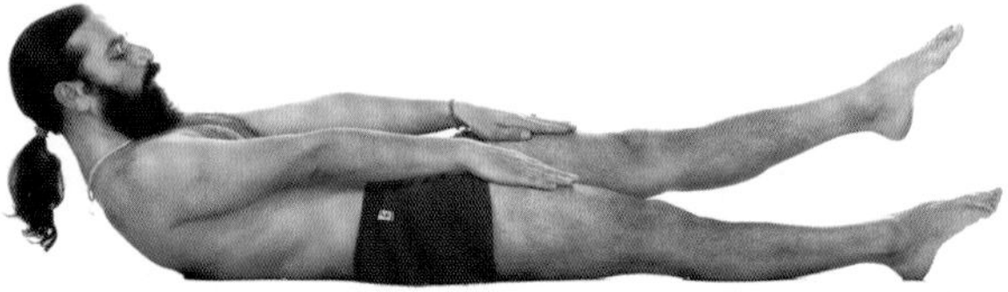

649
नाभि दर्शन आसन(उत्तान पाद)
Nābhi darśana āsana (uttāna pāda)
Navel gazing pose (lifted legs)

नाभिदर्शनासन (उत्तानपाद)
Nābhidarśanāsana (uttānapāda)

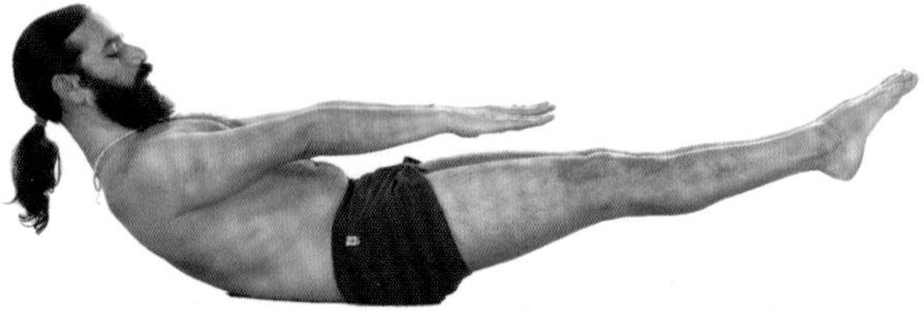

650
नाभि दर्शन आसन (उत्तान पाद, शिरः हस्त)
Nābhi darśana āsana (uttāna pāda, śiraḥ hasta)
Navel gazing pose (lifted legs, hands on head)

नाभिदर्शनासन (उत्तानपाद, शिरोहस्त)
Nābhidarśanāsana (uttānapāda, śirohasta)

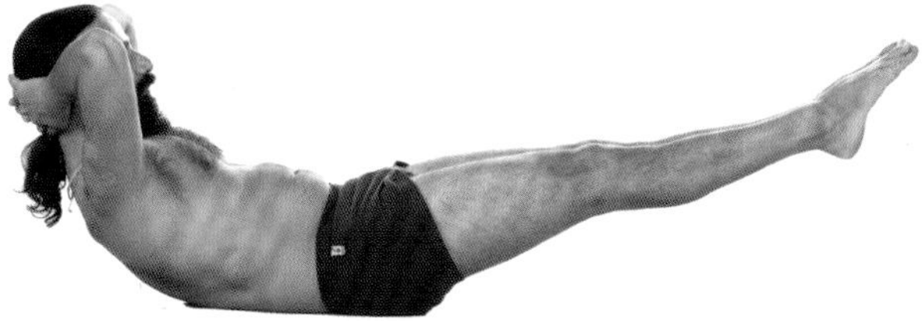

651
उत्तान पाद आसन (क्षितिज पाद)
Uttāna pāda āsana (kṣitija pāda)
Lifted leg pose (foot toward the horizon)

उत्तानपादासन (क्षितिजपाद)
Uttānapādāsana (kṣitijapāda)

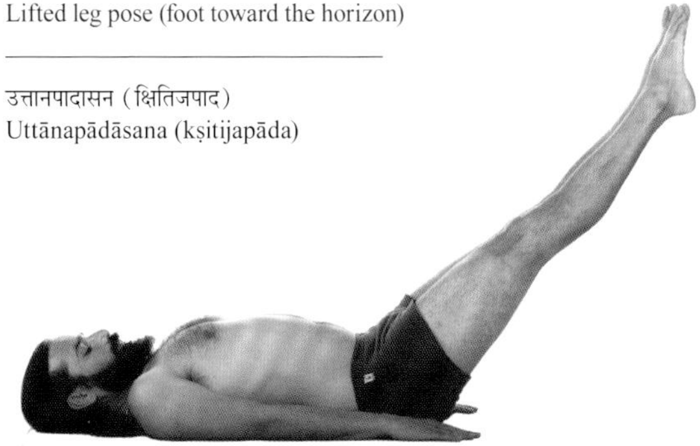

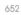

652
उत्तान पाद आसन (ऊर्ध्व पाद अङ्गुल)
Uttāna pāda āsana (ūrdhva pāda aṅgula)
Lifted leg pose (feet lifted, toes pointed)

उत्तानपादासन (ऊर्ध्वपादाङ्गुल)
Uttānapādāsana (ūrdhvapādāṅgula)

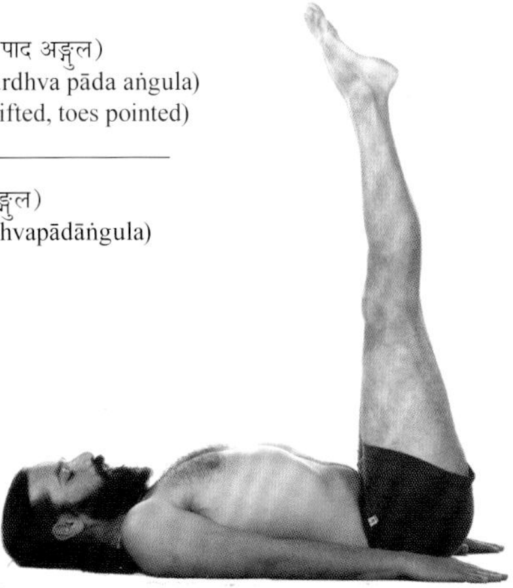

653
उत्तान पाद आसन (अधः पाद अङ्गुल)
Uttāna pāda āsana (adhaḥ pāda aṅgula)
Lifted leg pose (feet flexed)

उत्तानपादासन (अधोपादाङ्गुल)
Uttānapādāsana (adhopādāṅgula)

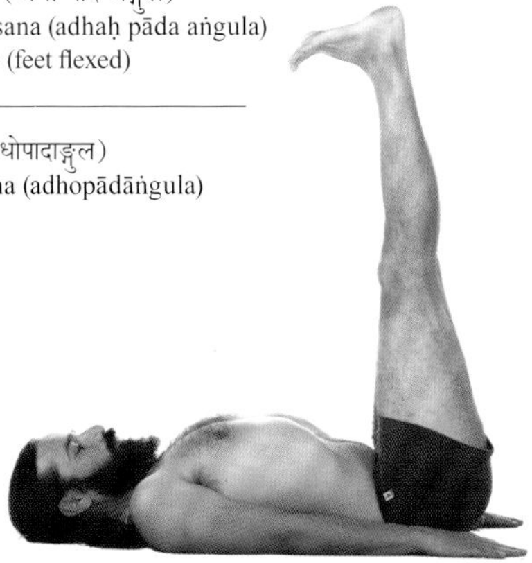

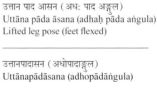

654
अनन्त आसन
Ananta āsana
Infinity pose

अनन्तासन
Anantāsana

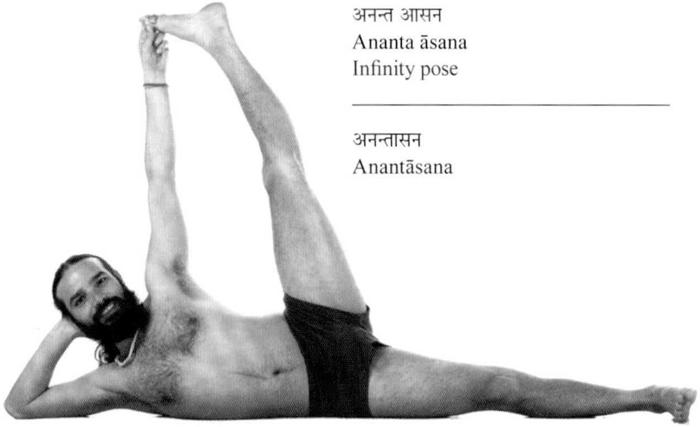

655
सूत्र सूची रन्ध्र आसन (उरु हस्त)
Sūtra sūcī randhra āsana (uru hasta)
Thread the needle pose (hands around thigh)

सूत्रसूचीरन्ध्रासन (उरुहस्त)
Sūtrasūcīrandhrāsana (uruhasta)

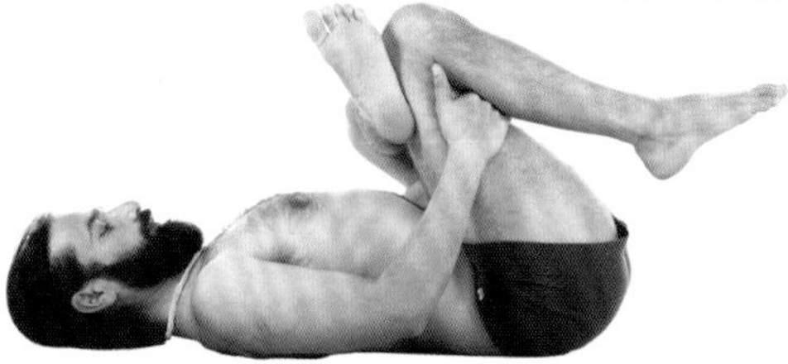

656
सूत्र सूची रन्ध्र आसन
Sūtra sūcī randhra āsana
Thread the needle pose

सूत्रसूचीरन्ध्रासन
Sūtrasūcīrandhrāsana

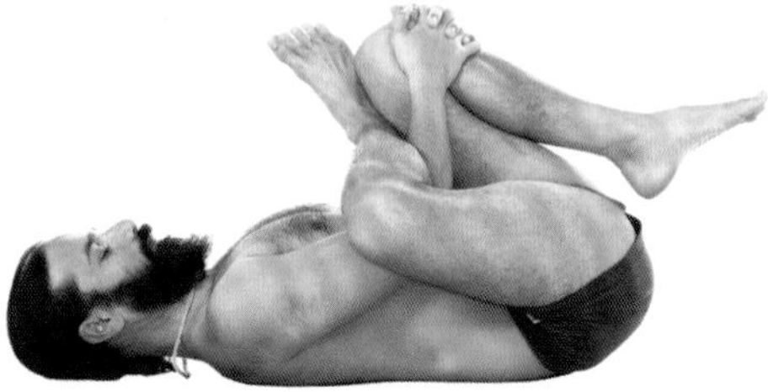

657
मुदित शिशु आसन
Mudita śiśu āsana
Blissful baby pose

मुदितशिशुासन
Muditaśiśuāsana

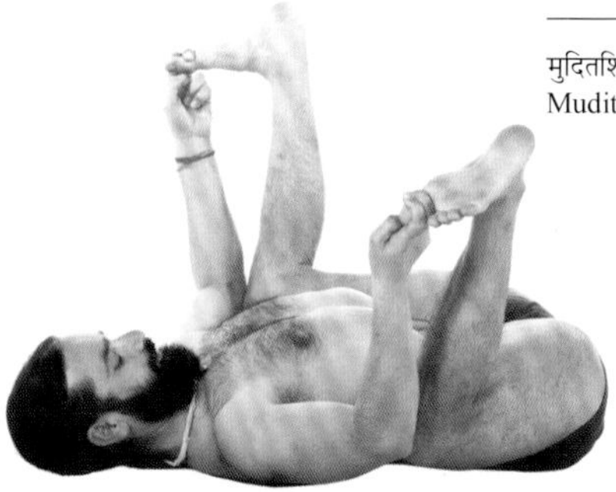

658
शिशु क्रीडा आसन
Śiśu krīḍā āsana
Playful baby pose

शिशुक्रीडासन
Śiśukrīḍāsana

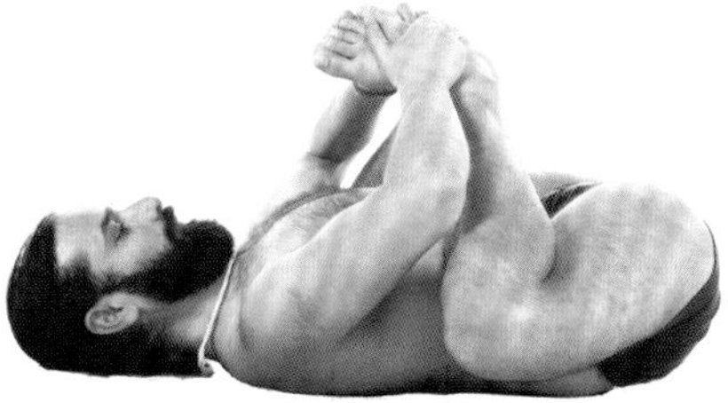

659
शिशु क्रीडा आसन (श्वास)
Śiśu krīḍā āsana (śvāsa)
Playful baby pose (playing with the breath)

शिशुक्रीडासन (श्वास)
Śiśukrīḍāsana (śvāsa)

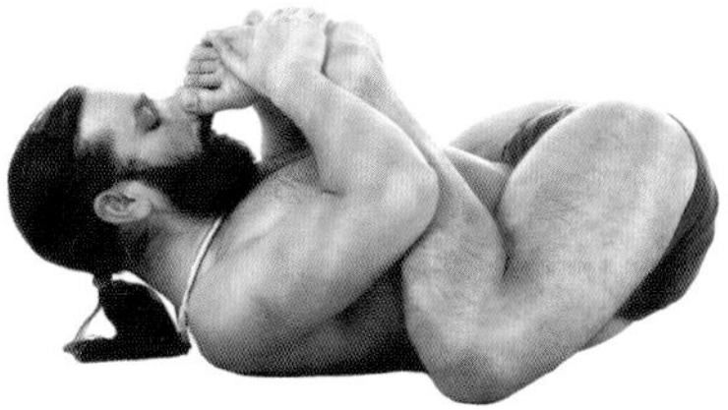

660
मुदित शिशु आसन (एक पाद)
Mudita śiśu āsana (eka pāda)
Blissful baby pose (one leg)

मुदितशिशुासन (एकपाद)
Muditaśiśāsana (ekapāda)

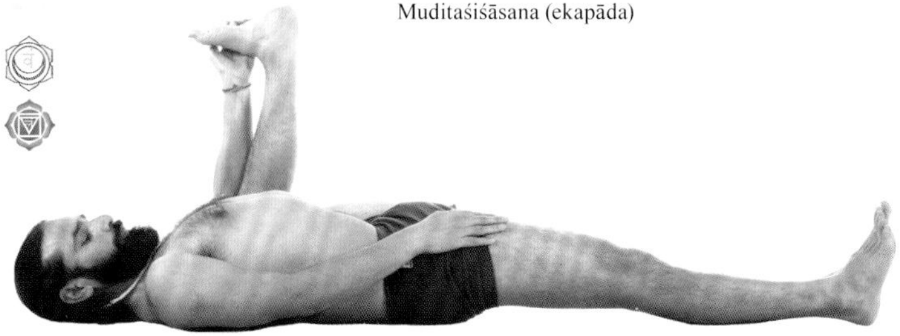

661
शिशु पाद तिलक आसन
Śiśu pāda tilaka āsana
Foot to forehead baby pose

शिशुपादतिलकासन
Śiśupādatilakāsana

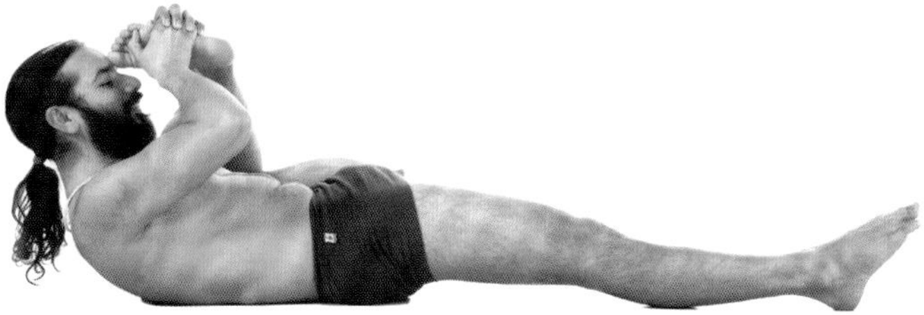

662
सुप्त नमस्कार भैरव आसन
Supta namaskāra bhairava āsana
Reclined praying fearless pose

सुप्तनमस्कारभैरवासन
Suptanamaskārabhairavāsana

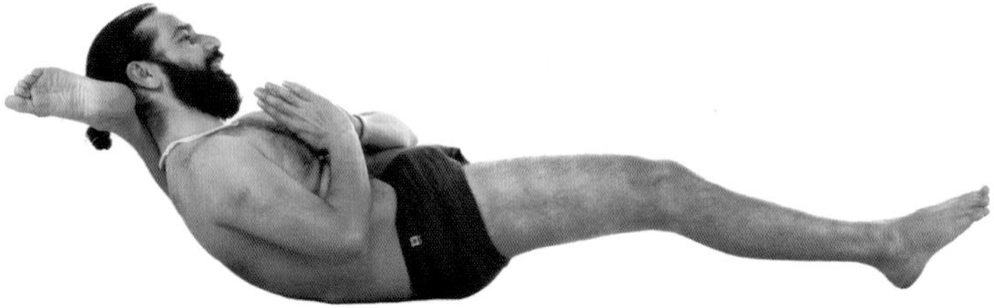

Believe in yourself and create your own path.

663
गर्भ आसन
Garbha āsana
Womb pose

गर्भासन
Garbhāsana

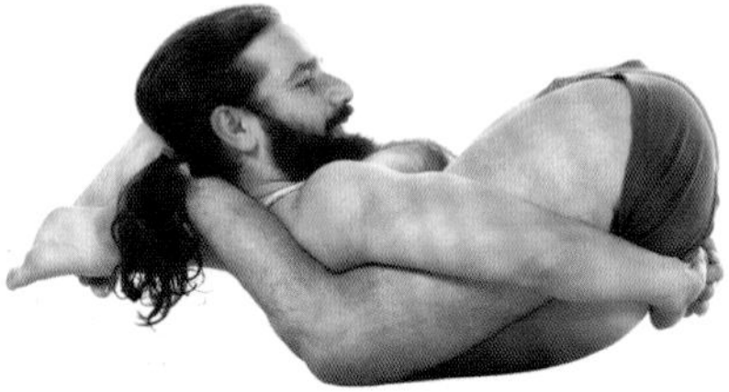

664
नमस्कार गर्भ आसन
Namaskāra garbha āsana
Praying womb pose

नमस्कारगर्भासन
Namaskāragarbhāsana

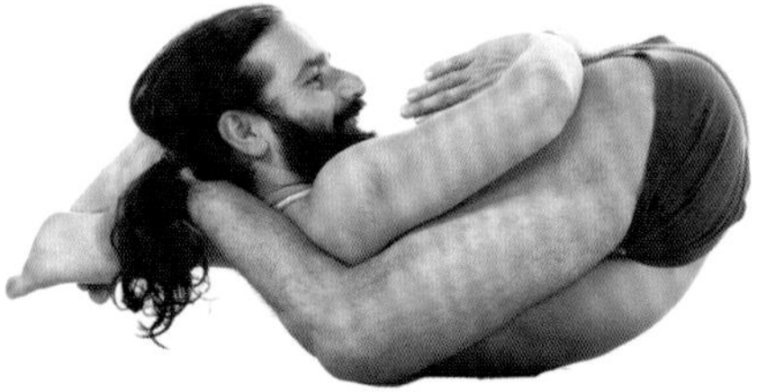

665
सुप्त हस्त पाद अङ्गुष्ठ आसन (सरज्जु)
Supta hasta pāda aṅguṣṭha āsana (sarajju)
Reclined hand to big toe pose (with strap)

सुप्तहस्तपादाङ्गुष्ठासन (सरज्जु)
Suptahastapādāṅguṣṭhāsana (sarajju)

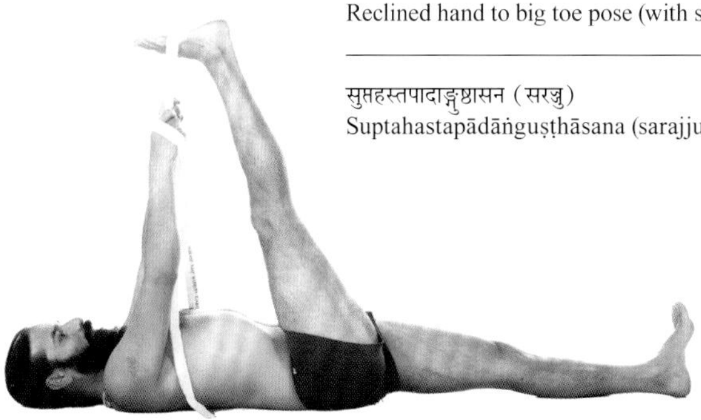

666
सुप्त हस्त पाद अङ्गुष्ठ आसन
Supta hasta pāda aṅguṣṭha āsana
Reclined hand to big toe pose

सुप्तहस्तपादाङ्गुष्ठासन
Suptahastapādāṅguṣṭhāsana

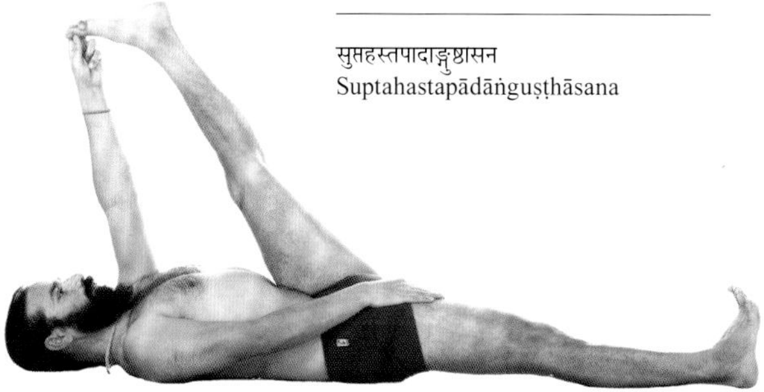

667
सुप्त हस्त पाद अङ्गुष्ठ आसन (जानु शिर)
Supta hasta pāda aṅguṣṭha āsana (jānu śira)
Reclined hand to big toe pose (knee to head)

सुप्तहस्तपादाङ्गुष्ठासन (जानुशिर)
Suptahastapādāṅguṣṭhāsana (jānuśira)

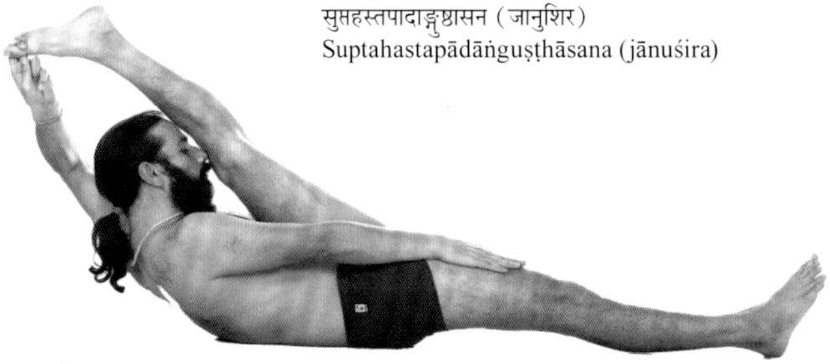

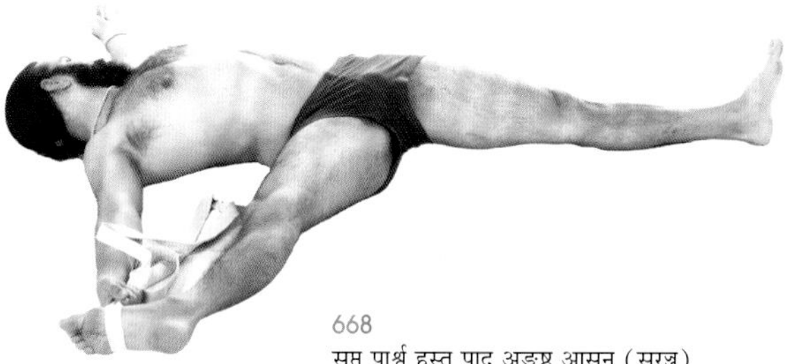

668
सुप्त पार्श्व हस्त पाद अङ्गुष्ठ आसन (सरज्जु)
Supta pārśva hasta pāda aṅguṣṭha āsana (sarajju)
Side reclined hand to big toe pose (with strap)

सुप्तपार्श्वहस्तपादाङ्गुष्ठासन (सरज्जु)
Suptapārśvahastapādāṅguṣṭhāsana (sarajju)

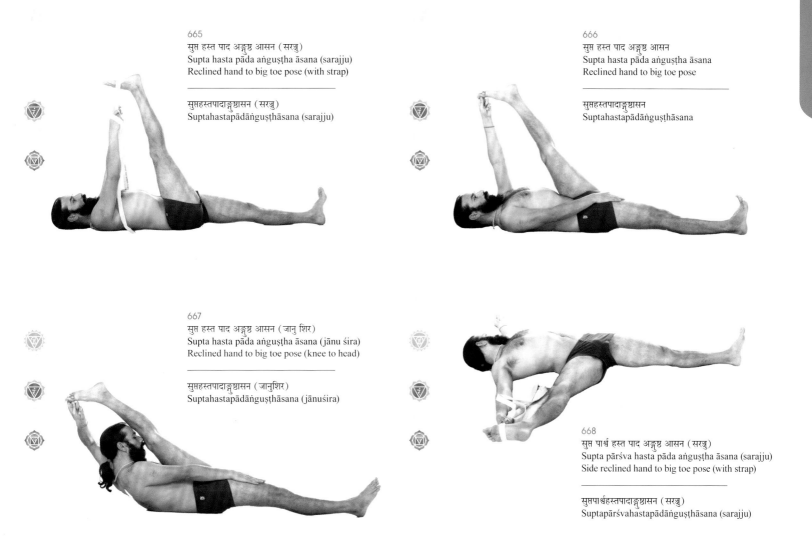

669
सुप्त पार्श्व हस्त पाद अङ्गुष्ठ आसन (हस्त गुल्फ)
Supta pārśva hasta pāda aṅguṣṭha āsana (hasta gulpha)
Side reclined hand to big toe pose (holding the ankle)

सुप्तपार्श्वहस्तपादाङ्गुष्ठासन (हस्तगुल्फ)
Suptapārśvahastapādāṅguṣṭhāsana (hastagulpha)

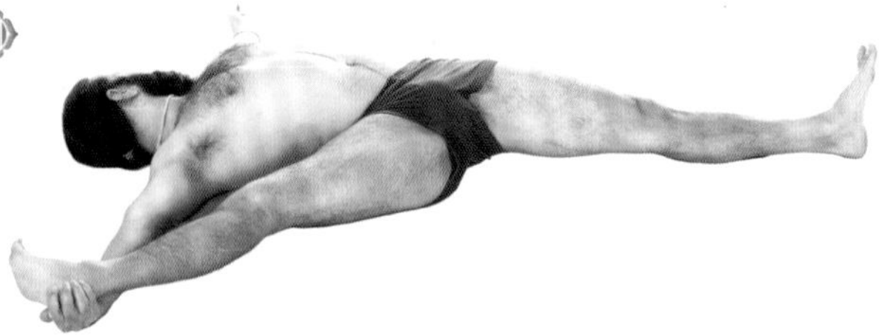

670
सुप्त परिवृत्त हस्त पाद अङ्गुष्ठ आसन
Supta parivṛtta hasta pāda aṅguṣṭha āsana
Twisted reclined hand to big toe pose

सुप्तपरिवृत्तहस्तपादाङ्गुष्ठासन
Suptaparivṛttahastapādāṅguṣṭhāsana

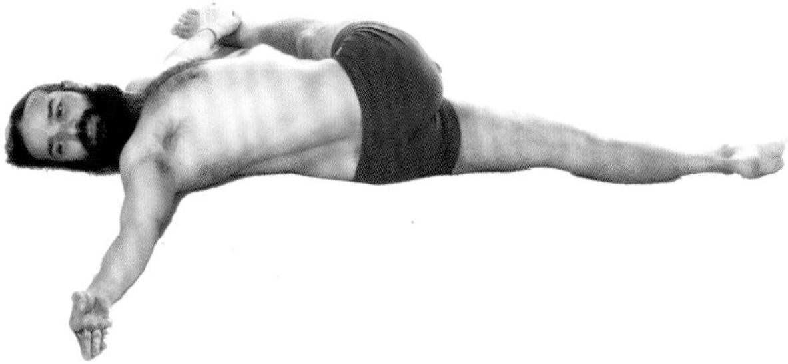

671
सुप्त परिवृत्त हस्त पाद अङ्गुष्ठ आसन (हृदय भू)
Supta parivṛtta hasta pāda aṅguṣṭha āsana (hṛdaya bhū)
Reclined twisted hand to big toe pose (heart on the earth)

सुप्तपरिवृत्तहस्तपादाङ्गुष्ठासन (हृदयभू)
Suptaparivṛttahastapādāṅguṣṭhāsana (hṛdayabhū)

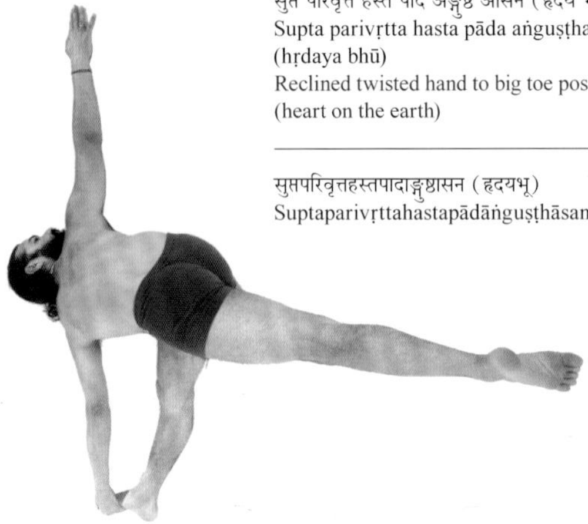

672
सुप्त जानु शिर त्रि विक्रम आसन
Supta jānu śira tri vikrama āsana
Reclined head to knee trinity wisdom pose

सुप्तजानुशिरत्रिविक्रमासन
Suptajānuśiratrivikramāsana

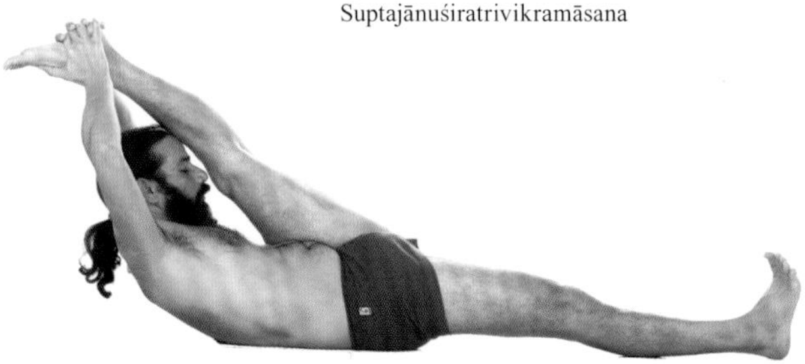

673
सुप्त पार्श्व त्रि विक्रम आसन
Supta pārśva tri vikrama āsana
Side reclined trinity wisdom pose

सुप्तपार्श्वत्रिविक्रमासन
Suptapārśvatrivikramāsana

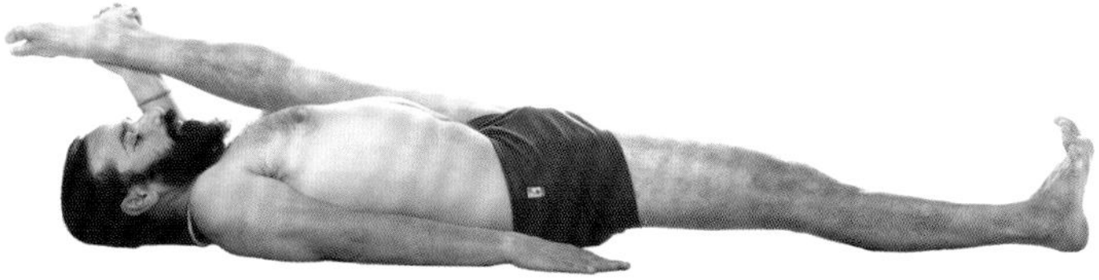

674
सुप्त समकोण पाद आसन (हस्त पाद अङ्गुष्ठ)
Supta samakoṇa pāda āsana (hasta pāda aṅguṣṭha)
Reclined side split pose (holding big toes)

सुप्तसमकोणपादासन (हस्तपादाङ्गुष्ठ)
Suptasamakoṇapādāsana (hastapādāṅguṣṭha)

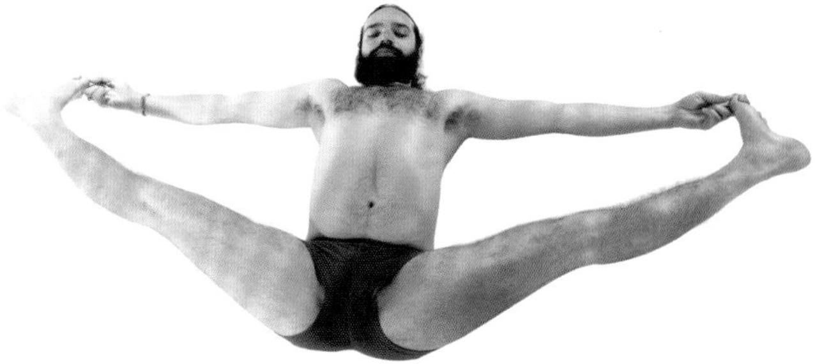

675
सुप्त समकोण पाद आसन (नमस्कार)
Supta samakoṇa pāda āsana (namaskāra)
Reclined side split pose (praying hands)

सुप्तसमकोणपादासन (नमस्कार)
Suptasamakoṇapādāsana (namaskāra)

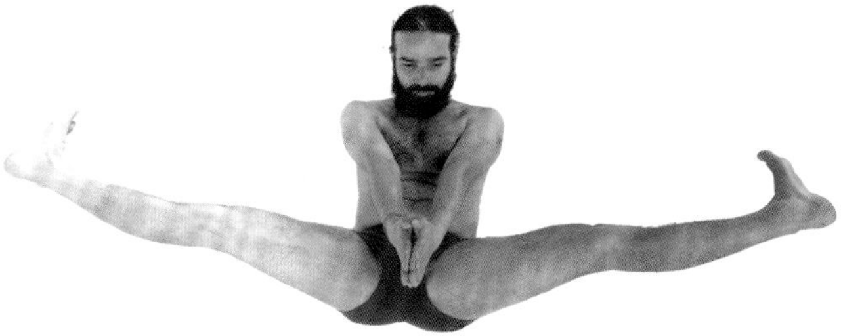

676
मेरु उदर आकुञ्चन आसन (एक जानु हस्त)
Meru udara ākuñcana āsana (eka jānu hasta)
Spinal and abdominal cleansing pose (holding one knee)

मेरूदराकुञ्चनासन (एकजानुहस्त)
Merūdarākuñcanāsana (ekajānuhasta)

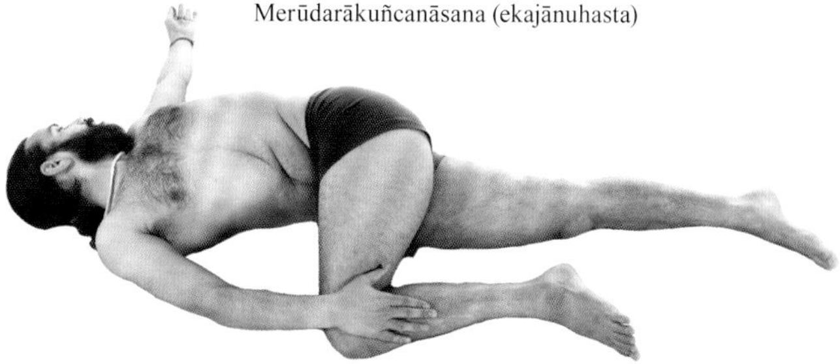

677
मेरु उदर आकुञ्चन आसन (जानु हस्त)
Meru udara ākuñcana āsana (jānu hasta)
Spinal and abdominal cleansing pose (holding knees)

मेरूदराकुञ्चनासन (जानुहस्त)
Merūdarākuñcanāsana (jānuhasta)

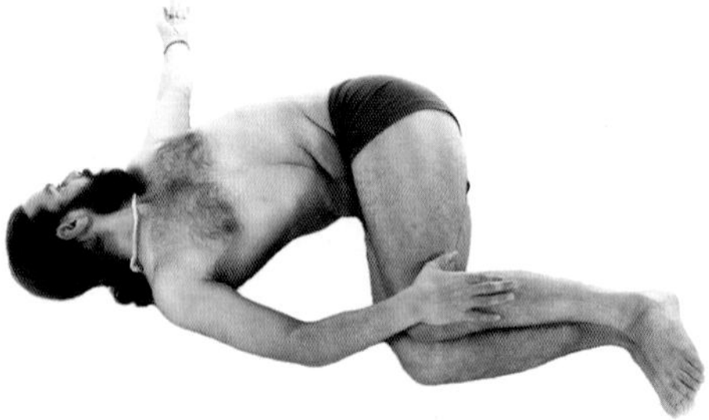

678
मेरु उदर आकुञ्चन आसन (गरुड पाद)
Meru udara ākuñcana āsana (garuḍa pāda)
Spinal and abdominal cleansing pose (cagle legs)

मेरूदराकुञ्चनासन (गरुडपाद)
Merūdarākuñcanāsana (garuḍapāda)

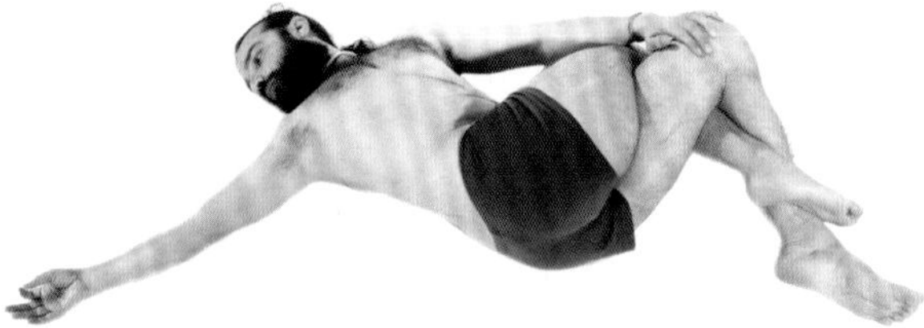

679
मेरु उदर आकुञ्चन आसन (हस्त पाद अङ्गुष्ठ)
Meru udara ākuñcana āsana (hasta pāda aṅguṣṭha)
Spinal and abdominal cleansing pose (holding big toe)

मेरूदराकुञ्चनासन (हस्तपादाङ्गुष्ठ)
Merūdarākuñcanāsana (hastapādaṅguṣṭha)

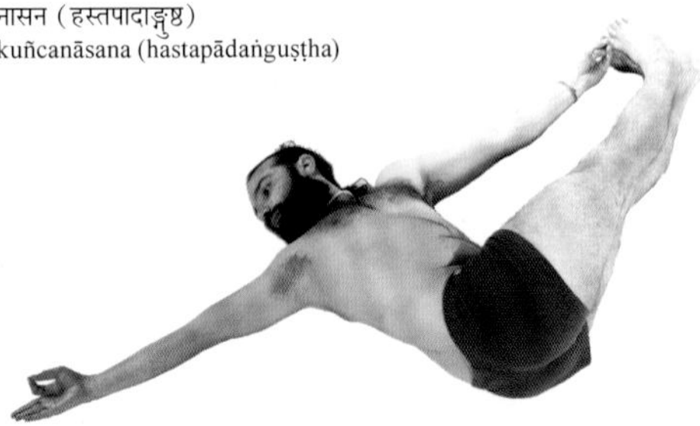

680
परिवृत्त चतुः कोण आसन (हृदय भू)
Parivṛtta catuḥ koṇa āsana (hṛdayaḥ bhū)
Twisted four angle pose (heart on the earth)

परिवृत्तचतुष्कोणासन (हृदयभू)
Parivṛttacatuṣkoṇāsana (hṛdayabhū)

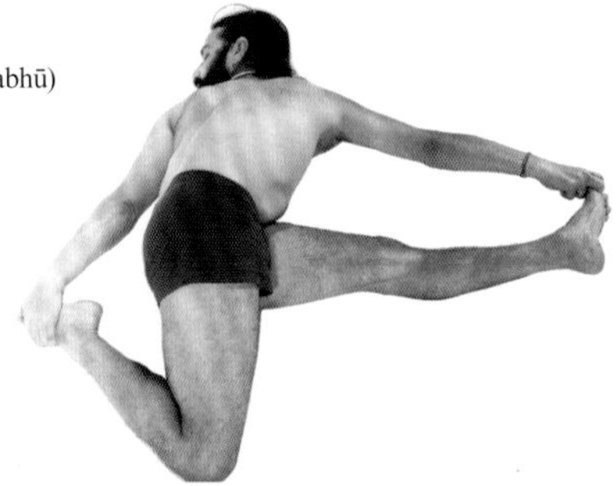

Lying on the Back

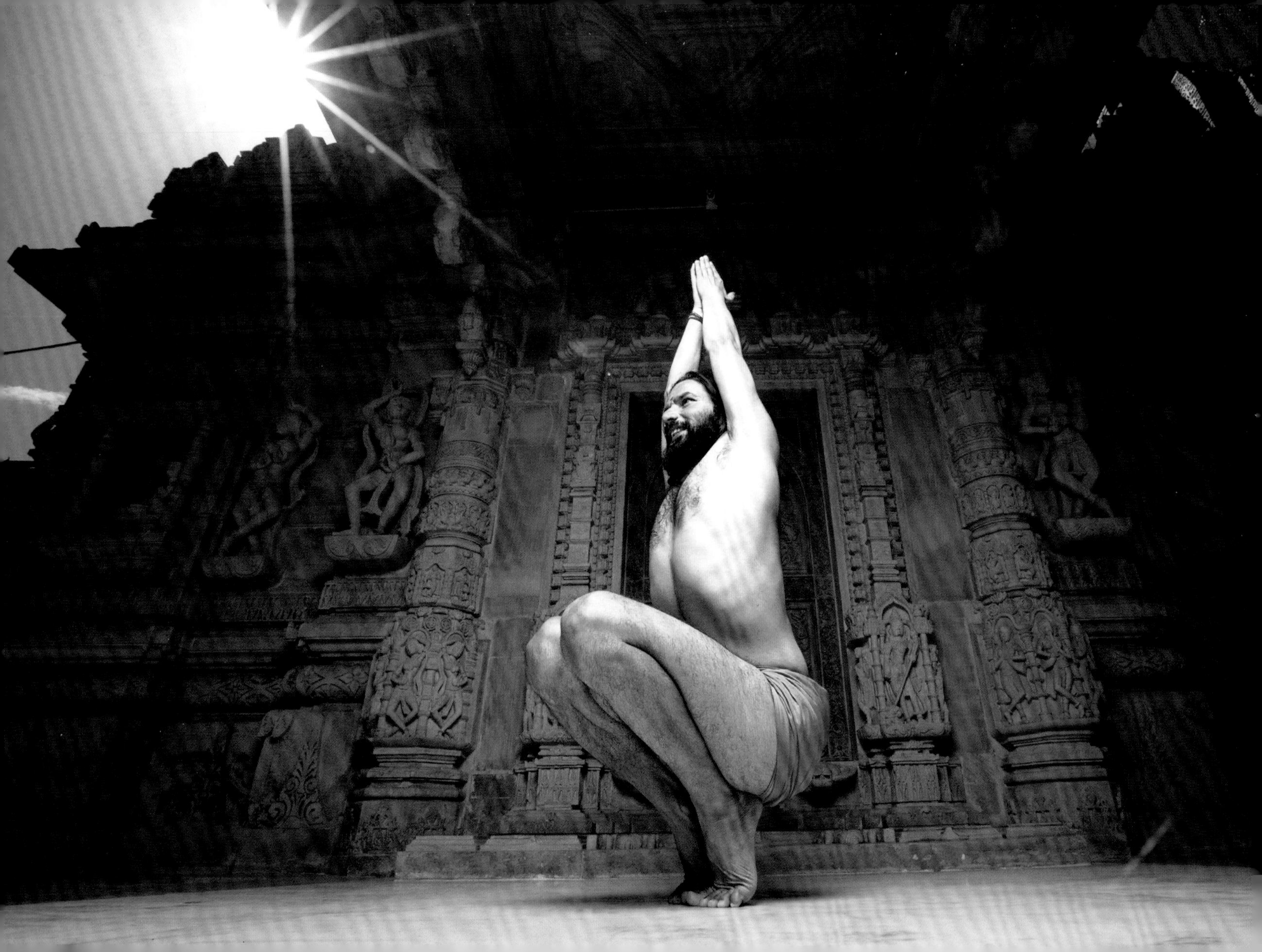

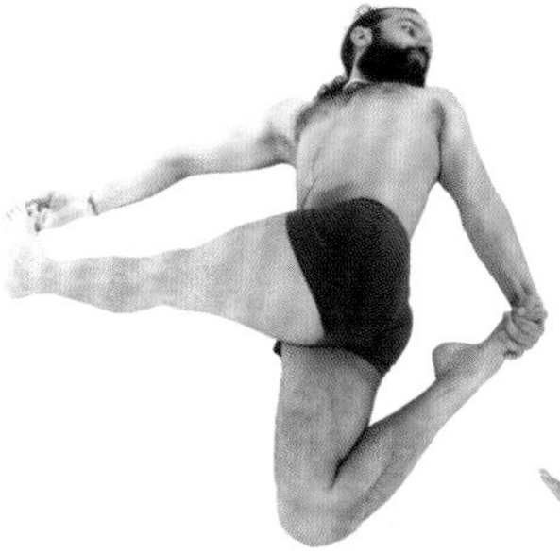

681
परिवृत्त चतुः कोण आसन (मेरु स्कन्ध भू)
Parivṛtta catuḥ koṇa āsana (meru skandha bhū)
Twisted four angle pose (spine and shoulders on the earth)

परिवृत्तचतुष्कोणासन (मेरुस्कन्धभू)
Parivṛttacatuṣkoṇāsana (meruskandhabhū)

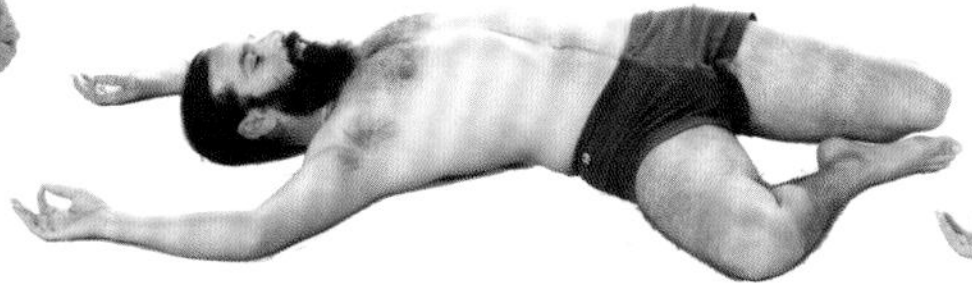

682
सुप्त चतुः अङ्ग आसन
Supta catuḥ aṅga āsana
Reclined four limb pose

सुप्तचतुरङ्गासन
Suptacaturaṅgāsana

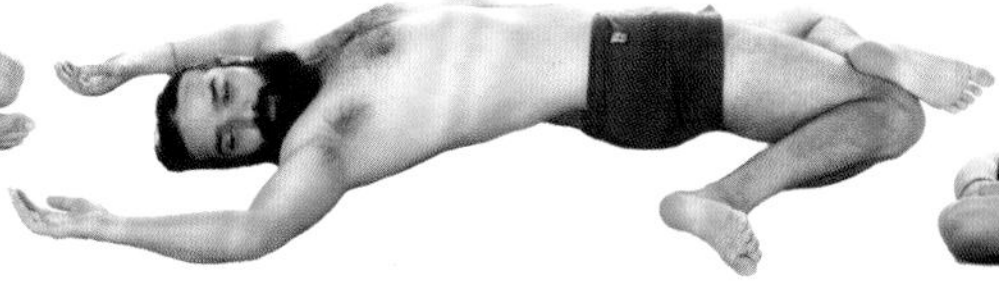

683
सुप्त चतुः अङ्ग आसन (जानु उपरि पाद)
Supta catuḥ aṅga āsana (jānu upari pāda)
Reclined four limb pose (foot on the knee)

सुप्तचतुरङ्गासन (जानूपरिपाद)
Suptacaturaṅgāsana (jānūparipāda)

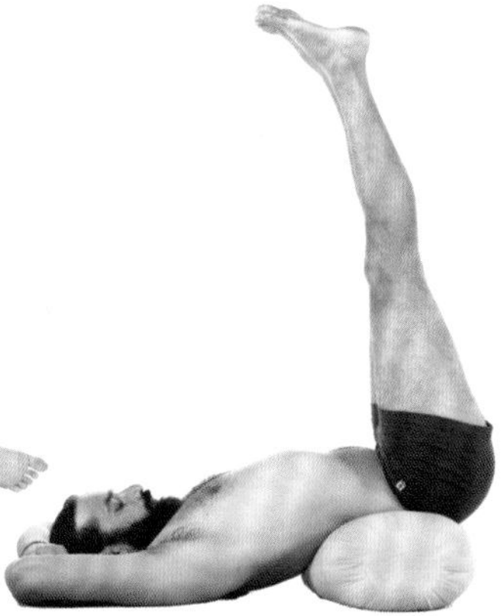

684
अर्ध विपरीतकरणी आसन (सालम्ब शिरोबद्ध कफोणि)
Ardha viparītakaraṇī āsana (sālamba śirobaddha kaphoṇi)
Half inversion pose (head supported on bound elbows)

अर्धविपरीतकरणीआसन (सालम्बशिरोबद्धकफोणि)
Ardhaviparītakaraṇīāsana (sālambaśirobaddhakaphoṇi)

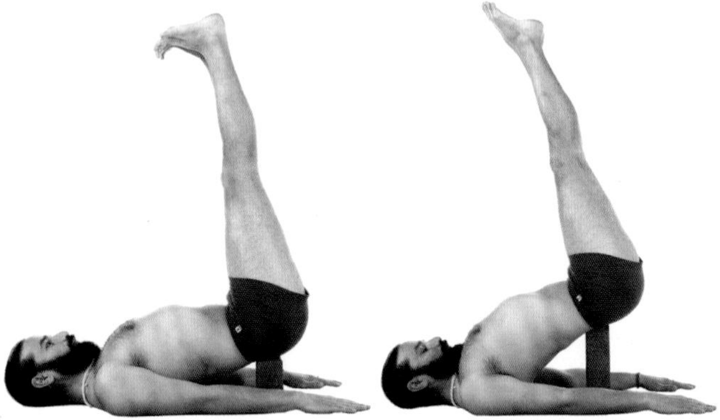

685
विपरीतकरणी (सालम्ब)
Viparītakaraṇī (sālamba)
Inversion (supported)

विपरीतकरणी (सालम्ब)
Viparītakaraṇī (sālamba)

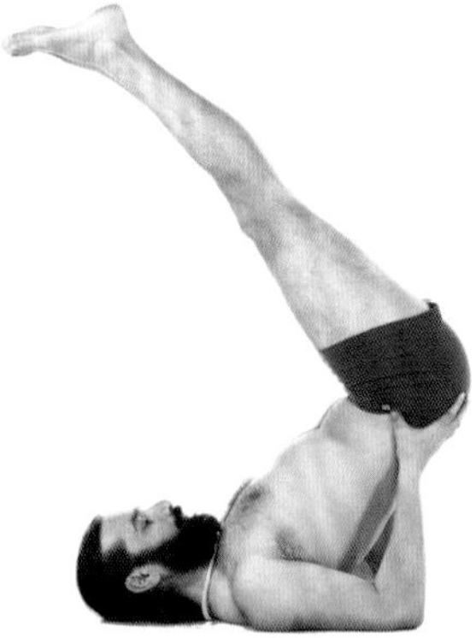

686
विपरीतकरणी
Viparītakaraṇī
Inversion

विपरीतकरणीमुद्रा
Viparītakaraṇī

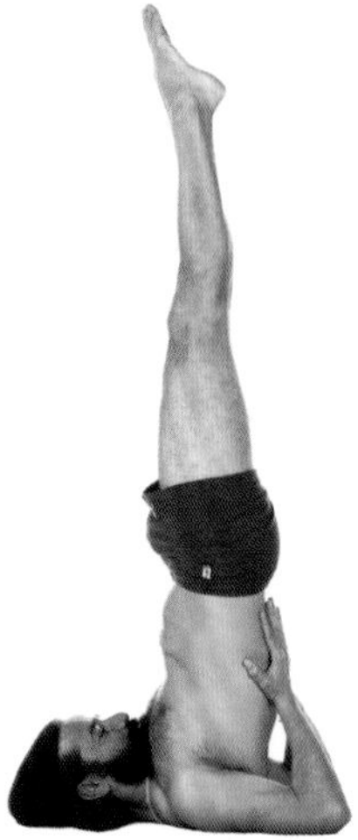

687
सर्व अङ्ग आसन
Sarva aṅga āsana
All limbs pose

सर्वाङ्गासन
Sarvāṅgāsana

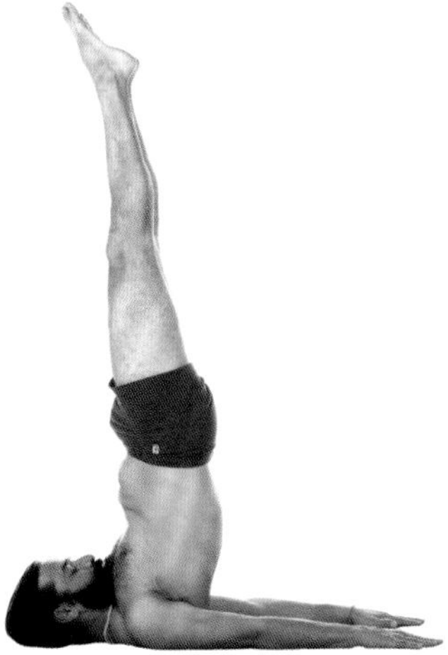

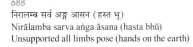

688
निरालम्ब सर्व अङ्ग आसन (हस्त भू)
Nirālamba sarva aṅga āsana (hasta bhū)
Unsupported all limbs pose (hands on the earth)

निरालम्बसर्वङ्गासन (हस्तभू)
Nirālambasarvāṅgāsana (hastabhū)

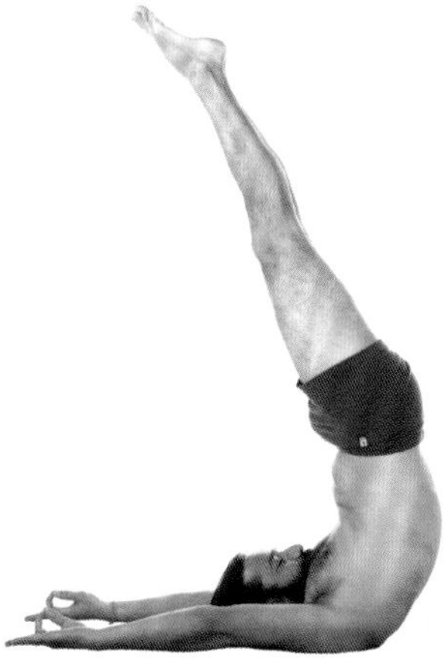

689
निरालम्ब सर्व अङ्ग आसन (पृष्ठ हस्त भू)
Nirālamba sarva aṅga āsana (pṛṣṭha hasta bhū)
Unsupported all limbs pose (hands on the earth behind head)

निरालम्बसर्वाङ्गासन (पृष्ठहस्तभू)
Nirālambasarvāṅgāsana (pṛṣṭhahastabhū)

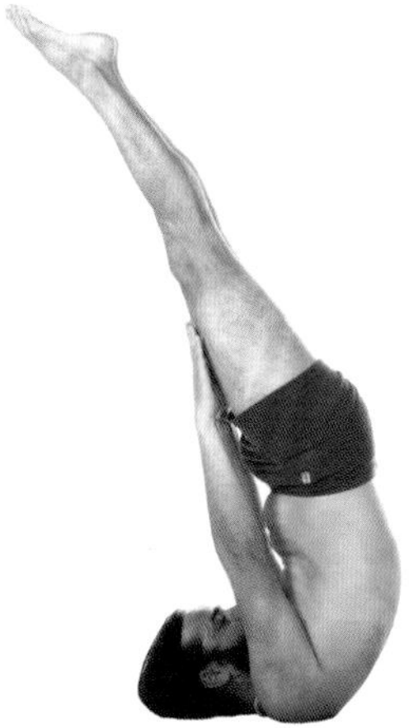

690
निरालम्ब सर्व अङ्ग आसन (उरु हस्त)
Nirālamba sarva āṅga āsana (uru hasta)
Unsupported all limbs pose (hands on thighs)

निरालम्बसर्वाङ्गासन (उरुहस्त)
Nirālambasarvāṅgāsana (uruhasta)

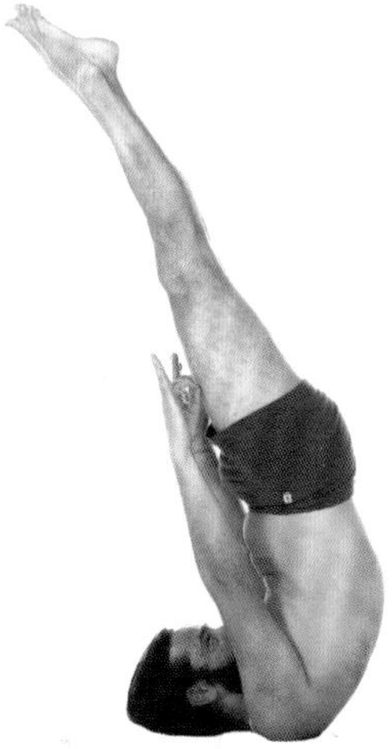

691
निरालम्ब सर्व अङ्ग आसन (उरु हस्त,ज्ञान मुद्रा)
Nirālamba sarva aṅga āsana (uru hasta, jñāna mudrā)
Unsupported all limbs pose (hands on thighs in jñāna mudrā)

निरालम्बसर्वाङ्गासन (उरुहस्त, ज्ञानमुद्रा)
Nirālambasarvāṅgāsana (uruhasta, jñānamudrā)

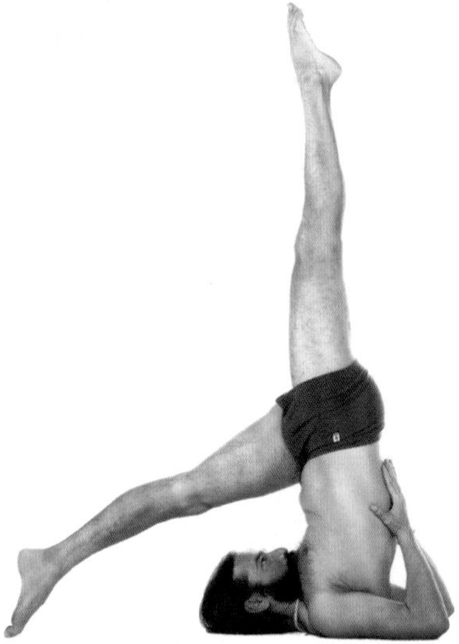

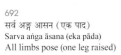

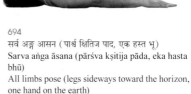

692
सर्व अङ्ग आसन (एक पाद)
Sarva aṅga āsana (eka pāda)
All limbs pose (one leg raised)

सर्वाङ्गासन(एकपाद)
Sarvāṇgāsana (ekapāda)

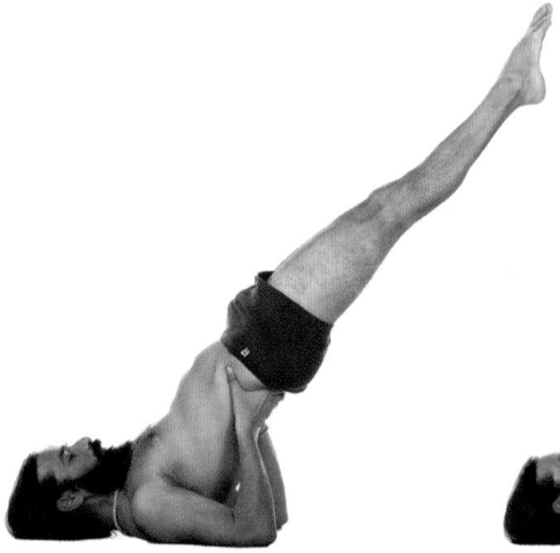

693
सर्व अङ्ग आसन (क्षितिज पाद)
Sarva aṅga āsana (kṣitija pāda)
All limbs pose (feet toward the horizon)

सर्वाङ्गासन (क्षितिजपाद)
Sarvāṅgāsana (kṣitijapāda)

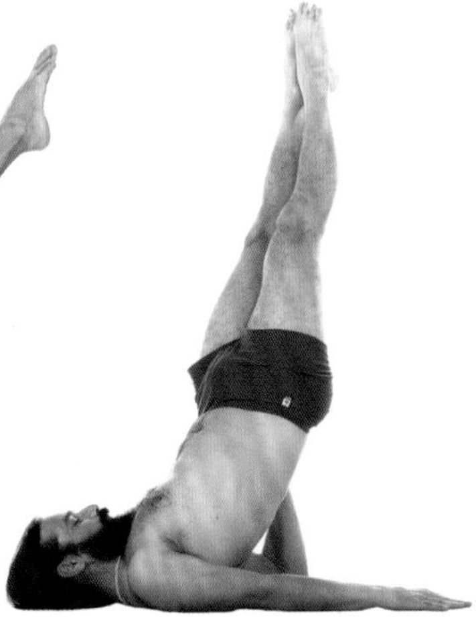

694
सर्व अङ्ग आसन (पार्श्व क्षितिज पाद, एक हस्त भू)
Sarva aṅga āsana (pārśva kṣitija pāda, eka hasta bhū)
All limbs pose (legs sideways toward the horizon, one hand on the earth)

सर्वाङ्गासन (पार्श्वक्षितिजपाद, एकहस्तभू)
Sarvāṅgāsana (pārśvakṣitijapāda, ekahastabhū)

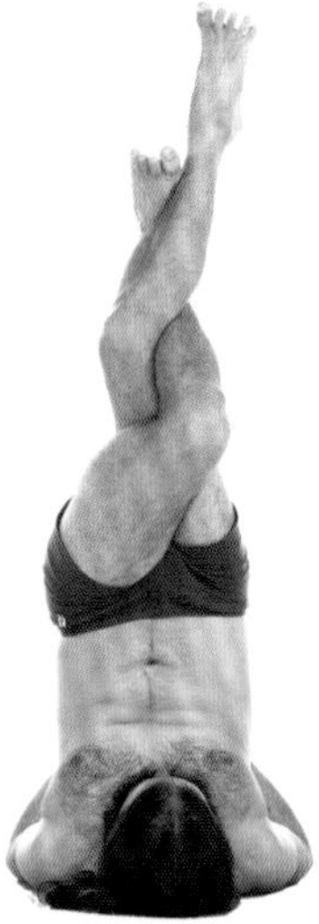

695
सर्व अङ्ग आसन (गरुड पाद)
Sarva aṅga āsana (garuḍa pāda)
All limbs pose (eagle legs)

सर्वाङ्गासन (गरुडपाद)
Sarvāṅgāsana (garuḍapāda)

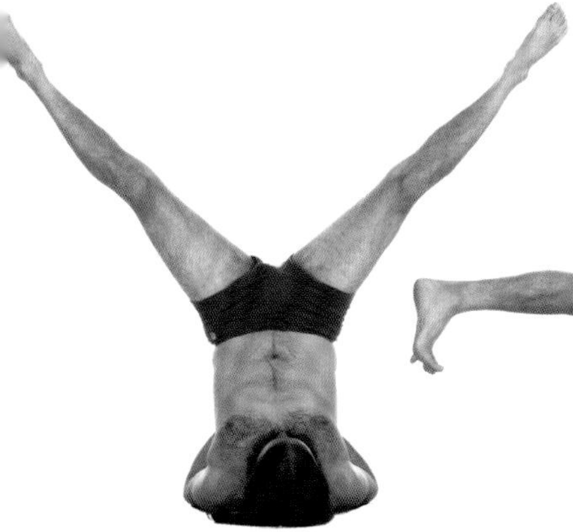

696
सर्व अङ्ग आसन (प्रसरित पाद)
Sarva aṅga āsana (prasarita pāda)
All limbs pose (legs wide open)

सर्वाङ्गासन (प्रसरितपाद)
Sarvāṅgāsana (prasaritapāda)

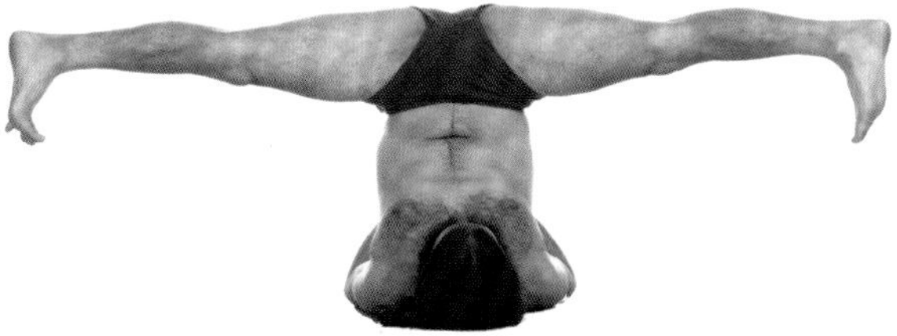

697
सर्व अङ्ग आसन (समकोण पाद)
Sarva aṅga āsana (samakoṇa pāda)
All limbs pose (side splits)

सर्वाङ्गासन (समकोणपाद)
Sarvāṅgāsana (samakoṇapāda)

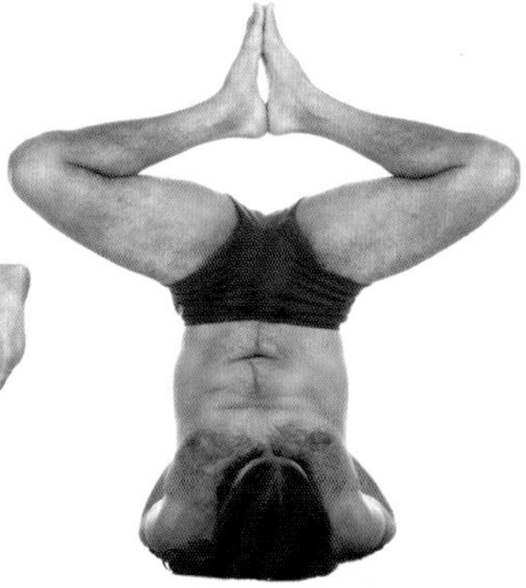

698
सर्व अङ्ग आसन (पार्वती पाद)
Sarva aṅga āsana (pārvatī pāda)
All limbs pose (soles of the feet together)

सर्वाङ्गासन (पार्वतीपाद)
Sarvāṅgāsana (pārvatīpāda)

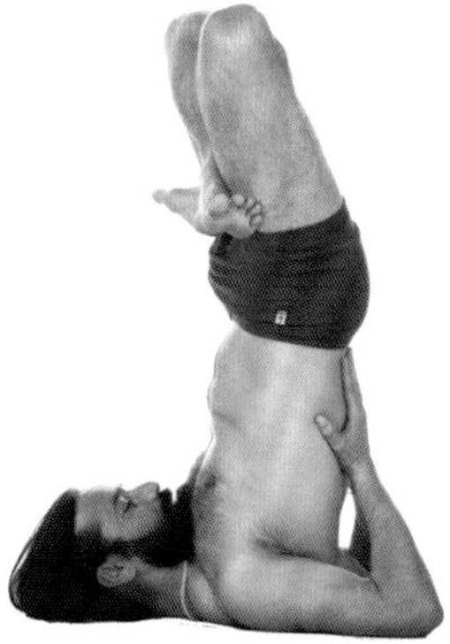

699
पद्म सर्व अङ्ग आसन
Padma sarva aṅga āsana
Lotus all limbs pose

पद्मसर्वाङ्गासन
Padmasarvāṅgāsana

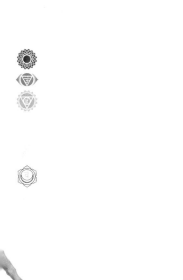

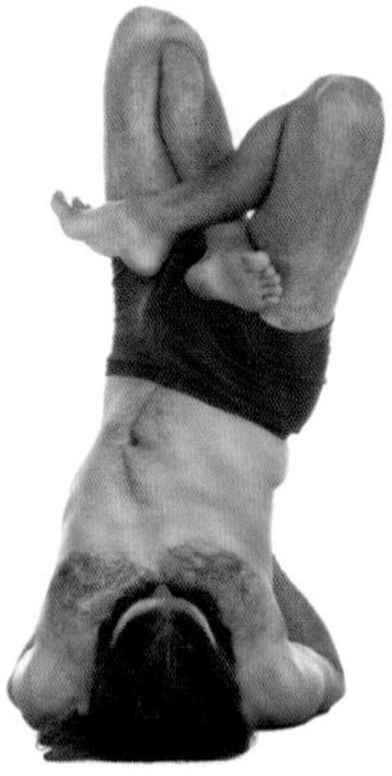

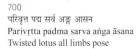

700
परिवृत्त पद्म सर्व अङ्ग आसन
Parivṛtta padma sarva aṅga āsana
Twisted lotus all limbs pose

परिवृत्तपद्मसर्वाङ्गासन
Parivṛttapadmasarvāṅgāsana

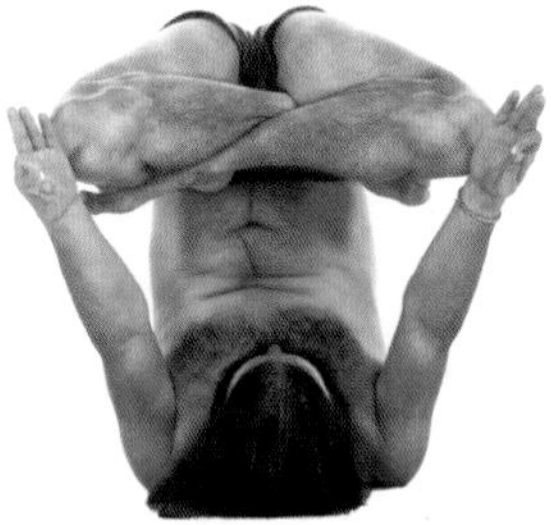

701
पद्म सर्व अङ्ग आसन (निरालम्ब)
Padma sarva aṅga āsana (nirālamba)
Lotus all limbs pose (unsupported)

पद्मसर्वाङ्गासन (निरालम्ब)
Padmasarvāṅgāsana (nirālamba)

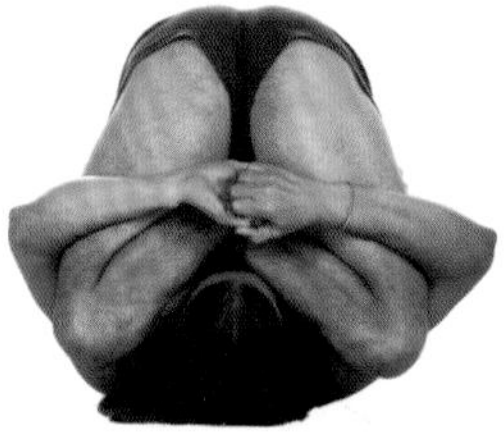

702
पद्म गर्भ पिण्ड आसन (रज्जु हस्त)
Padma garbha piṇḍa āsana (rajju hasta)
Lotus womb pose (hands clasped)

पद्मगर्भपिण्डासन (रज्जुहस्त)
Padmagarbhapiṇḍāsana (rajjuhasta)

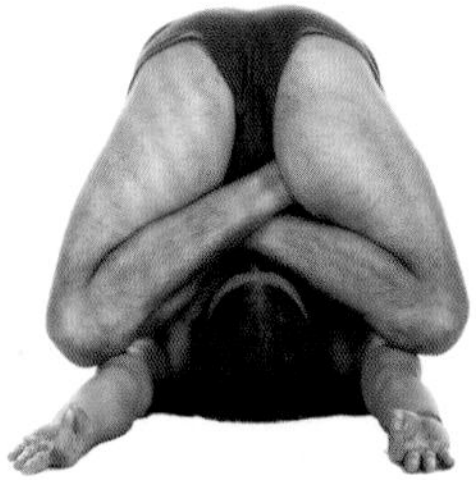

703
पद्म गर्भ पिण्ड आसन (पृष्ठ हस्त भू)
Padma garbha piṇḍa āsana (pṛṣṭha hasta bhū)
Lotus womb pose (hands on the earth behind)

पद्मगर्भपिण्डासन (पृष्ठहस्तभू)
Padmagarbhapiṇḍāsana (pṛṣṭhahastabhū)

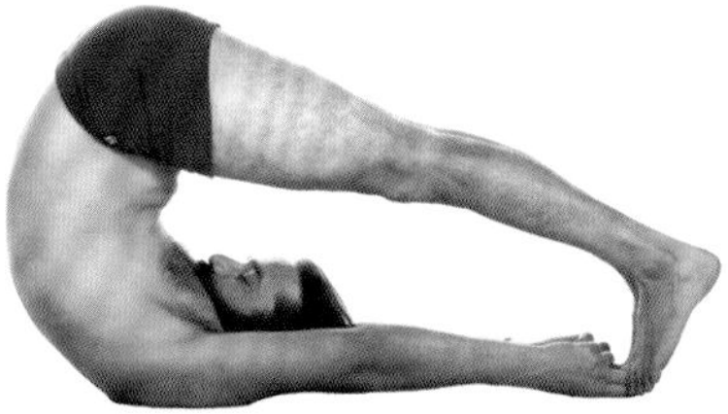

704
हल आसन (बद्ध पाद अङ्गुष्ठ)
Hala āsana (baddha pāda aṅguṣṭha)
Plough pose (holding big toes)

हलासन (बद्धपादाङ्गुष्ठ)
Halāsana (baddhapādāṅguṣṭha)

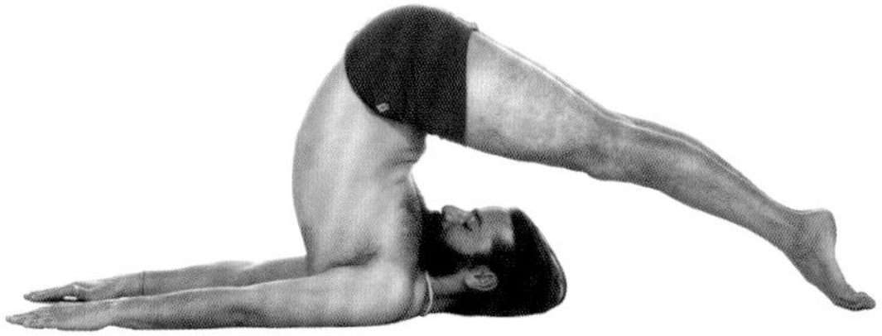

705
हल आसन (बहिर्पाद)
Hala āsana (bahirpāda)
Plough pose (feet outside)

हलासन (बहिर्पाद)
Halāsana (bahirpāda)

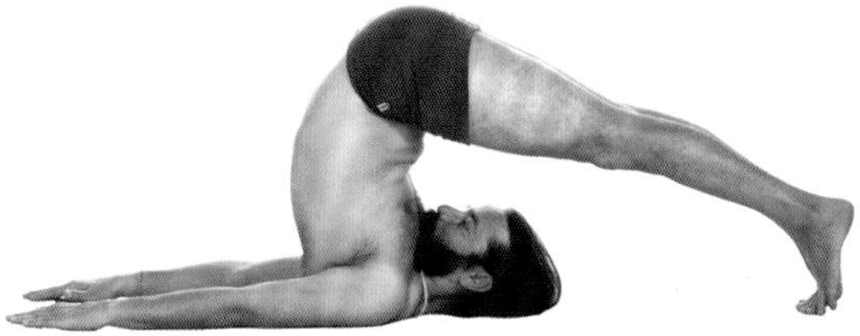

706
हल आसन (अन्तर्पाद)
Hala āsana (antarpāda)
Plough pose (feet inside)

हलासन (अन्तर्पाद)
Halāsana (antarpāda)

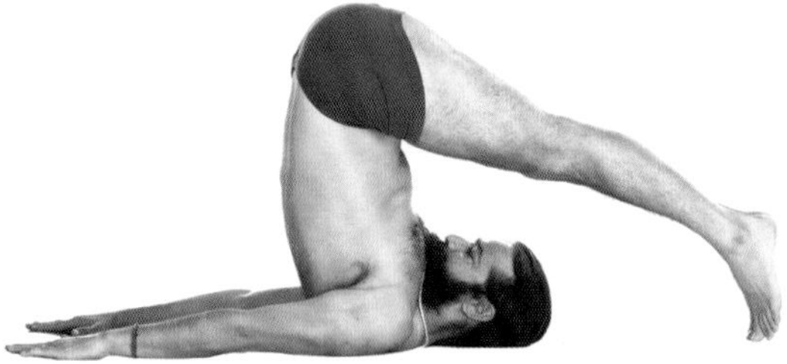

707
हल आसन (मेरु दण्ड ,अन्तर्पाद)
Hala āsana (meru daṇḍa, antarpāda)
Plough pose (spine straight, feet inside)

हलासन (मेरुदण्ड, अन्तर्पाद)
Halāsana (merudaṇḍa, antarpāda)

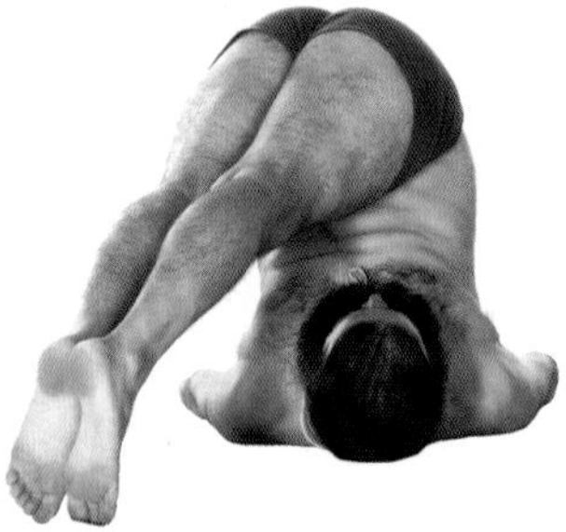

708
हल आसन (पार्श्व पाद)
Hala āsana (pārśva pāda)
Plough pose (feet to the side)

हलासन(पार्श्वपाद)
Halāsana (pārśvapāda)

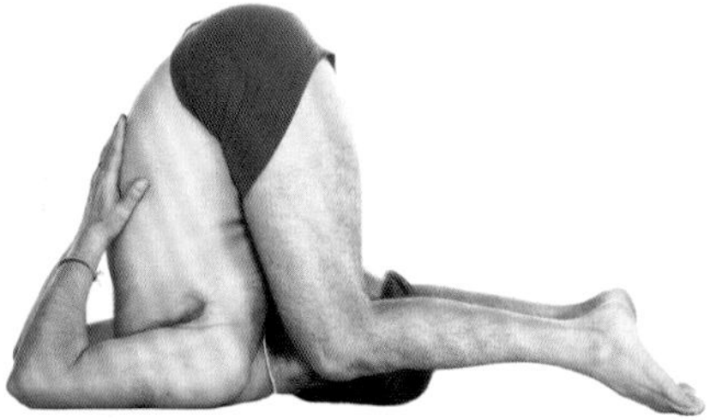

709
अर्ध कर्ण पीड हल आसन
Ardha karṇa pīḍa hala āsana
Half ear pressure plough pose

अर्धकर्णपीडहलासन
Ardhakarṇapīḍahalāsana

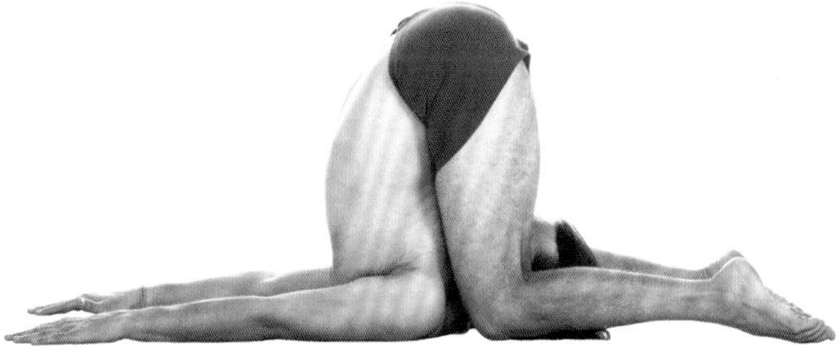

710
कर्ण पीड हल आसन
Karṇa pīḍa hala āsana
Ear pressure plough pose

कर्णपीडहलासन
Karṇapīḍahalāsana

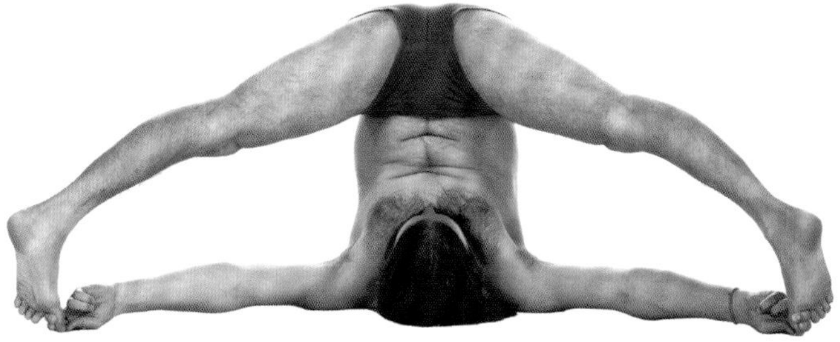

711
प्रसरित पाद हल आसन (बद्ध अङ्गुष्ठ)
Prasarita pāda hala āsana (baddha aṅguṣṭha)
Wide legs plough pose (holding big toes)

प्रसरितपादहलासन (बद्धाङ्गुष्ठ)
Prasaritapādahalāsana (baddhāṅguṣṭha)

712
अर्ध मत्स्य आसन (नाभि दर्शन)
Ardha matsya āsana (nābhi darśana)
Half fish pose (gazing at navel)

अर्धमत्स्यासन (नाभिदर्शन)
Ardhamatsyāsana (nābhidarśana)

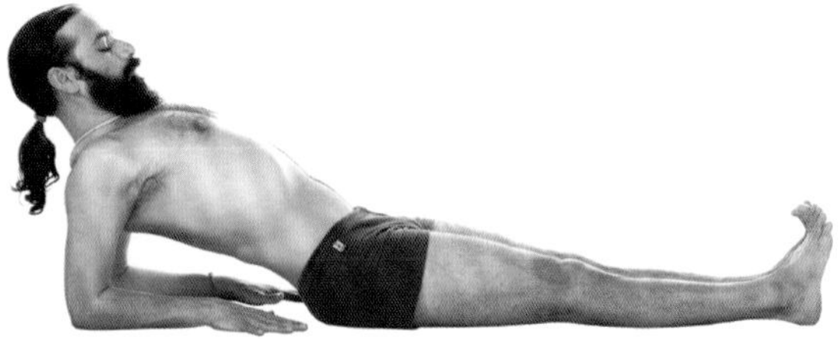

713
अर्ध मत्स्य आसन (अध: पाद अङ्गुल)
Ardha matsya āsana (adhaḥ pāda aṅgula)
Half fish pose (feet flexed)

अर्धमत्स्यासन (अधोपादाङ्गुल)
Ardhamatsyāsana (adhopādāṅgula)

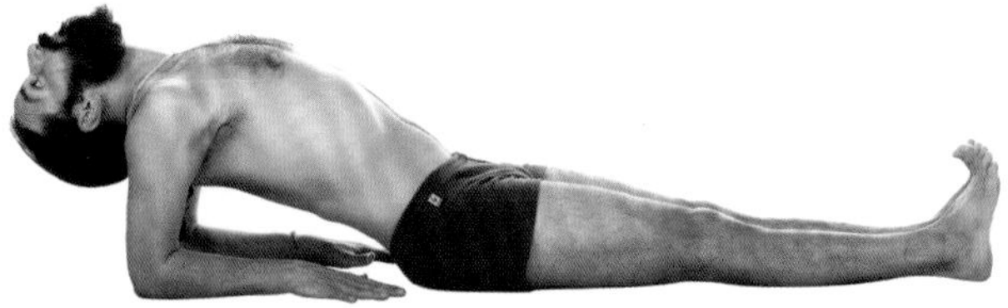

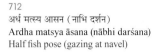

714
मत्स्य आसन (अध: पाद अङ्गुल)
Matsya āsana (adhaḥ pāda aṅgula)
Fish pose (feet flexed)

मत्स्यासन (अधोपादाङ्गुल)
Matsyāsana (adhopādāṅgula)

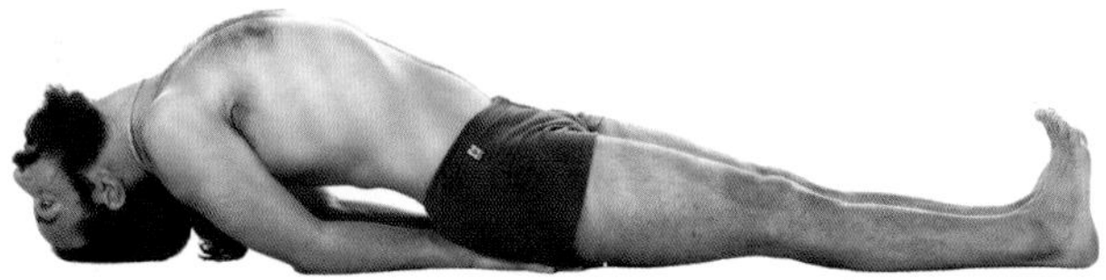

715
मत्स्य आसन (हृदय नमस्कार)
Matsya āsana (hṛdayaḥ namaskāra)
Fish pose (praying heart)

मत्स्यासन (हृदयनमस्कार)
Matsyāsana (hṛdayanamaskāra)

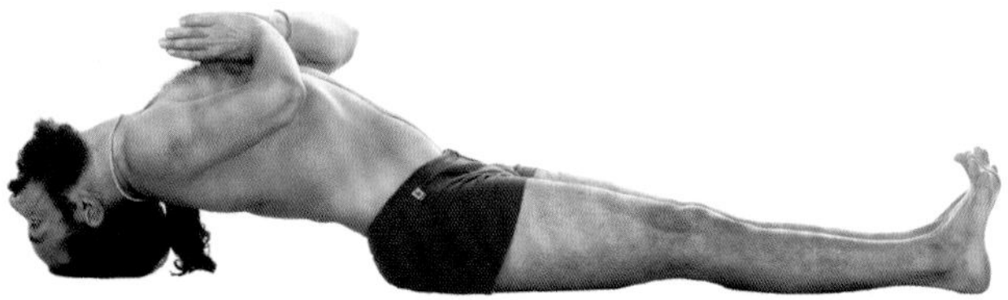

716
मत्स्य आसन (एक पाद क्षितिज)
Matsya āsana (eka pāda kṣitija)
Fish pose (one leg toward the horizon)

मत्स्यासन (एकपादक्षितिज)
Matsyāsana (ekapādakṣitija)

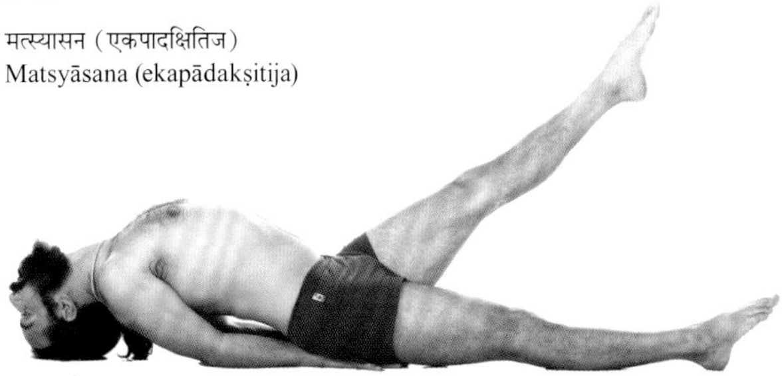

717
मत्स्य आसन (क्षितिज पाद)
Matsya āsana (kṣitija pāda)
Fish pose (legs toward the horizon)

मत्स्यासन (क्षितिजपाद)
Matsyāsana (kṣitijapāda)

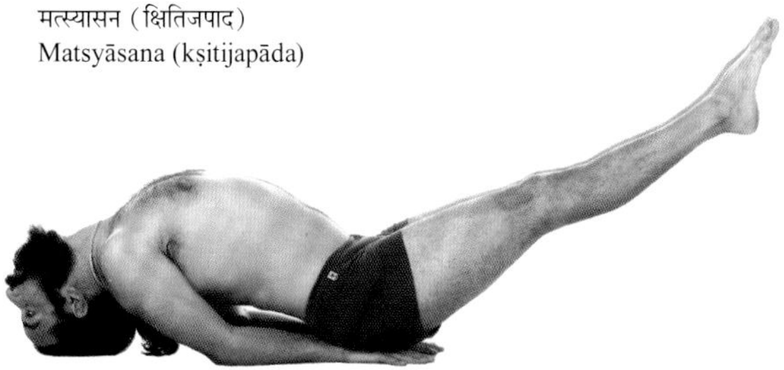

718
मत्स्य आसन (गरुड हस्त)
Matsya āsana (garuḍa hasta)
Fish pose (eagle arms)

मत्स्यासन (गरुडहस्त)
Matsyāsana (garuḍahasta)

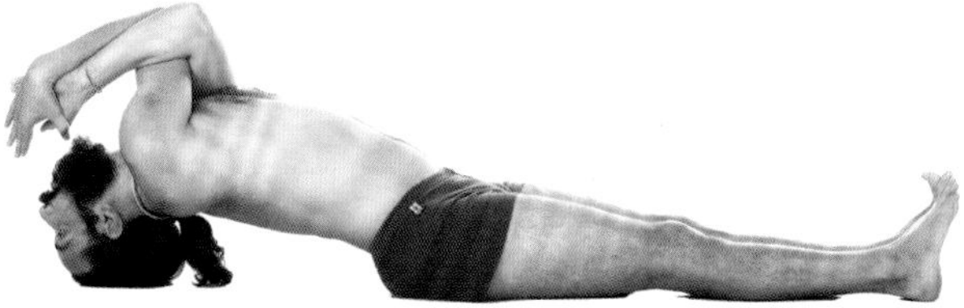

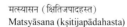

719
मत्स्य आसन (क्षितिज पाद हस्त)
Matsya āsana (kṣitija pāda hasta)
Fish pose (hands and legs toward the horizon)

मत्स्यासन (क्षितिजपादहस्त)
Matsyāsana (kṣitijapādahasta)

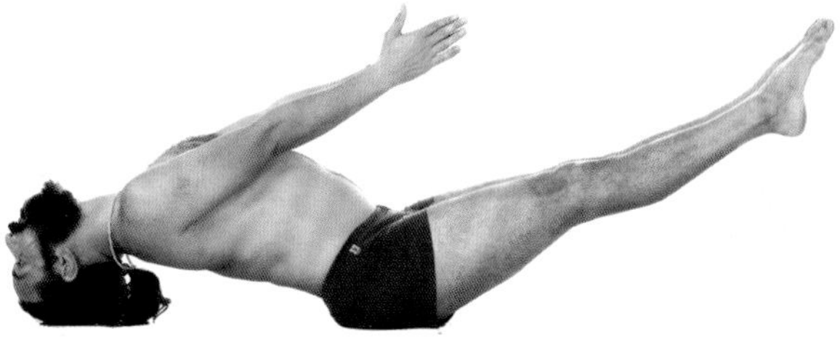

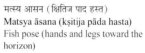

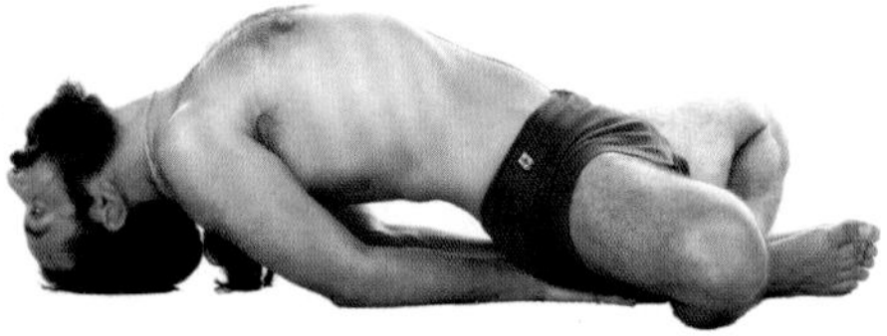

720
मत्स्य आसन (पार्वती पाद)
Matsya āsana (pārvatī pāda)
Fish pose (soles of the feet together)

मत्स्यासन (पार्वतीपाद)
Matsyāsana (pārvatīpāda)

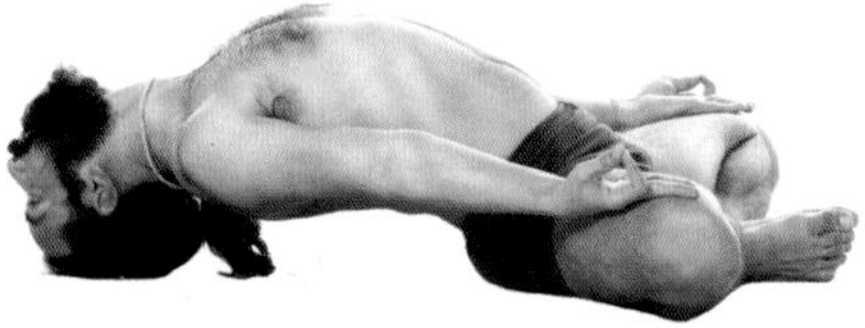

721
मत्स्य आसन (पार्वती, जानु हस्त)
Matsya āsana (pārvatī, jānu hasta)
Fish pose (soles of the feet together, hands on knees)

पार्वतीमत्स्यासन (जानुहस्त)
Matsyāsanā (pārvatijānuhasta)

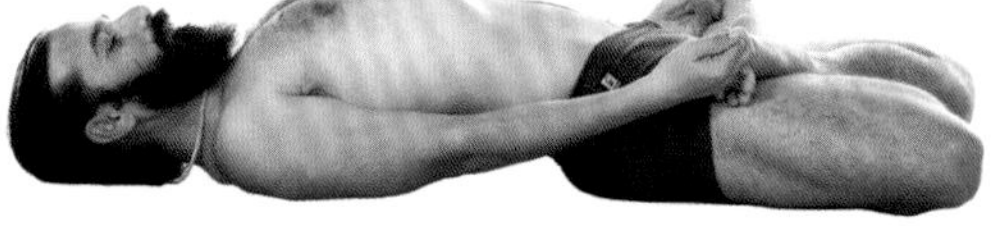

722
सुप्त पद्म मत्स्य आसन (आरम्भ अवस्था)
Supta padma matsya āsana (ārambha avasthā)
Reclined lotus fish pose (starting position)

सुप्तपद्ममत्स्यासन (आरम्भावस्था)
Suptapadmamatsyāsana (ārambhāvasthā)

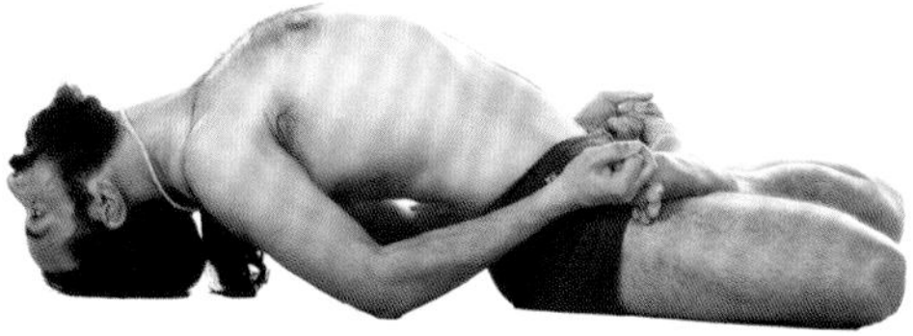

723
पद्म मत्स्य आसन
Padma matsya āsana
Lotus fish pose

पद्ममत्स्यासन
Padmamatsyāsana

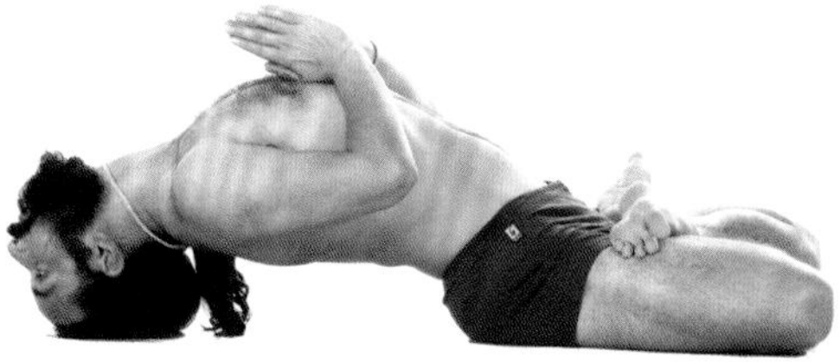

724
पद्म मत्स्य आसन (हृदय नमस्कार)
Padma matsya āsana (hṛdayaḥ namaskāra)
Lotus fish pose (hands in prayer at the heart)

पद्ममत्स्यासन (हृदयनमस्कार)
Padmamatsyāsana (hṛdayanamaskāra)

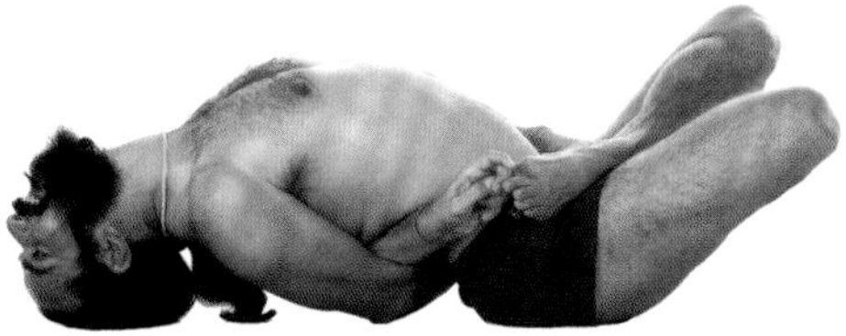

725
बद्ध पद्म मत्स्य आसन
Baddha padma matsya āsana
Bound lotus fish pose

बद्धपद्ममत्स्यासन
Baddhapadmamatsyāsana

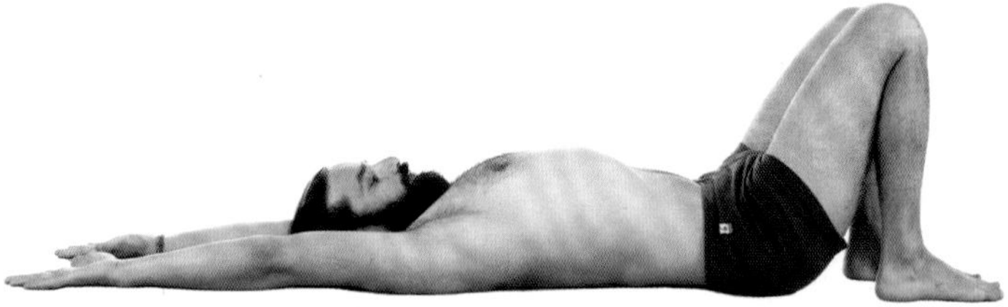

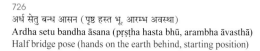

726
अर्ध सेतु बन्ध आसन (पृष्ठ हस्त भू, आरम्भ अवस्था)
Ardha setu bandha āsana (pṛṣṭha hasta bhū, arambha āvasthā)
Half bridge pose (hands on the earth behind, starting position)

अर्धसेतुबन्धासन (पृष्ठहस्तभू आरम्भावस्था)
Ardhasetubandhāsana (pṛṣṭhahastabhū, arambhāvasthā)

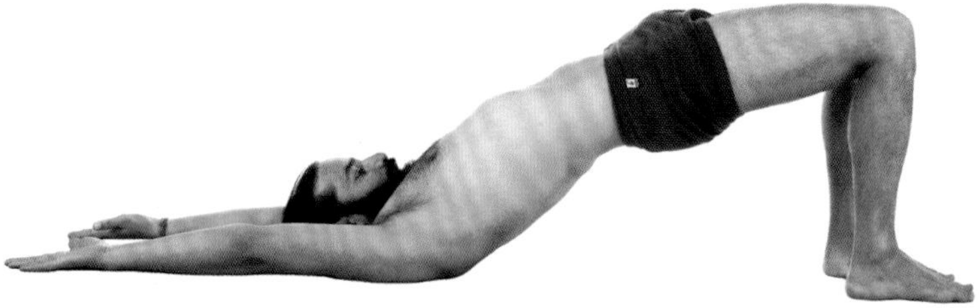

727
अर्ध सेतु बन्ध आसन (पृष्ठ हस्त भू)
Ardha setu bandha āsana (pṛṣṭha hasta bhū)
Half bridge pose (hands on the earth behind)

अर्धसेतुबन्धासन (पृष्ठहस्तभू)
Ardhasetubandhāsana (pṛṣṭhahastabhū)

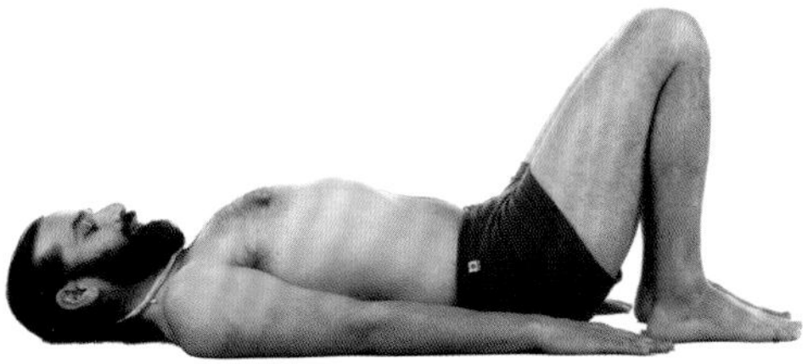

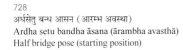

728
अर्धसेतु बन्ध आसन (आरम्भ अवस्था)
Ardha setu bandha āsana (ārambha avasthā)
Half bridge pose (starting position)

अर्धसेतुबन्धासन (आरम्भावस्था)
Ardhasetubandhāsana (ārambhāvasthā)

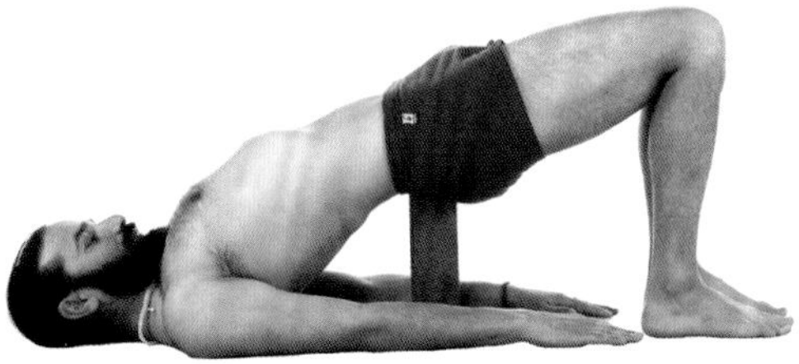

729
अर्ध सेतु बन्ध आसन (सालम्ब)
Ardha setu bandha āsana (sālamba)
Half bridge pose (supported)

अर्धसेतुबन्धासन (सालम्ब)
Ardhasetubandhāsana (sālamba)

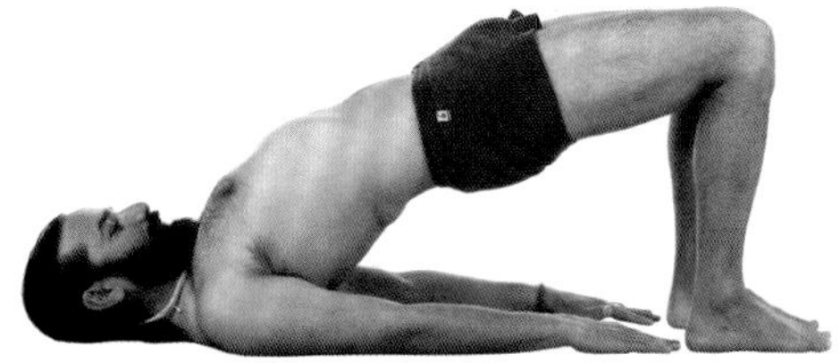

730
अर्ध सेतु बन्ध आसन (करतल भू)
Ardha setu bandha āsana (karatala bhū)
Half bridge pose (palms on the earth)

अर्धसेतुबन्धासन (करतलभू)
Ardhasetubandhāsana (karatalabhū)

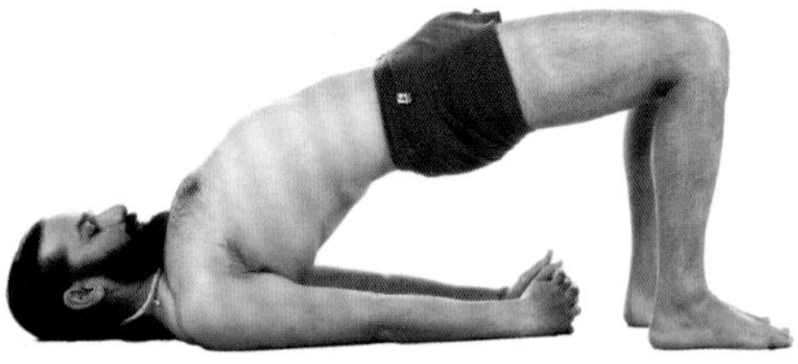

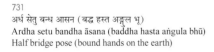

731
अर्ध सेतु बन्ध आसन (बद्ध हस्त अङ्गुल भू)
Ardha setu bandha āsana (baddha hasta aṅgula bhū)
Half bridge pose (bound hands on the earth)

अर्धसेतुबन्धासन (बद्धहस्ताङ्गुलभू)
Ardhasetubandhāsana (baddhahastāṅgulabhū)

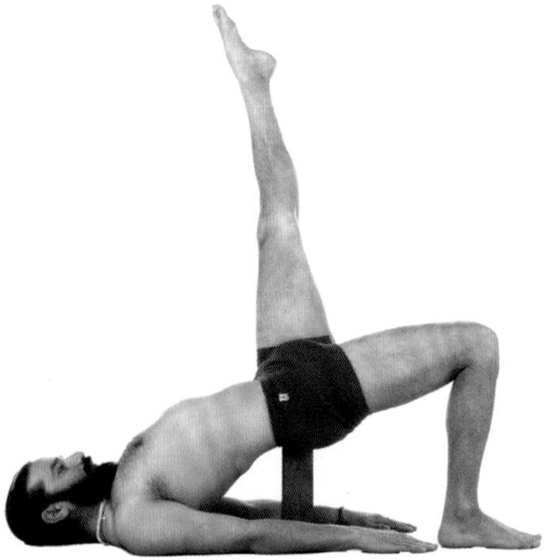

732
अर्ध सेतु बन्ध आसन (ऊर्ध्व एक पाद, सालम्ब)
Ardha setu bandha āsana (ūrdhva eka pāda, sālamba)
Half bridge pose (one leg lifted, supported)

अर्धसेतुबन्धासन (ऊर्ध्वैकपाद, सालम्ब)
Ardhasetubandhāsana (ūrdhvaikapāda, sālamba)

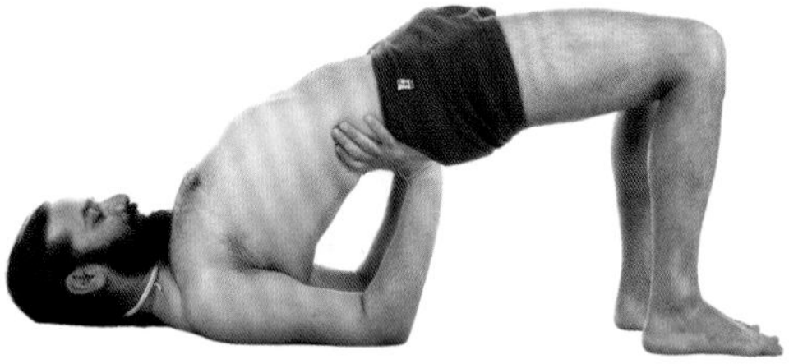

733
अर्ध सेतु बन्ध आसन (कटि हस्त)
Ardha setu bandha āsana (kati hasta)
Half bridge pose (hands on the waist)

अर्धसेतुबन्धासन (कटिहस्त)
Ardhasetubandhāsana (katihasta)

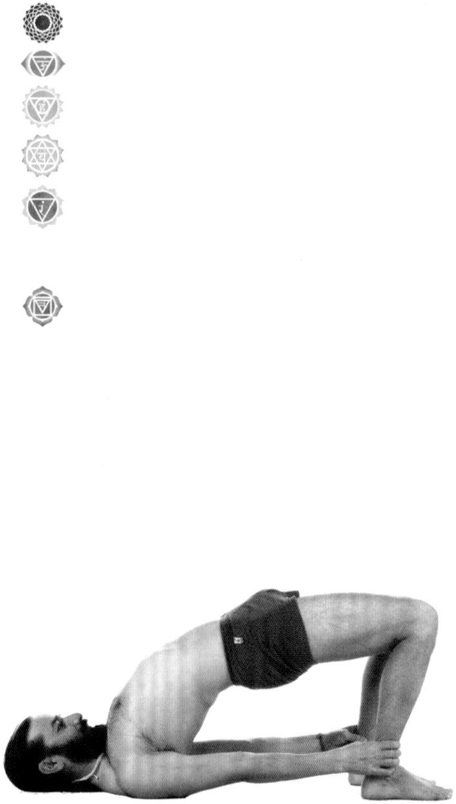

734
अर्ध सेतु बन्ध आसन (बद्ध हस्त गुल्फ)
Ardha setu baddha āsana (baddha hasta gulpha)
Half bridge pose (hands holding ankles)

अर्धसेतुबद्धासन (बद्धहस्तगुल्फ)
Ardhasetubaddhāsana (baddhahastagulpha)

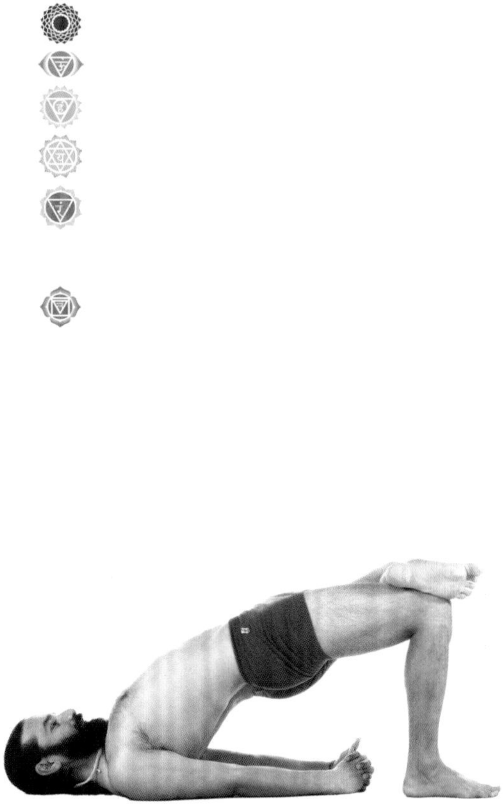

735
अर्ध सेतु बन्ध आसन (एक पाद जानु, बद्ध हस्त अङ्गुल भू)
Ardha setu bandha āsana (eka pāda jānu, baddha hasta aṅgula bhū)
Half bridge pose (one foot on knee, hands clasped on the earth)

अर्धसेतुबन्धासन (एकपादजानु, बद्धहस्ताङ्गुलभू)
Ardhasetubandhāsana (ekapādajānu, baddhahastāṅgulabhū)

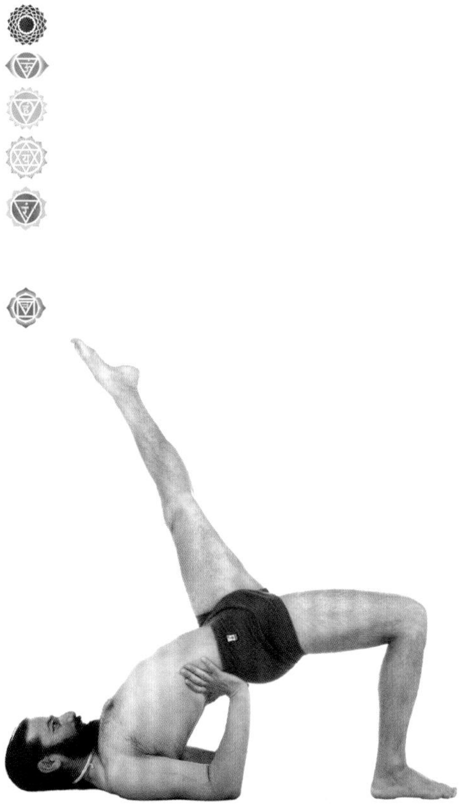

736
अर्ध सेतु बन्ध आसन (ऊर्ध्व एक पाद, कटि हस्त)
Ardha setu bandha āsana (ūrdhva eka pāda, kati hasta)
Half bridge pose (one leg lifted, hands on the waist)

अर्धसेतुबन्धासन (ऊर्ध्वैकपाद, कटिहस्त)
Ardhasetubandhāsana (ūrdhvaikapāda, katihasta)

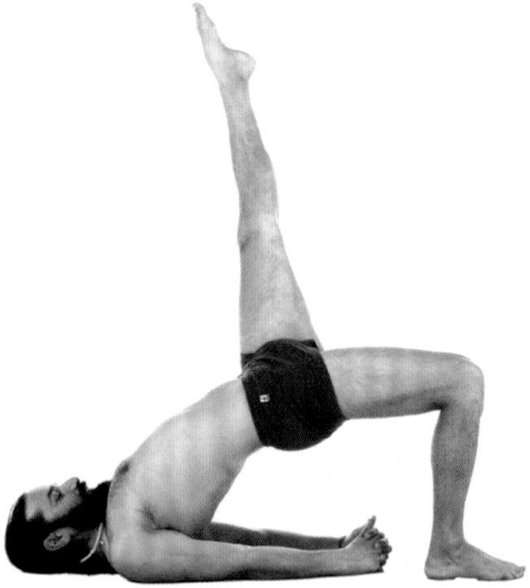

737
अर्ध सेतु बन्ध आसन (ऊर्ध्व एक पाद, बद्ध हस्त अङ्गुल भू)
Ardha setu bandha āsana (ūrdhva eka pāda, baddha hasta aṅgula bhū)
Half bridge pose (one leg lifted, bound hands)

अर्धसेतुबन्धासन (ऊर्ध्वैकपाद, बद्धहस्ताङ्गुलभू)
Ardhasetubandhāsana (ūrdhvaikapāda, baddhahastāṅgulabhū)

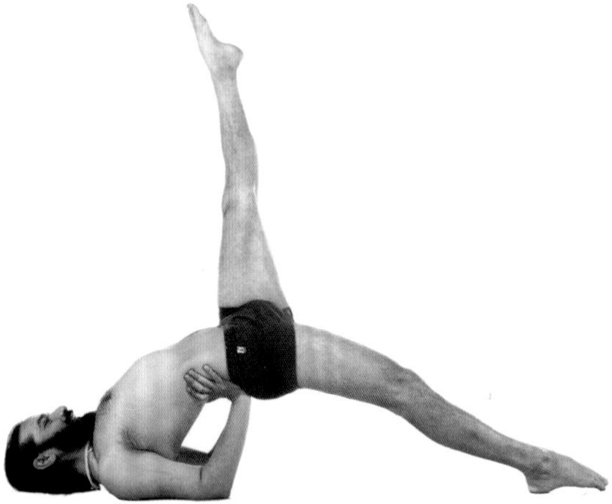

738
सेतु बन्ध आसन (ऊर्ध्व एक पाद, कटि हस्त)
Setu bandha āsana (ūrdhva eka pāda, kati hasta)
Bridge pose (one leg lifted, hands on the waist)

सेतुबन्धासन (ऊर्ध्वैकपाद, कटिहस्त)
Setubandhāsana (ūrdhvaikapāda, katihasta)

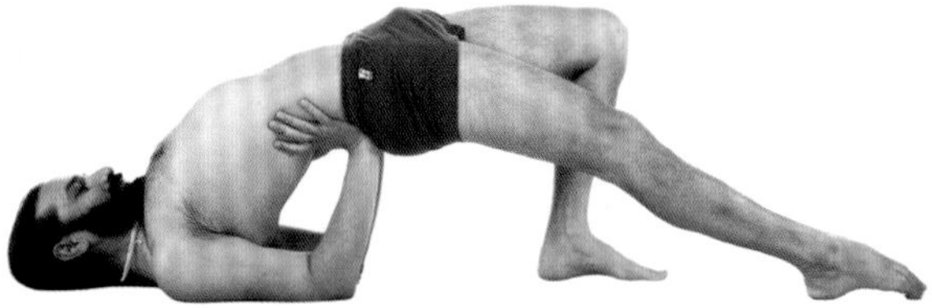

739
सेतु बन्ध आसन (एक पाद ,कटि हस्त)
Setu bandha āsana (eka pāda, kati hasta)
Bridge pose (one leg extended, hands on the waist)

सेतुबन्धासन (एकपाद, कटिहस्त)
Setubandhāsana (ekapāda, katihasta)

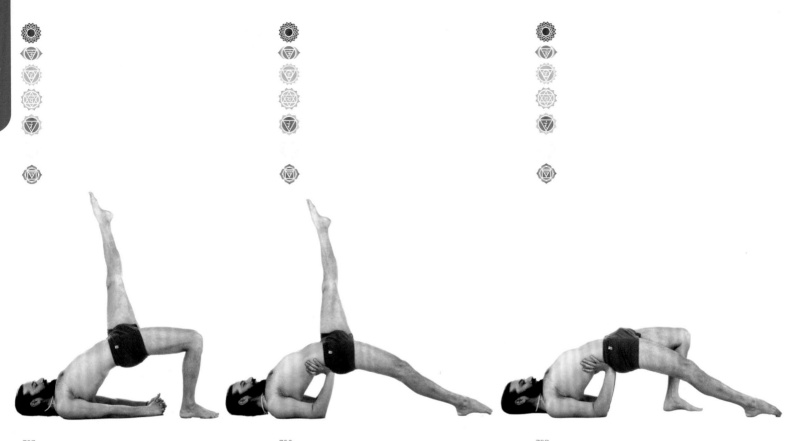

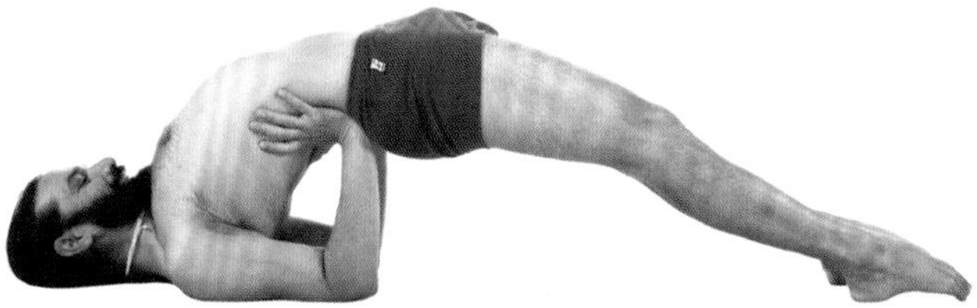

740
सेतु बन्ध आसन (कटि हस्त)
Setu bandha āsana (kati hasta)
Bridge pose (hands on the waist)

सेतुबन्धासन (कटिहस्त)
Setubandhāsana (katihasta)

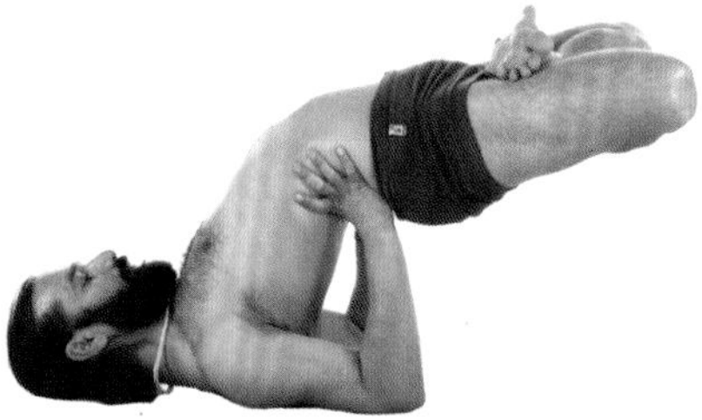

741
पद्म सेतु बन्ध आसन (आरम्भ अवस्था)
Padma setu bandha āsana (ārambha avasthā)
Lotus bridge pose (starting position)

पद्मसेतुबन्धासन (आरम्भावस्था)
Padmasetubandhāsana (ārambhāvasthā)

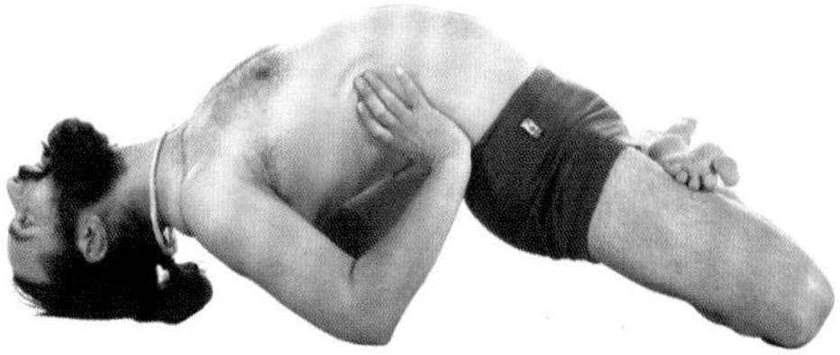

742
पद्म सेतु बन्ध आसन
Padma setu bandha āsana
Lotus bridge pose

पद्मसेतुबन्धासन
Padmasetubandhāsana

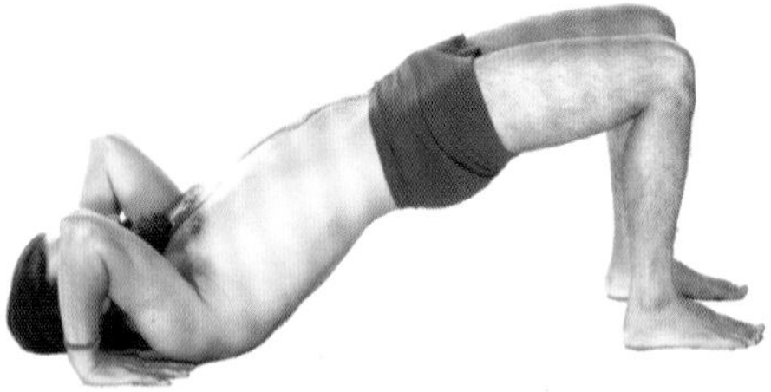

743
चक्र आसन (आरम्भ अवस्था)
Cakra āsana (ārambha avasthā)
Wheel pose (starting position)

चक्रासन (आरम्भावस्था)
Cakrāsana (ārambhāvasthā)

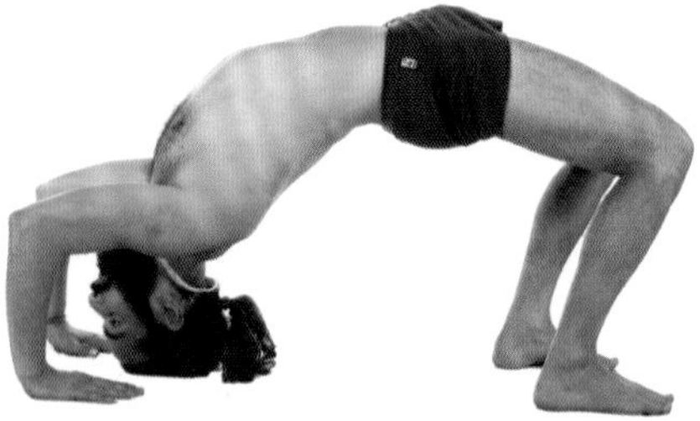

744
अर्ध चक्र आसन (शिर भू)
Ardha cakra āsana (śira bhū)
Half wheel pose (head on the earth)

अर्धचक्रासन (शिरभू)
Ardhacakrāsana (śirabhū)

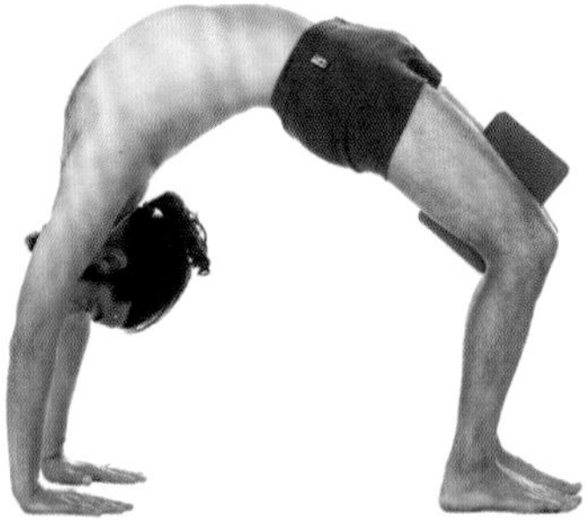

745
चक्र आसन (सालम्ब)
Cakra āsana (sālamba)
Wheel pose (supported)

चक्रासन (सालम्ब)
Cakrāsana (sālamba)

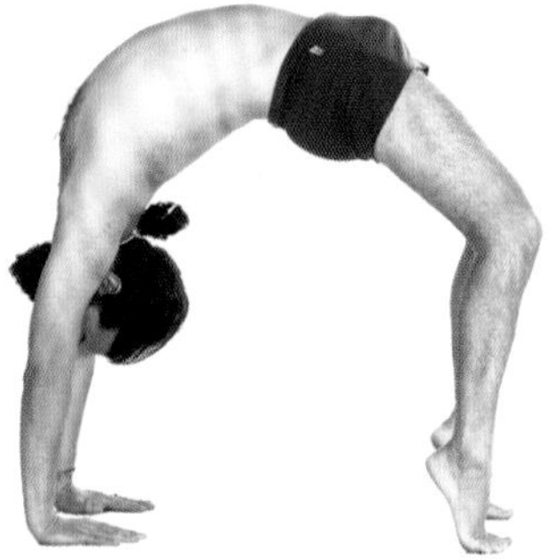

746
चक्र आसन (पाद अङ्गुल भू)
Cakra āsana (pāda aṅgula bhū)
Wheel pose (toes on the earth)

चक्रासन (पादाङ्गुलभू)
Cakrāsana (pādāṅgulabhū)

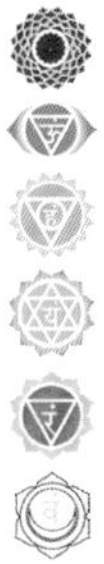

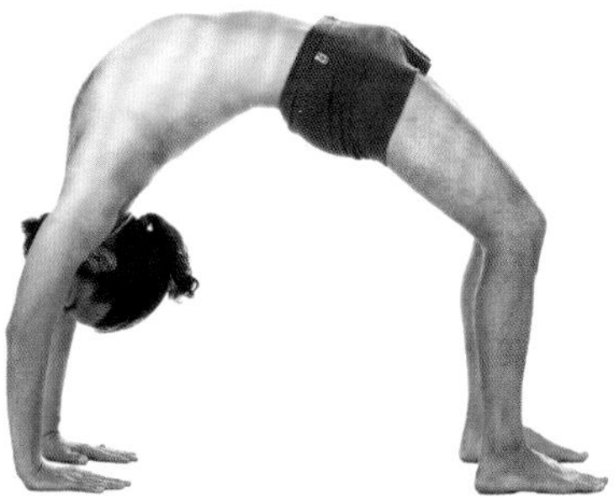

747
चक्र आसन
Cakra āsana
Wheel pose

चक्रासन
Cakrāsana

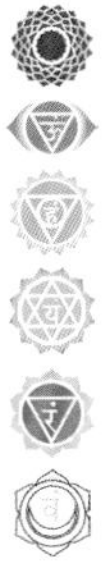

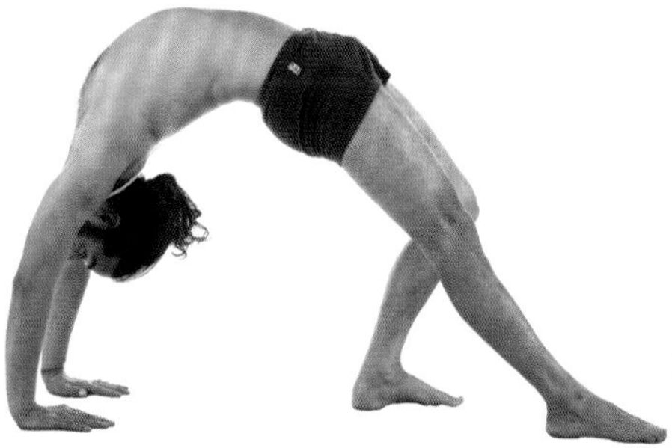

748
चक्र आसन (एक पाद अङ्गद)
Cakra āsana (eka pāda aṅgada)
Wheel pose (one leg extended)

चक्रासन (एकपादाङ्गद)
Cakrāsana (ekapādāṅgada)

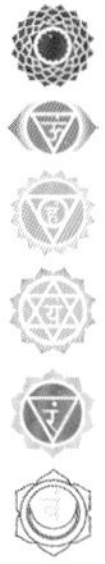

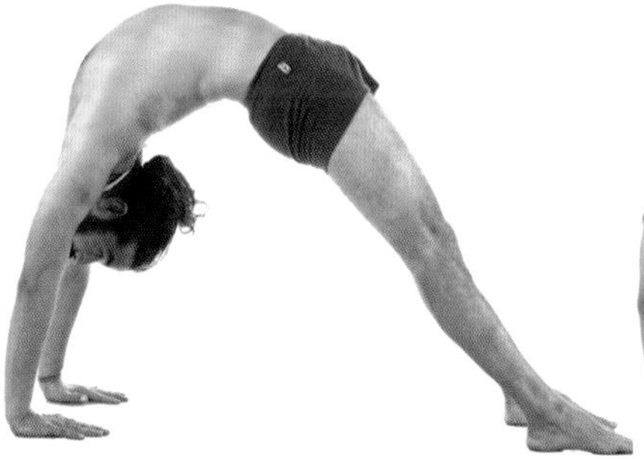

749
चक्र आसन (अङ्गद पाद)
Cakra āsana (aṅgada pāda)
Wheel pose (both legs extended)

चक्रासन (अङ्गदपाद)
Cakrāsana (aṅgadapāda)

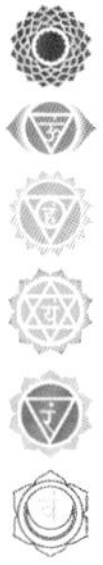

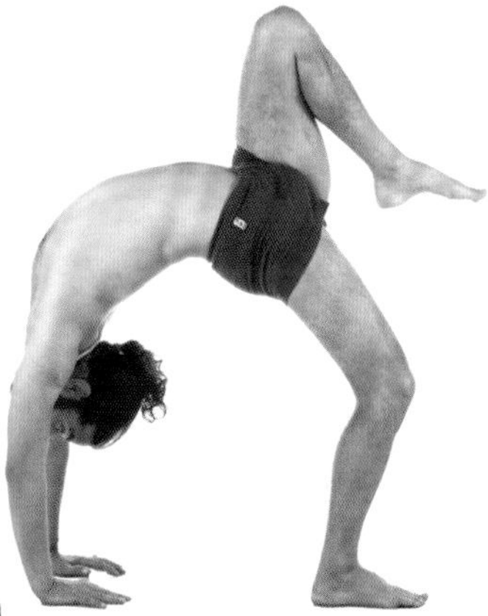

750
चक्र आसन (ऊर्ध्व एक जानु)
Cakra āsana (ūrdhva eka jānu)
Wheel pose (one knee lifted)

चक्रासन (ऊर्ध्वैकजानु)
Cakrāsana (ūrdhvaikajānu)

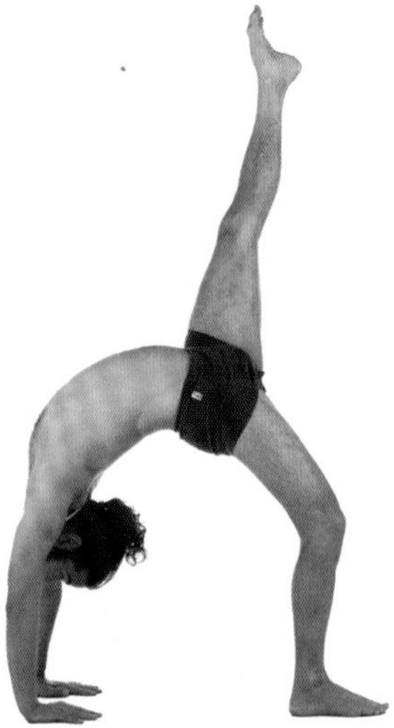

751
चक्र आसन (ऊर्ध्व एक पाद)
Cakra āsana (ūrdhva eka pāda)
Wheel pose (one leg lifted)

चक्रासन (ऊर्ध्वैकपाद)
Cakrāsana (ūrdhvaikapāda)

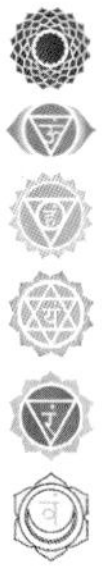

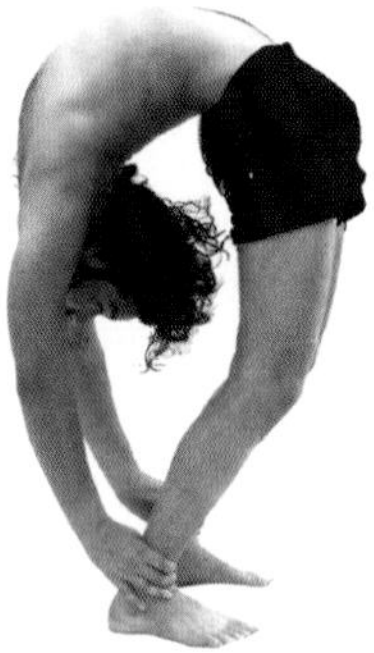

752
चक्र आसन (नाडी शोधन)
Cakra āsana (naḍi śodhana)
Wheel pose (energy channel purifying)

चक्रासन (नाडीशोधन)
Cakrāsana (naḍiśodhana)

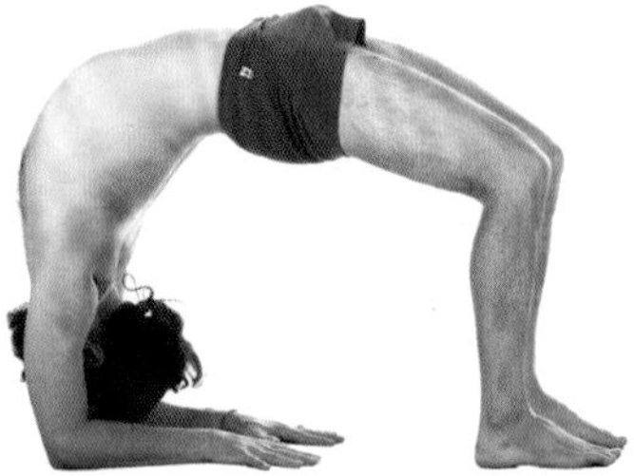

753
चक्र आसन (कफोणि भू)
Cakra āsana (kaphoṇi bhū)
Wheel pose (elbows on the earth)

चक्रासन (कफोणिभू)
Cakrāsana (kaphoṇibhū)

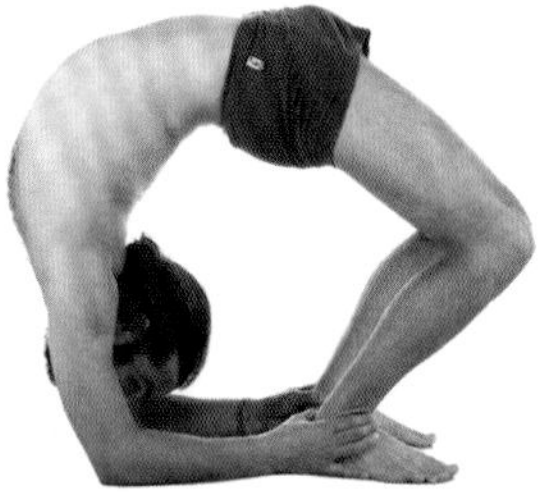

754
चक्र आसन (कफोणि भू, गुल्फ बद्ध)
Cakra āsana (kaphoṇi bhū, gulpha baddha)
Wheel pose (elbows on the earth, holding ankles)

चक्रासन (कफोणिभू, गुल्फबद्ध)
Cakrāsana (kaphoṇibhū, gulphabaddha)

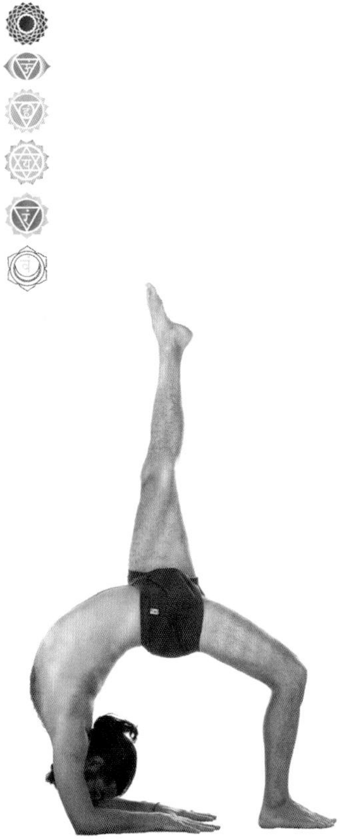

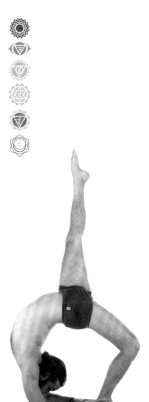

755
चक्र आसन (कफोणि भू, ऊर्ध्व एक पाद)
Cakra āsana (kaphoṇi bhū, ūrdhva eka pāda)
Wheel pose (elbows on the earth, one leg extended)

चक्रासन (कफोणिभू, ऊर्ध्वैकपाद)
Cakrāsana (kaphoṇibhū, ūrdhvaikapāda)

756
चक्र आसन (कफोणि भू, ऊर्ध्व एक पाद, बद्ध हस्त गुल्फ)
Cakra āsana (kaphoṇi bhū, ūrdhva eka pāda, baddha hasta gulpha)
Wheel pose (elbows on the earth, one leg extended, holding ankle)

चक्रासन (कफोणिभू, ऊर्ध्वैकपाद, बद्धहस्तगुल्फ)
Cakrāsana (kaphoṇibhū, ūrdhvaikapāda, baddhahastagulpha)

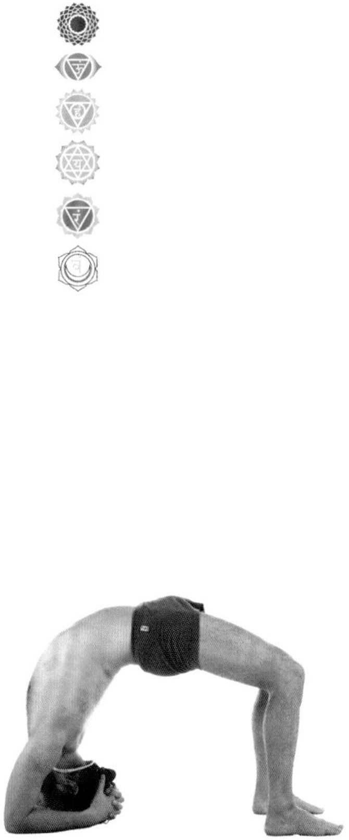

757
चक्र आसन (कफोणि भू)
Cakra āsana (kaphoṇi bhū)
Wheel pose (elbows on the earth)

चर्क्रासन (कफोणिभू)
Cakrāsana (kaphoṇibhū)

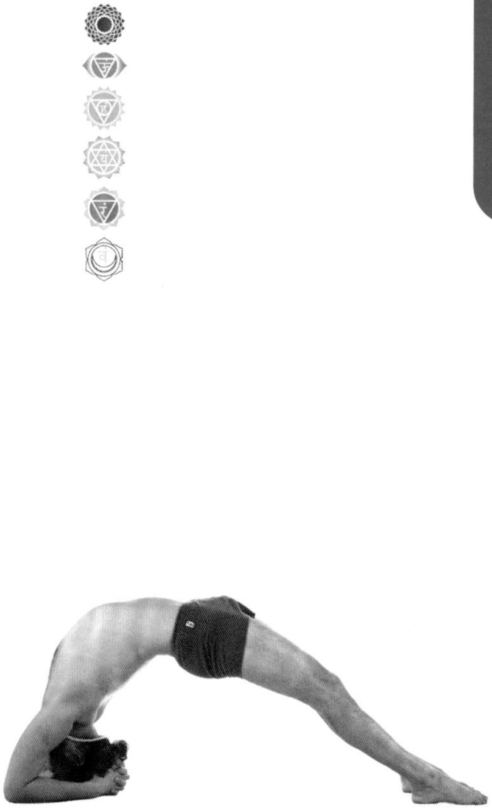

758
चक्र आसन (अङ्गद पाद ,कफोणि भू)
Cakra āsana (aṅgada pāda, kaphoṇi bhū)
Crown wheel pose (elbows on the earth, both legs extended)

चर्क्रासन (अङ्गदपाद, कफोणिभू)
Cakrāsana (aṅgadapāda, kaphoṇibhū)

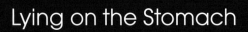

Lying on the Stomach

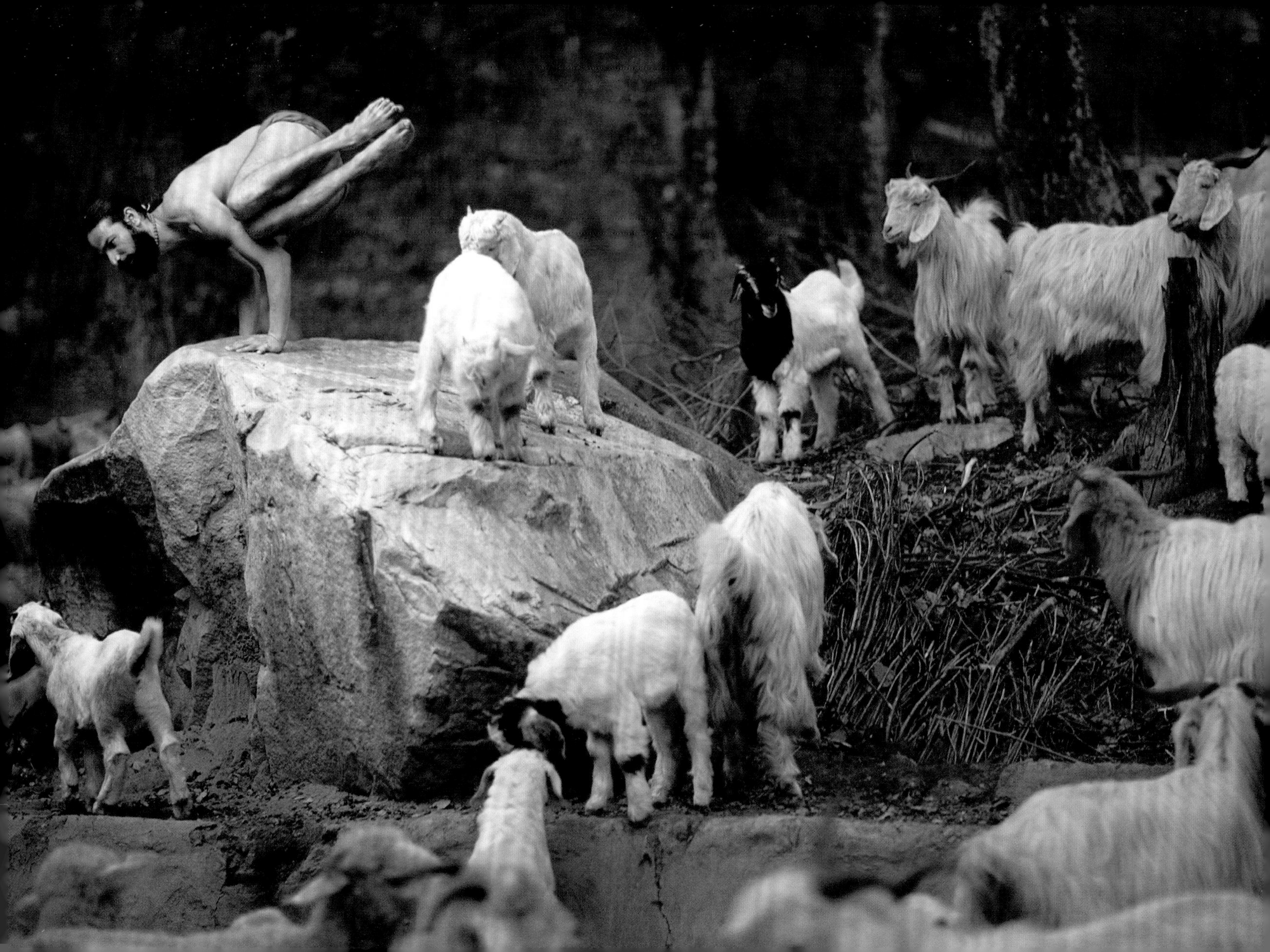

759
मकर आसन
Makara āsana
Crocodile pose

मकरासन
Makarāsana

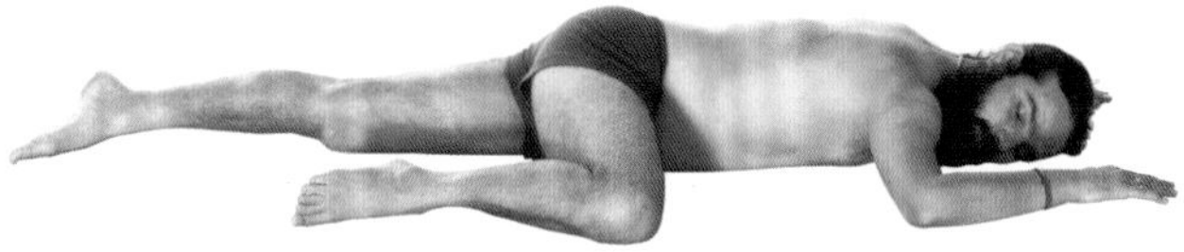

760
मण्डूक पाद मकर आसन
Maṇḍūka pāda makara āsana
Frog legs crocodile pose

मण्डूकपादमकरासन
Maṇḍūkapādamakarāsana

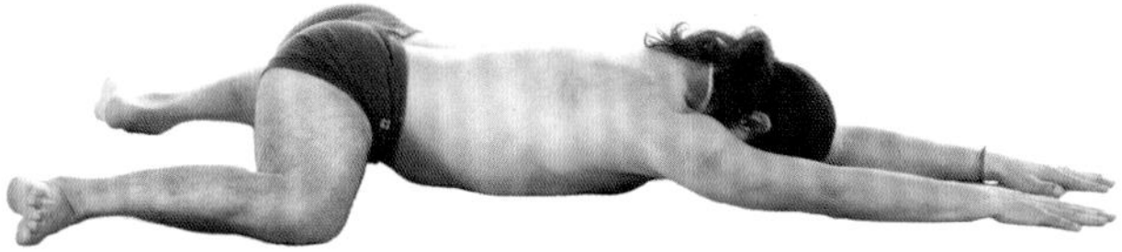

761
पद्म मकर आसन
Padma makara āsana
Lotus crocodile pose

पद्ममकरासन
Padmamakarāsana

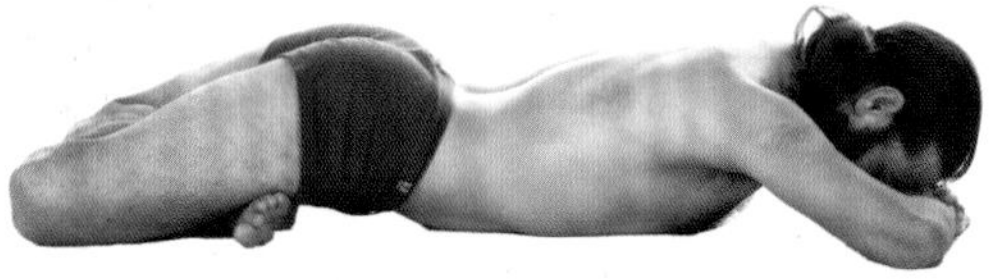

762
पद्म मकर आसन (पृष्ठ नमस्कार)
Padma makara āsana (pṛṣṭha namaskāra)
Lotus crocodile pose (hands in prayer behind)

पद्ममकरासन (पृष्ठनमस्कार)
Padmamakarāsana (pṛṣṭhanamaskāra)

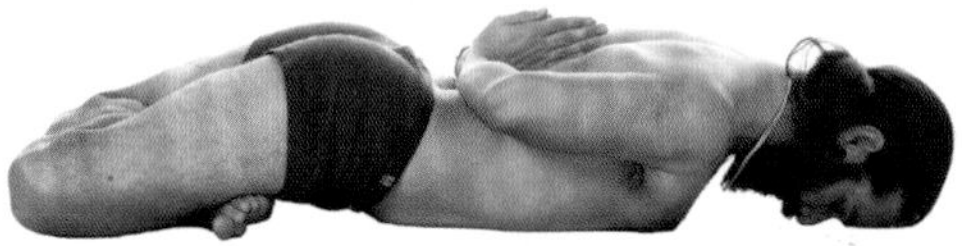

763
नाभि उत्तोलन आसन
Nābhi uttolana āsana
Navel balancing pose

नाभ्युत्तोलनासन
Nābhyuttolanāsana

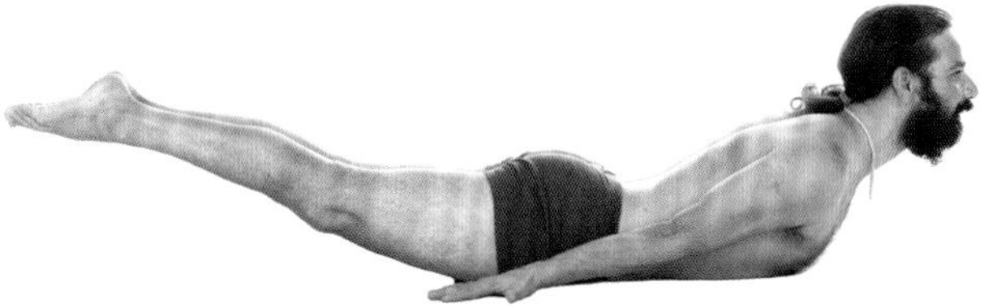

764
नाभि उत्तोलन उड्डियान आसन
Nābhi uttolana uḍḍiyāna āsana
Navel balancing flying bird pose

नाभ्युत्तोलनोड्डियानासन
Nābhyuttolanauḍḍiyānāsana

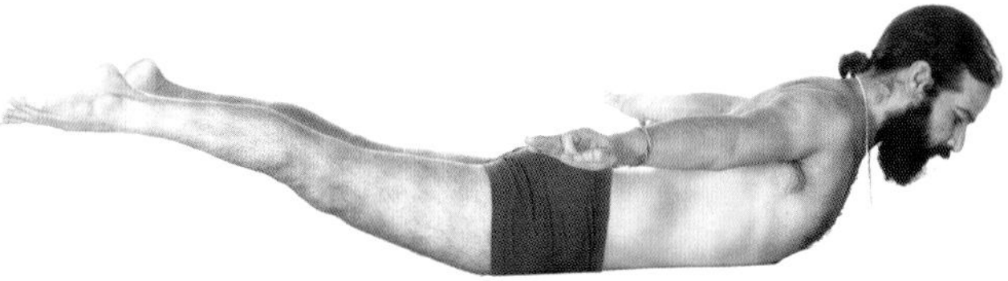

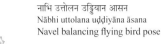

765
नाभि उत्तोलन आसन (विपरीत एक हस्त पाद)
Nābhi uttolana āsana (viparīta eka hasta pāda)
Navel balancing pose (opposite arm and leg lifted)

नाभ्युत्तोलनासन (विपरीतैकहस्तपाद)
Nābhyuttolanāsana (viparītaikahastapāda)

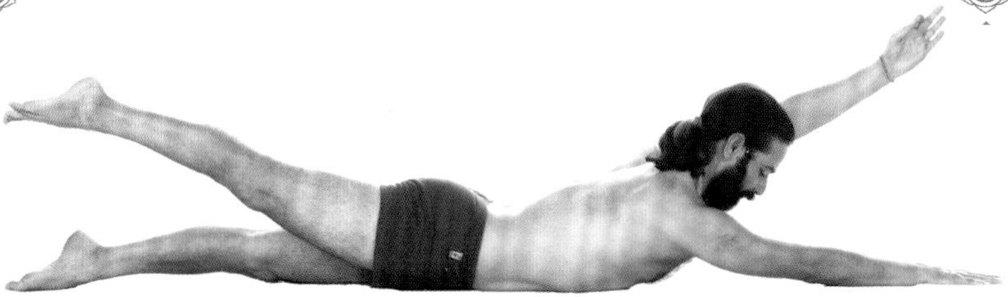

766
नाभि उत्तोलन आसन (पृष्ठ हस्त उत्तान)
Nābhi uttolana āsana (pṛṣṭha hasta uttāna)
Navel balancing pose (hands extended behind)

नाभ्युत्तोलनासन (पृष्ठहस्तोत्तान)
Nābhyuttolanāsana (pṛṣṭhahastottāna)

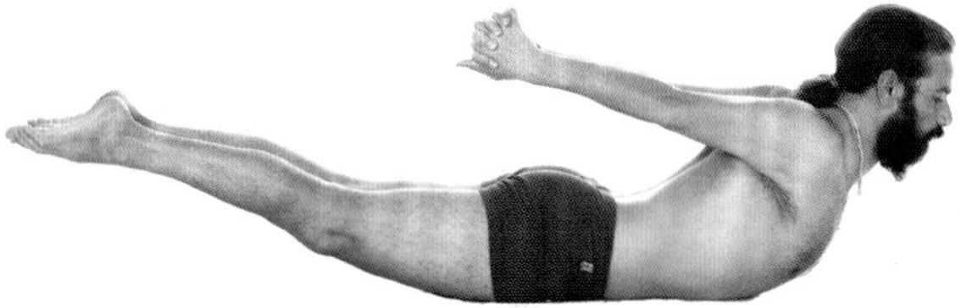

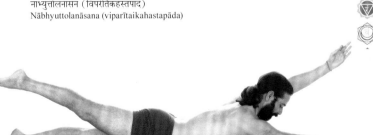

767
नाभि उत्तोलन आसन (नमस्कार हस्त)
Nābhi uttolana āsana (namaskāra hasta)
Navel balancing pose (hands in prayer)

नाभ्युत्तोलनासन (नमस्कारहस्त)
Nābhyuttolanāsana (namaskārahasta)

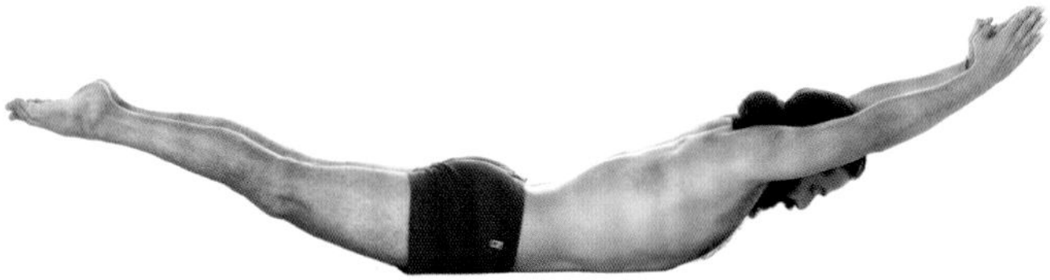

768
साष्टाङ्ग भू नमन आसन
Sāṣṭāṅga bhū namana āsana
Honoring the earth eight limbs pose

साष्टाङ्गभूनमनासन
Sāṣṭāṅgabhūnamanāsana

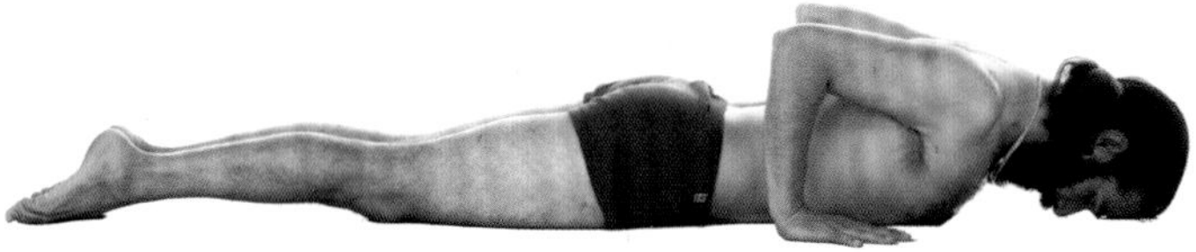

Life is a beautiful gift; every moment is rich with opportunity.

769
साष्टाङ्ग भू नमन आसन (एक पाद उत्तान)
Sāṣṭāṅga bhū namana āsana (eka pāda uttāna)
Honoring the earth eight limbs pose (one leg lifted)

साष्टाङ्गभूनमनासन (एकपादोत्तान)
Sāṣṭāṅgabhūnamanāsana (ekapādottāna)

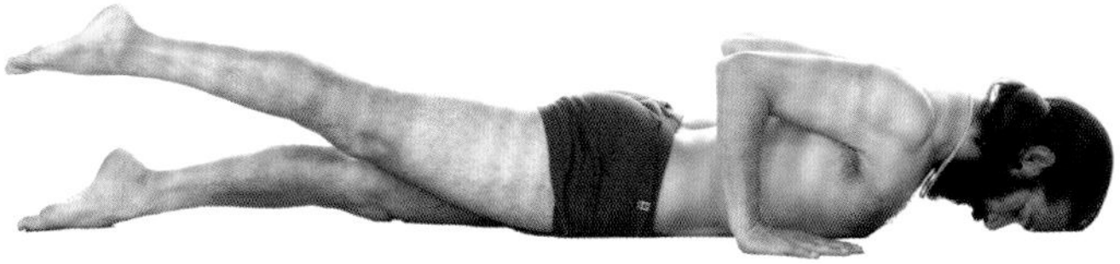

770
सर्प आसन (निरालम्ब हस्त)
Sarpa āsana (nirālamba hasta)
Snake pose (unsupported)

सर्पासन (निरालम्बहस्त)
Sarpāsana (nirālambahasta)

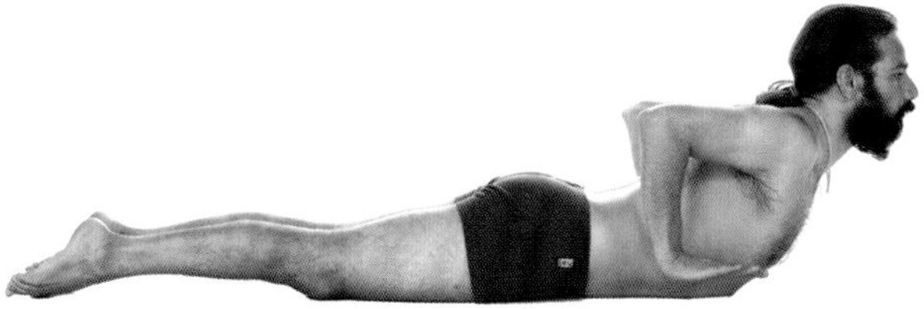

771
सर्प आसन (पृष्ठ हस्त उत्तान)
Sarpa āsana (pṛṣṭha hasta uttāna)
Snake pose (hands extended behind)

सर्पासन (पृष्ठहस्तोत्तान)
Sarpāsana (pṛṣṭhahastottāna)

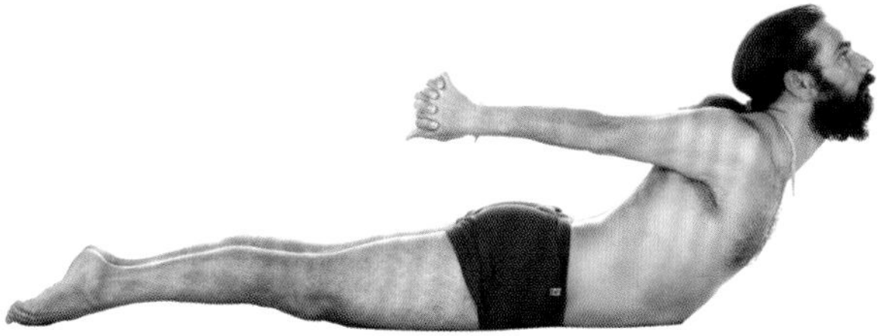

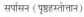

772
भुजङ्ग आसन (कफोणि भू)
Bhujaṅga āsana (kaphoṇi bhū)
Cobra pose (elbows on the earth)

भुजङ्गासन (कफोणिभू)
Bhujaṅgāsana (kaphoṇibhū)

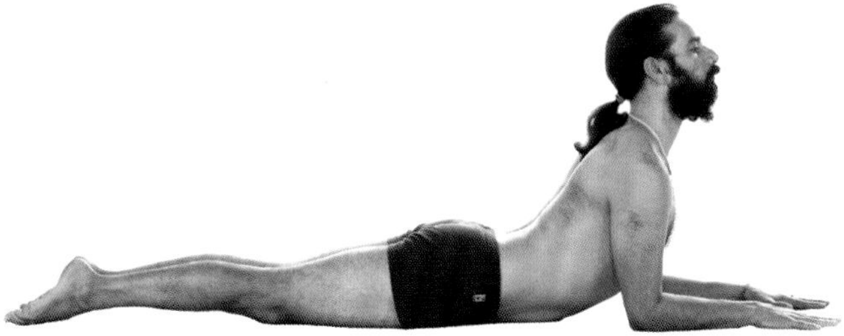

773
भुजङ्ग आसन (कफोणि भू, एक ऊर्ध्वपाद)
Bhujaṅga āsana (kaphoṇi bhū, eka ūrdhva pāda)
Cobra pose (elbows on the earth, one foot lifted)

भुजङ्गासन (कफोणिभू, एकोर्ध्वपाद)
Bhujaṅgāsana (kaphoṇibhū, ekordhvapāda)

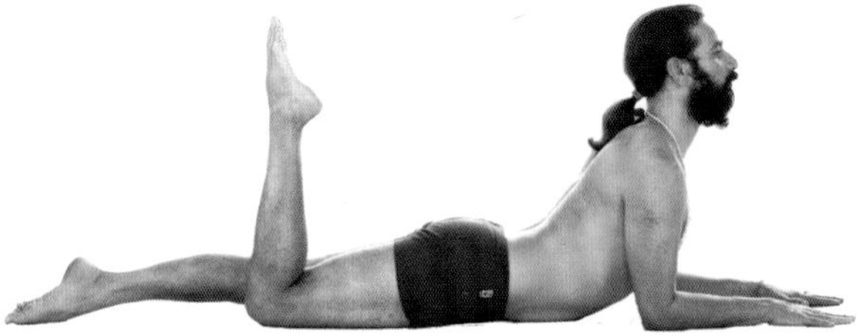

774
भुजङ्ग आसन (कफोणि भू,ऊर्ध्व पाद)
Bhujaṅga āsana (kaphoṇi bhū, ūrdhva pāda)
Cobra pose (elbows on the earth, legs lifted)

भुजङ्गासन (कफोणिभू ,ऊर्ध्वपाद)
Bhujaṅgāsana (kaphoṇibhū, ūrdhvapāda)

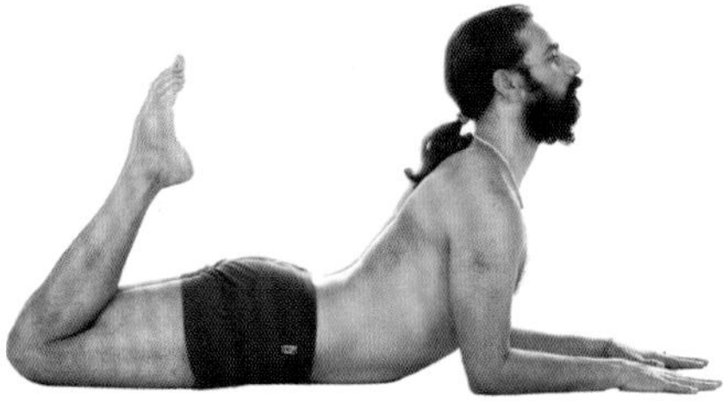

775
भुजङ्ग आसन
Bhujaṅga āsana
Cobra pose

भुजङ्गासन
Bhujaṅgāsana

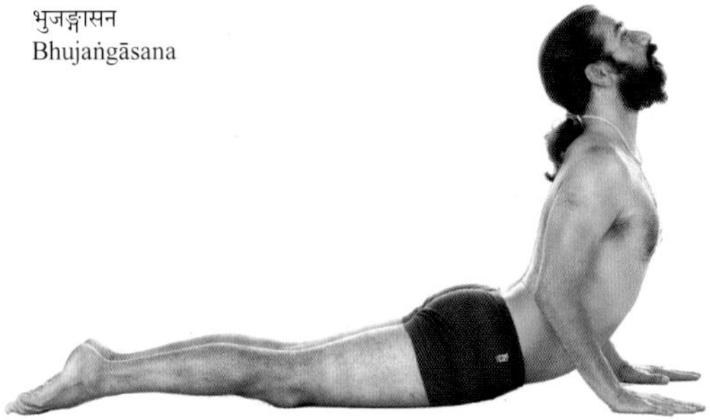

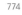

776
भुजङ्ग आसन (प्रसरित हस्त)
Bhujaṅga āsanạ (prasarita hasta)
Cobra pose (hands wide apart)

भुजङ्गासन (प्रसरितहस्त)
Bhujaṅgāsana (prasaritahasta)

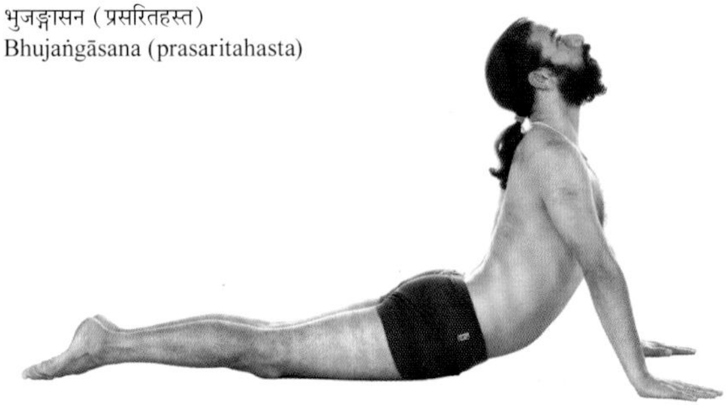

777
भुजङ्ग आसन (पाद दृष्टि)
Bhūjaṅga āsana (pāda dṛṣṭi)
Cobra pose (gazing at feet)

भुजङ्गासन (पाददृष्टि)
Bhūjaṅgāsana (pādadṛṣṭi)

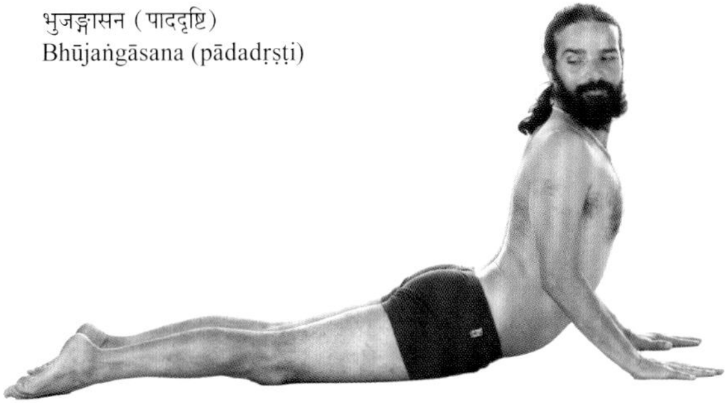

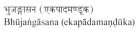

778
भुजङ्ग आसन (एक पाद मण्डूक)
Bhūjaṅga āsana (eka pāda maṇḍūka)
Cobra pose (one foot in frog)

भुजङ्गासन (एकपादमण्डूक)
Bhūjaṅgāsana (ekapādamaṇḍūka)

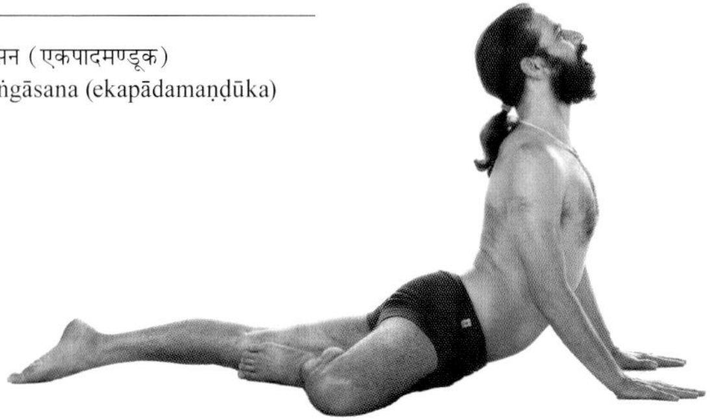

779
भुजङ्ग आसन (मण्डूक पाद)
Bhujaṅga āsana (maṇḍūka pāda)
Cobra pose (feet in frog)

भुजङ्गासन (मण्डूकपाद)
Bhujaṅgāsana (maṇḍūkapāda)

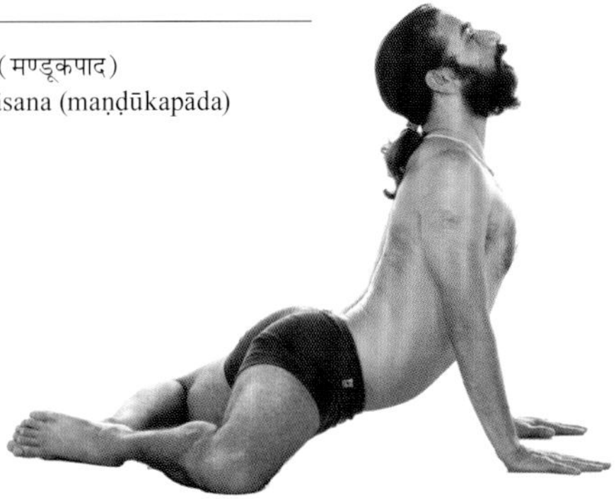

780
पूर्ण भुजङ्ग आसन
Pūrṇa bhujaṅga āsana
Full cobra pose

पूर्णभुजङ्गासन
Pūrṇabhujaṅgāsana

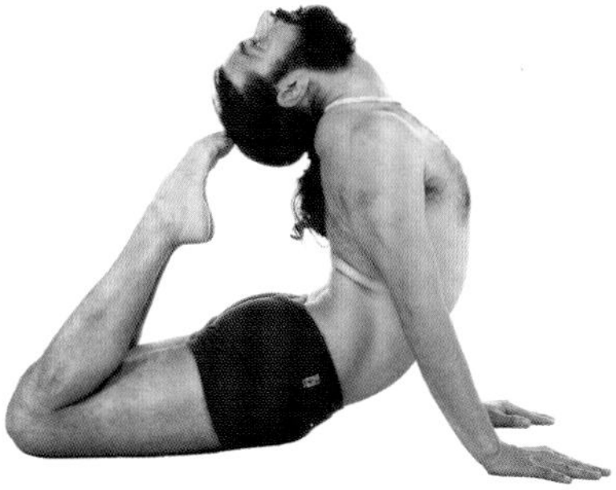

781
पद्म भुजङ्ग आसन
Padma bhujaṅga āsana
Lotus cobra pose

पद्मभुजङ्गासन
Padmabhujaṅgāsana

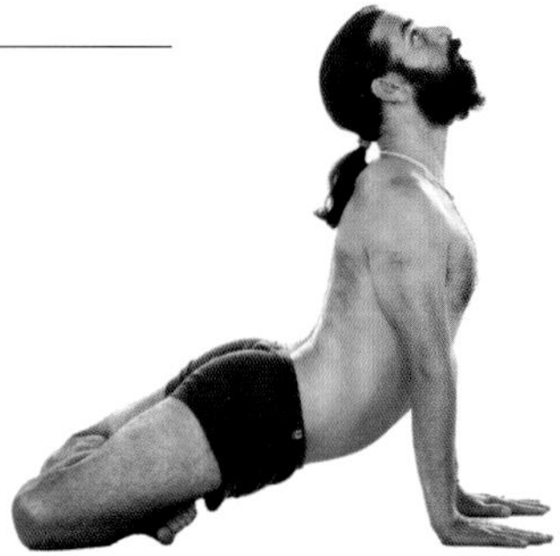

782
ऊर्ध्व मुख श्वान आसन (ऊर्ध्व दृष्टि)
Ūrdhva mukha śvāna āsana (ūrdhva dṛṣṭi)
Upward facing dog pose (facing up)

ऊर्ध्वमुखश्वानासन (ऊर्ध्वदृष्टि)
Ūrdhvamukhaśvānāsana (ūrdhvadṛṣṭi)

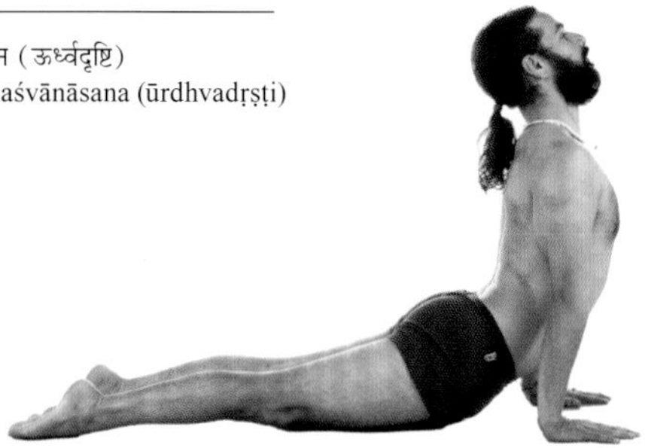

783
शलभ आसन (एक पाद उत्तान)
Śalabha āsana (eka pāda uttāna)
Locust pose (one leg lifted)

शलभासन (एकपादोत्तान)
Śalabhāsana (ekapādottāna)

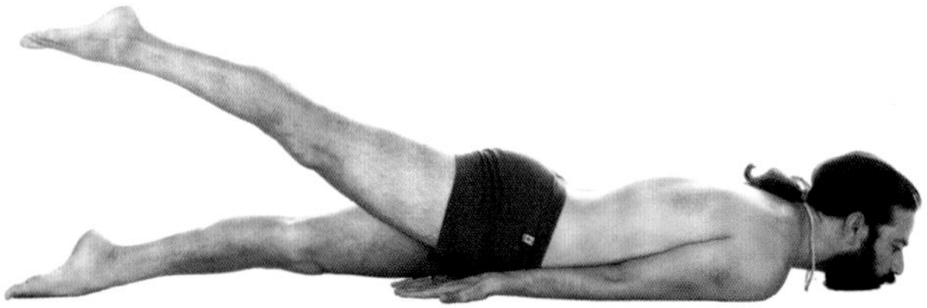

784
शलभ आसन (एक पाद उत्तान, बहिर्हस्त)
Śalabha āsana (eka pāda uttāna, bahirhasta)
Locust pose (one leg lifted, hands outside)

शलभासन (एकपादोत्तान, बहिर्हस्त)
Śalabhāsana (ekapādottāna, bahirhasta)

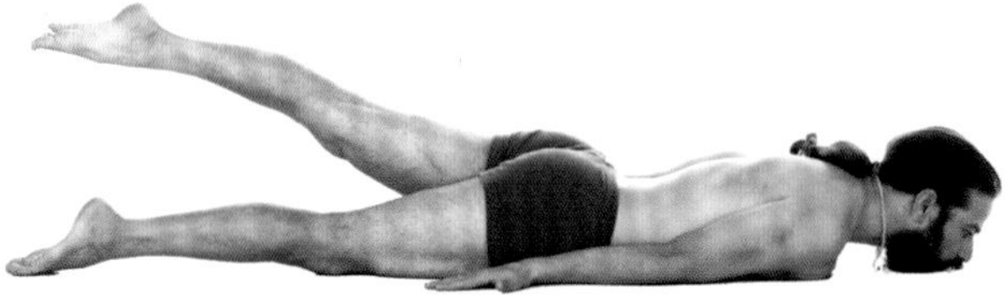

785
शलभ आसन (सालम्ब एक पाद)
Śalabha āsana (sālamba eka pāda)
Locust pose (one leg supported)

शलभासन (सालम्बैकपाद)
Śalabhāsana (sālambaikapāda)

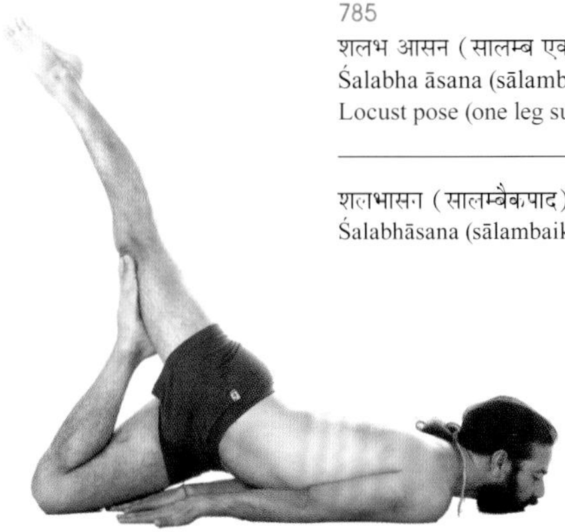

786
शलभ आसन
Śalabha āsana
Locust pose

शलभासन
Śalabhāsana

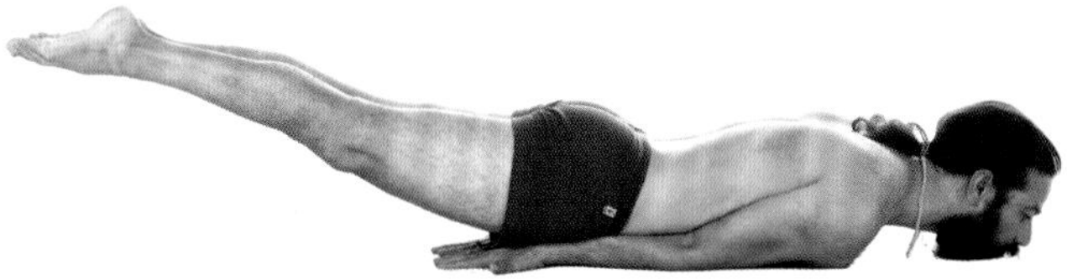

787
पुच्छ शलभ आसन
Puccha śalabha āsana
Locust feather pose

पुच्छशलभासन
Pucchaśalabhāsana

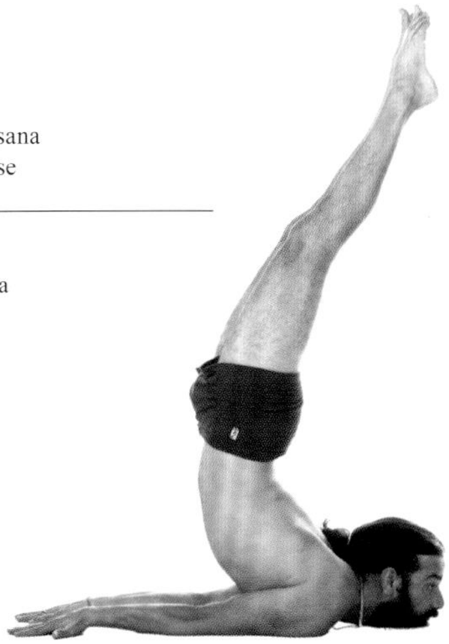

788
पूर्ण शलभ आसन
Pūrṇa śalabha āsana
Full locust pose

पूर्णशलभासन
Pūrṇaśalabhāsana

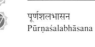

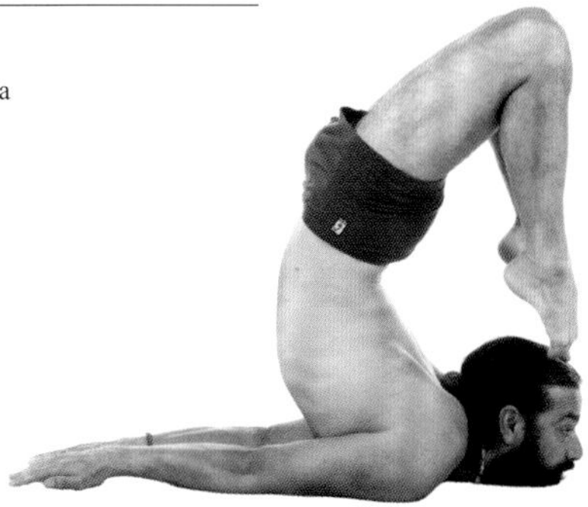

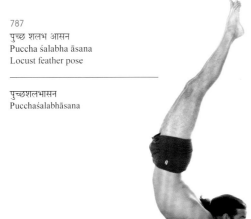

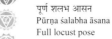

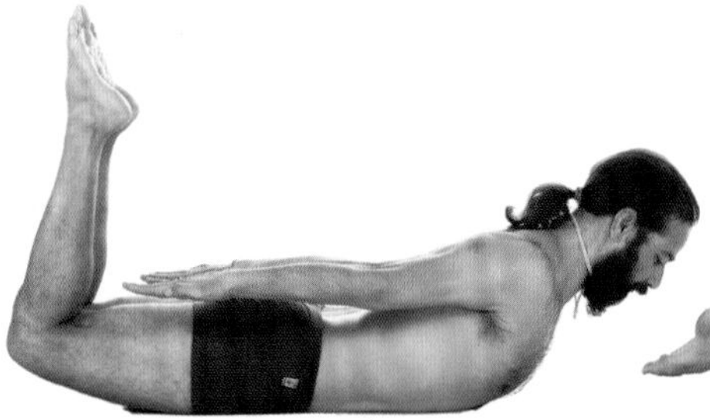

789
विमान पुच्छ आसन
Vimāna puccha āsana
Airplane tail pose

विमानपुच्छासन
Vimānapucchāsana

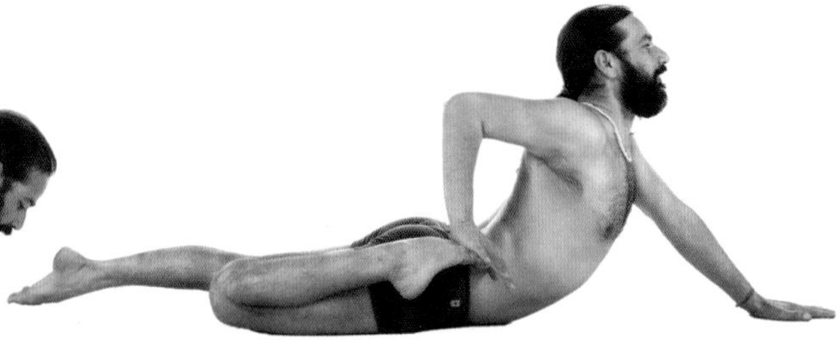

790
अर्ध भेक आसन
Ardha bheka āsana
Half frog pose

अर्धभेकासन
Ardhabhekāsana

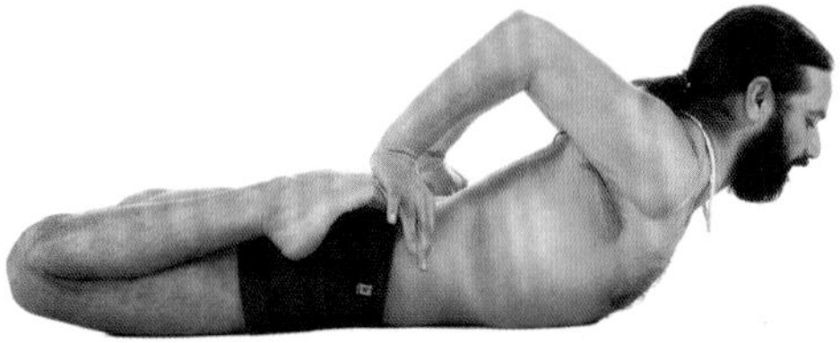

791
भेक आसन
Bheka āsana
Frog pose

भेकासन
Bhekāsana

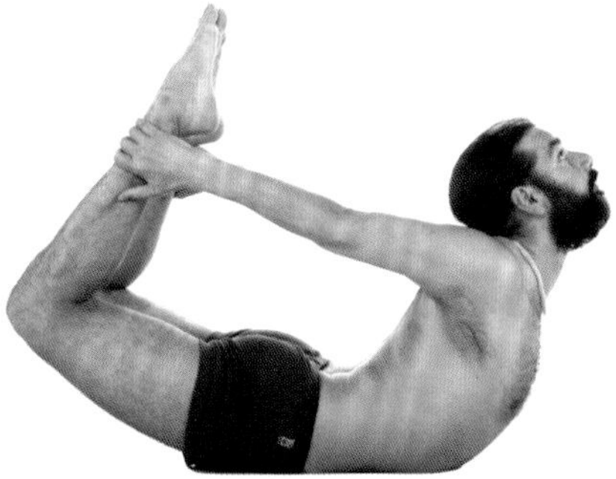

792
धनुः आसन
Dhanuḥ āsana
Bow pose

धनुरासन
Dhanuḥāsana

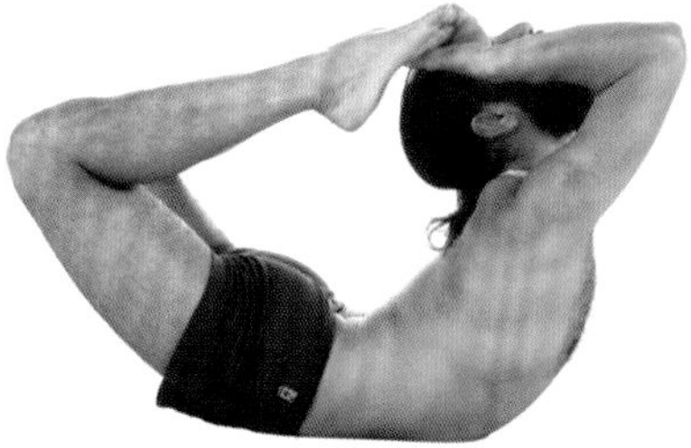

793
धनुः आसन (बद्ध पाद अङ्गुष्ठ)
Dhanuḥ āsana (baddha pāda aṅguṣṭha)
Bow pose (holding big toes)

धनुरासन (बद्धपादाङ्गुष्ठ)
Dhanuḥāsana (baddhapādāṅguṣṭha)

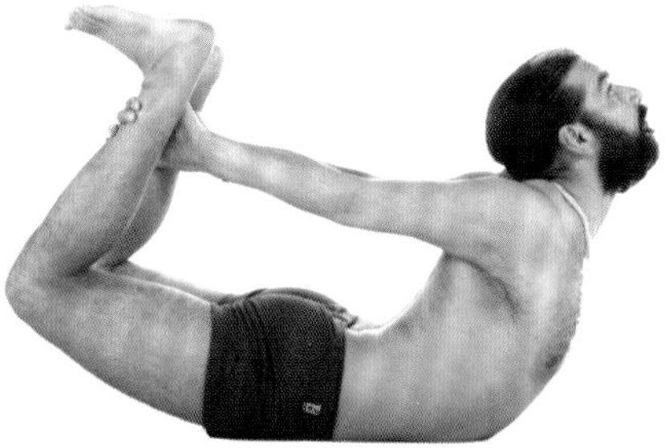

794
धनुः आसन (अन्तर्हस्त, अधोपाद अङ्गुल)
Dhanuḥ āsana (antarhasta, adhopāda aṅgula)
Bow pose (hands on inside, feet flexed)

धनुरासन (अन्तर्हस्त, अधोपादाङ्गुल)
Dhanuḥāsana (antarhasta, adhopādāṅgula)

Inversions

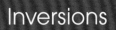

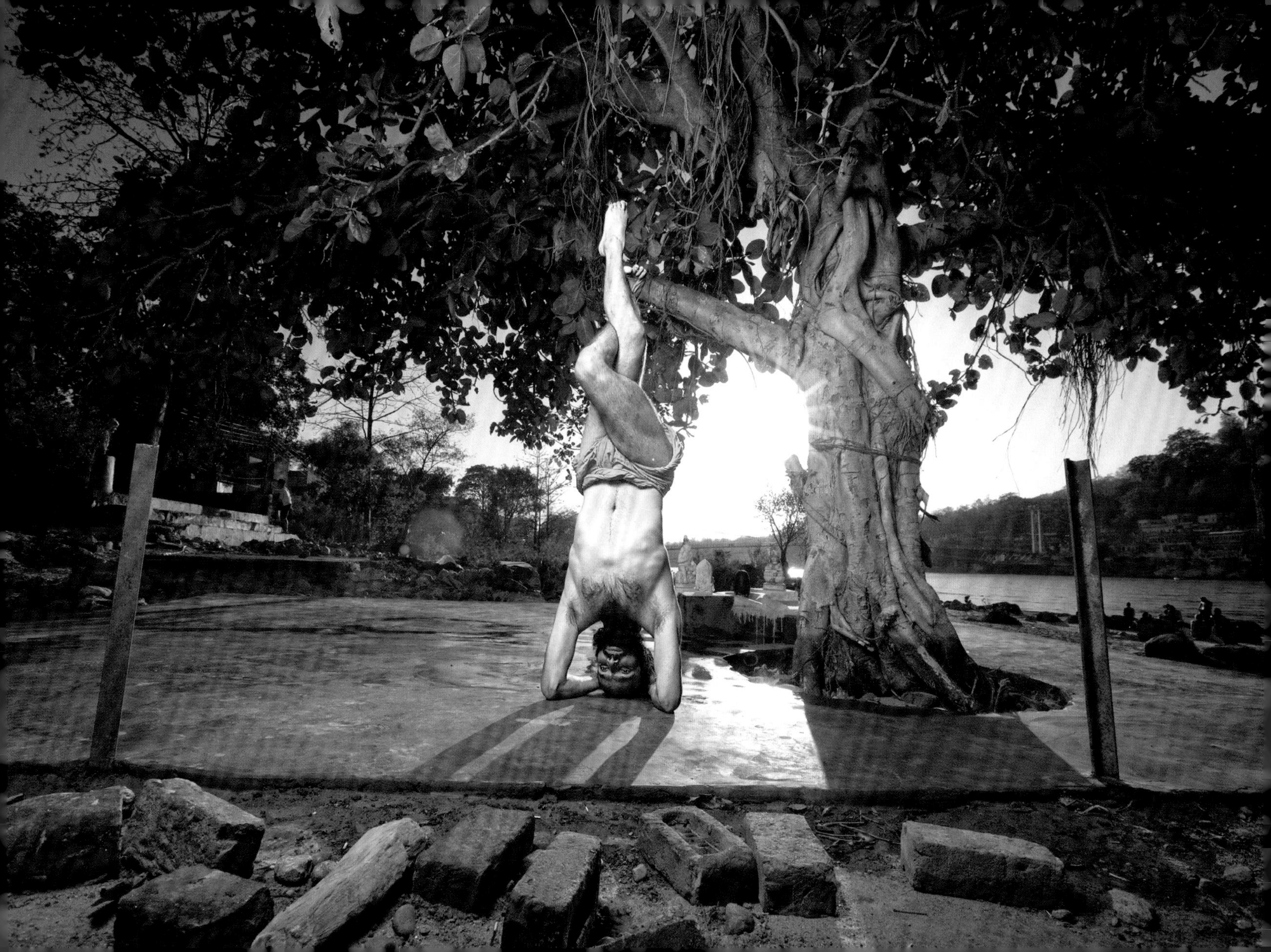

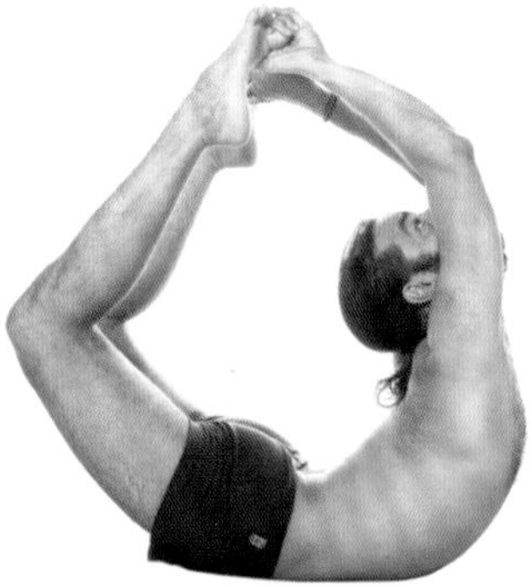

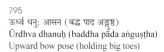

795
ऊर्ध्व धनुः आसन (बद्ध पाद अङ्गुष्ठ)
Ūrdhva dhanuḥ (baddha pāda aṅguṣṭha)
Upward bow pose (holding big toes)

ऊर्ध्वधनुरासन (बद्धपादाङ्गुष्ठ)
Ūrdhvadhanurāsana (baddhapādāṅguṣṭha)

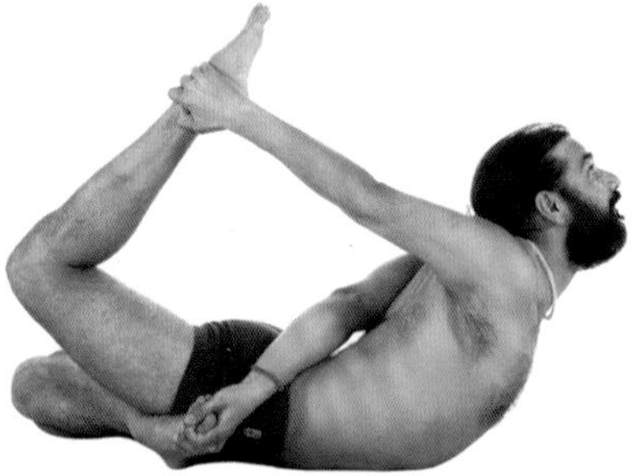

796
अर्धबद्ध पद्म धनुः आसन
Ardha baddha padma dhanuḥ āsana
Half bound lotus bow pose

अर्धबद्धपद्मधनुरासन
Ardhabaddhapadmadhanurāsana

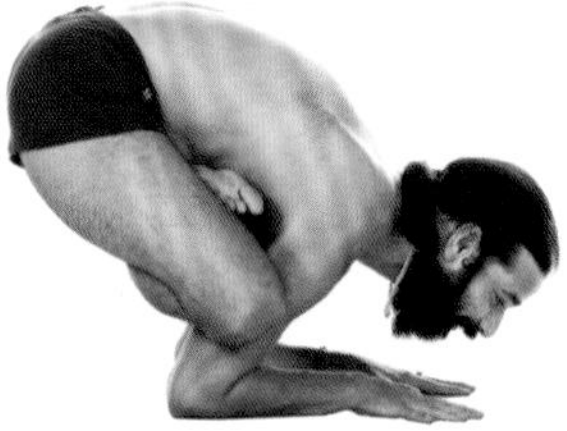

797
पद्म पिण्ड वृश्चिक आसन
Padma piṇḍa vṛścika āsana
Compact lotus scorpion pose

पद्मपिण्डवृश्चिकासन
Padmapiṇḍavṛścikāsana

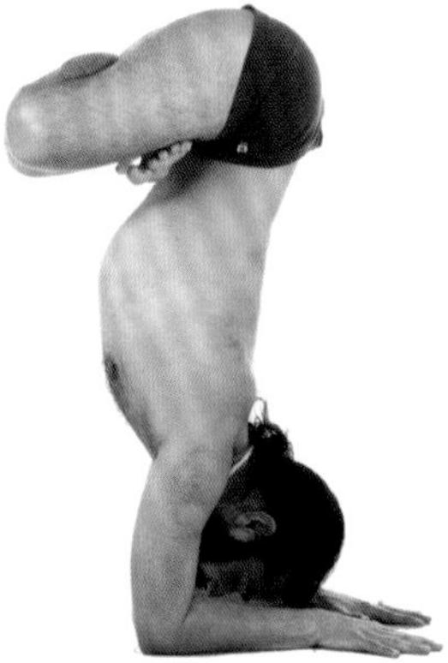

798
पद्म वृश्चिक आसन
Padma vṛścika āsana
Lotus scorpion pose

पद्मवृश्चिकासन
Padmavṛścikāsana

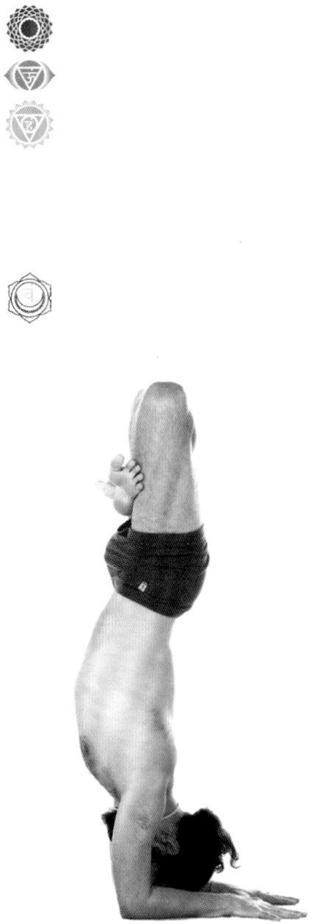

799
पुच्छ मयूर पद्म वृश्चिक आसन
Puccha mayūra padma vṛścika āsana
Peacock feather lotus scorpion pose

पुच्छमयूरपद्मवृश्चिकासन
Pucchamayūrapadmavṛścikāsana

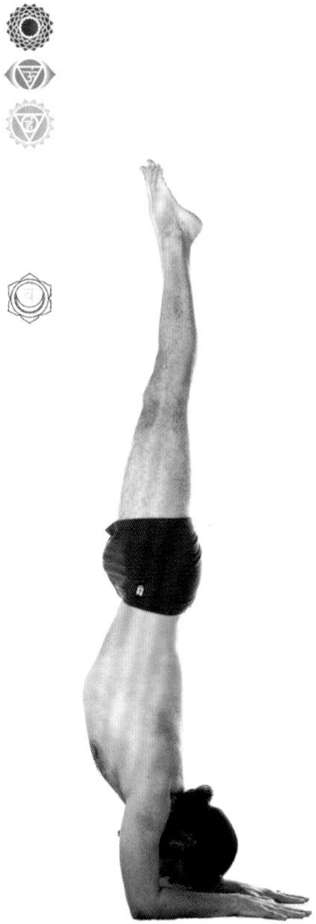

800
पुच्छ मयूर वृश्चिक आसन (ऊर्ध्व पाद)
Puccha mayūra vṛścika āsana (ūrdhva pāda)
Peacock feather scorpion pose (legs lifted)

पुच्छमयूरवृश्चिकासन (ऊर्ध्वपाद)
Pucchamayūravṛścikāsana (ūrdhvapāda)

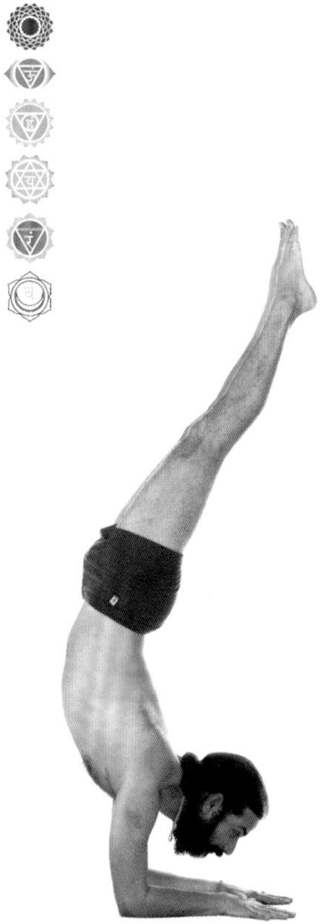

801
पुच्छ मयूर वृश्चिक आसन (क्षितिज पाद)
Puccha mayūra vṛścika āsana (kṣitija pāda)
Peacock feather scorpion pose (feet to the horizon)

पुच्छमयूरवृश्चिकासन (क्षितिजपाद)
Pucchamayūravṛścikāsana (kṣitijapāda)

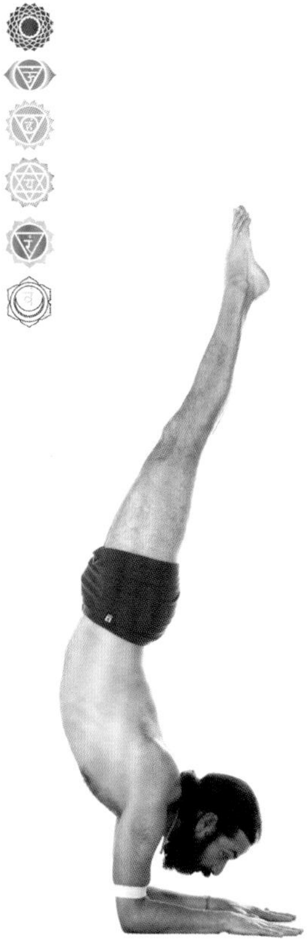

802
पुच्छ मयूर वृश्चिक आसन (सरज्जु)
Puccha mayūra vṛścika āsana (sarajju)
Peacock feather scorpion pose (with strap)

पुच्छमयूरवृश्चिकासन (सरज्जु)
Pucchamayūravṛścikāsana (sarajju)

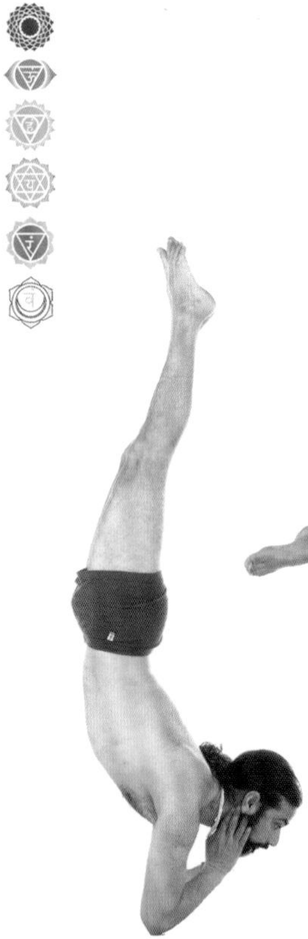

803
विकट पुच्छ मयूर वृश्चिक आसन
Vikaṭa puccha mayūra vṛścika āsana
Challenging peacock feather scorpion pose

विकटपुच्छमयूरवृश्चिकासन
Vikaṭapucchamayūravṛścikāsana

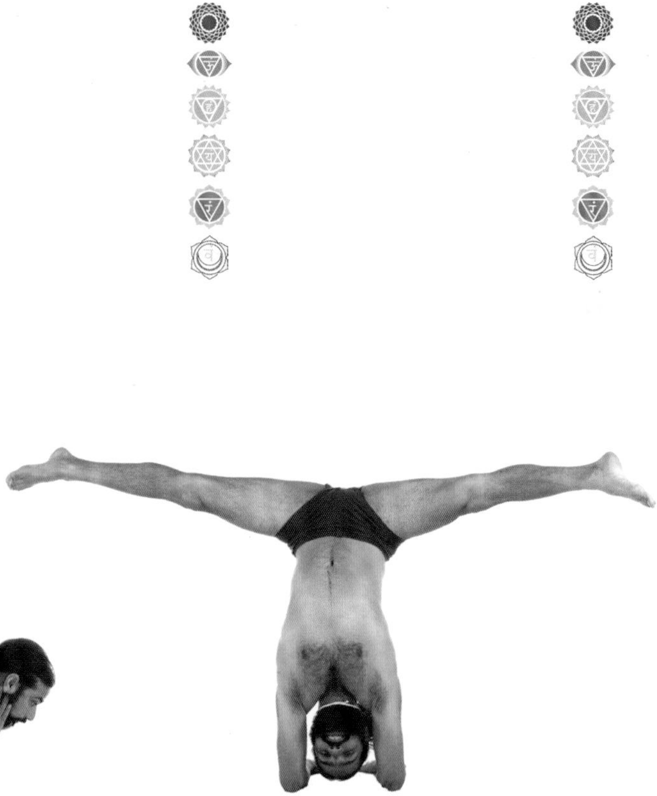

804
वृश्चिक आसन (समकोण पाद)
Vṛścika āsana (samakoṇa pāda)
Scorpion pose (split legs)

वृश्चिकासन(समकोणपाद)
Vṛścikāsana (samakoṇapāda)

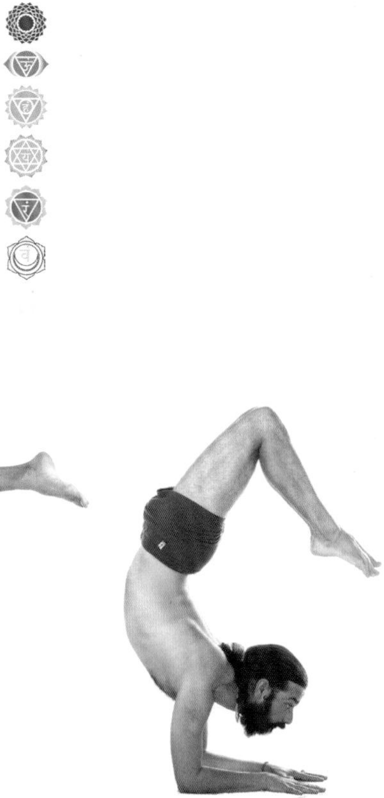

805
वृश्चिक आसन
Vṛścika āsana
Scorpion pose

वृश्चिकासन
Vṛścikāsana

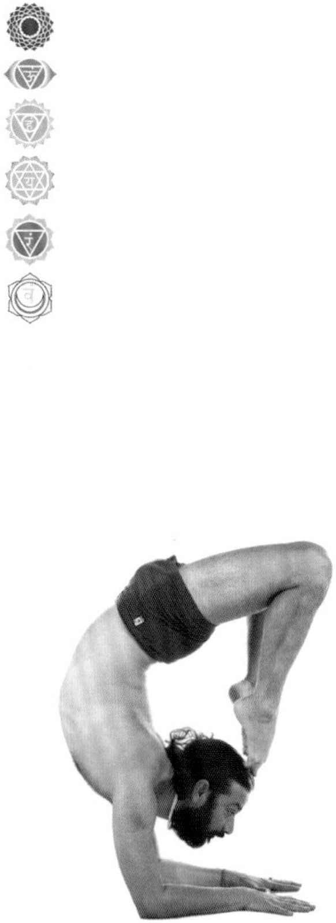

806
पूर्ण वृश्चिक आसन
Pūrṇa vṛścika āsana
Full scorpion pose

पूर्णवृश्चिकासन
Pūrṇavṛścikāsana

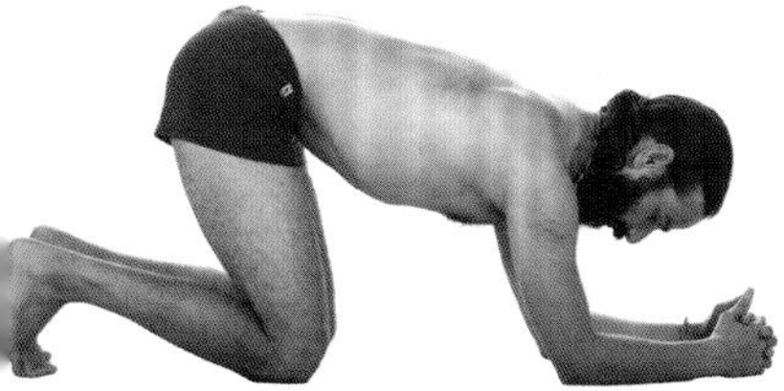

807
शीर्ष आसन (आरम्भ, कफोणि भू)
Śīrṣa āsana (ārambha, kaphoṇi bhū)
Headstand pose (starting position, elbows on earth)

शीर्षासन (आरम्भकफोणिभू)
Śīrṣāsana (ārambhakaphoṇibhū)

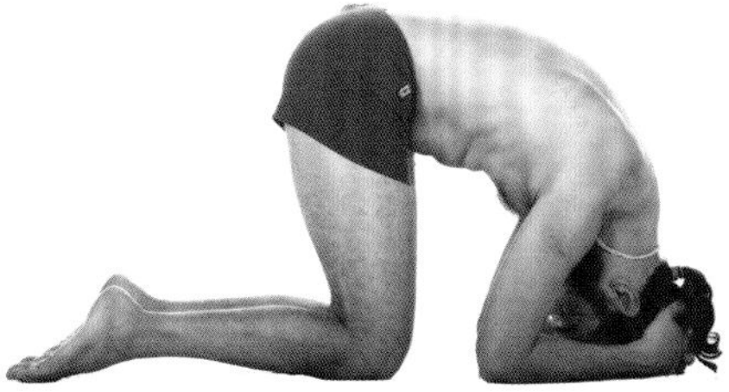

808
शीर्ष आसन (कफोणि भू)
Śīrṣa āsana (kaphoṇi bhū)
Headstand pose (elbows on the earth)

शीर्षासन (कफोणिभू)
Śīrṣāsana (kaphoṇibhū)

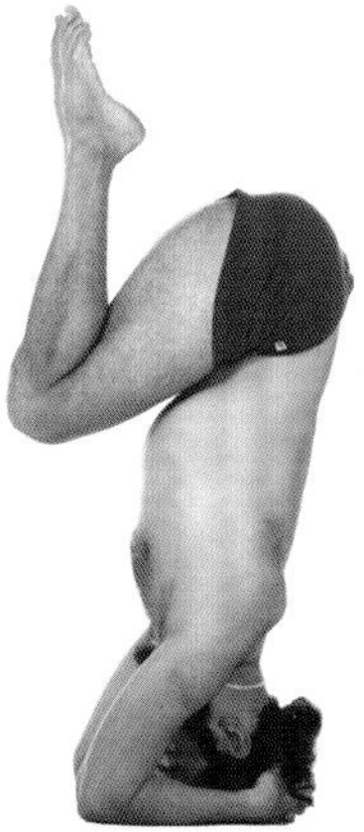

809
अर्ध शीर्ष आसन (कफोणि भू)
Ardha śīrṣa āsana (kaphoṇi bhū)
Half headstand pose (elbows on the earth)

अर्धशीर्षासन (कफोणिभू)
Ardhaśīrṣāsana (kaphoṇibhū)

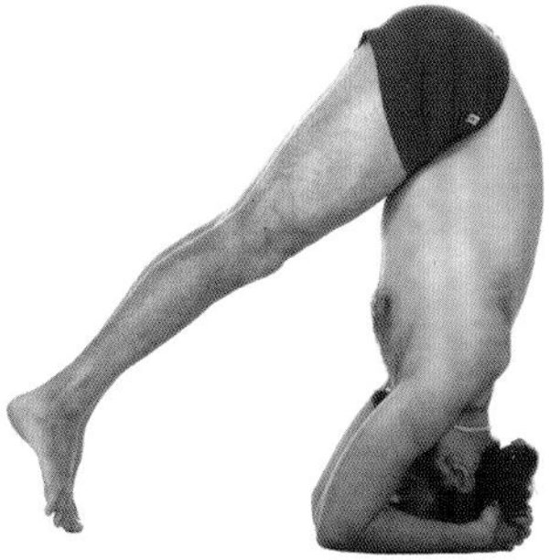

810
शीर्ष आसन (कफोणि भू, पाद अङ्गुल भू)
Śīrṣa āsana (kaphoṇi bhū, pāda aṅgula bhū)
Headstand pose (elbows on the earth,
toes on the earth)

शीर्षासन (कफोणिभू,पादाङ्गुलभू)
Śīrṣāsana (kaphoṇibhū, pādāṅgulabhū)

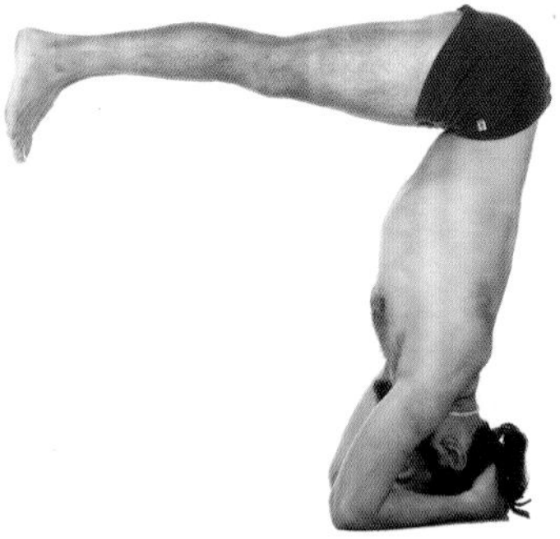

811
शीर्ष आसन (कफोणि भू, पाद दण्ड)
Śīrṣa āsana (kaphoṇi bhū, pāda daṇḍa)
Headstand pose (elbows on the earth, legs parallel in staff position)

शीर्षासन (कफोणिभू, पाददण्ड)
Śīrṣāsana (kaphoṇibhū, pādadaṇḍa)

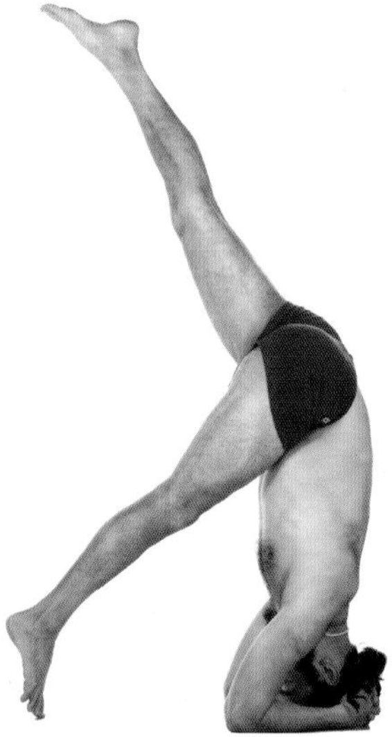

812
शीर्ष आसन (कफोणि भू, एक पाद अङ्गुल)
Śīrṣa āsana (kaphoṇi bhū, eka pāda aṅgula)
Headstand pose (elbows on the earth, one leg lifted)

शीर्षआसन (कफोणिभू, एकपादअङ्गुल)
Śīrṣāsana (kaphoṇibhū, ekapādaaṅgula)

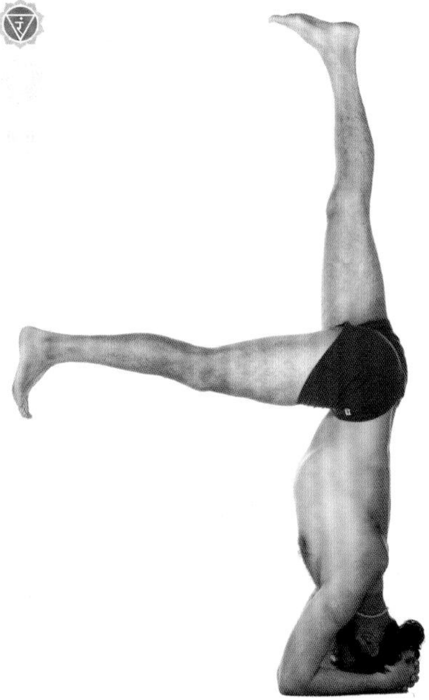

813
शीर्ष आसन (कफोणि भू, एक पाद दण्ड)
Śīrṣa āsana (kaphoṇi bhū, eka pāda daṇḍa)
Headstand pose (elbows on the earth, one leg in staff position)

शीर्षासन (कफोणिभू, एकपाददण्ड)
Śīrṣāsana (kaphoṇibhū, ekapādadaṇḍa)

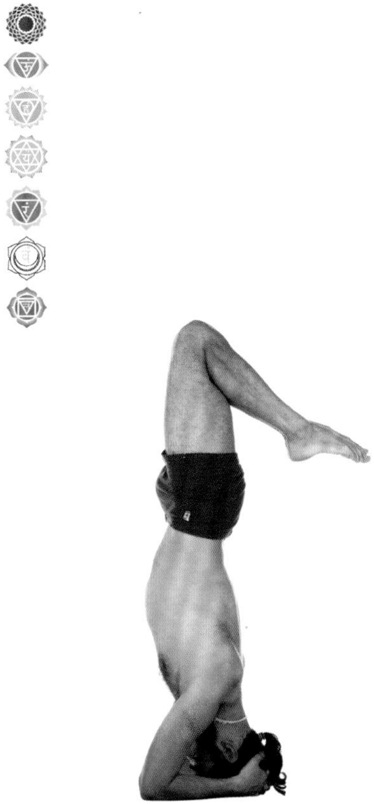

814
शीर्ष आसन (कफोणि भू, ऊर्ध्व जानु)
Śīrṣa āsana (kaphoṇi bhū, ūrdhva jānu)
Headstand pose (elbows on the earth, knees bent)

शीर्षासन (कफोणिभू, ऊर्ध्वजानु)
Śīrṣāsana (kaphoṇibhū, ūrdhvajānu)

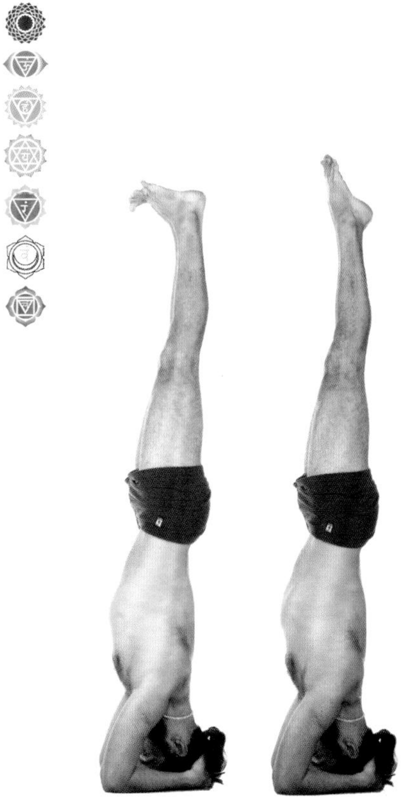

815
शीर्ष आसन (कफोणि भू)
Śīrṣa āsana (kaphoṇi bhū)
Headstand pose (elbows on the earth)

शीर्षासन (कफोणिभू)
Śīrṣāsana (kaphoṇibhū)

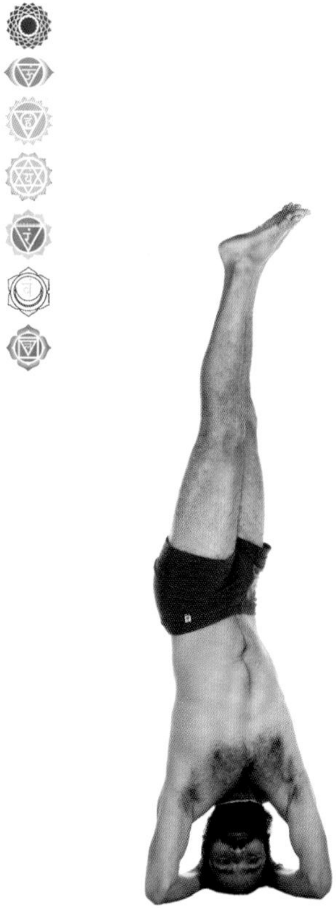

816
परिवृत्त शीर्ष आसन (कफोणि भू)
Parivṛtta śīrṣa āsana (kaphoṇi bhū)
Twisted headstand pose (elbows on the earth)

परिवृत्तशीर्षासन (कफोणिभू)
Parivṛttaśīrṣāsana (kaphoṇibhū)

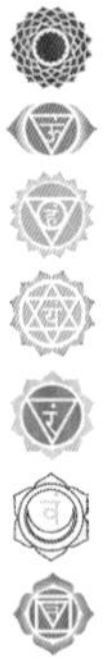

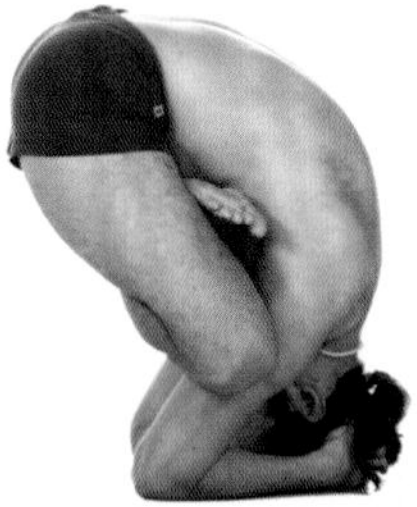

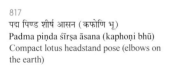

817
पद्म पिण्ड शीर्ष आसन (कफोणि भू)
Padma piṇda śīrṣa āsana (kaphoṇi bhū)
Compact lotus headstand pose (elbows on the earth)

पद्मपिण्डशीर्षआसन (कफोणिभू)
Padmapiṇḍaśīrṣāsana (kaphoṇibhū)

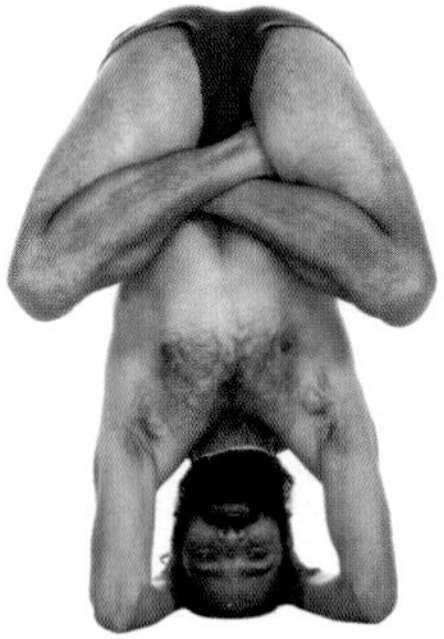

818
नाभि पद्म शीर्ष आसन (कफोणि भू)
Nābhi padma śīrṣa āsana (kaphoṇi bhū)
Navel lotus headstand pose (elbows on the earth)

नाभिपद्मशीर्षासन (कफोणिभू)
Nābhipadmaśīrṣāsana (kaphoṇibhū)

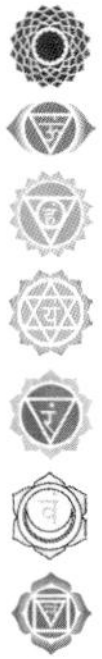

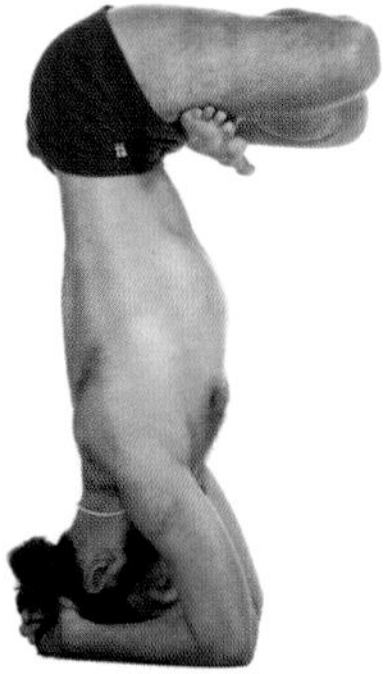

819
बुद्ध पद्म शीर्ष आसन (कफोणि भू)
Buddha padma śīrṣa āsana (kaphoṇi bhū)
Enlightened lotus headstand pose (elbows on the earth)

बुद्धपद्मशीर्षासन (कफोणिभू)
Buddhapadmaśīrṣāsana (kaphoṇibhū)

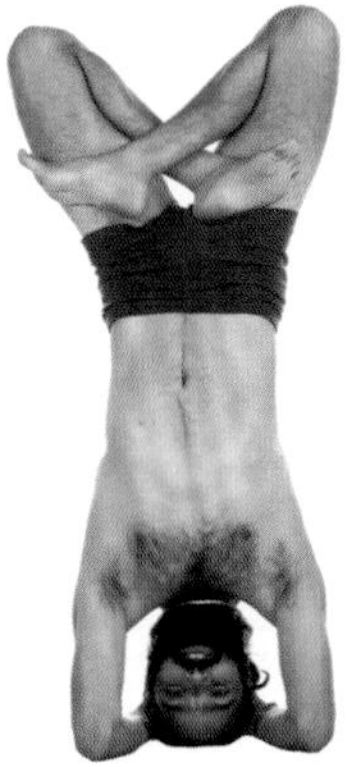

820
पद्म शीर्ष आसन (कफोणि भू)
Padma śīrṣa āsana (kaphoṇi bhū)
Lotus headstand pose (elbows on the earth)

पद्मशीर्षासन (कफोणिभू)
Padmaśīrṣāsana (kaphoṇibhū)

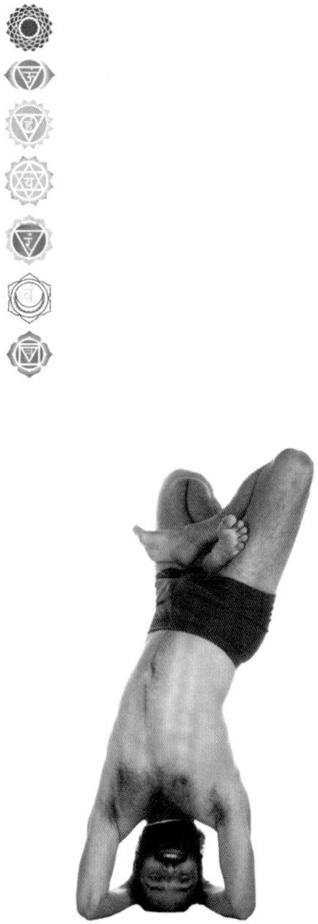

821
परिवृत्त पद्म शीर्ष आसन (कफोणि भू)
Parivṛtta padma śīrṣa āsana (kaphoṇi bhū)
Twisted lotus headstand pose (elbows on the earth)

परिवृत्तपद्मशीर्षासन (कफोणिभू)
Parivṛttapadmaśīrṣāsana (kaphoṇibhū)

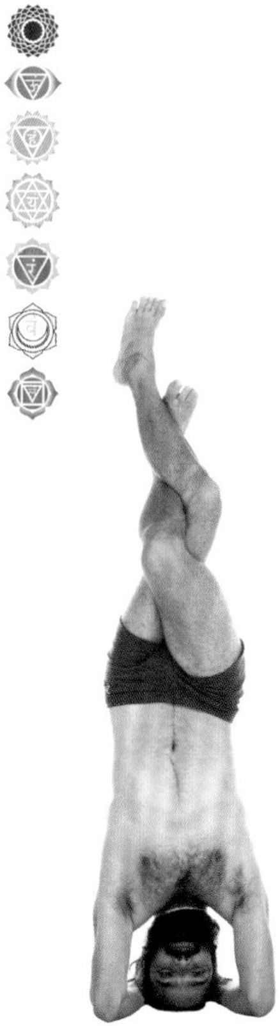

822
गरुड पाद शीर्ष आसन (कफोणि भू)
Garuḍa pāda śīrṣa āsana (kaphoṇi bhū)
Eagle legs headstand pose (elbows on the earth)

गरुडपादशीर्षासन (कफोणिभू)
Garuḍapādaśīrṣāsana (kaphoṇibhū)

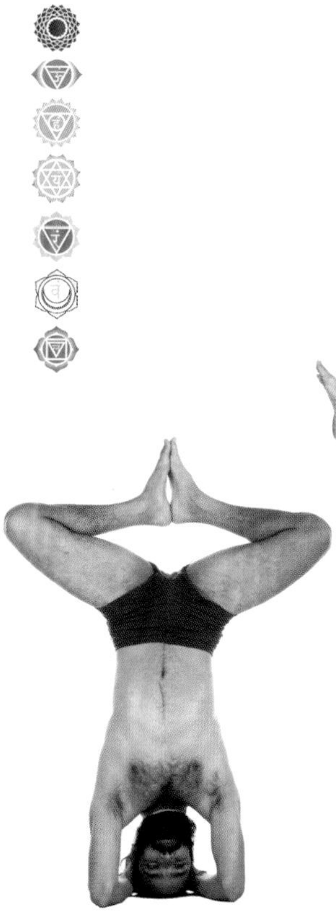

823
शीर्ष आसन (कफोणि भू, पार्वती पाद)
Śīrṣa āsana (kaphoṇi bhū, pārvatī pāda)
Headstand pose (elbows on the earth, soles of the feet together)

शीर्षासन (कफोणिभू, पार्वतीपाद)
Śīrṣāsana (kaphoṇibhū, pārvatīpāda)

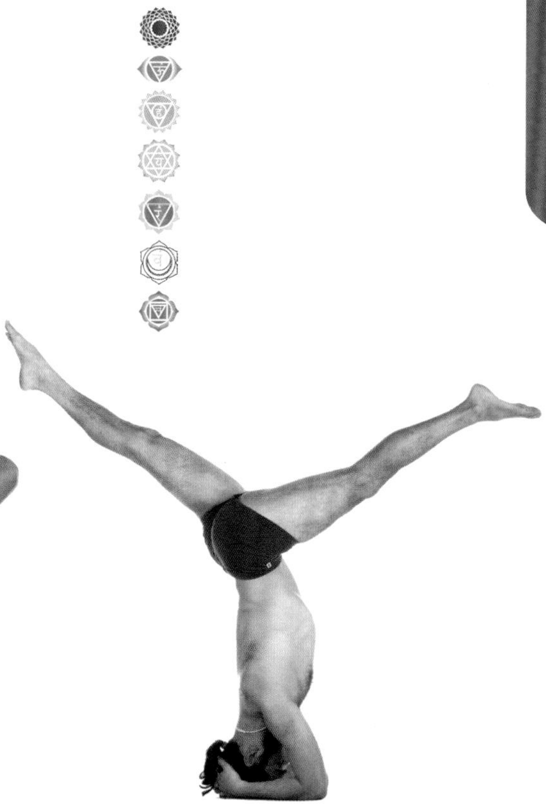

824
शीर्ष आसन (कफोणि भू, हनुमान पाद)
Śīrṣa āsana (kaphoṇi bhū, Hanumāna pāda)
Headstand pose (elbows on the earth, legs in Hanumāna splits)

शीर्षासन (कफोणिभू, हनुमानपाद)
Śīrṣaāsana (kaphoṇibhū, Hanumānapāda)

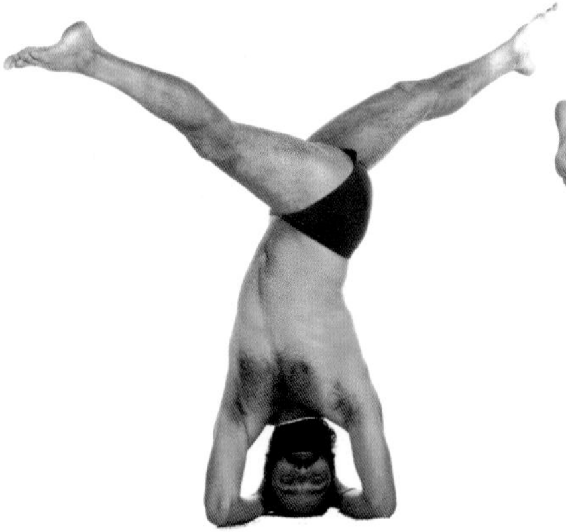

825
परिवृत्त शीर्ष आसन (कफोणि भू, हनुमान पाद)
Parivṛtta śīrṣa āsana (kaphoṇi bhū, Hanumāna pāda)
Twisted headstand pose (elbows on the earth, legs in Hanumāna splits)

परिवृत्तशीर्षासन (कफोणिभू, हनुमानपाद)
Parivṛttaśīrṣaāsana (kaphoṇibhūhanumānapāda)

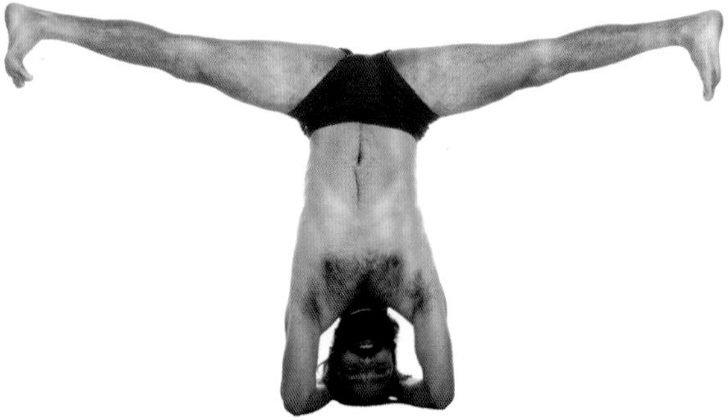

826
शीर्ष आसन (कफोणि भू, समकोण पाद)
Śīrṣa āsana (kaphoṇi bhū, samakoṇa pāda)
Headstand pose (elbows on the earth, legs in side splits)

शीर्षासन (कफोणिभू, समकोणपाद)
Śīrṣāsana (kaphoṇibhū, samakoṇapāda)

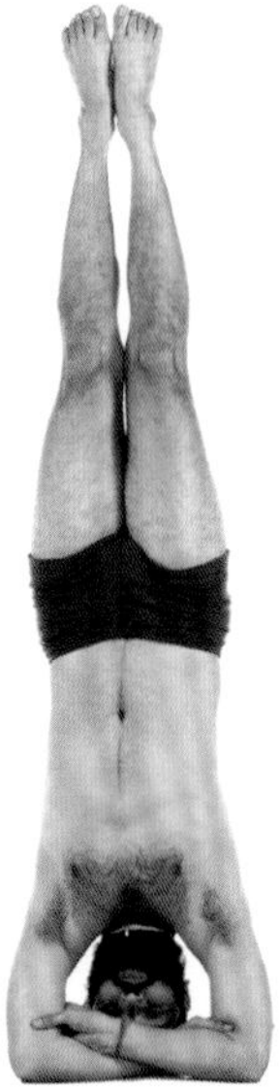

827
शीर्ष आसन (बद्ध कफोणि, सम्मुख)
Śīrṣa āsana (baddha kaphoṇi, sammukha)
Headstand pose (bound elbows in front of face)

शीर्षासन (बद्धकफोणि, सम्मुख)
Śīrsāsana (baddhakaphoṇi, sammukha)

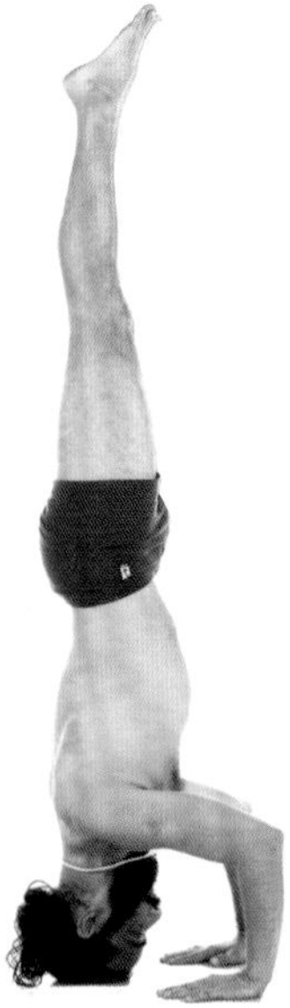

828
शीर्ष आसन (करतल भू)
Śīrṣa āsana (karatala bhū)
Headstand pose (palms on the earth)

शीर्षासन (करतलभू)
Śīrṣāsana (karatalabhū)

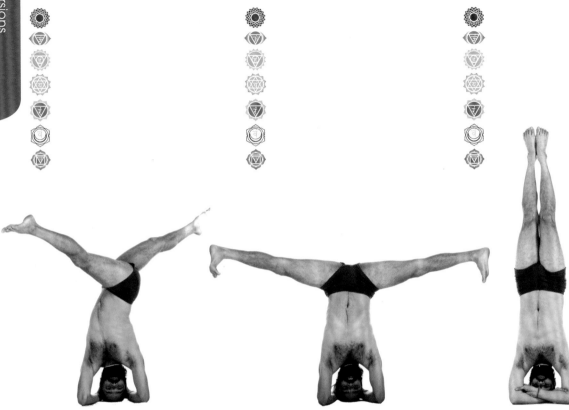

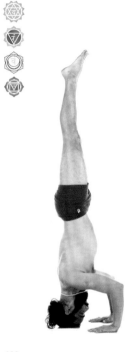

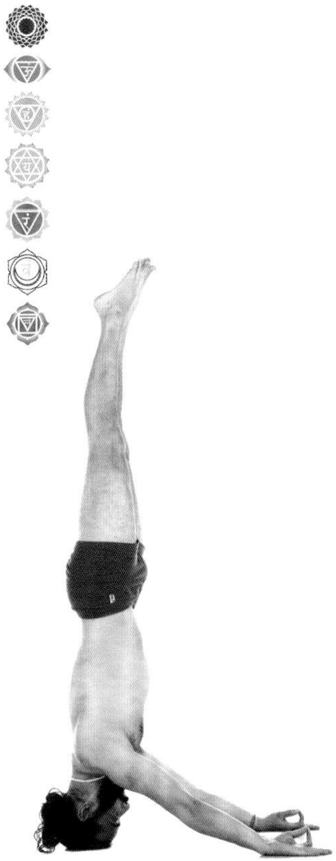

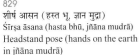

829
शीर्ष आसन (हस्त भू, ज्ञान मुद्रा)
Śīrṣa āsana (hasta bhū, jñāna mudrā)
Headstand pose (hands on the earth in jñāna mudrā)

शीर्षासन (हस्तभू, ज्ञानमुद्रा)
Śīrṣāsana (hastabhū, jñānamudrā)

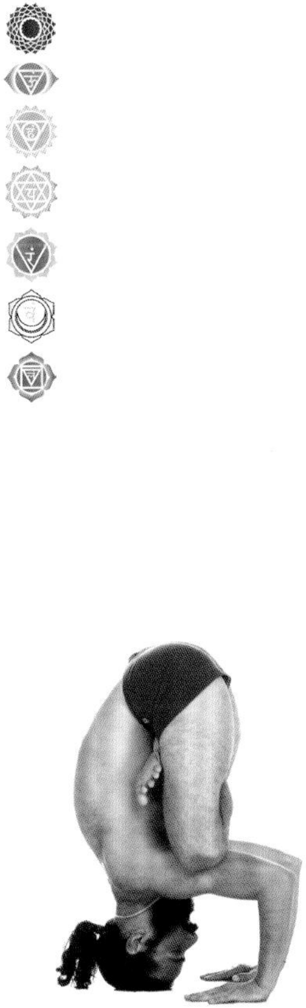

830
पद्म शीर्ष आसन (आरम्भ अवस्था)
Padma śīrṣa āsana (ārambha avasthā)
Lotus headstand pose (starting position)

पद्मशीर्षासन (आरम्भावस्था)
Padmaśīrṣāsana (ārambhāvasthā)

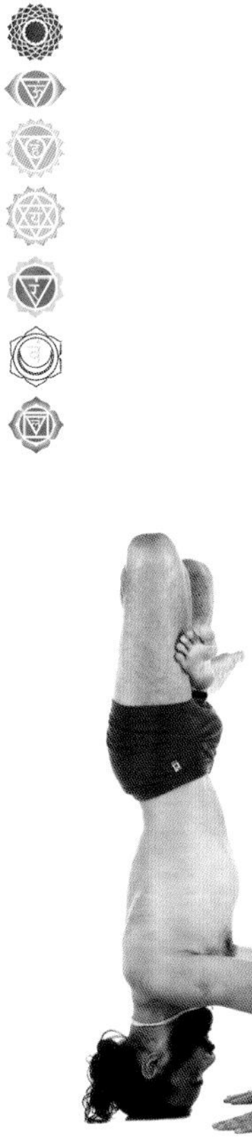

831
पद्म शीर्ष आसन (करतल भू, अन्तःअङ्गुल)
Padma śīrṣa āsana (karatala bhū, antaṛ aṅgula)
Lotus headstand pose (palms on the earth, fingers pointing in)

पद्मशीर्षासन (करतलभू, अन्तराङ्गुल)
Padmaśīrṣāsana (karatalabhū, antarāṅgula)

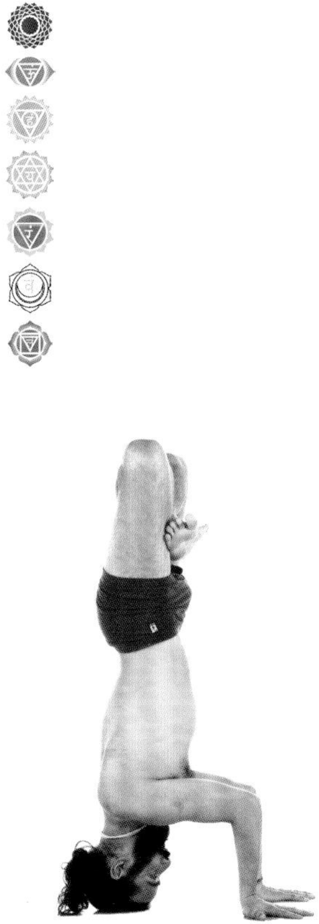

832
पद्म शीर्ष आसन (करतल भू बहिः अङ्गुल)
Padma śīrṣa āsana (karatala bhū bahir aṅgula)
Lotus headstand pose (palms on the earth, fingers pointing out)

पद्मशीर्षासन (करतलभूबहिराङ्गुल)
Padmaśīrṣāsana (karatalabhūbahirāṅgula)

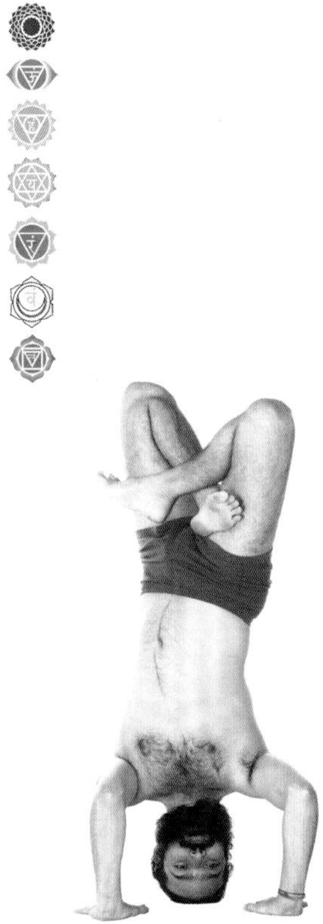

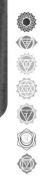

833
परिवृत्त पद्म शीर्ष आसन (करतल भू)
Parivṛtta padma śīrṣa āsana (karatala bhū)
Twisted lotus headstand pose (palms on the earth)

परिवृत्तपद्मशीर्षासन (करतलभू)
Parivṛttapadmaśīrṣāsana (karatalabhū)

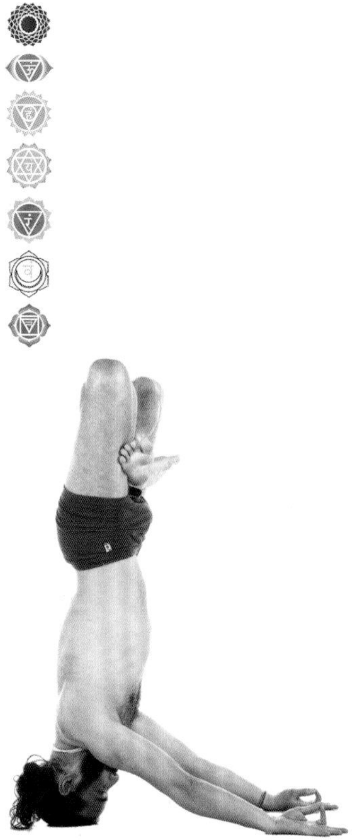

834
पद्म शीर्ष आसन (हस्त भू, ज्ञान मुद्रा)
Padma śīrṣa āsana (hasta bhū, jñāna mudrā)
Lotus headstand pose (hands on the earth in jñāna mudrā)

पद्मशीर्षासन (हस्तभू, ज्ञानमुद्रा)
Padmaśīrṣāsana (hastabhū, jñānamudrā)

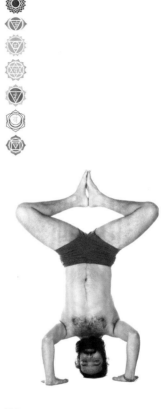

835
पार्वती पाद शीर्षा आसन (करतल भू)
Pārvatī pāda śīrṣa āsana (karatala bhū)
Feet together frog headstand pose (palms on the earth)

पार्वतीपादशीर्षासन (करतलभू)
Pārvatīpādaśīrṣāsana (karatalabhū)

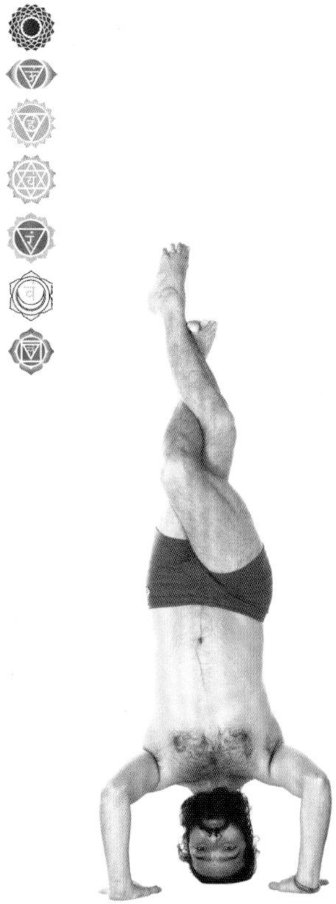

836
गरुड पाद शीर्ष आसन (करतल भू)
Garuḍa pāda śīrṣa āsana (karatala bhū)
Eagle legs headstand pose (palms on the earth)

गरुडपादशीर्षासन (करतलभू)
Garuḍapādaśīrṣāsana (karatalabhū)

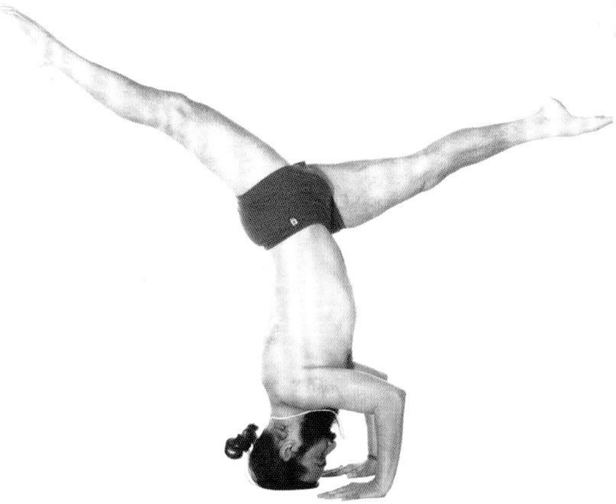

837
शीर्ष आसन (करतल भू, हनुमान पाद)
Śīrṣa āsana (karatala bhū, Hanumāna pāda)
Headstand pose (palms on the earth, legs in Hanumāna splits)

शीर्षासन (करतलभू,हनुमानपाद)
Śīrṣaāsana (karatalabhū, Hanumānapāda)

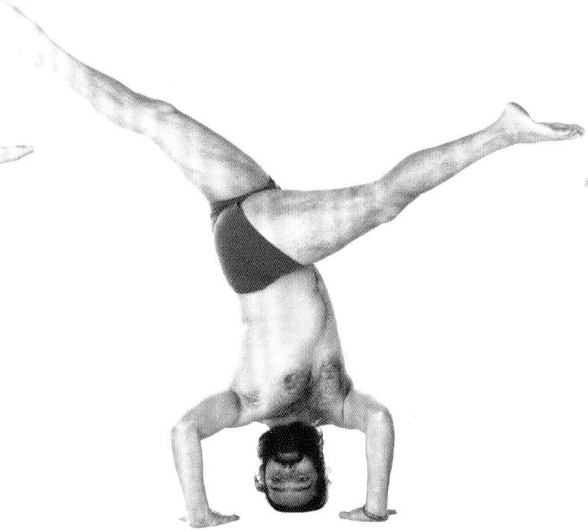

838
परिवृत्त शीर्षासन (करतल भू, हनुमान पाद)
Parivṛtta śīrṣa āsana (karatala bhū, Hanumāna pāda)
Twisted headstand pose (palms on the earth, legs in Hanumāna splits)

परिवृत्त शीर्षासन (करतलभू, हनुमानपाद)
Parivṛttaśīrṣaāsana (karatalabhū, Hanumānapāda)

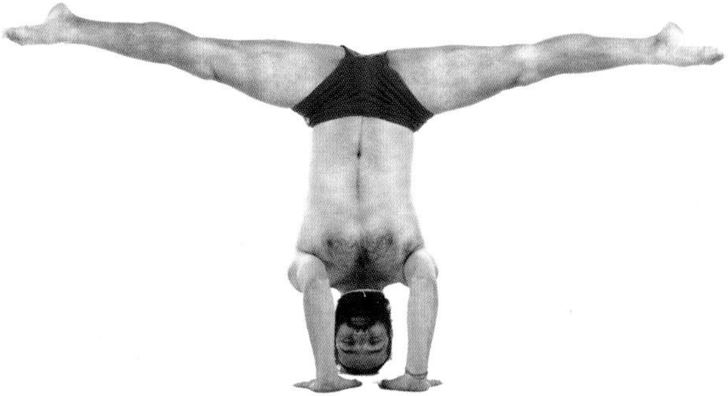

839
शीर्ष आसन (करतल भू, समकोण पाद)
Śīrṣa āsana (karatala bhū, samakoṇa pāda)
Headstand pose (palms on the earth, side splits)

शीर्षासन (करतलभू, समकोणपाद)
Śīrṣaāsana (karatalabhū, samakoṇapāda)

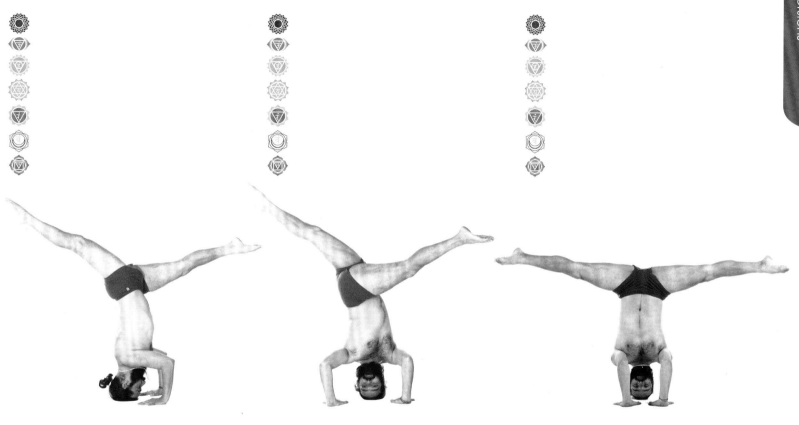

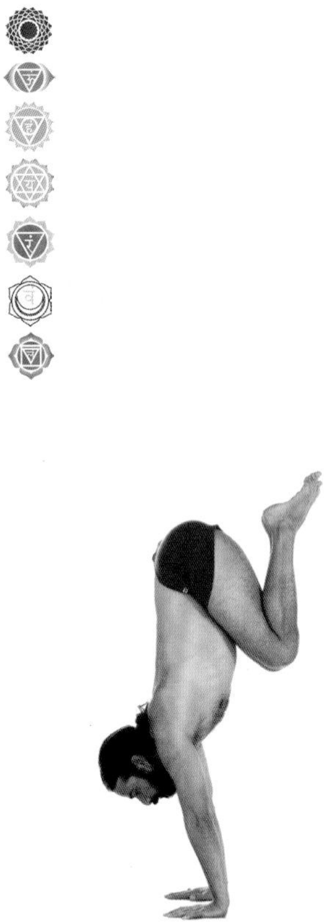

840
अधोमुख वृक्ष आसन (आरम्भ अवस्था)
Adhomukha vṛkṣa āsana (ārambha avasthā)
Downward facing tree pose (starting position)

अधोमुखवृक्षासन (आरम्भावस्था)
Adhomukhavṛkṣāsana (ārambhāvasthā)

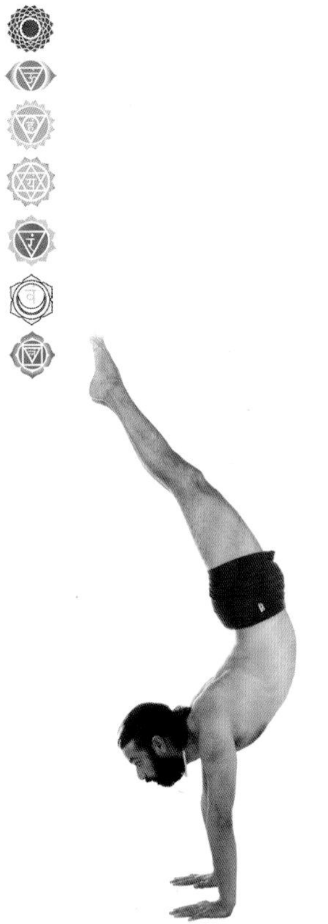

841
अधोमुख वृक्ष आसन
Adhomukha vṛkṣa āsana
Downward facing tree pose

अधोमुखवृक्षासन
Adhomukhavṛkṣāsana

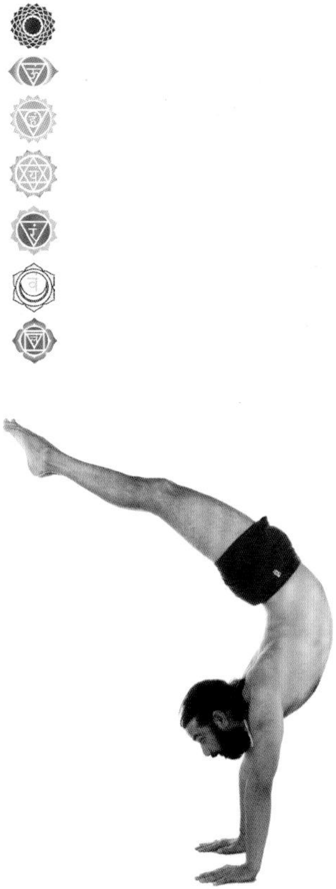

842
अधोमुख वृक्ष आसन (क्षितिज पाद)
Adhomukha vṛkṣa āsana (kṣitija pāda)
Downward facing tree pose (feet pointed toward the horizon)

अधोमुखवृक्षासन (क्षितिजपाद)
Adhomukhavṛkṣaāsana (ksitijapāda)

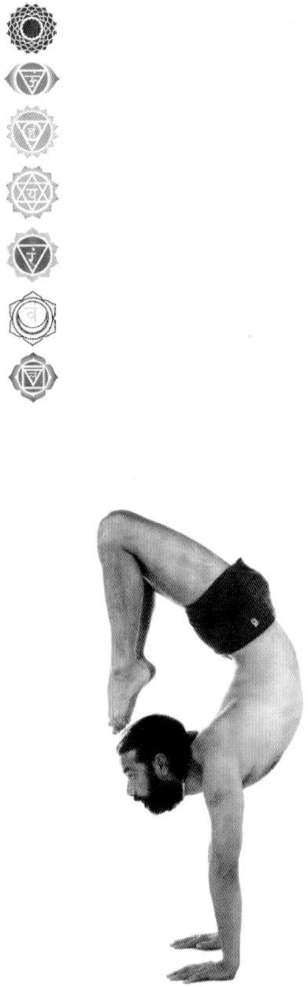

843
पूर्ण वृक्ष वृश्चिक आसन
Pūrṇa vṛkṣa vṛścika āsana
Full tree scorpion pose

पूर्णवृक्षवृश्चिकासन
Pūrṇavṛkṣavṛścikāsana

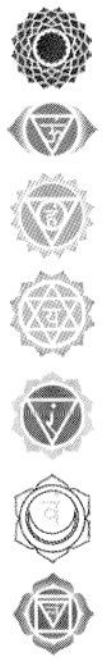

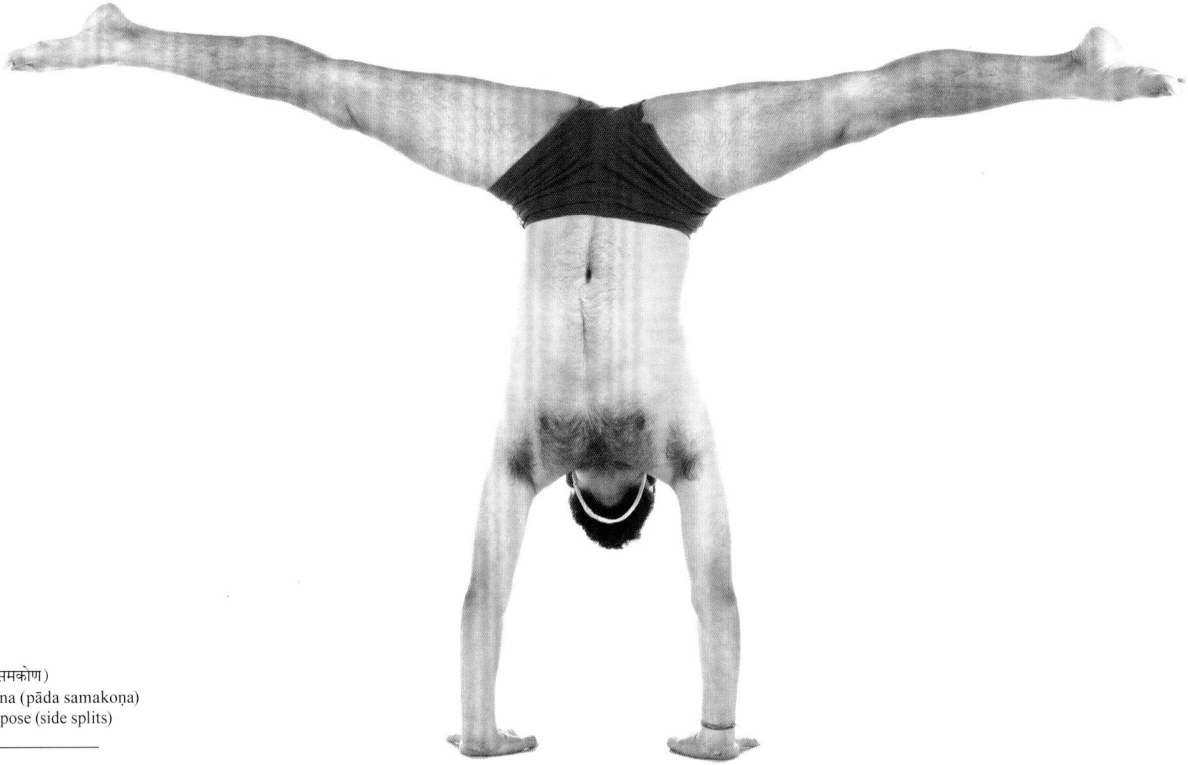

844
अधोमुख वृक्ष आसन (पाद समकोण)
Adhomukha vṛkṣa āsana (pāda samakoṇa)
Downward facing tree pose (side splits)

अधोमुखवृक्षासन (पादसमकोण)
Adhomukhavṛkṣāsana (pādasamakoṇa)

Resting

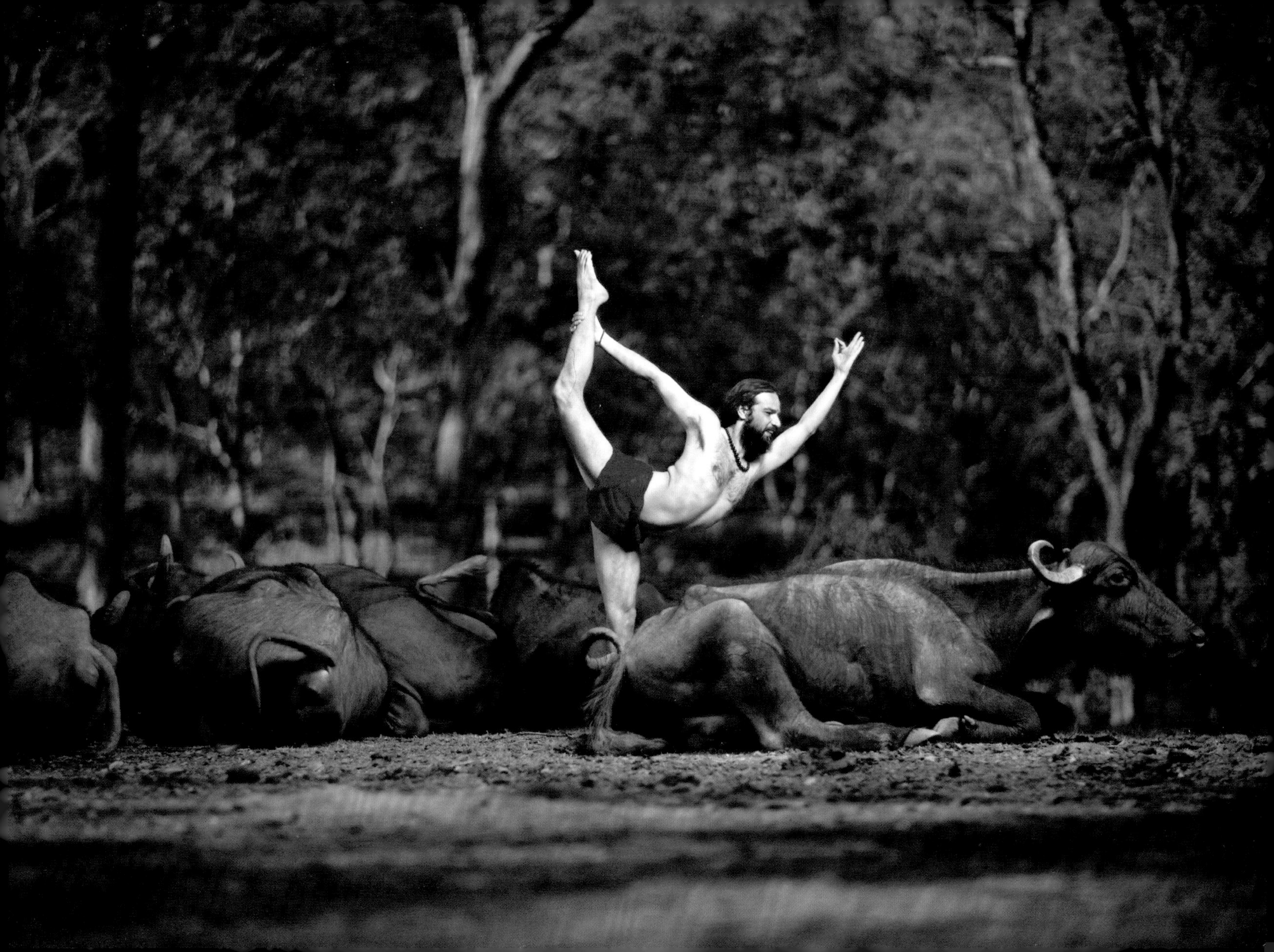

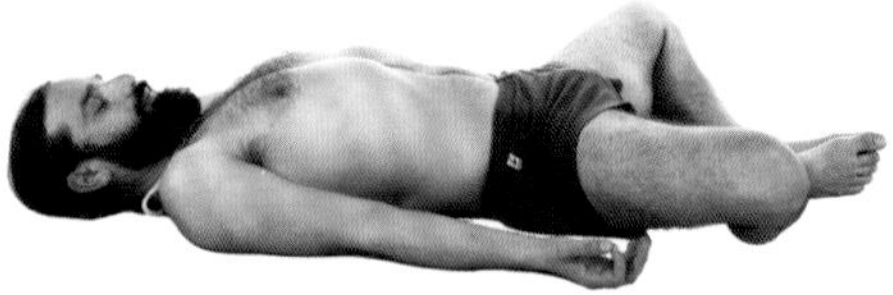

845
पार्वती पाद शव आसन
Pārvatī pāda śava āsana
Divine feminine corpse pose

पार्वतीपादशवासन
Pārvatīpādaśavāsana

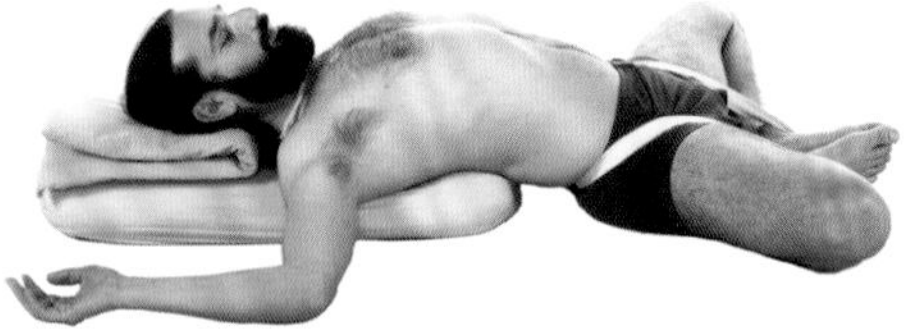

846
पार्वती पाद शव आसन (सरज्जु)
Pārvatī pāda śava āsana (sarajju)
Divine feminine corpse pose (with strap)

पार्वतीपादशवासन (सरज्जु)
Pārvatīpādaśavāsana (sarajju)

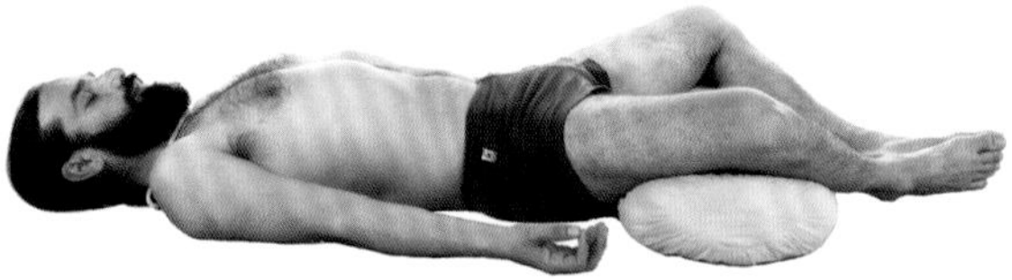

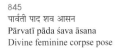

847
पार्वती पाद शव आसन (सालम्ब)
Pārvatī pāda śava āsana (sālamba)
Divine feminine corpse pose (supported)

पार्वतीपादशवासन (सालम्ब)
Pārvatīpādaśavāsana (sālamba)

Everyone needs a good rest.

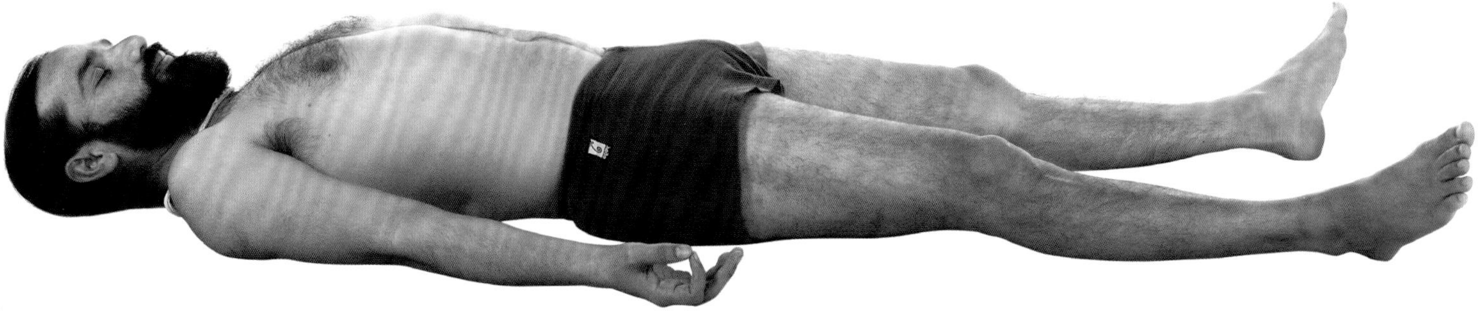

848
शव आसन
Śava āsana
Corpse pose

शवासन
Śavāsana

Classical Sun Salutation Sequence

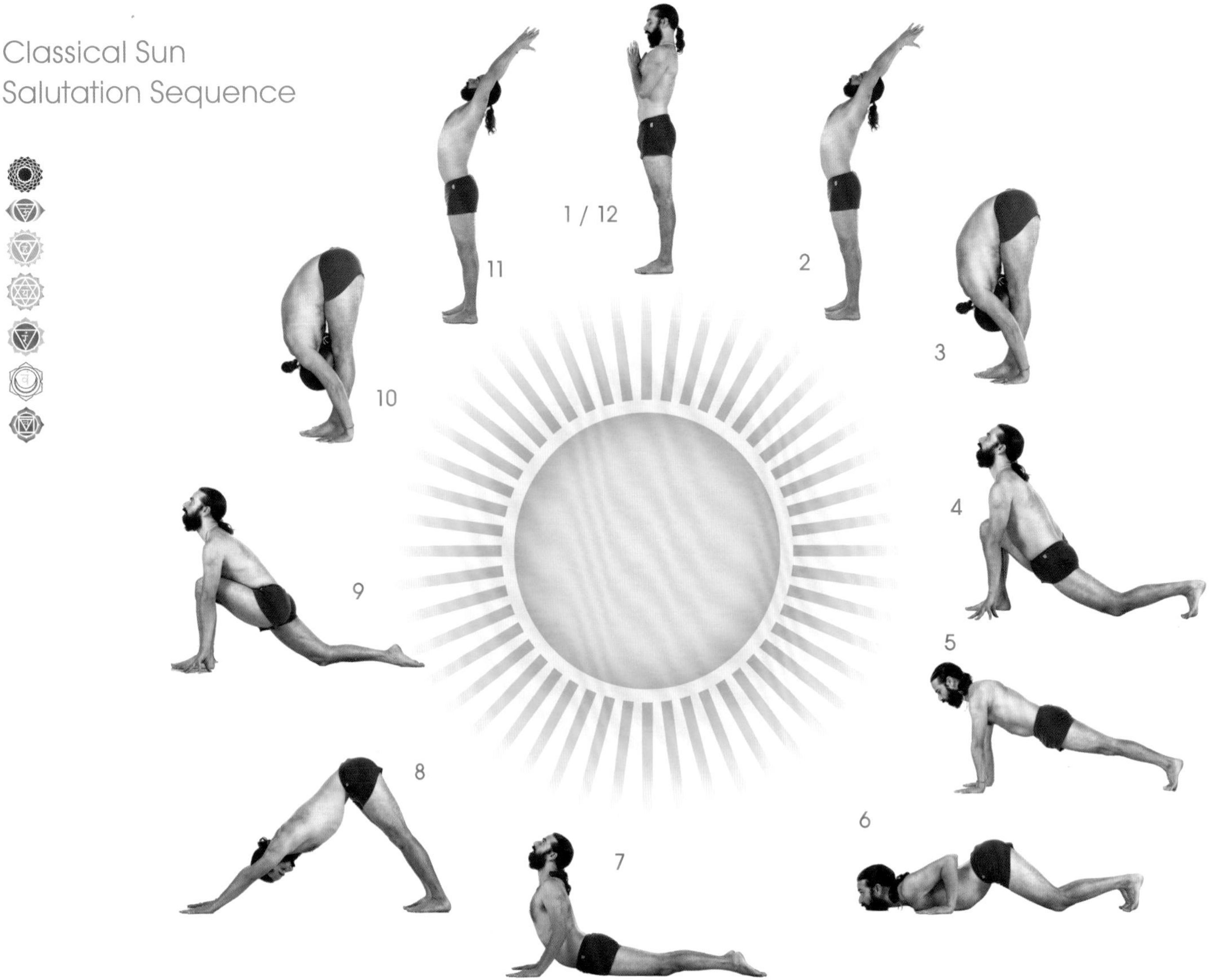

Classical Sun Salutation Sequence

1 / 12
नमस्कार ताड आसन
Namaskāra tāḍa āsana
Praying palm tree pose

2
ऊर्ध्व हस्त उत्तान आसन
Ūrdhva hasta uttāna āsana
Overhead hands stretch pose

3
पृष्ठ उत्तान आसन (पृष्ठ हस्त भू)
Pṛṣṭha uttāna āsana (pṛṣṭha hasta bhū)
Back stretch pose
(hands on the earth behind)

4
हस्त अङ्गुल भू चेतक आसन
Hasta aṅgula bhū cetaka āsana
Fingers on earth horse pose

5
चतुः अङ्ग दण्ड आसन
Catuḥ aṅga daṇḍa āsana
Four limb staff pose

6
साष्टाङ्ग नमस्कार आसन
Sāṣṭāṅga namaskāra āsana
Eight limb salutation pose

7
भुजङ्ग आसन
Bhujaṅga āsana
Cobra pose

8
पर्वत आसन
Parvata āsana
Mountain pose

9
हस्त अङ्गुल भू चेतक आसन
Hasta aṅgula bhū cetaka āsana
Fingers on earth horse pose

10
पृष्ठ उत्तान आसन (पृष्ठ हस्त भू)
Pṛṣṭha uttāna āsana (pṛṣṭha hasta bhū)
Back stretch pose (hands on the earth behind)

11
ऊर्ध्व हस्त उत्तान आसन
Ūrdhva hasta uttāna āsana
Overhead hands stretch pose

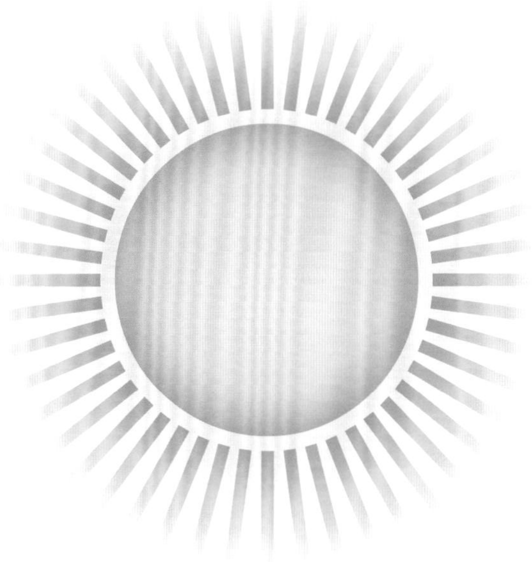

Handstand to Wheel Sequence

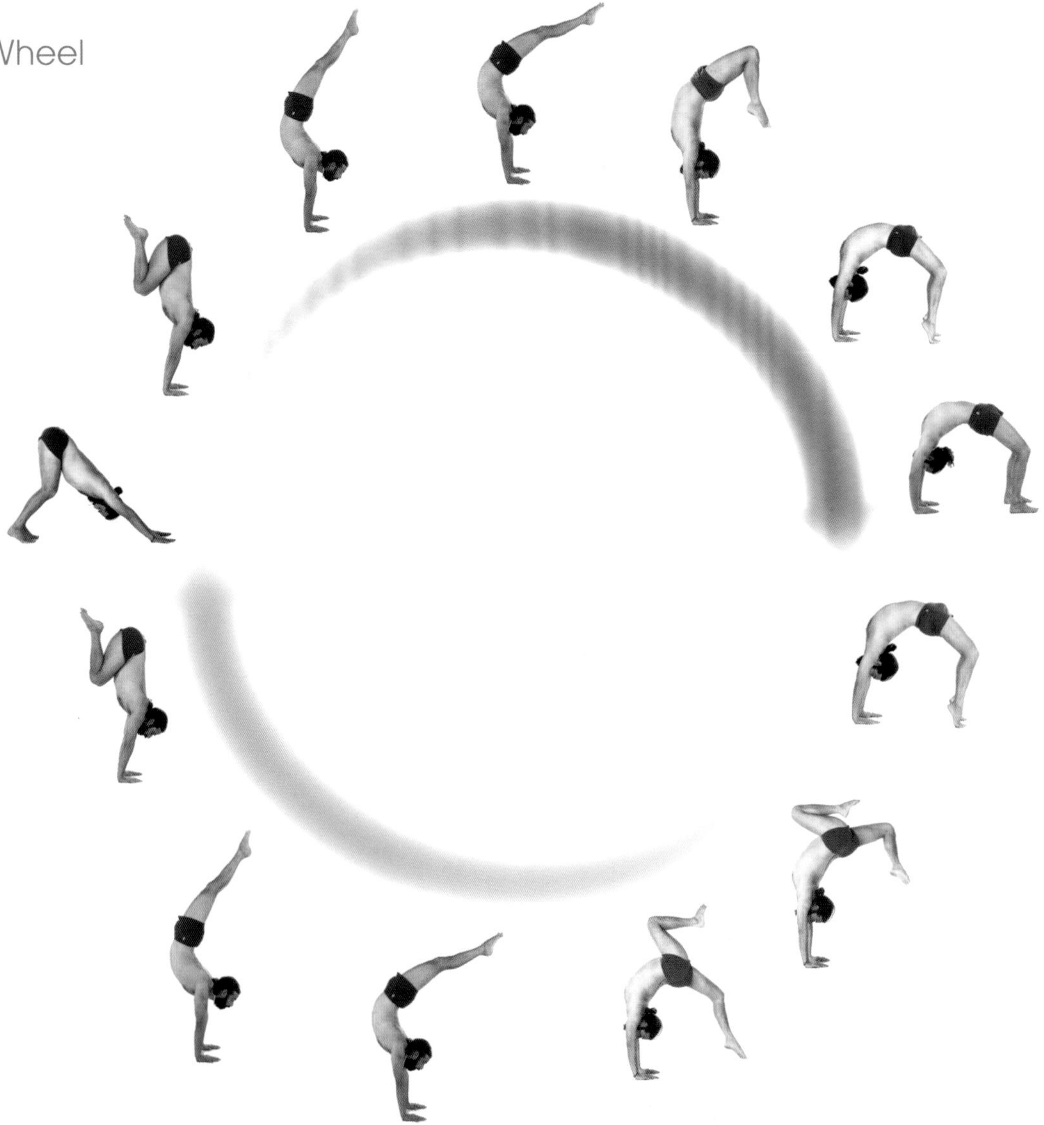

Drop Back Wheel Sequence

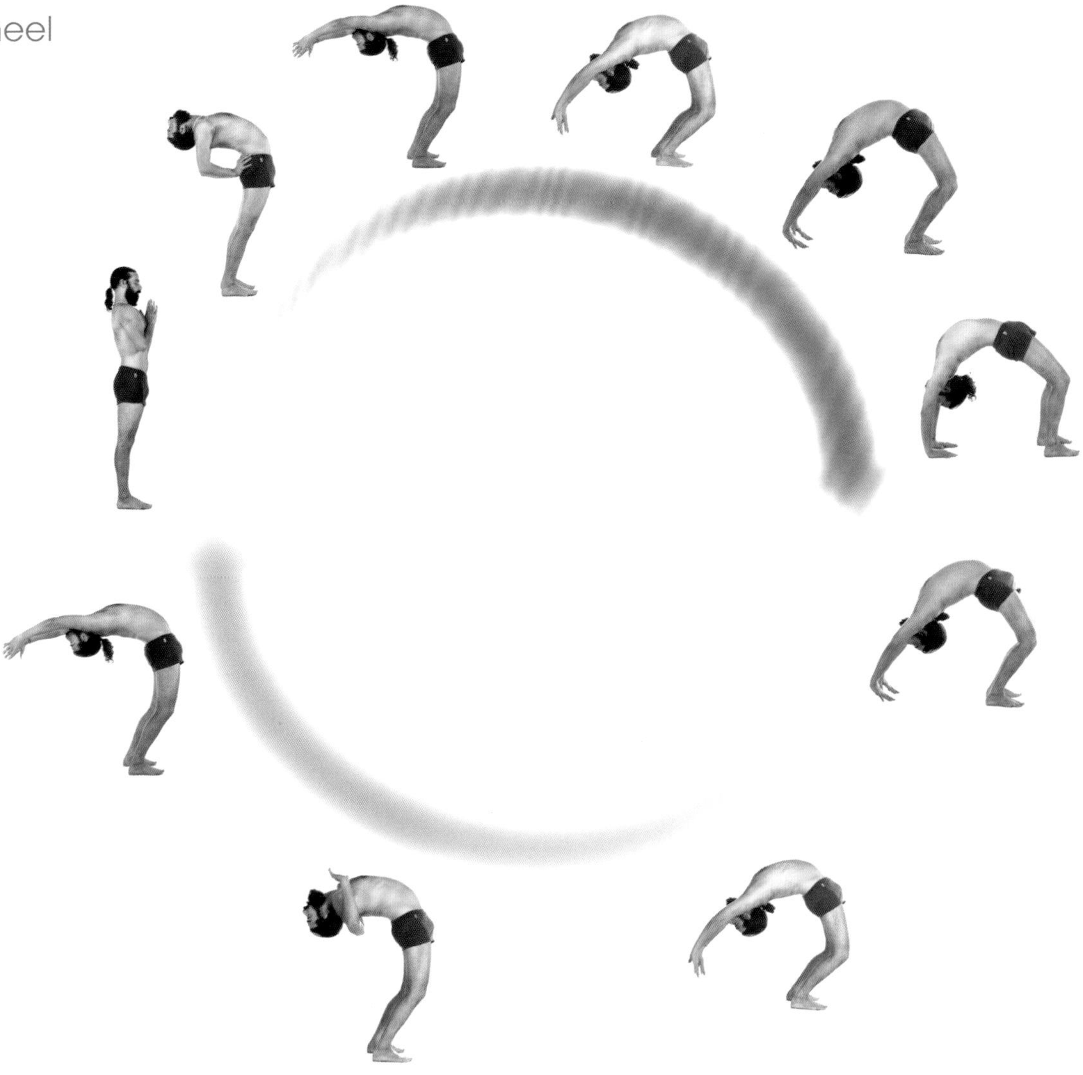

Scorpion Drop Back Sequence

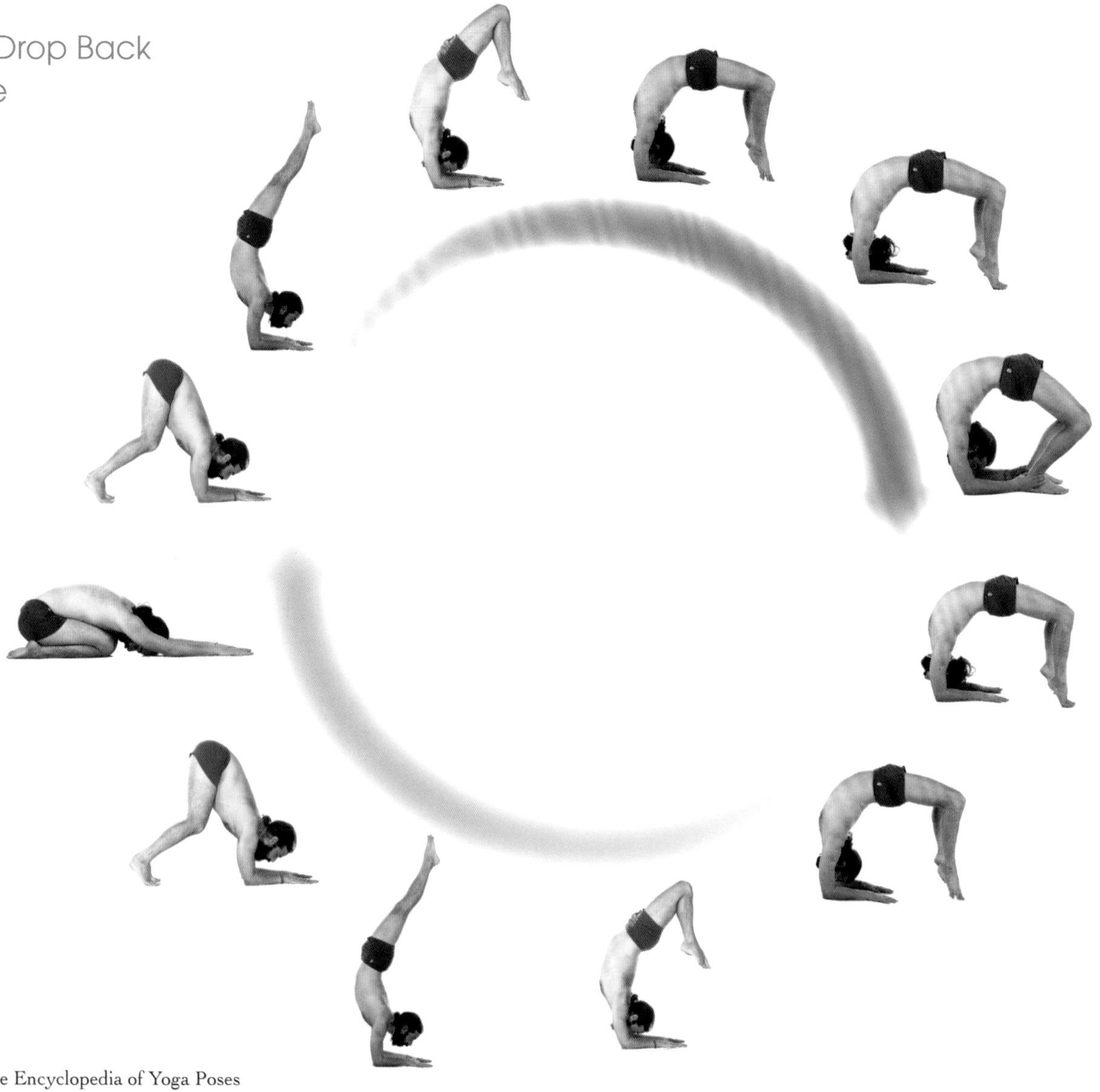

Shoulder Stand Bridge Sequence

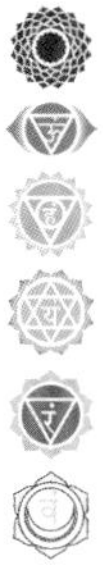

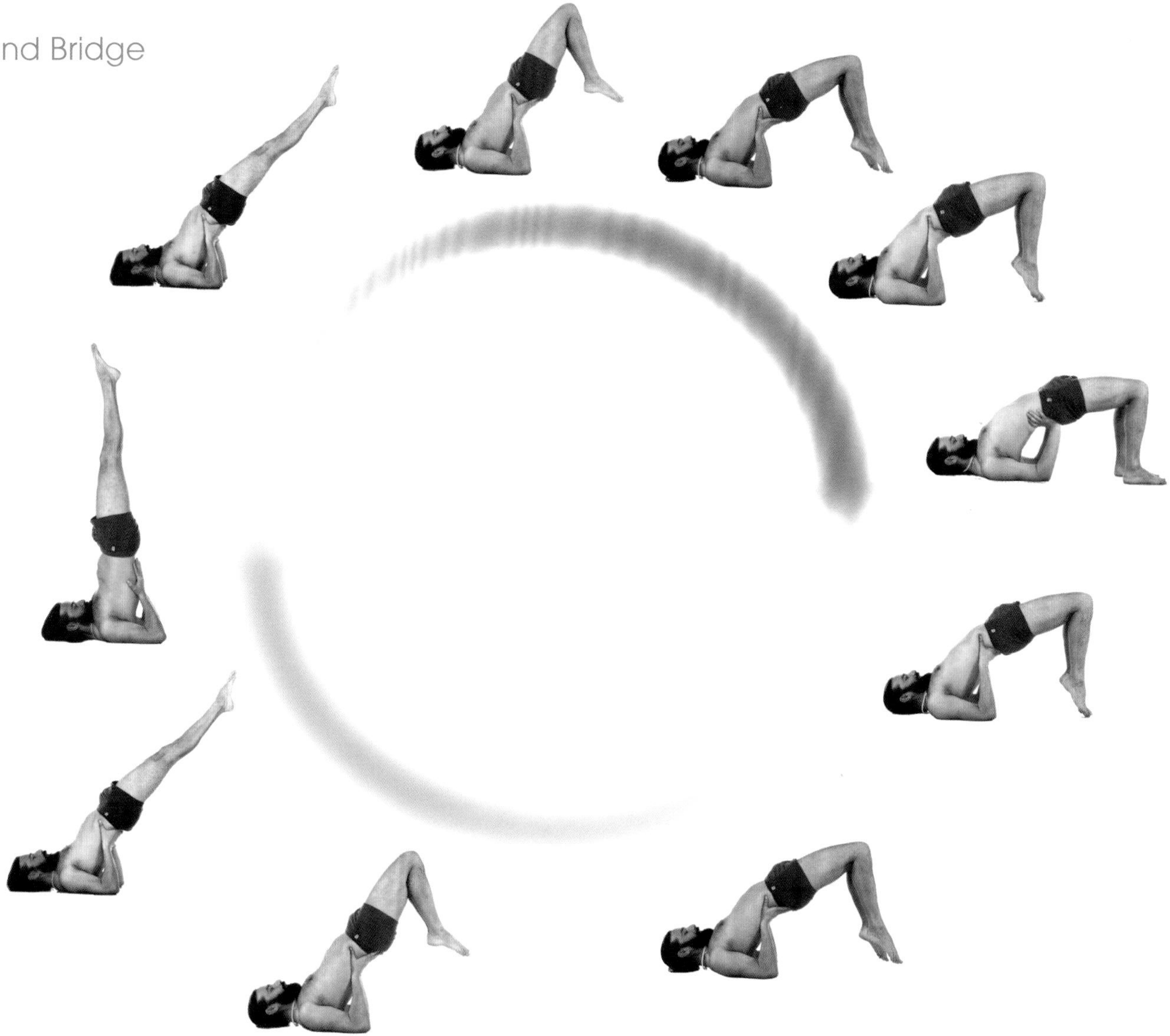

Yogrishi Vishvketu, PhD

Known for his infectious laughter and grounded approach to yogic spiritual life, Yogrishi Vishvketu is an international teacher who guides practitioners on the journey toward uncovering the blissful nature of the true self. Akhanda Yoga is his holistic approach, which integrates cleansing practices called kriyas, asana, pranayama, Vedic chanting, meditation, and yogic philosophy.

Born into a family of yogis and Ayurvedic practitioners, Yogrishi Vishvketu has been immersed in the wisdom and teachings of Yoga and the Vedic sciences his entire life. At the age of eight,

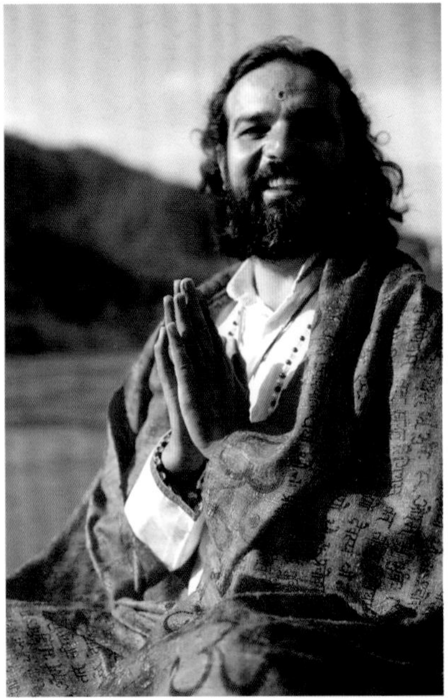

he began his formal studies at Gurukul Kanva Ashram in Uttarakhand, India. He went on to gain a scholarship to complete a five-year undergraduate degree in yoga and sports. After completing an MA in Yoga Philosophy as a gold-list scholar, he was awarded a PhD in Yoga Philosophy at Gurukula Kangri University in Haridwar, India. Although he was twice honored as the All-India Inter-University Yoga Asana Champion for Yogrishi Vishvketu, yoga is primarily an internal practice, and it is this understanding that is the focus of his teachings.

After Yogrishi Vishvketu completed his doctorate, his guru Baba Premnāth prophesied, "You will never have a job. You will create jobs for other people." Over the next several years, he taught yoga at the renowned Yoga Niketan Ashram in Rishikesh. In 2000, he moved to Canada and began to share his understanding of yoga and Vedic wisdom internationally through the Akhanda Yoga system. For the last ten years, he has trained more than two thousand yoga teachers internationally.

In 2007, along with Chetana Panwar, he co-founded the Anand Prakash Ashram Charitable Trust in Rishikesh, where he now spends much of the year. In addition to yoga training, he continues his father's legacy of charitable works by supporting animal welfare and environmental projects in the local community. In 2014, Anand Prakash Ashram founded a free school for over two hundred and fifty underserved children in rural Uttar Pradesh, India.

www.YouTube.com/akhandayoga

www.Facebook.com/YogiVishva

Twitter: @YogiVishvketu

Instagram: yogrishi_vishvketu

Akhanda Yoga®

Akhanda Yoga is a practice that aims to reconnect us with our true nature, which is boundless, blissful, and fearless. In Sanskrit, Akhanda means "whole," or "indivisible." This approach understands yoga as a complete system of movement, sound, breath, and meditation. It is an integrated path of practice that grounds Yogic and Vedic wisdom into our daily lives to create peace and harmony.

Through the World Conscious Yoga Family, Yogrishi Vishvketu offers workshops as well as Yoga Alliance— registered two-hundred- and five-hundred-hour Akhanda Yoga Teacher Training programs in India, Canada, and with affiliate studios worldwide.

To learn more about Yogrishi Vishvketu's community projects, or to view his international schedule of workshops, conferences, and teacher trainings, visit the websites listed below.

Akhanda Yoga: www.akhandayoga.com

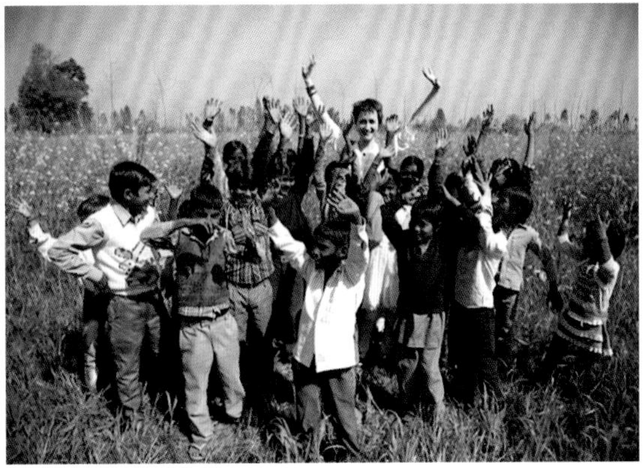

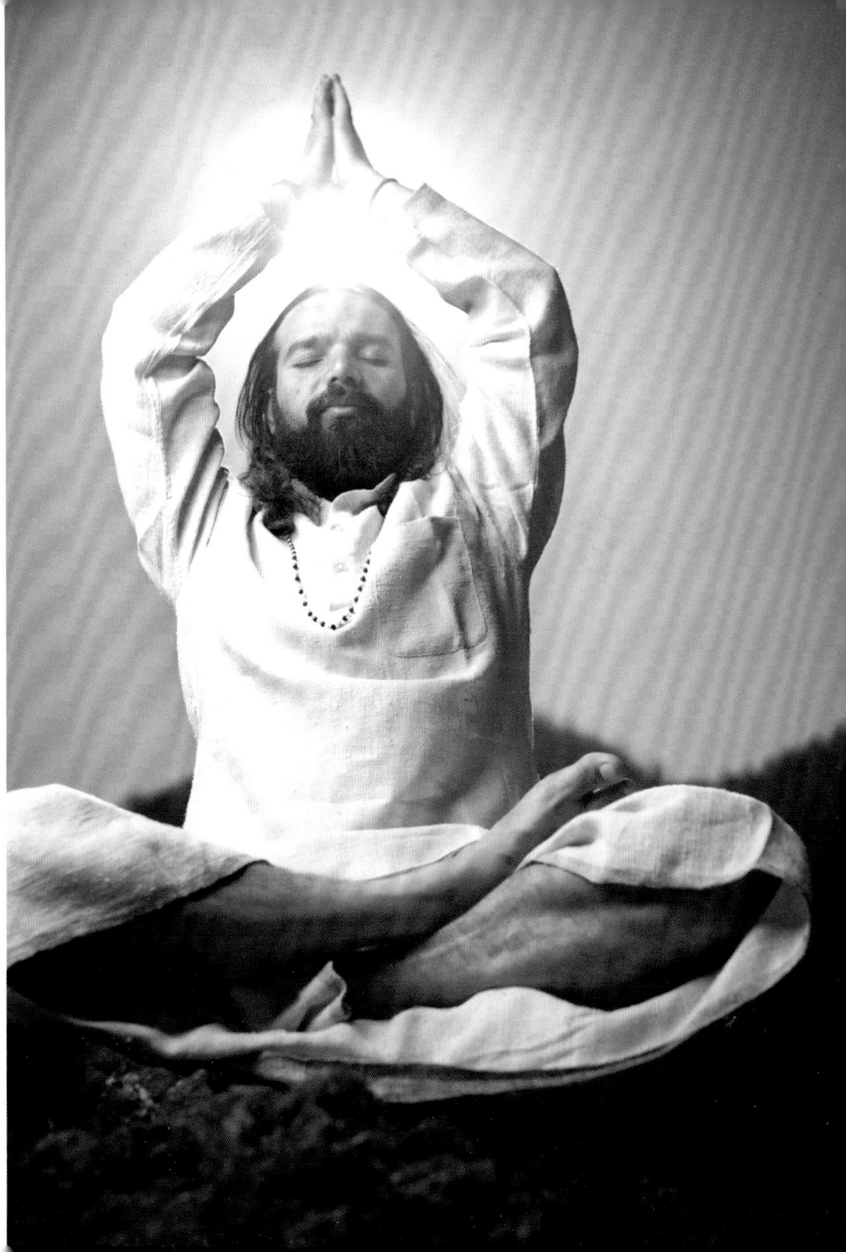

Glossary

A adhaḥ: flexed
adhomukha: downward facing
adhopāda: lower legs
ākarṇa: drawn
ākāśa: sky
ākuñcana: cleansing
ānanda: blissful
ananta: infinity
aṇga: body part, organ
aṇgada: extended
aṅgula: fingers
aṅguṣṭha: big toe, toes
antaṛ: inside
antara drishti, antaṛdṛṣti: focusing the gaze internally
apsarā: angel
ārambha: starting
ardha: half
arjuna bāṇa: focused arrow
āsana: pose
asthih: bones
avasthā: position

B baddha: clasped, bound, holding
bahaya drishti: a soft gaze with open eyes, helps to focus your concentration in the posture
bahiḥ: open
bahir: outside
bahirpāda: outside of feet
baka: crane
bālaka: baby
bhadra: beautiful
bhairava: fearless
bheka: frog
bhrūh: eyebrows
bhū: earth, earth goddess
bhuja: arm
bhujaṅga: cobra
brahmacarya: containment of vital energy
buddhi, manīṣā, prajñā: intelligence

C cakra: wheel
candra: moon
cātaka: skylark
catuḥ: four
cetaka: horse

D dakśiṇa: south
daṇḍa: stick/staff, straight
dantah, daśana: teeth
darśana: gazing
darshana: communion with blessing
deha, kāya, sarīra: body
devatas: deities that surrounded yogis
devī: god, goddess
dhanuḥ: bow
dhara: stacked
dhātri: giving
dhirga āntra: large intestine
dhruva: fig tree
dhyanam: meditation
drishti: vision and a focusing of awareness
dṛṣti: gazing
dvi: two

E eka: one

G garbha: womb
garuḍa: eagle
go: cow
grīvā: neck
gulpha: ankle
gupta: concealed
gurukula: a residential site of spiritual education

H ha: sun
hala: plough
hanu: chin
hasobha: joy
hasta: hands
hṛdayaḥ: heart

J jānu: knee
jatā: dreadlocks
jatāyu: vulture
jñāna mudrā: A posture where the index finger touches the thumb. Used for balancing energy and concentration.

K kāga: crow
kākhah, kukṣi: armpit
kalā: phase, time
Kālī: goddess
kanda pīḍa: energy releasing
kaṇth: throat
kāpāl: skull
kaphoṇi: elbow
kapolah: cheeks
kapota: pigeon
kara: hand
karatala: palm
karṇa, sroṇī: ear
karo: action
kartarī: scissors
kati: waist
keśa: hair
khañjana: wagtail
koṇa: angle
krauñca: curlew
krīḍā: playful
kriyas: spontaneous activity
kṛkalāsa: lizard
kṣitija: horizon
kukkuṭa: rooster practices
kūrma: tortoise

L laghu āntra: small intestine
lalāṭa, mastaka: forehead
liṇgam, siśna, meḍhrah: penis
lola: swinging

M mahā: great
makara: crocodile
mālā: garland
mana: mind
maṇdūka: frog
maṇgalā: auspiciousness
maṇi: jewel
maṇibandha: wrist
mantra: specific sounds used to activate energy centers, calm the mind, and aid in meditation
mārjārī: cat
mastiṣkam: brain
matsya: fish
mayūra: peacock
meru: spine

mṛdula: happy
mudita: blissful
mudrā: a body gesture that creates and maintains a certain energy
mukha: facing
mukham: face
mukta: relieving
mūla: root, sitting
muladhara: the root chakra
muṣṭika, muṣṭi: fist

N nābhi, nābha: navel
naḍi, snāyuh: energy channel
nakhah: nails
namana: bowing, humble, honoring
namaskāra: prayer
nāsikā: nose
nata rāja: Lord of the Dance
nātha: yogi
naukā: boat
netraloma: eyelashes
netram, locanam: eyes
nirālamba: unsupported
niraṅkāra: formless
nirbhaya: tranquil
nitamba: hips
nṛtya: dancing

O oṇkāra: the shape of OM

P pāda: legs, feet, toes
padma: lotus
pallava kṛmi: worm
parigha: gate
parivṛtta: twisted
pārśva: side
parvat, parvata: mountain
parvati pāda: soles of the feet together
pārvatī: divine feminine, the goddess
paścima: back
pavana: wind
pavitra: purity
phalakaṃ: table
phuphphusah: lungs
pīḍa: pressure
piṇḍa: compact, womb-like
prana: life-force energy
pranayama: increasing, balancing and transforming the solar and lunar energies within the body through breathing practices
prapāda: ball of the foot
prapadika: ball of toes on the earth
prasarita: wide
pṛṣṭha: back, behind
pṛṣṭhatah: from the back
puccha: feather, tail
pūrṇa: full
pūrva: forward, frontal
pūrvatah: from the front

R rāja: king
rajju: clasped, bound, holding
randhra: an opening
rasanā, jihvā: tongue
romah: pores

S śalabha: locust
sālamba: supported
sama sthiti: standing steady
samakoṇa pāda: side splits
samakṣa: in front, forward
samakṣatah: from the front
samidhā: sacred
sammukha: in front of face, facing forward
sandhi: joints
sankalpa: intention
sarajju: supported by strap
śārdūla: tiger
sarpa: snake
sarva: all
śaśāṅka: rabbit
sāṣṭāṅga: eight limbs
śava: corpse
setu bandha: bridge
śikhā: top of the head, crown
śīrṣa, śira: head
śīśu: baby
skandha: shoulder
śodhana: purifying
sparśa: touching
sthāpana: fire log
sūcī: needle
sukha: easy
supta: reclined
sūtra: thread
śvāna: dog
śvāsa: playing with the breath

T tāḍa: palm tree
tilaka: anointment of the third eye
ṭiṭṭibha: firefly
tri: trinity
trikoṇa: triangle
tulā: balancing, variation
tvak: skin

U udara: abdomen
uḍḍiyāna: lifted, flying bird
upari: on top
upaviṣṭa: sitting
ūrdhva: above, overhead, lifted, bent
uru: thigh
uṣṭra: camel
ut: up
utkaphoṇi: elbows up
utkaṭa: strong
uttāna: stretch, extended, lifted
utthita: standing
uttolana: balancing

V vajra: thunderbolt
vakra: seated
vakṣah: chest
vāma: left
vātāyana: window
vātsalya: cradle
vāyu yāna, vimāna: airplane
vika, vikaṭa: challenging
vikrama: wisdom
vinata: humble
viparīta: opposite
viparītakaraṇī: inversion
vīra: hero, warrior
virāṭa, vistṛta: extended
vṛkṣa: tree
vṛścika: scorpion

Y yantra: geometric symbols of the chakras
yoga daṇḍa: staff used by yogis to work with energy flow
yoni mudrā: source of life
yoni, bhagah: vagina

MANDALA
PUBLISHING

PO Box 3088
San Rafael, CA 94912
www.mandalaeartheditions.com

Find us on Facebook: www.facebook.com/mandalaearth
Follow us on Twitter: @mandalaearth

Library of Congress Cataloging-in-Publication Data available.
ISBN: 978-1-60887-656-3

INSIGHT EDITIONS
Publisher: Raoul Goff
Co-publisher: Michael Madden
Executive Editor: Vanessa Lopez
Project Editor: Courtney Andersson
Production Editor: Rachel Anderson
Production Manager: Jane Chinn

The following works were referenced during the creation of this book.

Bowditch, Bruce. *The Yoga Asana Index, A Complete Index of Hatha Yoga Postures*, 2nd ed. Nomentira Publishing, 2010.

Dhirendra, Bhramachari. *Yogasana Vijnana: The Science of Yoga*. India: Asia Publishing House, 1970.

Iyengar, B.K.S. *Light on Yoga*. London: Thorsons Classics Edition. HarperCollins, 2001.

Muktibodhananda, Swami. *Hatha Yoga Pradipika*, 3rd ed. India: Bihar School of Yoga, 1998.

Samvat, Vikram. *Yoga Asana*. Gorakhpur, India: Gita Press, 1993.

The Gheranda Samhita. Translated by James Mallinson. Woodstock, New York: YogaVidya.com, 2004.

Yogeshwaranand, Saraswati. *Bahiranga Yoga: First Steps to Higher Yoga*. Rishikesh, India: Yoga Niketan Trust, 2001.

ROOTS of PEACE REPLANTED PAPER

Insight Editions, in association with Roots of Peace, will plant two trees for each tree used in the manufacturing of this book. Roots of Peace is an internationally renowned humanitarian organization dedicated to eradicating land mines worldwide and converting war-torn lands into productive farms and wildlife habitats. Roots of Peace will plant two million fruit and nut trees in Afghanistan and provide farmers there with the skills and support necessary for sustainable land use.

Manufactured in China by Insight Editions

10 9 8 7 6 5 4 3 2